CRITICAL CONCEPT MASTERY SERIES

Acid-Base Disturbance Cases

CRITICAL CONCEPT MASTERY SERIES
Acid-Base Disturbance Cases

Zachary Healy, MD, PhD
Assistant Professor
Division of Pulmonary and Critical Care Medicine
Department of Medicine
Duke University Hospital
Durham, North Carolina

Mc
Graw
Hill

New York   Chicago   San Francisco   Athens   London   Madrid   Mexico City
Milan   New Delhi   Singapore   Sydney   Toronto

1 2 3 4 5 6 7 8 9   LCR   26 25 24 23 22 21

ISBN 978-1-260-45787-2
MHID 1-260-45787-7

This book was set in Minion Pro by KnowledgeWorks Global Ltd.
The editors were Amanda Fielding, Julie Grishaw, and Christina M. Thomas.
The production supervisor was Richard Ruzycka.
Project management was provided by Tasneem Kauser, KnowledgeWorks Global Ltd.
The cover designer was W2 Design.

This book is printed on acid-free paper.

Library of Congress Cataloging-in-Publication Data

Names: Healy, Zachary, author.
Title: Acid-base disturbance cases / Zachary Healy.
Other titles: Critical concept mastery series.
Description: New York : McGraw Hill LLC, [2020] | Series: Critical concept
    mastery series | Includes bibliographical references and index. |
    Summary: "The Critical Concept Mastery Series is meant to help advanced
    students and residents master concepts that are frequently seen but
    difficult to conquer using a case-based approach. The Acid-Base Disturbance
    Case book hones in on double and triple acid-base disturbances."— Provided by
    publisher.
Identifiers: LCCN 2020010526 | ISBN 9781260457872 (paperback) | ISBN
    9781260457889 (ebook)
Subjects: MESH: Acid-Base Imbalance | Case Report
Classification: LCC QP90.7 | NLM WD 220 | DDC 616.3/992—dc23
LC record available at https://lccn.loc.gov/2020010526

McGraw Hill books are available at special quantity discounts to use as premiums and sales promotions or for use in corporate training programs. To contact a representative, please visit the Contact Us pages at www.mhprofessional.com.

CONTENTS

PREFACE

This collection of clinical acid-base cases is meant to sharpen clinical skills in evaluating such disorders. We aim to do so by providing a structure for the evaluation of acute and chronic, primary and secondary acid-base disturbances, as well as approaches to identify the underlying etiologies. This series was conceived to provide cases with a level of complexity that would appeal not only to medical students, but also to residents and fellows, and it will intermittently include questions regarding the most appropriate treatment of patients after identifying the aforementioned acid-base disturbances. Although basic physiologic explanations are provided throughout, this text is not intended to replace essential physiology texts. References to such texts and supplemental peer-reviewed literature are provided throughout where appropriate. Following are a few notes prior to diving into the approach.

While the approach to analysis provided herein may appear rather black-and-white, real-world acid-base interpretation is often less clear, with plenty of gray area. This may be due to a number of issues, including the timing of laboratory studies, the growing use of point-of-care testing and venous blood gas data in the initial evaluation of patients, and limitations of the linear equations describing respiratory and metabolic compensation, among others. Importantly, we typically lack the necessary quantitative information to define the chronicity of acid-base disorders, which then makes interpretation of the acute disorders much more difficult. In such cases, we are required to make assumptions that potentially introduce additional error. For instance, in the first case in this series, you will see how *a priori* knowledge of a chronic respiratory acidosis can significantly alter the interpretation of metabolic acid-base disturbances (and underlying etiologies) in critically ill patients.

All of the cases presented here have been interpreted using the "bicarbonate" (or "Boston") approach introduced by Relman and Schwartz, as opposed to utilizing the base excess (BE) approach introduced by Siggard-Anderson, the standard base excess (SBE) introduced by Van Slyke, or the more complex Stewart approach to acid-base physiology. Each of these approaches will be briefly discussed. While there has much debate regarding which of the bicarbonate and Stewart approaches to acid-base physiology provides the greatest diagnostic and prognostic information, studies comparing the two methods have been largely inconsistent or shown clinical equivalence. As the bicarbonate approach remains the most popular approach taught in medical education and does not require simultaneously solving multiple equations, this approach will be utilized throughout the text. Additionally, we realize that there are multiple variations and short-hand versions of the equations used to determine the "delta-delta" as well as appropriate metabolic and respiratory compensation. While many of these variations or shorthand rules will produce the same or similar mathematical result, the physiologic principles underlying them are often lost or at least less transparent. This can often lead to transposition of terms or general confusion in less-experienced clinicians, and such shorthand should be reserved for more experienced practitioners. This text will utilize a consistent equation-based approach for all calculations, and all necessary equations will be provided in the introduction (as well as in the solutions to the case problems).

Next, one of the most important aspects of acid-base interpretation is the application of common sense, particularly with regard to taking the patient's medical and social history into account. This cannot be overstated. For instance, an otherwise-healthy, elderly patient presenting with an infiltrate on chest film, fever, productive cough, hypotension, and an elevated anion gap acidosis is most likely to have a lactic acidosis secondary to sepsis rather than toluene toxicity from inhalation drug abuse. And while it is always important to keep an open mind when formulating a differential diagnosis, common diagnoses will remain common; you will encounter lactic acidosis and diabetic ketoacidosis (DKA) much more frequently than cyanide or carbon-monoxide poisoning in practice. Finally, recall that most of the acid-base disorders encountered throughout medicine (and this text) are in critically ill patients; it is therefore not always possible to await confirmatory testing before instituting treatment decisions, and such decisions about diagnosis and treatment will often be based on imperfect information.

Zach Healy

INTRODUCTION

PROCESS OF EVALUATION

The first step in the evaluation of the acid-base status is the clinical evaluation. This should include a detailed history of the present illness, with particular attention to the timing/duration of the patient's symptom onset. In patients who are incapacitated or encephalopathic, this should also include a detailed history of the environment in which the patient was found (eg, prescription medications, over-the-counter [OTC] medications, bottles of industrial cleaner, running vehicle, etc) as well as any collateral history that is available. Additionally, it is important to include a detailed review of systems with particular attention to those symptoms that could contribute directly to an acid-base disorder (eg, emesis, diarrhea, pain, etc). A prior medical and surgical history is also critical, with particular attention to conditions associated with chronic acid-base disorders (eg, chronic renal insufficiency, chronic obstructive pulmonary disease [COPD], history of abdominal or pelvic surgery), and a history of prior suicidal ideation or suicide attempts. A complete medication list must also be obtained, including OTC medications and herbal or dietary supplements. An appropriate social and environmental history should include any history of substance abuse (alcohol, opioids, benzodiazepines, etc) and hobbies. A complete physical examination should also be included in the evaluation.

The next step in the evaluation process is to ensure that the appropriate or necessary data are available. This should include an arterial blood gas (ABG) analysis (including pH, $Paco_2$, and Pao_2), as well as a serum basic chemistry panel (sodium [Na], potassium [K], chloride [Cl], carbon dioxide [CO_2], blood urea nitrogen [BUN], creatinine [Cr]), and a serum albumin. These should be drawn at the same time or in very close proximity, and if possible prior to intervention. While a peripheral venous blood gas (VBG) or central venous blood gas analysis may also be used for evaluation of acid-base status, note that this can introduce error into your calculation. Table I-1 provides some general guidelines for correlating ABG and VBG values.

If the laboratory data do not match the clinical situation, check for potential laboratory errors in terms of the patient identification. Also, be alert to the potential for venous blood samples to be contaminated or diluted with intravenous fluids, particularly if a solution or medication is infusing distal to the site of venipuncture. The ABG can often be helpful here as arterial samples should not be affected by infusions and should therefore represent the clinical situation. Importantly, note that the reported bicarbonate (HCO_3) in an arterial or venous blood gas is a calculated rather than a measured value. Also note that the CO_2 from the serum chemistry panel represents the total CO_2 in the serum sample; since the majority (> 95%) of CO_2 is transported

TABLE I-1 • Differences between arterial, peripheral venous, and central venous blood gas values.			
Relative to ABG	pH	Pco$_2$, mm Hg	[HCO$_3^-$] (mEq/L)
Peripheral VBG	[0.03–0.04] **lower** than ABG	[2–10 mm Hg] **higher** than ABG	[1–2 mEq/L] **lower** than ABG
Mixed or central VBG	[0.02–0.06] **lower** than ABG	[3–6 mm Hg] **higher** than ABG	[−1 to 1 mEq/L] different (**no difference**)
ABG, arterial blood gas; HCO$_3^-$, bicarbonate; Pco$_2$, partial pressure of carbon dioxide; VBG, venous blood gas.			

in the form of HCO$_3$, we generally use the value reported for the CO$_2$ as the serum HCO$_3$. In the case of suspected pseudohyponatremia, remember to use the measured value rather than the corrected value in your studies. Finally, note that some substances can interfere with test results. Namely, hypertriglyceridemia or cell lysis can significantly alter lab values. Similarly, some metabolites of ethylene glycol and methanol can interfere with lactate determination, depending on the lab. Also, to check for internal consistency, one can use the Henderson-Hasselbach equation to ensure that the pH, partial pressure of carbon dioxide in arterial blood (Paco$_2$), and HCO$_3$ values are consistent:

$$pH = 6.1 + \log_{10}\left[\frac{[HCO_3]}{0.0307 * Paco_2}\right]; \text{ or } pH = 7.61 + \log_{10}\left[\frac{[HCO_3]}{Paco_2}\right]$$

While the normal value for arterial pH can range from 7.35 to 7.45, patients with appropriate compensation can have values within this range, and therefore acid-base disorders can often be missed. Consequently, for the purpose of the text, we will consider the normal range to be 7.38 to 7.42. Similarly, the normal values for HCO$_3$ range from 21 to 27 mEq/L, with a median value of 24 mEq/L; in order to prevent missing a potential acid-base disorder, we will use a normal range of 22 to 26 mEq/L. The normal range for Paco$_2$ is between 35 and 45 mm Hg with a median value of 40 mEq/L, although we will use a normal range of 38 to 42 mm Hg.

The next step in the evaluation process is an attempt to identify the patient's "baseline" acid-base status by defining any existing chronic acid-base disorders, if possible. This generally requires evaluation of a patient's prior laboratory data and/or an available blood gas when the patient was at baseline health. This is particularly important for patients with chronic respiratory acidosis, as, in addition to an elevated baseline Paco$_2$, the patient's "baseline" HCO$_3$ (and hence the chloride) can be significantly altered from that of "healthy" or "normal" patients. For example, assume you have a patient with advanced COPD who presents to the emergency department with blood gas values of pH 7.25, Paco$_2$ 65 mm Hg, and HCO$_3$ 27 mEq/L. The interpretation of this patient's blood gas, if we assume the patient has a "normal" baseline (eg, Paco$_2$ 40 mm Hg, HCO$_3$ 24 mEq/L) would be an acute respiratory acidosis with an appropriate renal compensation; however, if you know that the patient has a chronic respiratory acidosis with a baseline acid-base status of pH 7.30, $Paco_2$ 65 mm Hg, and HCO_3 36 mEq/L, you would be able to accurately diagnose that the patient has an acute metabolic acidosis, with an acute-on-chronic respiratory acidosis. In the first case, we were forced to assume a normal baseline, and this would have caused us to miss that patient's metabolic acidosis initially, which could potentially be catastrophic. This is particularly important in chronic respiratory acid-base disorders, where both the $Paco_2$ and the HCO_3 are altered. While some references suggest that the ratio $[HCO_3]/[Paco_2]$ can be used to determine if a respiratory process is acute or chronic, this ratio does not provide a 1:1 mapping to a particular set of acid-base disorders. For example, consider a patient presenting with a respiratory acidosis that has a ratio of 0.2. Based on Figure I-1, this patient may have an acute-on-chronic respiratory acidosis with or without a metabolic acidosis/alkalosis, an acute respiratory acidosis with a concomitant metabolic alkalosis, or a chronic respiratory acidosis with an acute metabolic alkalosis.

Unlike compensation in chronic respiratory acid-base disorders, the compensation in chronic metabolic acid-base disorders is poorly characterized and inefficient; therefore, it is less important to identify these conditions initially.

The next step is to determine if the primary issue is an acidemia or alkalemia. This is another instance where common sense must be utilized. While the normal value for the arterial pH may be between 7.35 and 7.45, multiple acid-base disturbances may still be present in a patient with a pH in this range. Therefore, it is important that one does not

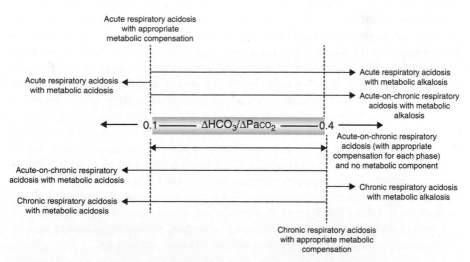

Figure I-1 • Potential combinations of acute and/or chronic metabolic and respiratory disorders that may be seen at different ratios of the change in serum bicarbonate (HCO_3) to the change in arterial CO_2.

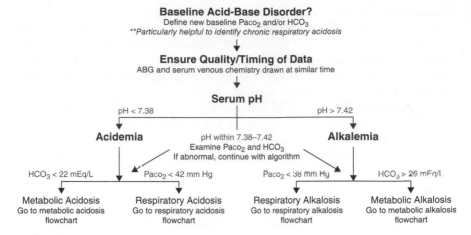

Healthy Patient:
Baseline HCO_3: 21-28 mEq/L, although we assume a median value of 24 mEq/L
Baseline $Paco_2$: 35-45 mm Hg, although we assume a median value of 40 mEq/L

Chronic Acid-Base Disorder:
Replace the values in red in the flow chart with the patient's baseline values

Figure I-2 • Initial algorithm for the evaluation of acid-base disorders.

examine the pH, see that it is 7.39, and assume that no acid-base disorder is present. For example, a patient recently presented to our emergency department with a pH of 7.39, $Paco_2$ of 25 mm Hg, and serum HCO_3 of 15 mEq/L and the diagnosis of an acute pulmonary embolus with cor pulmonale. Although the patient's pH was normal, this was due to the presence of an anion gap acidosis due to lactic acidosis secondary to cardiogenic shock and a concomitant respiratory alkalosis. Therefore, it is important to analyze the pH, $Paco_2$, and serum HCO_3 for every patient. Although we examine the pH first, this is simply to provide some guidance as to what the primary acid-base disorders are in any given patient. If the pH is in the range of 7.39 to 7.41, it may not be possible to determine which is the primary process. The next step is to determine the primary processes present, followed by examination for appropriate compensation and identification of any secondary acid-base disorders present. Recall that even with "complete" compensation, the arterial pH does not reach 7.40; this is a common misconception, and therefore we will use the term "appropriate" rather than "complete" compensation throughout the text. Respiratory compensation is driven by pH changes in the cerebrospinal fluid, leading to alterations in the respiratory centers. Metabolic compensation is driven by pH-sensitive cells in the renal tubules. Once one has identified all existing primary and secondary acid-base disorders present, one must go through each decision tree to attempt to identify the etiologies responsible for each disorder, as this will guide treatment decision making (see Figure I-2). Again, it is also important to identify patterns of disorders that are associated with particularly etiologies. For example, aspirin toxicity can be associated with a respiratory alkalosis and an anion gap acidosis.

METABOLIC ACIDOSIS

Figure I-3 represents the algorithm for a patient with a metabolic acidosis.

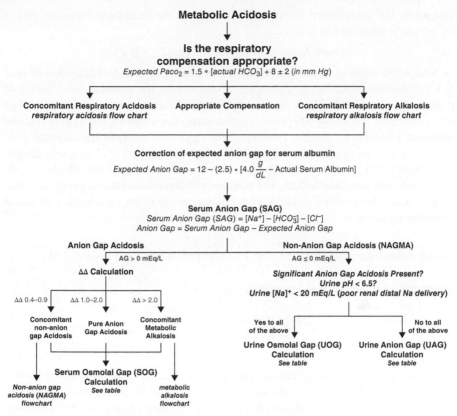

Metabolic Acidosis

Is the respiratory compensation appropriate?
Expected $Paco_2 = 1.5 * [actual\ HCO_3] + 8 \pm 2$ (in mm Hg)

Concomitant Respiratory Acidosis
respiratory acidosis flow chart

Appropriate Compensation

Concomitant Respiratory Alkalosis
respiratory alkalosis flow chart

Correction of expected anion gap for serum albumin
Expected Anion Gap = $12 - (2.5) * [4.0\ \frac{g}{dL} - $ Actual Serum Albumin]

Serum Anion Gap (SAG)
Serum Anion Gap (SAG) = $[Na^+] - [HCO_3] - [Cl^-]$
Anion Gap = Serum Anion Gap – Expected Anion Gap

Anion Gap Acidosis
AG > 0 mEq/L

ΔΔ Calculation

ΔΔ 0.4–0.9 | ΔΔ 1.0–2.0 | ΔΔ > 2.0

Concomitant non-anion gap Acidosis

Pure Anion Gap Acidosis

Concomitant Metabolic Alkalosis

Serum Osmolal Gap (SOG) Calculation
See table

Non-anion gap acidosis (NAGMA) flowchart

metabolic alkalosis flowchart

Non-Anion Gap Acidosis (NAGMA)
AG ≤ 0 mEq/L

Significant Anion Gap Acidosis Present?
Urine pH < 6.5?
Urine $[Na]^+$ < 20 mEq/L (poor renal distal Na delivery)

Yes to all of the above

Urine Osmolal Gap (UOG) Calculation
See table

No to all of the above

Urine Anion Gap (UAG) Calculation
See table

Figure I-3 • Algorithm for evaluation of a metabolic acidosis.

The first step in a patient with a metabolic acidosis is to determine if the compensation is appropriate. For a metabolic acidosis, we do not differentiate between acute and chronic when determining the compensation, as the respiratory compensation for a chronic metabolic acidosis is poorly defined and generally inefficient. The equation we will use, called the Winter equation, is generally accurate for a serum HCO_3 between 5 and 22 mEq/L:

$$Expected\ Paco_2 = 1.5 * [Actual\ HCO_3] + 8 \pm 2\ (in\ mm\ Hg).$$

Respiratory compensation for a metabolic acidosis begins within minutes and is "complete" within 12 to 24 hours. If the $Paco_2$ falls within this range, this is termed an "appropriate" or complete respiratory compensation, and no respiratory acid-base disorder is present. If the $Paco_2$ is lower than the expected range, there is a concomitant respiratory alkalosis, whereas if the $Paco_2$ is higher than the expected range, a concomitant respiratory acidosis is present. The limit of respiratory compensation is between 8 and 10 mm Hg. Once this has been determined, the next step is to determine if an anion gap acidosis is present. The first step in determining if an anion gap is present is to calculate the expected or "normal" anion gap. The serum anion gap represents the unmeasured anions in the serum. In the most basic form the serum anion gap is calculated as follows:

$$\text{Serum Anion Gap} = [Na^+] - [HCO_3^-] - [Cl^-],$$

In which the units of measure are milliequivalents per liter (mEq/L). Recall that the milliequivalent (mEq) is a measure of net charge (or valence), so 1 mmol of potassium is equal to 1 mEq, whereas 1 mmol of calcium, which carries a net charge of 2+, is equal to 2 mEq. Therefore, in this form, the unmeasured anions include albumin, phosphorus, lactate, bromide, and negatively charged monoclonal proteins. Phosphorus exists as an anion in the form of monohydrogen and dihydrogen phosphate (HPO_4^{2-} and $H_2PO_4^-$). There are also unmeasured cations, which include potassium, calcium, magnesium, and positively charged monoclonal proteins. Since magnesium, phosphorus, calcium, and potassium are often measured, one could write the equation as:

$$\text{Serum Anion Gap} = [Na^+] + [K^+] + [Ca^{2+}] + [Mg^{2+}] - [HCO_3^-] + [Cl^-] - [P^{-1}] \left(in \frac{mEq}{L} \right);$$

Alternatively, if the values are in mmol,

$$\text{Serum Anion Gap} = \begin{array}{l} [Na^+] + [K^+] + 2*[Ca^{2+}] \\ + 2*[Mg^{2+}] - [HCO_3^-] + [Cl^-] - 1.8*[P^{-1}] \end{array} \left(in \frac{mmol}{L} \right).$$

If the values are in milligrams per liter (mg/L), this can be converted using the molecular weights (mg/mmol or g/mol): for calcium, 40.1; and for phosphorus, 31. Recall that both phosphorus and calcium are typically expressed as mg/dL, so to convert from mg/dL to millimoles per liter (mmol/L), multiply the calcium value by 0.401 and the phosphorus by 0.31 to covert to mmol/L. In an otherwise healthy patient, these other unmeasured cations and anions generally cancel out; therefore, the major anion responsible for the anion gap is albumin. For the most common form of the serum anion gap equation (including only sodium, serum HCO_3, and chloride), we must correct the expected anion gap for the patient's serum albumin, using the following equation:

$$\text{Expected Anion Gap} = 12 - (2.5) * \left[4.0 \frac{g}{dL} - \text{Actual Serum Albumin} \right].$$

While the expected anion gap is ~12 mEq/L for an otherwise healthy patient with a serum albumin of 4.0 g/dL, this value will be lower in patients with hypoalbuminemia. There are conditions that can be associated with a low anion gap (< 3 mEq/L), as well as those associated with a negative anion gap. Some of these conditions are provided in Table I-2.

After determining the expected anion gap and calculating the serum anion gap, one can determine the anion gap (AG):

$$\text{Anion Gap} = \text{Serum Anion Gap (measured)} - \text{Expected Anion Gap} \left(in \frac{mEq}{L} \right).$$

TABLE I-2 • Unmeasured cations and anions, conditions associated with a low or negative serum anion gap, and other potential anions that may be present in a patient with one of these conditions.
Common Unmeasured Cations
• $[K^+]$ • $[Ca^{2+}]$ • $[Mg^{2+}]$ • Monoclonal protein accumulation (some IgG forms)
Common Unmeasured Anions
• Phosphorus • Lactate • Bromide/iodide • Albumin • Monoclonal protein (IgM)
Causes of a Low Serum Anion Gap (≤ 3 mEq/L)
• Laboratory error • Hypoalbuminemia • Severe NAGMA • Lithium toxicity • Monoclonal gammopathy, multiple myeloma • Bromide/iodine ingestion (interferes with serum $[Cl^-]$ measurement) • Pseudohyponatremia • HCO_3 infusion (chloride-deplete solution)
Causes of a Negative Serum Anion Gap
• Hyperlipidemia (falsely elevates serum $[Cl^-]$ measurement) • Bromide ingestion • Pyridostigmine use • Salicylate intoxication
NAGMA, non-anion gap metabolic acidosis.

If the anion gap is positive, this indicates that an anion gap acidosis is present, whereas if the value is zero or less than zero, there is no anion gap acidosis, and only a non-anion gap acidosis is present. At this point, it may be prudent to order some additional laboratory studies pending the patient's presentation and other clinical history (see Table I-3).

TABLE I-3 • Additional laboratory studies to consider for an anion gap and non-anion gap acidosis.	
Anion Gap Acidosis	**Non-Anion Gap Acidosis**
• Complete blood count with differential • Serum lactate (either arterial or venous) • Urine drug screen • Serum drug screen, which should include ethanol, salicylates, and acetaminophen levels • Liver function testing • Serum osmolality • Serum acetone or ketones (beta-hydroxybutyrate)	• Urine electrolytes (Na, K, Cl) • Urinalysis • Urine osmolality • Urine urea

DELTA-DELTA CALCULATION

For a patient with an anion gap acidosis, the next step is to determine if the patient has a pure anion gap acidosis, or there is also a concomitant non-anion gap acidosis or a metabolic alkalosis. This is determined by using the delta-delta ($\Delta\Delta$):

$$\Delta\Delta = \frac{(\text{Calculated Anion Gap}) - (\text{Expected Anion Gap})}{(\text{Expected Serum CO}_2) - (\text{Actual Serum CO}_2)}.$$

The delta-delta equation compares the size of the anion gap to the magnitude of change in the serum HCO_3. Recall that one should use the serum HCO_3 as a surrogate for the serum CO_2. Additionally, for the expected serum HCO_3, one should use the patient's baseline serum HCO_3 if it is known to be different than 24 mEq/L. For patients with a pure anion gap, the ratio is generally between 1.0 and 2.0. Recall that a strong acid dissolves in blood to an anion and a hydrogen molecule. The hydrogen molecule reacts with an HCO_3 molecule to yield a water molecule and a molecule of carbon dioxide. Therefore, for each molecule of acid, the change in anion gap would be balanced by the loss of an HCO_3 molecule, yielding a 1:1 ratio. However, this requires that renal function is maintained, and that the excretion of anion and the acid component of strong acid are equal overall. Additionally, the hydrogen ion released from the strong acid can also be buffered by bone or within cells, and therefore the anion gap will be higher than the reduction in the serum HCO_3. Obviously, as the serum HCO_3 level is further reduced, more of the acid will be buffered by other means. Therefore, the delta-delta ratio can be elevated up to a value of 2.0 and still represent a pure anion gap acidosis. A value of 1.6 is commonly seen in patients with a pure type A lactic acidosis. It is important to note here that the body does not produce lactic acid; rather, hydrogen ions are produced as part of the anaerobic metabolism pathways that lead to lactate anion production. Therefore, the ratio here is not 1:1. Additionally, many of the conditions leading to a lactic acidosis (type A lactic acidosis) are also associated with reduced renal function (leading to an imbalance in anion and acid excretion) and more severe acidosis (which pushes more H^+ to be buffered in the bone and intracellularly).

Patients with a value less than 0.4, despite having an elevated anion gap are more likely to have a pure non-anion gap acidosis without an actual anion gap acidosis. This is simply due to the limits of the equations we use to describe much more complex physiology. In this case, the reduction in the serum HCO_3 significantly outweighs the increase in the anion gap. This scenario is usually seen in patients with a very small but positive anion gap, but a significant reduction in serum HCO_3, such as a type 1 renal tubular acidosis (RTA).

Patients with a value between 0.4 and 0.9 are diagnosed with a mixed anion gap and non-anion gap acidosis. Patients with a value greater than 2.0 are diagnosed with an anion gap acidosis and a metabolic alkalosis. For each additional acid-base disorder present, one must pursue a diagnostic workup based on the provided algorithms. Table I-4 summarizes the interpretation of delta-delta values.

TABLE I-4 • Interpretation of the delta-delta equation valuesle.	
Delta-Delta Value	Condition Present
< 0.4	Non-anion gap only
0.4–0.9	Anion gap *and* non-anion gap acidosis
1.0–2.0	Anion gap acidosis only
> 2.0	Anion gap acidosis and metabolic alkalosis

SERUM OSMOLAL GAP

Once the delta-delta evaluation is completed, a serum osmolal gap should be calculated. While this is not necessary in patients with a clearly identifiable cause and consistent clinical history, we generally include this as part of the algorithm to prevent this step from being missed, as the timely identification of an anion gap acidosis with a serum osmolal gap is critical to preventing significant morbidity. The serum osmolal gap is important for determining whether toxic alcohol ingestions have occurred. First, we calculate the serum osmolality (equivalent to the expected anion gap calculation). Again, as with the serum anion gap calculations, there are a number of ways this can be written, which can include additional variables. The most significant solutes in plasma are sodium, HCO_3, chloride, glucose, urea, and ethanol. Therefore, the most common form is written as follows:

$$\text{Calculated Serum Osmolality} = 2 * [\text{Na}^+] + \frac{[\text{Glucose}]}{18} + \frac{[\text{BUN}]}{2.8} + \frac{[\text{Ethanol}]}{3.8},$$

where the units are as follows: serum osmolality, mOsm/kg (which is equivalent to the serum osmolality when written mOsm/L of water, as 1 L of water weights 1 kg); Na, mmol/L; glucose, mg/dL; BUN, mg/dL; ethanol, mg/dL. The conversion factors for glucose, BUN, and ethanol shown in the preceding equation convert the units from mg/dL to mOsm/kg. The sodium value is doubled to use as a surrogate for the chloride and HCO_3 values. The following are additional terms (with conversion factors) that may be used in the equation if the values are measured in milligrams per deciliter (mg/dL): methanol, 3.2; isopropyl alcohol, 6.0; ethylene glycol, 6.2; acetone, 5.8. Finally, if the beta-hydroxybutyrate or lactate are measured, they may be included directly (without conversion) in units of mmol/L.

Using the more common formulation for the calculated serum osmolality, we can determine the serum osmolal gap by measuring the serum osmolality:

Serum Osmolal Gap = Measured Serum Osmolality – Calculated Serum Osmolality.

The serum osmolal gap, when normal, should fall in the range of –10 to +10 mOsm/kg. Anything greater than +10 mOsm/kg is considered a positive serum osmolal gap, and a value greater than +15 mOsm/kg is generally considered a critical value. Table I-5 includes conditions that can lead to an increased serum osmolal gap with and without a concomitant serum anion gap acidosis.

TABLE I-5 • Conditions associated with an elevated serum osmolal gap with or without an associated anion gap acidosis.

With an Elevated Serum Anion Gap

1. Ethanol ingestion with alcohol ketoacidosis (acetone is an unmeasured osmole, in addition to ethanol)—the osmolality is usually elevated more so by the increased ethanol concentration, so the osmolal "gap" depends on whether the term for ethanol is included in the osmolality calculation*
2. Organic alcohol ingestions (methanol, ethylene glycol, diethylene glycol, propylene glycol)
3. DKA—similar to ethanol ingestion, earlier, glucose and acetone contribute to the osmolality, since the glucose term is always included in the calculation
4. Salicylate toxicity
5. Renal failure—the BUN is nearly always included in the osmolality

Without an Elevated Serum Anion Gap

1. Hyperosmolar therapy (mannitol, glycerol)
2. Other organic solvent ingestion (eg, acetone)
3. Isopropyl alcohol ingestion (produces only acetone rather than an organic acid, so no anion gap is seen)
4. Hypertriglyceridemia
5. Hyperproteinemia

*A mildly elevated osmolal gap has been reported in the literature in patients with lactic acidosis in critical illness, particularly severe distributive shock. The pathology is not quite clear, although it likely is related to multiorgan failure—particularly involving the liver and kidneys—and the release of cellular components known to contribute to the osmolal gap. This is typically around 10 mOsm/L, although it may be as high as 20–25 mOsm/L.

ANION GAP ACIDOSIS

Once all the calculations for the anion gap acidosis portion of the algorithm have been performed, one can attempt to determine the underlying etiology. Common and less common causes of an anion gap acidosis are provided in Tables I-6 and I-7.

Lactic acidosis, DKA, and chronic renal insufficiency/failure remain the most common forms of anion gap acidosis seen clinically. Lactate, which is produced from anaerobic metabolism, can then be converted back to glucose in the liver via the Cori cycle, excreted as an anion in kidney, or used in the Kreb cycle via conversion to pyruvate. L-Lactic acidosis can be classified into type A and type B; a separate form of acidosis,

TABLE I-6 • Causes of anion gap metabolic acidosis.

Common	Less Common
Lactic acidosis (including transient)	Cyanide poisoning
Renal failure ("uremia")	Carbon monoxide poisoning
DKA	Aminoglycosides
Alcohol ketoacidosis	Phenformin use
Starvation ketoacidosis	D-Lactic acidosis
Salicylate poisoning (ASA)	Paraldehyde
Acetaminophen poisoning (paracetamol)	Iron
Organic alcohol poisoning (ethylene glycol, methanol, propylene glycol)	Isoniazid
Toluene poisoning ("glue-sniffing")	Inborn errors of metabolism

TABLE I-7 • Anions/metabolites associated with different causes of an anion gap acidosis.

Methanol → Formic acid
Ethylene glycol → Oxalic acid
Propylene glycol* → D-Lactic acid (potential metabolite)
Toluene → Hippuric acid
Ketoacidosis → Ketones (acetoacetone, beta-hydroxybutyrate)
Aspirin → Salicylates
Acetaminophen → 5-Oxoproline (pyroglutamic acid)
Cyanide → 2-Aminothiazoline-4-carboxylic acid (ATC)

*Pharmacologic Agents Potentially Utilizing Propylene Glycol

- Lorazepam
- Phenobarbital
- Bactrim
- Esmolol
- Nitroglycerin

termed *D-lactic acidosis*, occurs as a by-product of bacterial metabolism in patients with specific risk factors. Type A lactic acidosis is seen more commonly, and is associated with evidence of poor tissue perfusion or oxygenation, whereas type B lactic acidosis is typically associated with delayed clearance or tissue utilization of lactate. Causes of a type A lactic acidosis includes shock, limb ischemia, carbon monoxide, and severe hypoxemia. Causes of a type B lactic acidosis include liver/renal failure, malignancy, drug toxicity, and inborn errors of metabolism. Type D-lactic acidosis can result from bacterial metabolism in patients with reduced small bowel absorption (short-gut syndrome, gastric bypass with small bowel resection). It usually occurs after a large carbohydrate load but may also be seen in patients with DKA (via metabolism of methylglyoxal) or patients receiving infusions of medications containing propylene glycol. D-Lactate is filtered freely and is not well resorbed in the proximal tubule.

Patients with a ketoacidosis usually have preserved renal function. The anions are excreted as salts with sodium or potassium rather than with ammonium. The administration of glucose (and insulin in DKA) reduces the production of ketone bodies, while the administration of isotonic fluids leads to increased anion and acid excretion (along with sodium, but not chloride). The anion gap is therefore usually "closed" or resolved by a shift to a non-anion gap acidosis.

Chronic kidney disease (CKD) may be associated with a non-anion gap acidosis, a pure anion gap acidosis, or a mixed anion and non-anion gap acidosis. Early in the disease process, acid excretion is more significantly impacted than anion excretion, leading to a non-anion gap acidosis. As the disease progresses, there is more impact on anion excretion, leading to a mixed or pure anion gap acidosis.

NON-ANION GAP ACIDOSIS

The primary etiologies for a non-anion gap acidosis include acid ingestion/infusion, RTA, and gastrointestinal (GI) losses of HCO_3. Aside from the history, the primary tools for determining the etiology of a non-anion gap acidosis are urine studies, including the urine pH, presence of kidney stones, the urine anion or osmolal gap, and the serum potassium. Approximately 50 mEq of non-volatile acid is excreted by the kidneys on a daily basis, although they are capable of handling up to 10-fold increase in acid load. Renal acid excretion occurs predominantly via conjugation of hydrogen ions to ammonia, forming ammonium (NH_4^+). Therefore, the normal response to a metabolic acidosis is to increase NH_4^- excretion, thus reducing the urine pH (typically < 5.5). This acid excretion primarily occurs in the distal tubules and collecting duct. In a type 1 (distal) RTA, type 4 RTA, and CKD, patients will have reduced ammonium excretion in response to an acid load. It is important to differentiate these conditions from those diagnoses associated with a loss of HCO_3 via either the GI tract or the kidney. In a proximal RTA, there is defective resorption of HCO_3 in the proximal tubule, which may be accompanied by other abnormalities in the proximal tubule. In diarrhea, HCO_3 and potassium are lost via the GI tract.

In order to differentiate between GI losses of HCO_3 and reduced renal acid excretion, one may use a surrogate measure of serum ammonium excretion, in addition to the urinary pH. Although some facilities can directly measure the urinary ammonium, many cannot. Therefore, there are two primary options for estimating the urinary NH_4^- excretion: the urine anion gap and the urine osmolal gap.

The urine anion gap provides an indirect estimate of the urine ammonium excretion. The urine anion gap is calculated as follows:

$$\text{Urine Anion Gap} = Na^+_{urine} + K^+_{urine} - Cl^-_{urine}$$

The typical value of the urine anion gap is between +10 and +100 mEq/L in patients consuming a Western diet. Urinary chloride is most commonly excreted in complex with sodium, potassium, or ammonium ions. Therefore, in a patient with intact urinary acidification, as urinary ammonium excretion increases, more chloride is excreted, and the urine anion gap will become more negative. In patients with a GI source of HCO_3 loss such as diarrhea, the urine anion gap will be considerably negative, typically between −20 mEq/L and −50 mEq/L. Alternatively, in patients with dysfunctional urinary acidification, the urine ammonium excretion will not increase significantly, and the urine anion gap will remain positive, usually within the normal range (+10 to +100 mEq/L). A value between −20 and +10 is generally inconclusive.

There are several limitations to the use of the urine anion gap. First, the urine anion gap can also be impacted by the excretion of other unmeasured anions not usually present in the urine, so it should be used with significant caution in patients with a concomitant anion gap acidosis. In these patients, the unmeasured anion (eg, lactate, hippurate, 5-oxoproline, etc) will serve to falsely elevate the urine anion gap. Additionally, the presence of polyuria or a urine sodium level less than ~10 to 20 mEq/L can also make the urine anion gap less reliable.

An alternative to the urine anion gap is the urine osmolal gap. The urine osmolal gap is calculated in a manner similar to the serum osmolal gap:

$$\text{Calculated Urine Osmolality} = 2*([Na^+]+[K^+])+\frac{[Urea]}{2.8}+\frac{[Glucose]}{18}$$

$$\text{Urine Osmolal Gap} = \text{Measured Urine Osmolality} - \text{Calculated Urine Osmolality}$$

The urine osmolal gap should be proportionate to the urinary ammonium, as this is the only other major urinary solute not included in the above-calculated urine osmolality (recall that vast majority of unmeasured anions will be complexed with either sodium or potassium, which are included here). Therefore, the urine osmolal gap is a more direct measure of the urine ammonium excretion. A normal value in a patient with a normal acid-base balance falls between 10 and 100 mOsm/kg, although in patients with an RTA these values are usually on the low end of this spectrum (< 20 mOsm/kg). When faced with an acid load, a patient with intact urinary acidification (ie, diarrhea) will significantly increase the urine ammonium excretion, and hence the urine osmolal gap will also increase significantly (> 400 mOsm/kg). Since the ammonium must be also be complexed to an anion for excretion, the urine ammonium concentration can be estimated as one-half of the urine osmolal gap (ie, for a urine osmolal gap of 400 mOsm/L, the urine ammonium concentration would be estimated as 200 mOsm/L). Generally, the urine osmolal gap will not exceed ~600 mOsm/L. Alternatively, in a patient with dysfunctional urinary acidification (ie, type 1 or type 4 RTA), the serum osmolal gap will not exceed 150 mOsm/kg.

Similar to the urine anion gap, there are limitations to the use of the urine osmolal gap. First, the urine osmolal gap should not be used in a patient with increased urinary excretion of non-ammonium solutes (eg, mannitol, methanol), which would yield a potentially inappropriate elevation in the urine osmolal gap. Additionally, a urinary tract infection with a urease-producing bacteria can lead to inappropriate elevation of the urine osmolal gap, as urea can react with water to produce ammonium and HCO_3, depending on the urine pH.

Once the urine anion gap or urine osmolal gap have been determined, the urine pH, serum potassium, presence of renal stones, and other abnormalities of the urinalysis can be used to determine the most likely diagnosis and underlying etiology. However, it should also be noted that the urine pH is not helpful in differentiating the etiology in chronic or prolonged metabolic acidosis that is also associated with hypokalemia (eg, chronic diarrhea), in severe volume depletion, or in patients with urinary tract infections secondary to urease-producing organisms.

A distal or type 1 RTA is classically associated with a more significant drop in the serum HCO_3 (usually < 12 mEq/L), an elevated urine anion gap, a reduced urine osmolal gap, an elevated urinary pH, the possible presence of renal stones, and a low or normal serum potassium. Causes of a distal RTA are listed in Table I-8. The diagnosis of a proximal RTA requires a high degree of clinical suspicion, as it cannot be diagnosed based on the urine anion gap or the urine osmolal gap (see Table I-9). In addition to abnormalities in urinary HCO_3 resorption, patients may have abnormalities in the absorption of other solutes from the proximal tubule (eg, phosphate, uric acid, amino acids, glucose). This more generalized proximal tubule dysfunction is termed *Fanconi syndrome*. The urine pH and urine anion/osmolal gap calculations are not helpful unless the patient is receiving a HCO_3, or the disease process is caught very early. Once the process becomes chronic, the patient reaches a steady state in terms of the serum HCO_3 (12 to 18 mEq/L), and therefore

TABLE I-8 • Evaluation of non-anion gap acidosis.

Evaluation Strategy

1. History (acute or chronic issues, medications, altered GI anatomy, genetic diseases, etc). Also, is the patient receiving an acid load, such as TPN?

2. Does the patient have chronic renal insufficiency? If so, this alone may be responsible for the non-anion gap acidosis.

3. Calculate urine anion gap and urine osmolal gap. The urine anion gap may be of limited value in patients with severe serum anion gap acidosis, as it may be falsely elevated. Similarly, the urine osmolal gap may be inappropriately elevated in patients with a significant serum osmolal gap (particularly due to mannitol).

4. Note the serum potassium as well as the urine pH.

5. If proximal RTA is suspected, look for evidence of other inappropriate compounds in the urine (amino acids, elevated phosphate, glucosuria), and calculate the fractional resorption of sodium bicarbonate (should be > 15%). Also check serum for evidence of dysfunction of the PTH–vitamin D–calcium axis.

Cause of NAGMA

Low Serum Potassium
GI: Diarrhea, pancreaticoduodenal fistula, urinary intestinal diversion
Renal: Type 1 RTA (distal), type 2 RTA (proximal)
Medications/exposures: Carbonic anhydrase inhibitors, toluene
Other: D-Lactic acidosis
High (or Normal) Serum Potassium
GI: Elevated ileostomy output
Renal: Type 4 RTA or CKD
Medications: NSAIDs; antibiotics (trimethoprim, pentamidine); heparin; ACE inhibitors, ARBs, aldosterone antagonists (spironolactone); acid administration (TPN)

Evaluation of RTA

	Type 1 RTA	Type 2 RTA	Type 4 RTA
Severity of metabolic acidosis, [HCO_3]	Severe (< 10–12 mEq/L typically)	Intermediate (12–20 mEq/L)	Mild (15–20 mEq/L)
Associated urine abnormalities	Urinary phosphate, calcium increased; bone disease often present	Urine glucose, amino acids, phosphate, calcium may be elevated	
Urine pH	HIGH (> 5.5)	Low (acidic), until serum HCO_3 level exceeds resorptive ability of proximal tubule; then becomes alkalotic once reabsorptive threshold is crossed	Low (acidic)
Serum K^+	Low to normal; should correct with oral HCO_3 therapy	Classically low, although may be normal or even high with rare genetic defects; worsens with oral HCO_3 therapy	HIGH
Renal stones	Often	No	No

(Continued)

TABLE I-8 • Evaluation of non-anion gap acidosis. (*continued*)			
	Type 1 RTA	Type 2 RTA	Type 4 RTA
Renal tubular defect	Reduced NH_4 secretion in distal tubule	Reduced HCO_3 resorption in proximal tubule	Reduced H^+/K^+ exchange in distal and collecting tubules due to decreased aldosterone or aldosterone resistance
Urine anion gap	> 10	Negative initially; then positive when receiving serum HCO_3; then negative after therapy	> 10
Urine osmolal gap	Reduced (< 150 mOsm/L) during acute acidosis	At baseline < 100 mEq/L; unreliable during acidosis	Reduced (< 150 mOsm/L) during acute acidosis

ACE, angiotensin-converting enzyme; ARB, angiotensin receptor blocker; CKD, chronic kidney disease; GI, gastrointestinal; HCO_3, bicarbonate; NSAID, nonsteroidal anti-inflammatory drug; PTH, parathyroid hormone; RTA, renal tubular acidosis; TPN, total parenteral nutrition.

the urine pH and anion gap will be inconclusive and appropriate for the patient's diet. If the patient is placed on a HCO_3 infusion, and the serum HCO_3 level surpasses the patient's absorptive capabilities, the urine pH will increase rapidly. Alternatively, one can calculate the fractional excretion (FE) of HCO_3. A value greater than 15% indicates that a proximal RTA is likely.

$$FE_{HCO_3^-} = \frac{[\text{Urine } HCO_3^-] * \text{Serum Cr}}{[\text{Serum } HCO_3^-] * \text{Urine Cr}}$$

A distal RTA is generally associated with a mild reduction in serum HCO_3 (~18 to 22 mEq/L), an elevated urine anion gap, a reduced urine osmolal gap, a normal urine pH, and an elevated serum potassium level.

Finally, for patients with any type of anion gap acidosis, the serum HCO_3 deficit can also be calculated. While HCO_3 therapy is administered only in severe acidemia in patients with lactic acidosis, serum HCO_3 does have a role in the treatment of certain toxicities and in the management of non-anion gap acidosis. First, one must calculate the HCO_3 space, which can then be used to determine the total HCO_3 deficit.

$$HCO_3^- \text{ space} = \left[0.4 * \left(\frac{2.6}{HCO_3^-} \right) \right] * \text{Lean Body Weight (in kg)}$$

$$HCO_3^- \text{ Deficit} = HCO_3^- \text{ space} * HCO_3^- \text{ Deficit/L}$$

TABLE I-9 • Causes of renal tubular acidosis.
Causes of Type 1 (Distal) RTA
Primary   • Idiopathic or familial (may be recessive or dominant)   ***Secondary***   • Medications: Lithium, amphotericin, ifosfamide, NSAIDs   • Rheumatologic disorders: Sjögren syndrome, SLE, RA   • Hypercalciuria (idiopathic) or associated with vitamin D deficiency or hyperparathyroidism   • Sarcoidosis   • Obstructive uropathy   • Wilson disease   • Rejection of renal transplant allograft   • Toluene toxicity
Causes of Type 2 (Proximal) RTA
Primary   • Idiopathic   • Familial (primarily recessive disorders)   • Genetic: Fanconi syndrome, cystinosis, glycogen storage disease (type 1), Wilson disease, galactosemia   ***Secondary***   • Medications: Acetazolamide, topiramate, aminoglycoside antibiotics, ifosfamide, reverse transcriptase inhibitors (tenofovir)   • Heavy metal poisoning: Lead, mercury, copper   • Multiple myeloma or amyloidosis (secondary to light chain toxicity)   • Sjögren syndrome   • Vitamin D deficiency   • Rejection of renal transplant allograft
Causes of Type 4 RTA (Hypoaldosteronism or Aldosterone Resistance)
Primary   • Primary adrenal insufficiency   • Inherited disorders associated with hypoaldosteronism   • Pseudohypoaldosteronism (types 1 and 2)   ***Secondary***   • Causes of hyporeninemic hypoaldosteronism such as renal disease (diabetic nephropathy), NSAID use, calcineurin inhibitors, volume expansion/volume overload   • Causes of distal tubule voltage defects such as sickle cell disease, obstructive uropathy, SLE   • Severe illness/septic shock   • Angiotensin II-associated medications: ACE inhibitors, ARBs, direct renin inhibitors   • Potassium-sparing diuretics: Spironolactone, amiloride, triamterene   • Antibiotics: Trimethoprim, pentamidine
ACE, angiotensin-converting enzyme; ARB, angiotensin receptor blocker; NSAID, nonsteroidal anti-inflammatory drug; RA, rheumatoid arthritis; RTA, renal tubular acidosis; SLE, systemic lupus erythematosus.

RESPIRATORY ACIDOSIS

The algorithm for the evaluation of a respiratory acidosis is shown in Figure I-4. It is particularly helpful to determine whether a patient has a baseline respiratory acidosis prior to evaluation as it will greatly aid in determining the acute acid-base disorders present. The first step in the evaluation is to determine if the metabolic compensation is appropriate. This requires a decision as to whether the respiratory process is acute or chronic in nature.

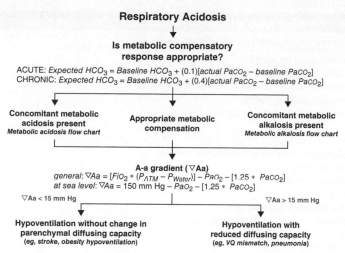

Figure I-4 • Algorithm for the evaluation of a respiratory acidosis.

Equation for the metabolic compensation for *acute* respiratory acidosis:

$$\text{Expected HCO}_3 = \text{Baseline HCO}_3 + (0.1)[\text{Actual Paco}_2 - \text{Baseline Paco}_2];$$

Equation for the metabolic compensation for *chronic* respiratory acidosis:

$$\text{Expected HCO}_3 = \text{Baseline HCO}_3 + (0.4)[\text{Actual Paco}_2 - \text{Baseline Paco}_2];$$

where the baseline HCO_3 and the baseline $Paco_2$ should be determined from prior laboratory studies, or if not known, values of 24 mEq/L and 40 mm Hg should be used. If the actual value of the HCO_3 is less than the expected value, then a concomitant metabolic acidosis is present. If the actual HCO_3 is greater than expected, then a metabolic alkalosis is present. If the actual value is as expected, then no metabolic acid-base disorder is present, and the change in the HCO_3 is appropriate. Once this has been determined, one may use the alveolar-arterial partial pressure of oxygen gradient (A-a gradient) to help differentiate the underlying conditions. The A-a gradient is elevated if it is greater than ~15 mm Hg:

$$\nabla\text{A-a} = [\text{Fio}_2 * (P_{ATM} - P_{water})] - \text{Pao}_2 - (1.25) * \text{Paco}_2$$

At sea level, the atmospheric pressure is 1 ATM or 760 mm Hg, the partial pressure of water is 47 mm Hg, and the fraction of inspired oxygen (Fio_2) is 0.21, so the A-a oxygen gradient reduces the following:

$$\nabla\text{A-a}_{\text{sea level}} = 150 \text{ mm Hg} - \text{Pao}_2 - (1.25) * \text{Paco}_2$$

However, many conditions may be associated with an A-a gradient, and the normal A-a gradient can vary with a number of factors, including age. Additionally, patients may have a baseline A-a gradient that is elevated and unknown (and does not cause the patient to require supplemental oxygen), which may also complicate the picture. Overall, the history and clinical presentation are generally adequate to narrow the differential diagnoses (see Table I-10).

TABLE I-10 · Potential causes of respiratory acidosis.

Central Nervous System and Neuromuscular Disease

- Stroke/cerebrovascular accident
- Head trauma, increased intracranial pressure
- General or moderate anesthesia
- Opioid or other sedative toxicity
- Spinal cord injury (above the C6 level)
- Seizure
- Botulism
- Organophosphate or other anticholinergic toxicity
- Bulbar neuropathies
- Hypokalemic myopathy
- Myasthenia gravis
- Guillain-Barré syndrome (or variants)
- ALS (and other neuromuscular disorders, including muscular dystrophies and mitochondrial disorders)
- Multiple sclerosis
- Myxedema

Chest Wall

- Trauma (flail chest)
- Pneumothorax, pleural effusion or other pleural space occupying lesions
- Kyphosis or other chest wall abnormality leading to abnormal respiratory mechanics
- Diaphragmatic dysfunction or paralysis
- Thymoma or other structure/tumor causing external airway compression

Pulmonary or Airway

- Upper or lower airway obstruction (including tracheomalacia and obstructive sleep apnea)
- Tracheal stenosis
- Central sleep apnea
- Aspiration of foreign body with obstruction or massive aspiration event
- Angioedema
- Allergic reaction with airway involvement

Pulmonary or Airway (cont.)

- Laryngospasm
- Bronchospasm
- Vocal cord paralysis
- Status asthmaticus
- COPD
- Bronchiolitis
- Interstitial lung disease with severe restriction
- Massive pulmonary edema
- ARDS (particularly in the fibrotic or fibroproliferative phase)
- Bronchiectasis, including end-stage cystic fibrosis

Vascular

- Pulmonary embolism
- Fat embolism
- Cardiac arrest

Other

- Esophageal intubation (or other misplacement of airway device)
- Air-trapping during mechanical ventilation
- Snakebite with neurotoxin envenomation

ALS, amyotrophic lateral sclerosis; ARDS, acute respiratory distress syndrome; COPD, chronic obstructive pulmonary disease.

METABOLIC ALKALOSIS

The algorithm for the evaluation of a metabolic alkalosis is shown in Figure I-5. The first step in evaluation is to determine whether the respiratory compensation is appropriate. Similar to the case for metabolic acidosis, we have the following equation to determine appropriate compensation:

$$\text{Expected } Paco_2 = \text{Baseline } Paco_2 - (0.7)[\text{Actual } HCO_3 - \text{Baseline } HCO_3]$$

Once it has been determined that the respiratory compensation is appropriate or there is a concomitant respiratory acid-base disorder, the next step is to review the history for any potential causes, including an alkali load, genetic conditions such as a cystic fibrosis (CF), or the recent use of laxative (see Table I-11). A thorough review of the medications is also necessary at this point. The physical examination is also critical as it may point to evidence of hypertension (HTN) or a hyperaldosterone state. The next step in evaluation is to determine if the condition is a chloride- or fluid-responsive condition (such as hyperemesis) or a chloride-resistant process. This is accomplished by evaluating the urine chloride. Once this has been established, one may use a combination of the presence or absence of HTN, the urine and serum potassium, and the plasma renin and aldosterone levels.

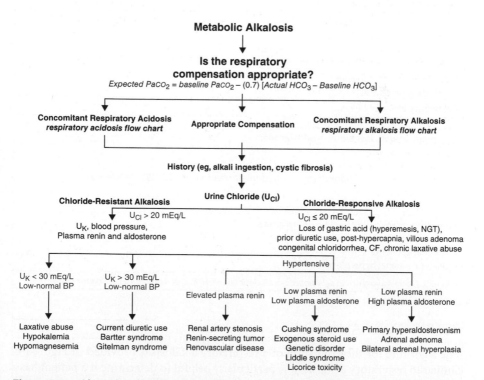

Figure I-5 • Algorithm for the evaluation of a metabolic alkalosis.

TABLE I-11 • Causes of metabolic alkalosis.
History
Rule Out the Following as Causes
• Alkali load ("milk-alkali" or calcium-alkali syndrome, oral sodium bicarbonate, intravenous sodium bicarbonate) • Genetic causes (CF) • Presence of hypercalcemia • Intravenous β-lactam antibiotics • Laxative abuse (may also cause a metabolic acidosis depending on diarrheal HCO_3 losses)
If None of the Above, Then…
Urine Chloride < 20 mEq/L (*chloride-responsive causes*) • Loss of gastric acid (hyperemesis, NGT suctioning) • Prior diuretic use (in hours to days following discontinuation) • Post-hypercapnia • Villous adenoma • Congenital chloridorrhea • Chronic laxative abuse (may also cause a metabolic acidosis depending on diarrheal HCO_3 losses) • CF
OR: Urine Chloride > 20 mEq/L (*chloride-resistant causes*):
Urine Chloride > 20 mEq/L, Lack of HTN, Urine Potassium < 30 mEq/L
• Hypokalemia or hypomagnesemia • Laxative abuse (if dominated by hypokalemia)
Urine Chloride > 20 mEq/L, Lack of HTN, Urine Potassium Variable
• Current diuretic use • Bartter syndrome • Gitelman syndrome
Urine Chloride > 20 mEq/L, Presence of HTN, Urine Potassium Variable but Usually > 30 mEq/L
Elevated plasma renin level: • Renal artery stenosis • Renin-secreting tumor • Renovascular disease
Low plasma renin, low plasma aldosterone: • Cushing syndrome • Exogenous mineralocorticoid use • Genetic disorder (11-hydoxylase or 17-hydrolyase deficiency, 11β-HSD deficiency) • Liddle syndrome • Licorice toxicity
Low plasma renin, high plasma aldosterone: • Primary hyperaldosteronism • Adrenal adenoma • Bilateral adrenal hyperplasia
11β-HSD, 11beta-hydroxysteroid dehydrogenase; CF, cystic fibrosis; HTN, hypertension; NGT, nasogastric tube.

RESPIRATORY ALKALOSIS

The algorithm for the evaluation of a respiratory alkalosis is provided in Figure I-6. Similar to respiratory acidosis, it is particularly helpful to determine if a patient has a baseline respiratory alkalosis prior to evaluation as it will greatly aid in determining

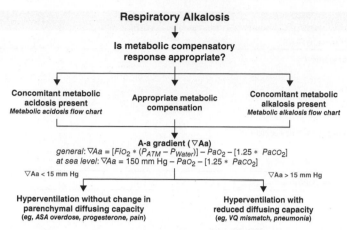

Figure I-6 • Algorithm for the evaluation of respiratory alkalosis.

the acute acid-base disorders present. The first step in the evaluation is to determine if the metabolic compensation is appropriate. This requires a decision as to whether the respiratory process is acute or chronic in nature.

Equation for metabolic compensation for acute respiratory alkalosis:

$$\text{Expected HCO}_3 = \text{Baseline HCO}_3 - (0.2)[\text{Actual Paco}_2 - \text{Baseline Paco}_2].$$

Equation for metabolic compensation for chronic respiratory alkalosis:

$$\text{Expected HCO}_3 = \text{Baseline HCO}_3 - (0.4)[\text{Actual Paco}_2 - \text{Baseline Paco}_2].$$

Once it has been determined if a concomitant metabolic acid-base disorder is present, the A-a gradient may be used to aid in determining the etiology of the respiratory alkalosis (see Table I-12).

This effectively rounds out the process for evaluation for acid-base disorders. Before proceeding to the cases, we will briefly address the other methods for evaluation of acid-base disorders.

THE STEWART APPROACH TO ACID-BASE DISORDERS

The underlying physiochemical principles of the Stewart approach are as follows: (1) There is continual maintenance of electrical neutrality in the serum; (2) weak acids are partially dissociated in water governed by dissociation equilibria; and (3) mass must always be conserved in a closed system. In contrast to the "bicarbonate" approach we employ in this text, the Stewart approach is founded on the principle that the serum HCO_3 is a dependent rather than an independent variable, and the primary independent determinants of the acid-base status (and hence pH) are the $Paco_2$, the concentration of weak acids (A_{TOT}; primarily

TABLE I-12 • Causes of respiratory alkalosis.
Central Nervous System
• Anxiety or panic
• Pain
• Volitional
• Psychosis
• Fever
• Stroke/cerebrovascular accident
• Trauma
• Tumor
Pulmonary and Airways
• High altitude
• Pneumonia/pneumonitis
• Aspiration of foreign body or other substance
• Severe hypoxemia due to atelectasis, ARDS, edema, carboxy/met-hemoglobinemia, etc
• Pulmonary embolism
• Asthma
• Chest wall trauma
• Pulmonary edema
Other Causes
• Drug toxicity (nicotine, progesterone, catecholaminergic vasoactive drugs, salicylates, xanthines, doxapram)
• Pregnancy
• Liver failure/cirrhosis
• Excess mechanical ventilation
• Heat exposure/stroke
• Compensation and/or recovery from metabolic acidosis
ARDS, acute respiratory distress syndrome.

albumin), and the concentration of strong ions (SID_{APP}). The primary advantage of this method is that is allows for consideration of a more complete number of variables impacting the acid-base status and provides a more physiologic explanation for hyperchloremic metabolic acidosis. However, it is a far more complex method of approaching acid-base evaluation, requires more laboratory studies, and has not shown a consistent benefit in terms of diagnosing acid-base status or impacting clinical outcomes compared with the more widely applied bicarbonate approach.

THE BASE EXCESS (BE) AND STANDARD BASE EXCESS (SBE) APPROACHES

Proposed as an alternative to the use of an HCO_3 estimate of ABG measurements, the base excess (BE) is a parameter derived by Siggard-Andersen in 1960. The BE is the concentration of a strong acid or strong base (mmoL/L) required to return the pH of a whole blood sample to pH 7.40, assuming a Pco_2 of 40 mm Hg and normal temperature, thus eliminating the respiratory component from the equation and focusing on the metabolic component alone. Normal values range from −3 to

+3 mmol/L (positive BE = alkalotic pH; negative BE = acidotic pH). The equation used to calculate the BE is as follows:

$$BE = \{[HCO_3^-] - 24.4\} + \{(2.3 * [Hb] + 7.7) * (pH - 7.4) * (1 - 0.023 \times [Hb]).$$

However, this equation is not truly invariant of changes in the P_{CO_2}, as it only accounts for buffering intravascularly, and does not take into account the entire extracellular space. A modified version of the Van Slyke equation, called, the SBE, attempts to account for this by assuming the buffering capacity of hemoglobin (Hb) is distributed throughout the extracellular fluid (ECF), so the Hb concentration is assumed to be one-third the normal value (of 13 to 15 g/dL) rather than the patient's actual Hb to ensure it is not dependent on the P_{aCO_2}. The downside to each of these approaches is that they ignore the respiratory components of acid-base status and provide no means to differentiate between anion gap and non-anion gap causes of a metabolic acidosis.

References

All of the following texts and/or publications were used in the preparation of this text, including the introduction and cases. Additional publications may be cited on a case-by-case basis as well, depending on the specific topics addressed.

Acetaminophen Toxicity

Flanagan RJ, Mant TG. Coma and metabolic acidosis early in severe acute paracetamol poisoning. Hum Toxicol. 1986;5:179.

Mazer M, Perrone J. Acetaminophen-induced nephrotoxicity: pathophysiology, clinical manifestations, and management. J Med Toxicol. 2008;4:2.

McBride, PV, Rumack, BH. Acetaminophen intoxication. Semin Dial. 1992;5:292.

Vale JA, Proudfoot AT. Paracetamol (acetaminophen) poisoning. Lancet. 1995;346:547.

Zein JG, Wallace DJ, Kinasewitz G, et al. Early anion gap metabolic acidosis in acetaminophen overdose. Am J Emerg Med. 2010;28:798.

Alcoholic and Starvation Ketoacidosis

Jenkins DW, Eckle RE, Craig JW. Alcoholic ketoacidosis. JAMA. 1971;217:177.

Levy LJ, Duga J, Girgis M, Gordon EE. Ketoacidosis associated with alcoholism in nondiabetic subjects. Ann Intern Med. 1973;78:213.

Palmer BF, Clegg DJ. Electrolyte disturbances in patients with chronic alcohol-use disorder. N Engl J Med. 2017;377:1368.

Reichard GA Jr, Owen OE, Haff AC, et al. Ketone-body production and oxidation in fasting obese humans. J Clin Invest. 1974;53:508.

Schelling JR, Howard RL, Winter SD, Linas SL. Increased osmolal gap in alcoholic ketoacidosis and lactic acidosis. Ann Intern Med. 1990;113:580.

Toth HL, Greenbaum LA. Severe acidosis caused by starvation and stress. Am J Kidney Dis. 2003;42:E16.

Anion Gap

Bern M. Clinically significant pseudohyponatremia. Am J Hematol. 2006;81:558.

Corey HE. Stewart and beyond: new models of acid-base balance. Kidney Int. 2003;64:777.

Faradji-Hazan V, Oster JR, Fedeman DG, et al. Effect of pyridostigmine bromide on serum bromide concentration and the anion gap. J Am Soc Nephrol. 1991;1:1123.

Feldman M, Soni N, Dickson B. Influence of hypoalbuminemia or hyperalbuminemia on the serum anion gap. J Lab Clin Med. 2005;146:317.

Fenves AZ, Kirkpatrick HM 3rd, Patel VV, et al. Increased anion gap metabolic acidosis as a result of 5-oxoproline (pyroglutamic acid): a role for acetaminophen. Clin J Am Soc Nephrol. 2006;1:441.

Fernandez PC, Cohen RM, Feldman GM. The concept of bicarbonate distribution space: the crucial role of body buffers. Kidney Int. 1989;36:747.

Forni LG, McKinnon W, Lord GA, et al. Circulating anions usually associated with the Krebs cycle in patients with metabolic acidosis. Crit Care. 2005;9:R591.

Komaru Y, Inokuchi R, Ueda Y, et al. Use of the anion gap and intermittent hemodialysis following continuous hemodiafiltration in extremely high dose acute-on-chronic lithium poisoning: a case report. Hemodial Int. 2018;22:E15.

Kraut JA, Kurtz I. Toxic alcohol ingestions: clinical features, diagnosis, and management. Clin J Am Soc Nephrol. 2008;3:208.

Kraut JA, Mullins ME. Toxic alcohols. N Engl J Med. 2018;378:270.

Kraut JA, Nagami GT. The serum anion gap in the evaluation of acid-base disorders: what are its limitations and can its effectiveness be improved? Clin J Am Soc Nephrol. 2013;8:2018.

Kraut JA, Xing SX. Approach to the evaluation of a patient with an increased serum osmolal gap and high-anion-gap metabolic acidosis. Am J Kidney Dis. 2011;58:480.

Lu J, Zello GA, Randell E, et al. Closing the anion gap: contribution of D-lactate to diabetic ketoacidosis. Clin Chim Acta. 2011;412:286.

Madias NE, Ayus JC, Adrogué HJ. Increased anion gap in metabolic alkalosis: the role of plasma-protein equivalency. N Engl J Med. 1979;300:1421.

Murray T, Long W, Narins RG. Multiple myeloma and the anion gap. N Engl J Med. 1975;292:574.

Pierce NF, Fedson DS, Brigham KL, et al. The ventilatory response to acute base deficit in humans. Time course during development and correction of metabolic acidosis. Ann Intern Med. 1970;72:633.

Relman AS. What are acids and bases? Am J Med. 1954;17:435.

Schwartz WB, Relman AS. A critique of the parameters used in the evaluation of acid-base disorders. "Whole-blood buffer base" and "standard bicarbonate" compared with blood pH and plasma bicarbonate concentration. N Engl J Med. 1963;268:1382.

Zimmer BW, Marcus RJ, Sawyer K, Harchelroad F. Salicylate intoxication as a cause of pseudohyperchloremia. Am J Kidney Dis. 2008;51:346.

Arterial-Venous Differences in Blood Gases

Chu YC, Chen CZ, Lee CH, et al. Prediction of arterial blood gas values from venous blood gas values in patients with acute respiratory failure receiving mechanical ventilation. J Formos Med Assoc. 2003;102:539.

Kelly AM, Kyle E, McAlpine R. Venous pCO(2) and pH can be used to screen for significant hypercarbia in emergency patients with acute respiratory disease. J Emerg Med. 2002;22:15.

Malatesha G, Singh NK, Bharija A, et al. Comparison of arterial and venous pH, bicarbonate, PCO2 and PO2 in initial emergency department assessment. Emerg Med J. 2007;24:569.

Malinoski DJ, Todd SR, Slone S, et al. Correlation of central venous and arterial blood gas measurements in mechanically ventilated trauma patients. Arch Surg. 2005;140:1122.

Walkey AJ, Farber HW, O'Donnell C, et al. The accuracy of the central venous blood gas for acid-base monitoring. J Intensive Care Med. 2010; 25:104.

Aspirin Overdose

Eichenholz A, Mulhausen RO, Redleaf PS. Nature of acid-base disturbance in salicylate intoxication. Metabolism. 1963;12:164.

Gabow PA, Anderson RJ, Potts DE, Schrier RW. Acid-base disturbances in the salicylate-intoxicated adult. Arch Intern Med. 1978;138:1481.

Hill JB. Salicylate intoxication. N Engl J Med. 1973;288:1110.

Temple AR. Acute and chronic effects of aspirin toxicity and their treatment. Arch Intern Med. 1981;141:364.

Thisted B, Krantz T, Strøom J, Sørensen MB. Acute salicylate self-poisoning in 177 consecutive patients treated in ICU. Acta Anaesthesiol Scand. 1987;31:312.

BE and SBE Calculation

Morgan TJ, Clark C, Endre Z. Accuracy of base excess – an in vitro evaluation of the Van Slyke equation. Crit Care Med. 2000;28:2932.

Siggaard-Andersen O. The Van Slyke equation. Scand J Clin Lab Invest. 1977;146:15.

Siggaard-Andersen O, Engel K, Jorgensen K, et al. A micro method for determination of pH carbon dioxide tension, base excess and standard bicarbonate in capillary blood. Scand J Clin Lab Invest. 1960;12:172.

Siggaard-Anderson O, Fogh-Andersen N. Base excess or buffer base (strong ion difference) as measure of a non-respiratory acid-base disturbance. Acta Anesth Scand. 1995;39(suppl 107):123.

Chronic Kidney Disease

Bailey JL. Metabolic acidosis: an unrecognized cause of morbidity in the patient with chronic kidney disease. Kidney Int Suppl. 2005;S15.

Halperin ML, Ethier JH, Kamel KS. Ammonium excretion in chronic metabolic acidosis: benefits and risks. Am J Kidney Dis. 1989;14:267.

Kraut JA, Kurtz I. Metabolic acidosis of CKD: diagnosis, clinical characteristics, and treatment. Am J Kidney Dis. 2005;45:978.

Krieger NS, Frick KK, Bushinsky DA. Mechanism of acid-induced bone resorption. Curr Opin Nephrol Hypertens. 2004;13:423.

Warnock DG. Uremic acidosis. Kidney Int. 1988;34:278.

Widmer B, Gerhardt RE, Harrington JT, Cohen JJ. Serum electrolyte and acid base composition. The influence of graded degrees of chronic renal failure. Arch Intern Med. 1979;139:1099.

Delta-Delta

Farwell WR, Taylor EN. Serum anion gap, bicarbonate and biomarkers of inflammation in healthy individuals in a national survey. CMAJ. 2010;182:137.

Feldman M, Soni N, Dickson B. Influence of hypoalbuminemia or hyperalbuminemia on the serum anion gap. J Lab Clin Med. 2005;146:317.

Rastegar A. Use of the deltaAG/deltaHCO3- ratio in the diagnosis of mixed acid-base disorders. J Am Soc Nephrol. 2007;18:2429.

Rose BD, Post TW. Clinical Physiology of Acid-Base and Electrolyte Disorders, 5e. New York, NY: McGraw-Hill; 2001:583.

Wang F, Butler T, Rabbani GH, Jones PK. The acidosis of cholera. Contributions of hyperproteinemia, lactic acidemia, and hyperphosphatemia to an increased serum anion gap. N Engl J Med. 1986;315:1591.

Diabetic Ketoacidosis

DeFronzo RA, Matzuda M, Barret E. Diabetic ketoacidosis: a combined metabolic-nephrologic approach to therapy. Diabetes Rev. 1994;2:209.

Fulop M, Murthy V, Michilli A, et al. Serum beta-hydroxybutyrate measurement in patients with uncontrolled diabetes mellitus. Arch Intern Med. 1999;159:381.

Porter WH, Yao HH, Karounos DG. Laboratory and clinical evaluation of assays for beta-hydroxybutyrate. Am J Clin Pathol. 1997;107:353.

Rose BD, Post TW. Clinical Physiology of Acid-Base and Electrolyte Disorders, 5e. New York, NY: McGraw Hill; 2001:809815.

Shen T, Braude S. Changes in serum phosphate during treatment of diabetic ketoacidosis: predictive significance of severity of acidosis on presentation. Intern Med J. 2012;42:1347.

Wachtel TJ, Tetu-Mouradjian LM, Goldman DL, et al. Hyperosmolarity and acidosis in diabetes mellitus: a three-year experience in Rhode Island. J Gen Intern Med. 1991;6:495.

General Acid-Base Disorders

Berend K, de Vries AP, Gans RO. Physiological approach to assessment of acid-base disturbances. N Engl J Med. 2014;371:1434.

General Compensation

Adrogué HJ, Madias NE. Secondary responses to altered acid-base status: the rules of engagement. J Am Soc Nephrol. 2010;21:920.

Isopropyl Alcohol

Abramson S, Singh AK. Treatment of the alcohol intoxications: ethylene glycol, methanol and isopropanol. Curr Opin Nephrol Hypertens. 2000;9:695.

Bekka R, Borron SW, Astier A, et al. Treatment of methanol and isopropanol poisoning with intravenous fomepizole. J Toxicol Clin Toxicol. 2001;39:59.

Gaudet MP, Fraser GL. Isopropanol ingestion: case report with pharmacokinetic analysis. Am J Emerg Med. 1989;7:297.

Gaulier JM, Lamballais F, Yazdani F, Lachâtre G. Isopropyl alcohol concentrations in postmortem tissues to document fatal intoxication. J Anal Toxicol. 2011;35:254.

Monaghan MS, Ackerman BH, Olsen KM, et al. The use of delta osmolality to predict serum isopropanol and acetone concentrations. Pharmacotherapy. 1993;13:60.

Pappas AA, Ackerman BH, Olsen KM, Taylor EH. Isopropanol ingestion: a report of six episodes with isopropanol and acetone serum concentration time data. J Toxicol Clin Toxicol. 1991;29:11.

Trullas JC, Aguilo S, Castro P, Nogue S. Life-threatening isopropyl alcohol intoxication: is hemodialysis really necessary? Vet Hum Toxicol. 2004;46:282.

Zaman F, Pervez A, Abreo K. Isopropyl alcohol intoxication: a diagnostic challenge. Am J Kidney Dis. 2002;40:E12.

Lactic Acidosis

Adeva-Andany M, López-Ojén M, Funcasta Calderón R, et al. Comprehensive review on lactate metabolism in human health. Mitochondrion. 2014;17:76.

Coronado BE, Opal SM, Yoburn DC. Antibiotic-induced D-lactic acidosis. Ann Intern Med. 1995;122:839.

Halperin ML, Kamel KS. D-lactic acidosis: turning sugar into acids in the gastrointestinal tract. Kidney Int. 1996;49:1.

Jorens PG, Demey HE, Schepens PJ, et al. Unusual D-lactic acid acidosis from propylene glycol metabolism in overdose. J Toxicol Clin Toxicol. 2004;42:163.

Levy B. Lactate and shock state: the metabolic view. Curr Opin Crit Care. 2006;12:315.

Madias NE. Lactic acidosis. Kidney Int. 1986;29:752.

Mikkelsen ME, Miltiades AN, Gaieski DF, et al. Serum lactate is associated with mortality in severe sepsis independent of organ failure and shock. Crit Care Med. 2009;37:1670.

Stolberg L, Rolfe R, Gitlin N, et al. D-Lactic acidosis due to abnormal gut flora: diagnosis and treatment of two cases. N Engl J Med. 1982;306:1344.

Tsao YT, Tsai WC, Yang SP. A life-threatening double gap metabolic acidosis. Am J Emerg Med 2008;26:385.e5.

Uchida H, Yamamoto H, Kisaki Y, et al. D-lactic acidosis in short-bowel syndrome managed with antibiotics and probiotics. J Pediatr Surg. 2004;39:634.

Uribarri J, Oh MS, Carroll HJ. D-lactic acidosis. A review of clinical presentation, biochemical features, and pathophysiologic mechanisms. Medicine (Baltimore). 1998;77:73.

Metabolic Alkalosis

Abreo K, Adlakha A, Kilpatrick S, et al. The milk-alkali syndrome. A reversible form of acute renal failure. Arch Intern Med. 1993;153:1005.

Barton CH, Vaziri ND, Ness RL, et al. Cimetidine in the management of metabolic alkalosis induced by nasogastric drainage. Arch Surg. 1979;114:70.

Bear R, Goldstein M, Phillipson E, et al. Effect of metabolic alkalosis on respiratory function in patients with chronic obstructive lung disease. Can Med Assoc J. 1977;117:900.

Galla JH, Gifford JD, Luke RG, Rome L. Adaptations to chloride-depletion alkalosis. Am J Physiol. 1991;261:R771.

Garella S, Chang BS, Kahn SI. Dilution acidosis and contraction alkalosis: review of a concept. Kidney Int. 1975;8:279.

Gennari FJ, Weise WJ. Acid-base disturbances in gastrointestinal disease. Clin J Am Soc Nephrol. 2008;3:1861.

Hamm LL, Nakhoul N, Hering-Smith KS. Acid-base homeostasis. Clin J Am Soc Nephrol. 2015;10:2232.

Hulter HN, Sebastian A, Toto RD, et al. Renal and systemic acid-base effects of the chronic administration of hypercalcemia-producing agents: calcitriol, PTH, and intravenous calcium. Kidney Int. 1982;21:445.

Khanna A, Kurtzman NA. Metabolic alkalosis. J Nephrol. 2006;19(suppl 9):S86.

Laski ME, Sabatini S. Metabolic alkalosis, bedside and bench. Semin Nephrol. 2006;26:404.

Luke RG, Galla JH. It is chloride depletion alkalosis, not contraction alkalosis. J Am Soc Nephrol. 2012;23:204.

Miller PD, Berns AS. Acute metabolic alkalosis perpetuating hypercarbia. A role for acetazolamide in chronic obstructive pulmonary disease. JAMA. 1977;238:2400.

Oster JR, Materson BJ, Rogers AI. Laxative abuse syndrome. Am J Gastroenterol. 1980;74:451.

Patel AM, Goldfarb S. Got calcium? Welcome to the calcium-alkali syndrome. J Am Soc Nephrol. 2010;21:1440.

Rose BD, Post TW. Clinical Physiology of Acid-Base and Electrolyte Disorders, 5e. New York, NY: McGraw Hill; 2001:559.

Schwartz WB, Van Ypersele de Strihou, Kassirer JP. Role of anions in metabolic alkalosis and potassium deficiency. N Engl J Med. 1968;279:630.

Sweetser LJ, Douglas JA, Riha RL, Bell SC. Clinical presentation of metabolic alkalosis in an adult patient with cystic fibrosis. Respirology. 2005;10:254.

Taki K, Mizuno K, Takahashi N, Wakusawa R. Disturbance of CO_2 elimination in the lungs by carbonic anhydrase inhibition. Jpn J Physiol. 1986;36:523.

Turban S, Beutler KT, Morris RG, et al. Long-term regulation of proximal tubule acid-base transporter abundance by angiotensin II. Kidney Int. 2006;70:660.

Methanol and Ethylene Glycol Poisoning

Church AS, Witting MD. Laboratory testing in ethanol, methanol, ethylene glycol, and isopropanol toxicities. J Emerg Med. 1997;15:687.

Eder AF, Dowdy YG, Gardiner JA, et al. Serum lactate and lactate dehydrogenase in high concentrations interfere in enzymatic assay of ethylene glycol. Clin Chem. 1996;42:1489.

Hoffman RS, Smilkstein MJ, Howland MA, Goldfrank LR. Osmol gaps revisited: normal values and limitations. J Toxicol Clin Toxicol. 1993;31:81.

Höjer J. Severe metabolic acidosis in the alcoholic: differential diagnosis and management. Hum Exp Toxicol. 1996;15:482.

Liesivuori J, Savolainen H. Methanol and formic acid toxicity: biochemical mechanisms. Pharmacol Toxicol. 1991;69:157.

Lynd LD, Richardson KJ, Pursell RA, et al. An evaluation of the osmole gap as a screening test for toxic alcohol poisoning. BMC Emerg Med. 2008;8:5.

Malandain H, Cano Y. Interferences of glycerol, propylene glycol, and other diols in the enzymatic assay of ethylene glycol. Eur J Clin Chem Clin Biochem. 1996;34:651.

Purssell RA, Pudek M, Brubacher J, Abu-Laban RB. Derivation and validation of a formula to calculate the contribution of ethanol to the osmolal gap. Ann Emerg Med. 2001;38:653.

Shirey T, Sivilotti M. Reaction of lactate electrodes to glycolate. Crit Care Med. 1999;27:2305.

Sivilotti ML. Methanol intoxication. Ann Emerg Med. 2000;35:313.

Milk-Alkali Syndrome

Abreo K, Adlakha A, Kilpatrick S, et al. The milk-alkali syndrome. A reversible form of acute renal failure. Arch Intern Med. 1993;153:1005.

Burnett CH, Commons RR. Hypercalcemia without hypercalcuria or hypophosphatemia, calcinosis and renal insufficiency; a syndrome following prolonged intake of milk and alkali. N Engl J Med. 1949;240:787.

Felsenfeld AJ, Levine BS. Milk alkali syndrome and the dynamics of calcium homeostasis. Clin J Am Soc Nephrol. 2006;1:641.

Medarov BI. Milk-alkali syndrome. Mayo Clin Proc. 2009;84:261.

Orwoll ES. The milk-alkali syndrome: current concepts. Ann Intern Med. 1982;97:242.

Patel AM, Goldfarb S. Got calcium? Welcome to the calcium-alkali syndrome. J Am Soc Nephrol. 2010;21:1440.

Picolos MK, Lavis VR, Orlander PR. Milk-alkali syndrome is a major cause of hypercalcaemia among non-end-stage renal disease (non-ESRD) inpatients. Clin Endocrinol (Oxf). 2005;63:566.

Multiple Myeloma

Bridoux F, Kyndt X, Abou-Ayache R, et al. Proximal tubular dysfunction in primary Sjögren's syndrome: a clinicopathological study of 2 cases. Clin Nephrol. 2004;61:434.

Bridoux F, Sirac C, Hugue V, et al. Fanconi's syndrome induced by a monoclonal Vkappa3 light chain in Waldenstrom's macroglobulinemia. Am J Kidney Dis. 2005;45:749.

Decourt C, Bridoux F, Touchard G, Cogné M. A monoclonal V kappa l light chain responsible for incomplete proximal tubulopathy. Am J Kidney Dis. 2003;41:497.

Déret S, Denoroy L, Lamarine M, et al. Kappa light chain-associated Fanconi's syndrome: molecular analysis of monoclonal immunoglobulin light chains from patients with and without intracellular crystals. Protein Eng. 1999;12:363.

Figge J, Rossing TH, Fencl V. The role of serum proteins in acid-base equilibria. J Lab Clin Med. 1991;117:453.

Fonseka CL, Galappaththi SR, Karunarathna JD, et al. A case of multiple myeloma presenting as a distal renal tubular acidosis with extensive bilateral nephrolithiasis. BMC Hematol. 2016;16:8.

Gumprecht T, O'Connor DT, Rearden A, Wolf PL. Negative anion gap in a young adult with multiple myeloma. Clin Chem. 1976;22:1920.

Kobayashi T, Muto S, Nemoto J, et al. Fanconi's syndrome and distal (type 1) renal tubular acidosis in a patient with primary Sjögren's syndrome with monoclonal gammopathy of undetermined significance. Clin Nephrol. 2006;65:427.

Messiaen T, Deret S, Mougenot B, et al. Adult Fanconi syndrome secondary to light chain gammopathy. Clinicopathologic heterogeneity and unusual features in 11 patients. Medicine (Baltimore). 2000;79:135.

Minemura K, Ichikawa K, Itoh N, et al. IgA-kappa type multiple myeloma affecting proximal and distal renal tubules. Intern Med. 2001;40:931.

Sachs J, Fredman B. The hyponatremia of multiple myeloma is true and not pseudohyponatremia. Med Hypotheses. 2006;67:839.

Non-Anion Gap Metabolic Acidosis and Renal Tubular Acidosis

Batlle D, Chin-Theodorou J, Tucker BM. Metabolic acidosis or respiratory alkalosis? Evaluation of a low plasma bicarbonate using the urine anion gap. Am J Kidney Dis. 2017;70:440.

Batlle D, Grupp M, Gaviria M, Kurtzman NA. Distal renal tubular acidosis with intact capacity to lower urinary pH. Am J Med. 1982;72:751.

Batlle D, Haque SK. Genetic causes and mechanisms of distal renal tubular acidosis. Nephrol Dial Transplant. 2012;27:3691.

Batlle DC, Hizon M, Cohen E, et al. The use of the urinary anion gap in the diagnosis of hyperchloremic metabolic acidosis. N Engl J Med. 1988;318:594.

Batlle DC, von Riotte A, Schlueter W. Urinary sodium in the evaluation of hyperchloremic metabolic acidosis. N Engl J Med. 1987;316:140.

Buckalew VM Jr, McCurdy DK, Ludwig GD, et al. Incomplete renal tubular acidosis. Physiologic studies in three patients with a defect in lowering urine pH. Am J Med. 1968;45:32.

Karet FE. Mechanisms in hyperkalemic renal tubular acidosis. J Am Soc Nephrol. 2009;20:251.

Kraut JA, Madias NE. Differential diagnosis of nongap metabolic acidosis: value of a systematic approach. Clin J Am Soc Nephrol. 2012;7:671.

Rastegar M, Nagami GT. Non-anion gap metabolic acidosis: a clinical approach to evaluation. Am J Kidney Dis. 2017;69:296.

Rodríguez Soriano J. Renal tubular acidosis: the clinical entity. J Am Soc Nephrol. 2002;13:2160.

Polyethylene Glycol

Jahn A, Bodreau C, Farthing K, Elbarbry F. Assessing propylene glycol toxicity in alcohol withdrawal patients receiving intravenous benzodiazepines: a one-compartment pharmacokinetic model. Eur J Drug Metab Pharmacokinet. 2018;43:423.

Kraut JA, Kurtz I. Toxic alcohol ingestions: clinical features, diagnosis, and management. Clin J Am Soc Nephrol. 2008;3:208.

Kraut JA, Xing SX. Approach to the evaluation of a patient with an increased serum osmolal gap and high-anion-gap metabolic acidosis. Am J Kidney Dis. 2011;58:480.

Parker MG, Fraser GL, Watson DM, Riker RR. Removal of propylene glycol and correction of increased osmolar gap by hemodialysis in a patient on high dose lorazepam infusion therapy. Intensive Care Med. 2002;28:81.

Wilson KC, Reardon C, Theodore AC, Farber HW. Propylene glycol toxicity: a severe iatrogenic illness in ICU patients receiving IV benzodiazepines: a case series and prospective, observational pilot study. Chest. 2005;128:1674.

Zar T, Graeber C, Perazella MA. Recognition, treatment, and prevention of propylene glycol toxicity. Semin Dial. 2007;20:217.

Zar T, Yusufzai I, Sullivan A, Graeber C. Acute kidney injury, hyperosmolality and metabolic acidosis associated with lorazepam. Nat Clin Pract Nephrol. 2007;3:515.

Propofol Infusion Syndrome

Cannon ML, Glazier SS, Bauman LA. Metabolic acidosis, rhabdomyolysis, and cardiovascular collapse after prolonged propofol infusion. J Neurosurg. 2001;95:1053.

Mirrakhimov AE, Voore P, Halytskyy O, et al. Propofol infusion syndrome in adults: a clinical update. Crit Care Res Pract. 2015;2015:260385.

Sabsovich I, Rehman Z, Yunen J, Coritsidis G. Propofol infusion syndrome: a case of increasing morbidity with traumatic brain injury. Am J Crit Care. 2007;6:82.

Wong JM. Propofol infusion syndrome. Am J Ther. 2010;17:487.

Respiratory Compensation for Metabolic Acidosis

Bushinsky DA, Coe FL, Katzenberg C, et al. Arterial PCO2 in chronic metabolic acidosis. Kidney Int. 1982;22:311.

Daniel SR, Morita SY, Yu M, Dzierba A. Uncompensated metabolic acidosis: an underrecognized risk factor for subsequent intubation requirement. J Trauma. 2004;57:993.

Fulop M. A guide for predicting arterial CO2 tension in metabolic acidosis. Am J Nephrol. 1997;17:421.

Javaheri S, Kazemi H. Metabolic alkalosis and hypoventilation in humans. Am Rev Respir Dis. 1987;136:1011.

Javaheri S, Shore NS, Rose B, Kazemi H. Compensatory hypoventilation in metabolic alkalosis. Chest. 1982;81:296.

Pierce NF, Fedson DS, Brigham KL, et al. The ventilatory response to acute base deficit in humans. Time course during development and correction of metabolic acidosis. Ann Intern Med. 1970;72:633.

Wiederseiner JM, Muser J, Lutz T, et al. Acute metabolic acidosis: characterization and diagnosis of the disorder and the plasma potassium response. J Am Soc Nephrol. 2004;15:1589.

Respiratory Acidosis: Causes

Weinberger SE, Schwartzstein RM, Weiss JW. Hypercapnia. N Engl J Med. 1989;321:1223.

West JB. Causes of carbon dioxide retention in lung disease. N Engl J Med. 1971;284:1232.

Williams MH Jr, Shim CS. Ventilatory failure. Etiology and clinical forms. Am J Med. 1970;48:477.

Respiratory Acidosis: Metabolic Compensation

Arbus GS, Herbert LA, Levesque PR, et al. Characterization and clinical application of the "significance band" for acute respiratory alkalosis. N Engl J Med. 1969;280:117.

Brackett NC Jr, Wingo CF, Muren O, Solano JT. Acid-base response to chronic hypercapnia in man. N Engl J Med. 1969;280:124.

Gledhill N, Beirne GJ, Dempsey JA. Renal response to short-term hypocapnia in man. Kidney Int. 1975;8:376.

Howard RS, Rudd AG, Wolfe CD, Williams AJ. Pathophysiological and clinical aspects of breathing after stroke. Postgrad Med J. 2001;77:700.

Kelly AM, Kyle E, McAlpine R. Venous pCO(2) and pH can be used to screen for significant hypercarbia in emergency patients with acute respiratory disease. J Emerg Med. 2002;22:15.

Krapf R, Beeler I, Hertner D, Hulter HN. Chronic respiratory alkalosis. The effect of sustained hyperventilation on renal regulation of acid-base equilibrium. N Engl J Med. 1991;324:1394.

Lee MC, Klassen AC, Heaney LM, Resch JA. Respiratory rate and pattern disturbances in acute brain stem infarction. Stroke. 1976;7:382.

Martinu T, Menzies D, Dial S. Re-evaluation of acid-base prediction rules in patients with chronic respiratory acidosis. Can Respir J. 2003;10:311.

Polak A, Haynie GD, Hays RM, Schwartz WB. Effects of chronic hypercapnia on electrolyte and acid-base equilibrium. I. Adaptation. J Clin Invest. 1961;40:1223.

Van Yperselle de Striho, Brasseur L, De Coninck JD. The "carbon dioxide response curve" for chronic hypercapnia in man. N Engl J Med. 1966;275:117.

Respiratory Alkalosis: Causes

Demeter SL, Cordasco EM. Hyperventilation syndrome and asthma. Am J Med. 1986;81:989.

Gardner WN. The pathophysiology of hyperventilation disorders. Chest. 1996;109:516.

Nardi AE, Freire RC, Zin WA. Panic disorder and control of breathing. Respir Physiol Neurobiol. 2009;167:133.

Saisch SG, Wessely S, Gardner WN. Patients with acute hyperventilation presenting to an inner-city emergency department. Chest. 1996;110:952.

Serum Osmolar Gap

Arroliga AC, Shehab N, McCarthy K, Gonzales JP. Relationship of continuous infusion lorazepam to serum propylene glycol concentration in critically ill adults. Crit Care Med. 2004;32:1709.

Braden GL, Strayhorn CH, Germain MJ, et al. Increased osmolal gap in alcoholic acidosis. Arch Intern Med. 1993;153:2377.

Gabow PA. Ethylene glycol intoxication. Am J Kidney Dis. 1988;11:277.

Gennari FJ. Current concepts. Serum osmolality. Uses and limitations. N Engl J Med. 1984;310:102.

Glasser L, et. al. Serum osmolality and its applicability to drug overdose. Am J Clin Pathol. 1973;60:695.

Kraut JA, Kurtz I. Toxic alcohol ingestions: clinical features, diagnosis, and management. Clin J Am Soc Nephrol. 2008;3:208.

Kraut JA, Xing SX. Approach to the evaluation of a patient with an increased serum osmolal gap and high-anion-gap metabolic acidosis. Am J Kidney Dis. 2011;58:480.

Lynd LD, Richardson KJ, Purssell RA, et al. An evaluation of the osmole gap as a screening test for toxic alcohol poisoning. BMC Emerg Med. 2008;8:5.

Marraffa JM, Holland MG, Stork CM, et al. Diethylene glycol: widely used solvent presents serious poisoning potential. J Emerg Med. 2008;35:401.

Purssell RA, Pudek M, Brubacher J, Abu-Laban RB. Derivation and validation of a formula to calculate the contribution of ethanol to the osmolal gap. Ann Emerg Med. 2001;38:653.

Robinson AG, Loeb JN Ethanol ingestion—commonest cause of elevated plasma osmolality? N Engl J Med. 1971;284:1253.

Schelling JR, Howard RL, Winter SD, Linas SL. Increased osmolal gap in alcoholic ketoacidosis and lactic acidosis. Ann Intern Med. 1990;113:580.

Stewart Approach

Corey HE. Stewart and beyond: new models of acid-base balance. Kidney Int. 2003;64:777.

Doberer D, Funk GC, Kirchner K, Schneeweiss B. A critique of Stewart's approach: the chemical mechanism of dilutional acidosis. Intensive Care Med. 2009;35:2173.

Ježek F, Kofránek J. Modern and traditional approaches combined into an effective gray-box mathematical model of full-blood acid-base. Theor Biol Med Model. 2018;15:14.

Kellum JA. Disorders of acid-base balance. Crit Care Med. 2007;35:2630.

Kurtz I, Kraut J, Ornekian V, Nguyen MK. Acid-base analysis: a critique of the Stewart and bicarbonate-centered approaches. Am J Physiol Renal Physiol. 2008;294:F1009.

Ho KM, Lan NS, Williams TA, et al. A comparison of prognostic significance of strong ion gap (SIG) with other acid-base markers in the critically ill: a cohort study. J Intensive Care. 2016;4:43.

Kimura S, Shabsigh M, Morimatsu H. Traditional approach versus Stewart approach for acid-base disorders: Inconsistent evidence. SAGE Open Med. 2018;6:2050312118801255.

Knight C, Voth GA. The curious case of the hydrated proton. Acc Chem Res. 2012;45:101.

Kurtz I, Kraut J, Ornekian V, Nguyen MK. Acid-base analysis: a critique of the Stewart and bicarbonate-centered approaches. Am J Physiol Renal Physiol. 2008;294:F100931.

Masevicius FD, Dubin A. Has Stewart approach improved our ability to diagnose acid-base disorders in critically ill patients? World J Crit Care Med. 2015;4:62.

Morgan TJ. The meaning of acid-base abnormalities in the intensive care unit: part III — effects of fluid administration. Crit Care. 2005;9:204.

Morgan TJ. The Stewart approach–one clinician's perspective. Clin Biochem Rev. 2009;30:41.

Stewart P. How to Understand Acid-Base, New York, NY: Elsevier; 1981.

Stewart PA. Independent and dependent variables of acid-base control. Respir Physiol. 1978;33:9.

Stewart PA. Modern quantitative acid-base chemistry. Can J Physiol Pharmacol 1983;61:1444.

Story DA, Poustie S, Bellomo R. Quantitative physical chemistry analysis of acid-base disorders in critically ill patients. Anaesthesia. 2001;56:530.

Toluene Toxicity

Cámara-Lemarroy CR, Gónzalez-Moreno EI, Rodriguez-Gutierrez R, González-González JG. Clinical presentation and management in acute toluene intoxication: a case series. Inhal Toxicol. 2012;24:434.

Carlisle EJ, Donnelly SM, Vasuvattakul S, et al. Glue-sniffing and distal renal tubular acidosis: sticking to the facts. J Am Soc Nephrol. 1991;1:1019.

Streicher HZ, Gabow PA, Moss AH, et al. Syndromes of toluene sniffing in adults. Ann Intern Med. 1981;94:758.

Taher SM, Anderson RJ, McCartney R, et al. Renal tubular acidosis associated with toluene "sniffing". N Engl J Med. 1974;290:765.

Yücel M, Takagi M, Walterfang M, Lubman DI. Toluene misuse and long-term harms: a systematic review of the neuropsychological and neuroimaging literature. Neurosci Biobehav Rev. 2008; 32:910.

Urine Anion Gap

Batlle DC, Hizon M, Cohen E, et al. The use of the urinary anion gap in the diagnosis of hyperchloremic metabolic acidosis. N Engl J Med. 1988;318:594.

Lee Hamm L, Hering-Smith KS, Nakhoul NL Acid-base and potassium homeostasis. Semin Nephrol. 2013;33:257.

Oh M, Carroll HJ. Value and determinants of urine anion gap. Nephron. 2002;90:252.

Urine Osmolar Gap

Dyck RF, Asthana S, Kalra J, et al. A modification of the urine osmolal gap: an improved method for estimating urine ammonium. Am J Nephrol. 1990;10:359.

Kim GH, Han JS, Kim YS, et al. Evaluation of urine acidification by urine anion gap and urine osmolal gap in chronic metabolic acidosis. Am J Kidney Dis. 1996;27:42.

Meregalli P, Lüthy C, Oetliker OH, Bianchetti MG. Modified urine osmolal gap: an accurate method for estimating the urinary ammonium concentration? Nephron. 1995;69:98.

CASE 1

A 68-year-old man presents to the emergency department (ED) with encephalopathy that has gradually been worsening over the past 2 days. He has advanced COPD, GOLD class D, with very severe expiratory airflow obstruction (FEV$_1$ < 30% predicted). He uses 3 to 4 L/min supplemental O$_2$ via nasal cannula (NC). He uses BiPAP intermittently at night as he feels it is "too claustrophobic" overall. He uses a LAMA/LABA combination inhaler daily, in addition to albuterol PRN. He is unable to provide significant history, but his wife notes that he developed worsening shortness of breath and productive cough a week ago. A physician at his local clinic ordered an antibiotic and steroid taper, but the patient did not experience much of an improvement. He has been using albuterol nebulizers up to every 2 hours over the past 2 days. Over that time, he has appeared more groggy during the day, eating and drinking less, and not performing his iADLs as he typically does. His wife became very concerned about his breathing pattern and brought him to the ED. The patient also has a history of gout and coronary artery disease, for which he takes aspirin, carvedilol, and losartan. His vital signs on admission were 37.6°C, RR 33, HR 119, BP 166/69, and SaO$_2$ 88% on 6 L/min NC. His examination is notable for the following findings: a very thin, elderly man in obvious distress, arousable only to sternal rub. He has diminished air movement in all lung fields. Laboratory values are drawn before interventions are started. No prior laboratory values are available for this patient in your computer system. Laboratory results are as follows.

Laboratory data			
ABGs		Basic Metabolic Panel	
pH	7.14	Na	142 mEq/L
Paco$_2$	122 mm Hg	K	5.6 mEq/L
Pao$_2$	59 mm Hg	Cl	89 mEq/L
HCO$_3$	41 mEq/L	CO$_2$	41 mEq/L
		BUN	38 mg/dL
		Cr	1.2 mg/dL
		Lactate	2.3 mmol/L
		Albumin	4.0 g/dL

QUESTIONS

Q1-1: What is/are the primary acid-base disturbance(s) occurring in this case?

A. Metabolic acidosis only
B. Respiratory acidosis only
C. Metabolic acidosis and a respiratory acidosis
D. Metabolic alkalosis and a respiratory alkalosis
E. Metabolic alkalosis
F. Respiratory alkalosis

Q1-2: This patient has a respiratory acidosis, but you are unsure if it is acute, chronic, or acute on chronic. What would you expect the patient's pH and serum HCO_3 to be if this entire respiratory process was *acute*?

A. pH 7.20, HCO_3 20 mEq/L
B. pH 7.11, HCO_3 30 mEq/L
C. pH 7.52, HCO_3 44 mEq/L
D. pH 6.91, HCO_3 33 mEq/L

Q1-3: For this question, let us assume the preceding information is true, and the patient's respiratory acidosis is entirely an acute process. What other acid-base abnormality must be present?

A. Anion gap metabolic acidosis
B. Non-anion gap metabolic acidosis
C. Respiratory alkalosis
D. Metabolic alkalosis

Q1-4: What would you expect the patient's pH and serum HCO_3 to be if the entire respiratory process was *chronic*?

A. pH 7.25, HCO_3 53 mEq/L
B. pH 7.31, HCO_3 60 mEq/L
C. pH 7.07, HCO_3 40 mEq/L
D. pH 6.92, HCO_3 22 mEq/L

Q1-5: For this question, let us assume that the patient's respiratory acidosis is entirely a *chronic* process. What other acid-base disorder must be present?

A. Metabolic alkalosis
B. Anion-gap metabolic acidosis
C. Non-anion gap metabolic acidosis
D. Respiratory alkalosis

Q1-6: Now, let us assume this is a *pure respiratory acidosis* with no other ongoing metabolic process (ie, no metabolic acidosis or alkalosis): How would you classify the patient's respiratory acidosis?

A. Acute respiratory acidosis
B. Chronic respiratory acidosis
C. Acute-on-chronic respiratory acidosis

ANSWERS

Q1-1: B
Respiratory acidosis only.

Rationale:

1. The pH is 7.14; therefore, the primary disorder is an **acidosis.**
2. The $Paco_2$ of 122 mm Hg is **higher** than 40 mm Hg, so there is a **respiratory acidosis.**
3. The HCO_3 of 41 is **more** than 24, so this is **not likely to be a primary metabolic acidosis.**

The difficult issue in this case is that we do not have any baseline information of the patient. Patients with chronic hypoxemic respiratory failure such as this patient are also at risk for possible chronic hypercarbic failure, which could mean the patient's baseline (or **normal** values) for the $Paco_2$ and the HCO_3 are elevated. **This can make interpretation of acute issues occurring on top of chronic issues more difficult. We will explore this topic in a bit more detail in the following questions.**

Q1-2: D
pH 6.91, HCO_3 33 mEq/L.

Rationale: First, we need to determine the expected serum HCO_3 if we assume (1) this is an acute process only, so the patient's baseline values for $Paco_2$ is 40 mm Hg and the HCO_3 is 24 mEq/L, and (2) there is appropriate (complete) renal compensation (~24 hours). For the serum HCO_3, you need the following equation:

Metabolic Compensation for Acute Respiratory Acidosis:

$$\text{Expected } HCO_3 = \text{Baseline } HCO_3 + (0.10) [\text{Actual } Paco_2 - \text{Baseline } Paco_2].$$

Therefore, for this patient,

$$\text{Expected } HCO_3 = 24 + [0.10 * (122 - 40 \text{ mm Hg})] = 24 + (0.1) * (84) \sim \textbf{33 mEq/L.}$$

Now, with the $Paco_2$ and the HCO_3, we can calculate the expected pH, using the Henderson-Hasselbach equation:

Henderson-Hasselbalch Equation:

$$ph = 6.10 + \log \left(\frac{[HCO_3]}{0.03 * Pco_2} \right)$$

Therefore, for this patient,

$$pH = 6.10 + \log ([33]/(0.03 * 122)) = 6.91.$$

Q1-3: D
Metabolic alkalosis.

Rationale: Assuming the patient's process is entirely *acute*, we would expect the patient's serum HCO_3 to be 33 mEq/L, but it is 41 mEq/L, indicating that there is another process ongoing. Since the actual measured HCO_3 is higher than the expected, there is a concomitant alkalosis ongoing, and that process must be a metabolic process.

Therefore, if we assume the patient has an acute respiratory acidosis, the patient must also have a concomitant metabolic alkalosis.

The next questions will assume an alternative approach with drastically different diagnoses as a result.

Q1-4: B
pH 7.31, HCO_3 60 mEq/L.

Rationale: First, we calculate the serum HCO_3 in a completely compensated, chronic respiratory acidosis as follows:

Metabolic Compensation for Chronic Respiratory Acidosis:

$$\text{Expected } HCO_3 = \text{Baseline } HCO_3 + (0.4) [\text{Actual } Paco_2 - \text{Baseline } Paco_2]$$
$$\text{Expected } HCO_3 = 24 + ((0.4 \text{ mEq/mm Hg} * L) * 88 \text{ mm Hg}) = \textbf{60 mEq/L.}$$

Recall that renal compensation for an acute respiratory acidosis requires about 24 hours, while several days (4 to 7) are required to develop a complete **chronic** compensation. We would then use the Henderson-Hasselbach equation to determine the pH, using the values of $Paco_2$ 122 mm Hg and HCO_3 of 60 mEq/L.

Henderson-Hasselbalch Equation:

$$ph = 6.10 + \log \left(\frac{[HCO_3]}{0.03 * Pco_2} \right)$$

This would yield a pH of 7.31.

Q1-5: C
Non-anion gap metabolic acidosis.

Rationale: If we assume the respiratory acidosis is entirely *chronic*, as we did in Q1-3, earlier, then we would expect the HCO_3 to 60 mEq/L, but it is 41 mEq/L, and therefore a concomitant metabolic acidosis must be present. The anion gap in this case would be less than zero (142 – 89 – 60 = –7 < 12; remember the baseline HCO_3

is now assumed to be 60 mEq/L), and therefore, we would assume that the process would be a non-anion gap metabolic acidosis.

Now, as previously stated, we are assuming that the metabolic compensation for the chronic respiratory acidosis is 100% efficient all the way up to the patient's $Paco_2$ of 122 mm Hg. However, in practice renal compensation becomes less efficient as the $Paco_2$ rises above 80 mm Hg. For the sake of these cases, however, we will assume 100% efficiency to reduce the complexity.

Now:

1. If we assume an *acute* respiratory acidosis only, then the patient has a **concomitant metabolic alkalosis.**
2. If we assume a *chronic* respiratory acidosis only, then the patient has a **concomitant non-anion gap metabolic acidosis.**

In the next question, we will consider a third possible scenario.

Q1-6: C
Acute-on-chronic respiratory acidosis.

Rationale: This patient's pH and HCO_3 fall between the extremes of pure acute respiratory acidosis (pH 6.91 with HCO_3 of 33) and a chronic respiratory acidosis (pH 7.25, HCO_3 53), so it is most likely that this patient has a baseline chronic respiratory acidosis and had a more acute respiratory acidosis that brought him to the hospital.

Determining the patient's *baseline* Pco_2 and serum HCO_3 is bit more complicated but can be done using the following equation:

Equation for Acute-on-Chronic Respiratory Disorder:

$$\text{Baseline } Paco_2 = 4 * ([\text{Current } HCO_3] - 10 - 0.10 * [\text{Current } Paco_2])$$
$$\text{Baseline } Paco_2 = 4 * (41 - 10 - (0.10 * [122]))$$
$$\text{Baseline } Paco_2 = 4 * (41 - 10 - 12.2) = 4 * (18.8) = 75 \text{ mm Hg.}$$

Therefore, if the process were a *pure* acute-on-chronic respiratory acidosis, we would expect the patient's baseline $Paco_2$ to be about 75 mm Hg. We can now calculate what the patient's baseline HCO_3 would be, as well, using the equation for complete renal compensation in chronic hypercarbic respiratory failure.

Metabolic Compensation for Chronic Respiratory Alkalosis:

$$\text{Expected } HCO_3 = \text{Baseline } HCO_3 - (0.40) [\text{Actual } Paco_2 - \text{Baseline } Paco_2]$$
$$\text{Expected } HCO_3 = 24 + 4 * [0.10 * (\text{baseline } Paco_2 - 40 \text{ mm Hg})]$$
$$\text{Expected } HCO_3 = 24 + (4 * 3.5) = 38 \text{ mEq/L.}$$

And the patient's baseline pH would be 7.32 (determined with the Henderson-Hasselbach equation).

Recall that we made two important assumptions to arrive at this answer. First, we assumed that the patient's acidosis is purely a respiratory acidosis, and that no other acid-base disorders are present outside of the acute-on-chronic respiratory failure. Second, we are assuming that the compensation for both the acute and the chronic processes are "complete" or appropriate. Again, this requires that the acute respiratory acidosis has been present for approximately 24 hours, and that the chronic process had been present for a least several days prior to the onset of the acute process. However, this patient could also have a purely acute respiratory acidosis with a concomitant metabolic alkalosis. Or the patient could have a pure chronic respiratory acidosis with an acute metabolic acidosis. This case demonstrates how important knowledge of a baseline or chronic acid-base disorder is when assessing an acute change in a patient. This knowledge can significantly alter diagnostic and treatment plans.

Now:

1. If we assume an *acute* respiratory acidosis only, then the patient has a **concomitant metabolic alkalosis**.
2. If we assume a *chronic* respiratory acidosis only, then the patient has a **concomitant non-anion gap metabolic acidosis**.
3. If we assume there is no metabolic process ongoing, and the changes in the HCO_3 represent only renal compensation for respiratory acidosis, then the patient has an acute-on-chronic acidosis, and at baseline the patient's chronic respiratory acidosis yields pH 7.32, $Paco_2$ 75 mm Hg, and HCO_3 38 mm Hg.

Clearly, having knowledge of the patient's baseline acid-base status can significantly aid in interpreting acid-base cases.

References

Brackett NC Jr, Wingo CF, Muren O, Solano JT. Acid-base response to chronic hypercapnia in man. N Engl J Med. 1969;280:124.

Brown LK. Hypoventilation syndromes. Clin Chest Med. 2010;31:249.

Epstein SK, Singh N. Respiratory acidosis. Respir Care. 2001;46:366.

Kelly AM, Kyle E, McAlpine R. Venous pco(2) and pH can be used to screen for significant hypercarbia in emergency patients with acute respiratory disease. J Emerg Med. 2002;22:15.

Polak A, Haynie GD, Hays RM, Schwartz WB. Effects of chronic hypercapnia on electrolyte and acid-base equilibrium. I. Adaptation. J Clin Invest. 1961;40:1223.

Rosen RL. Acute respiratory failure and chronic obstructive lung disease. Med Clin North Am. 1986;70:895.

Van Yperselle de Striho, Brasseur L, De Coninck JD. The "carbon dioxide response curve" for chronic hypercapnia in man. N Engl J Med. 1966;275:117.

Visconti L, Santoro D, Cernaro V, et al. Kidney-lung connections in acute and chronic diseases: current perspectives. J Nephrol. 2016;29:341.

CASE 2

An 88-year-old man with Gold class D COPD (FEV$_1$ 0.57 L, 21% predicted) presents to the emergency department with worsening dyspnea, productive cough, and mild lethargy. His symptoms began approximately 3 days ago, and he subsequently started a short course of prednisone without improvement. He has been using his nebulizers frequently. He also started on an antibiotic 3 days ago, and has been experiencing significant nausea and diarrhea since then. He is not able to take any food or medication PO due to nausea. He is tachypneic, with an RR of 34, and on examination there is minimal air movement bilaterally. He is somewhat cachectic. There is no peripheral edema or cyanosis. A CXR shows flattening of the diaphragms bilaterally, hyperinflation, but no evidence of an acute infiltrate. He is given methylprednisolone 125 mg IV once, three nebulizers, and placed on noninvasive ventilation. His RR is 34, HR 110, BP 164/78, and SaO$_2$ 92% on 3 L/min bleed-in to the BiPAP. His home oxygen prescription is for 2 L/min at rest and with activity. His laboratory findings are shown below. A review of the patient's prior lab studies shows his baseline serum HCO$_3$ is approximately 30 mEq/L and has been steady for the past year.

Laboratory data			
ABGs		Basic Metabolic Panel	
pH	6.97	Na	131 mEq/L
Paco$_2$	80 mm Hg	K	2.8 mEq/L
Pao$_2$	70 mm Hg	Cl	110 mEq/L
HCO$_3$	18 mEq/L	CO$_2$	18 mEq/L
		BUN	29 mg/dL
		Cr	1.1 mg/dL
		Glucose	144 mg/dL
		Albumin	2.4 g/dL
		EtOH	0 mg/dL

QUESTIONS

Q2-1: Define the patient's baseline acid-base status: Does this patient have an underlying chronic acid-base disorder that we need to account for in order to appropriately interpret the acute acid-base disorders?

A. There is no evidence for an underlying, chronic respiratory or metabolic acid-base disorder in this patient, so we would assume a baseline $Paco_2$ of 40 mm Hg and an HCO_3 of 24 mEq/L.

B. While the patient has a condition that predisposes him to a chronic acid-base disorder, there is insufficient information to estimate the patient's baseline $Paco_2$ and HCO_3 values; therefore, we will assume a baseline $Paco_2$ of 40 mm Hg and a baseline HCO_3 of 24 mEq/L.

C. The patient has an underlying acid-base condition, and we have sufficient information to estimate the patient's baseline $Paco_2$ and HCO_3 values.

Q2-2: A review of the patient's prior laboratory studies shows his baseline serum HCO_3 is approximately 30 mEq/L. Given this information, what is the patient's expected baseline $Paco_2$ (assuming that there is appropriate compensation for a chronic respiratory acidosis)?

A. $Paco_2$ 45 mm Hg
B. $Paco_2$ 50 mm Hg
C. $Paco_2$ 55 mm Hg
D. $Paco_2$ 70 mm Hg

Q2-3: Now that we have defined the baseline acid-base status, what is/are the primary acid-base disturbance(s) occurring in this case?

A. Metabolic acidosis only
B. Respiratory acidosis only
C. Metabolic alkalosis only
D. Respiratory alkalosis only
E. Metabolic acidosis and a respiratory acidosis
F. Metabolic alkalosis and a respiratory alkalosis

Q2-4: For a perfectly healthy patient, a normal anion gap is assumed to be 12. What should be considered a normal anion gap in this patient?

A. 10
B. 8
C. 7
D. 4

Q2-5: What would one expect the patient's serum HCO_3 to be if he is appropriately compensating for both the *acute* and *chronic* portions of the current respiratory acidosis (assume no metabolic acidosis is present for this portion of the case)?

A. 28 mEq/L
B. 32 mEq/L
C. 38 mEq/L
D. 44 mEq/L

Q2-6: How would the metabolic acidosis component be classified in this case?

A. Anion gap acidosis
B. Non-anion gap acidosis
C. Anion and non-anion gap acidosis
D. Anion gap acidosis and a metabolic alkalosis
E. There is no metabolic acidosis; the change in the patient's serum HCO_3 from baseline represents an appropriate compensation for the patient's respiratory acid-base process.

Q2-7: You decide to investigate the patient's non-anion gap acidosis. The patient's urine studies are as follows:

Urine Na	11 mEq/L
Urine K	13 mEq/L
Urine Cl	45 mEq/L

What is the cause of the patient's non-anion gap acidosis?

A. Type 1 (distal) RTA
B. Type 2 (proximal) RTA
C. GI losses of HCO_3
D. Type 4 RTA

ANSWERS

Q2-1: C

The patient has a predisposing condition (COPD) with a baseline elevated HCO_3. There is sufficient information from the prompt to estimate the patient's baseline $Paco_2$. The next step will be to estimate the patient's baseline values.

Rationale: Ignoring these underlying chronic acid-base disorders can significantly alter the interpretation of a patient's acute acid-base status. This was demonstrated in the first case of the series. However, often, we do not have the necessary information (eg, prior ABG or VBG, or prior serum chemistry with an HCO_3) and are forced to assume the ongoing processes are all acute in nature. We are primarily concerned about chronic respiratory acid-base disorders, as these can significantly alter the patient's baseline or expected values for the serum HCO_3 and $Paco_2$, and we have reliable equations to predict the expected baseline values. The respiratory compensation for both chronic metabolic acidosis and alkalosis is generally poor, so there are no equations or rules to predict what the $Paco_2$ should be in these cases. While the baseline serum HCO_3 may be significantly off from our standard value of 24 mEq/L in these patients, we would assume a baseline $Paco_2$ of 40 mm Hg in patients with chronic metabolic processes. Once we identify the patient's baseline $Paco_2$ and HCO_3 values, we will need to use these values in the appropriate equations to identify the ongoing acute processes.

Q2-2: C

$Paco_2$ 55 mm Hg.

Rationale: We can calculate an expected baseline $Paco_2$ for this patient by using his baseline serum HCO_3, assuming the normal HCO_3 of 24 mEq/L, and that the baseline HCO_3 represents appropriate compensation for a *chronic* respiratory acidosis.

Metabolic Compensation for Chronic Respiratory Acidosis:

$$\text{Baseline } HCO_3 = \text{Normal } HCO_3 + (0.4)\,[\text{Baseline } Paco_2 - \text{Normal } Paco_2]$$
$$[\text{Baseline } HCO_3 - \text{Normal } HCO_3] = (0.4)\,[\text{Baseline } Paco_2 - \text{Normal } Paco_2]$$
$$(2.5) * [\text{Baseline } HCO_3 - \text{Normal } HCO_3] = \text{Baseline } CO_2 - \text{Normal } Paco_2$$
$$(2.5) * [\text{Baseline } HCO_3 - \text{Normal } HCO_3] = \text{Normal } Paco_2 - \text{Baseline } Paco_2$$

where the "normal" HCO_3 and $Paco_2$ values are 24 mEq/L and 40 mm Hg, respectively.

Actual $Paco_2 = 2.5 * [30 - 24] + 40$ mm Hg $= 2.5 * [6] + 40$ mm Hg $= 55$ mm Hg.

Therefore, at baseline, we would anticipate the patient has a $Paco_2$ of 55 mm Hg. The patient's pH at baseline would then be ~7.35. The patient therefore has an acute-on-chronic respiratory failure, with a current $Paco_2$ of 80 mm Hg.

Q2-3: E
Metabolic acidosis and a respiratory acidosis.

Rationale:

1. The pH is 6.97; therefore, the primary disorder is an **acidosis.**
2. The $Paco_2$ of 80 mm Hg is greater than 40 mm Hg, so there is a **respiratory acidosis.**
3. The HCO_3 of 18 mEq/L is less than 24 mEq/L, so there is also a **metabolic acidosis.**

Q2-4: B
8.

Rationale: The normal anion gap is 12. The term *anion gap* refers to those ions (negatively charged molecules) in the bloodstream that we do not routinely measure, including phosphates, sulfates, organic acids, and negatively charged plasma proteins. One of the most abundant negatively charged ions in the blood is serum albumin. A normal serum albumin level is 4.0 g/dL. For patients with hypoalbuminemia (low serum albumin), the normal or expected anion gap is smaller.

Expected Anion Gap:

$$\text{Expected Anion Gap} = 12 - (2.5) * \left[4.0\frac{g}{dL} - \text{Actual Serum Albumin} \right].$$

Therefore, for this patient,

$$\text{Expected Anion Gap} = 12 - [2.5 * (4 - 2.4)] = 12 - (2.5 * 1.6) = 8 \text{ mEq/L}.$$

This is an important concept as patients with hypoalbuminemia may "hide" an anion gap acidosis if this correction is not performed.

Q2-5: B
32 mEq/L.

Rationale: We dealt with the *chronic* portion of the patient's respiratory acidosis in the prior question. We know that the patient's baseline $Paco_2$ is 55 mm Hg, with a baseline HCO_3 of 30 mEq/L. We also know that, due to the *acute* portion of the respiratory acidosis, the patient's new $Paco_2$ is 80 mm Hg. Therefore, we can use the equation for compensation in *acute* respiratory acidosis, using the following values:

Metabolic Compensation for Acute Respiratory Acidosis:

$$\text{Expected HCO}_3 = \text{Baseline HCO}_3 + (0.10) [\text{Actual Paco}_2 - \text{Baseline Paco}_2]$$
$$\text{Expected HCO}_3 = 30 + [0.10 * (80 \text{ mm Hg} - 55 \text{ mm Hg})] = 32 \text{ mEq/L}.$$

If we assumed that the patient's respiratory failure was all *chronic*, the expected HCO_3 would be 40 mEq/L, with a pH of 7.32. Rather, if we assumed that the patient's respiratory failure was all acute (italic bolded), the expected HCO_3 would be 28 mEq/L, with a pH of 7.17.

Q2-6: C
Anion and non-anion gap acidosis.

Rationale: The patient's serum HCO_3 is 18, far below that expected for compensation in his respiratory acidosis. Therefore, a metabolic acidosis is present.

1. Is there evidence for a chronic respiratory acid-base disorder that requires adjustment of the patient's "normal" HCO_3? Here, we have already determined that the patient has a chronic respiratory acidosis, as his baseline $Paco_2$ is 55 mm Hg and the HCO_3 is 30 mEq/L. We would need to use this value (30 mEq/L) for the patient's baseline HCO_3 in the delta-delta equation if needed.
2. Expected anion gap:

$$\text{Expected Anion Gap} = 12 - (2.5) * \left[4.0 \frac{g}{dL} - \text{Actual Serum Albumin} \right]$$

$$= 12 - (2.5 * [4.0 - 2.4])$$

$$= 12 - (2.5 * [1.6]) = \textbf{8 mEq/L.}$$

3. Anion gap calculation:

$$\text{Serum Anion Gap} = [Na^+] - [HCO_3^-] - [Cl^-]$$

$AG = 131 - (110 + 18) = 3$ mEq/L, which is < 8 mEq/L, so **no anion gap acidosis present.**

Therefore, the patient must have a non-anion gap acidosis, and the delta-delta calculation is not required.

Q2-7: C
GI losses of HCO_3.

Rationale: We have somewhat limited information at present and can only calculate a urine anion gap, as follows:

Urine Anion Gap:

$$\text{Urine Anion Gap (UAG)} = [U_{Na}] + [U_K] - [U_{Cl}]$$

Interpretation:

- A UAG that is greater than ~20 → reduced renal acid excretion (RTA).
- A UAG that is −20 → GI loss of bicarbonate (eg, diarrhea), although type 2 RTA is possible.
- A UAG between −20 and +10 is generally considered inconclusive.

The patient presented with complaints of diarrhea for several days as a result of starting antibiotics. The urine anion gap is less than −20 mEq/L, consistent with a GI cause for the acidosis as opposed to renal issue with urinary acidification. This acute metabolic acidosis completely disrupts the patient's ability to compensate for his both acute and chronic respiratory failure issues. This is a common issue encountered in patients with acute-on-chronic hypercarbic respiratory failure who also develop concomitant renal failure, as the kidneys are no longer able to compensate.

CASE 3

A 44-year old homeless man with schizophrenia and alcoholism presents to the emergency department with altered mental status and renal failure. He is intubated shortly after arrival due to an inability to protect his airway. No collateral history is available. He is tachypneic with RR in the 30s prior to intubation. His other vital signs are HR 122, BP 99/60, and SaO$_2$ 95% on RA. His examination is otherwise unremarkable.

Laboratory data.			
ABGs		Basic Metabolic Panel	
pH	7.06	Na	131 mEq/L
Paco$_2$	30 mm Hg	K	5.6 mEq/L
Pao$_2$	80 mm Hg	Cl	98 mEq/L
HCO$_3$	7 mEq/L	CO$_2$	7 mEq/L
		BUN	68 mg/dL
		Cr	3.8 mg/dL
		Glucose	80 mg/dL
		Albumin	2.0 g/dL
		EtOH	0 mg/dL

QUESTIONS

Q3-1: Define the patient's baseline acid-base status: Does this patient have an underlying chronic acid-base disorder that we need to account for in order to appropriately interpret the acute acid-base disorders?

A. There is no evidence of an underlying chronic respiratory or metabolic acid-base disorder in this patient, so we would assume a baseline $Paco_2$ of 40 mm Hg and an HCO_3 of 24 mEq/L.

B. While the patient has a condition predisposing him to a chronic acid-base disorder, there is insufficient information to estimate the patient's baseline $Paco_2$ and HCO_3 values; therefore, we will assume a baseline $Paco_2$ of 40 mm Hg and a baseline HCO_3 of 24 mEq/L.

C. The patient has an underlying acid-base condition, and we have sufficient information to estimate the patient's baseline $Paco_2$ and HCO_3 values.

Q3-2: What is/are the primary acid-base disturbance(s) occurring in this case?

A. Metabolic acidosis only
B. Respiratory acidosis only
C. Metabolic alkalosis only
D. Respiratory alkalosis only
E. Metabolic acidosis and a respiratory acidosis
F. Metabolic alkalosis and a respiratory alkalosis

Q3-3: For a perfectly healthy patient, a normal anion gap is assumed to be 12. What should be considered a normal anion gap in this patient?

A. 12
B. 10
C. 7
D. 4

Q3-4: How would the metabolic acidosis component be classified in this case?

A. Anion gap acidosis
B. Non-anion gap acidosis
C. Anion and non-anion gap acidosis
D. Anion gap acidosis and a metabolic alkalosis

Q3-5: What laboratory testing would you order next in this patient to determine the source of the metabolic acidosis?

A. Serum drug screen, osmolality, beta-hydroxybuturate, lactate
B. Urine electrolytes, urinalysis
C. Serum cortisol

Q3-6: Your laboratory testing returns the following values:

Serum EtOH	< 3 mg/dL
Serum acetaminophen level	< 5 mg/dL (ULN for therapeutic use 20 mg/dL)
Serum salicylate level	< 5 mg/dL (ULN for therapeutic use 30 mg/dL)
Serum osmolality	350 mOsm/kg
Serum L-lactate	1.3 mmol/L (ULN 2.0 mmol/L venous)
Beta-hydroxybutyrate (acetone)	< 0.18 mmol/L (ULN 0.18 mmol/L)
Serum glucose	80 mg/dL

What is the serum osmolal gap?

A. 0
B. 4
C. 22
D. 59

Q3-7: Does the patient in this case demonstrate appropriate respiratory compensation?

A. Yes, the respiratory compensation is appropriate.
B. No, a concomitant respiratory alkalosis is present.
C. No, a concomitant respiratory acidosis is present.
D. Yes, the metabolic compensation is appropriate.
E. No, a concomitant metabolic acidosis is present.
F. No, a concomitant metabolic alkalosis is present.

Q3-8: What is the next step in this patient's management?

A. Intravenous bicarbonate infusion
B. Intravenous ethanol infusion
C. Methylene blue
D. Fomepizole
E. Continuous renal replacement therapy (CRRT)
F. Intermittent hemodialysis
G. A and E
H. B and F
I. D and E
J. D and F

ANSWERS

Q3-1: A

There is no evidence of an underlying chronic respiratory or metabolic acid-base disorder in this patient. Although the patient has a history of alcoholism, which may predispose to cirrhosis (and a chronic respiratory alkalosis), there is no documented history of cirrhosis. Additionally, while the patient presents with renal failure there is no mention of CKD/end-stage renal disease (ESRD), so we would assume this is an acute process.

Rationale: Ignoring these underlying chronic acid-base disorders can significantly alter the interpretation of a patient's acute acid-base status. This was demonstrated in the first case of this series. However, often we do not have the necessary information (eg, prior ABG or VBG, or prior serum chemistry with an HCO_3) and are forced to assume the ongoing processes are all acute in nature. We are primarily concerned about chronic respiratory acid-base disorders as these can significantly alter the patient's baseline or expected values for the serum HCO_3 and $Paco_2$, and we have reliable equations to predict the expected baseline values. The respiratory compensation for both chronic metabolic acidosis and alkalosis is generally poor, so there are no equations or rules to predict what the $Paco_2$ should be in these cases. While the baseline serum HCO_3 may be significantly off from our standard value of 24 mEq/L in these patients, we would assume a baseline $Paco_2$ of 40 mm Hg in patients with chronic metabolic processes. Once we identify the patient's baseline $Paco_2$ and HCO_3 values, we will need to use these values in the appropriate equations to identify the ongoing acute processes.

Q3-2: A

Metabolic acidosis only.

Rationale:

1. The pH is 7.06; therefore, the primary disorder is an **acidosis**.
2. The $Paco_2$ of 30 mm Hg is less than 40 mm Hg, so this is not the cause of acidosis.
3. The HCO_3 of 7 is less than 24, so there is a **primary metabolic acidosis.**

Q3-3: C

7.

Rationale: The normal anion gap is 12. The term *anion gap* refers to those ions (negatively charged molecules) in the bloodstream that we do not routinely measure, including phosphates, sulfates, organic acids, and negatively charged plasma proteins. One of the most abundant negatively charged ions in the blood is serum albumin. A normal serum albumin is 4.0 g/dL. For patients with hypoalbuminemia (low serum albumin), the normal or expected anion gap is smaller.

Expected Anion Gap (AG):

$$\text{Expected AG} = 12 - (2.5) * \left[4.0 \frac{g}{dL} - \text{Actual Serum Albumin} \right].$$

So for this patient,

$$\text{Expected AG} = 12 - [2.5 * (4 - 2)] = 12 - (2.5 * 2) = 7.$$

This is an important concept, as patients with hypoalbuminemia may "hide" an anion gap acidosis if this correction is not performed.

Q3-4: A
Anion gap acidosis.

Rationale:

1. Expected anion gap: We calculated this in the previous question, and the expected anion gap is 7.
2. Anion gap calculation:

$$\text{AG} = \text{Na} - (\text{Cl} + \text{HCO}_3)$$

$131 - (98 + 7) = 26$, which is $> 7 \rightarrow$ **anion gap acidosis is present.**

3. Delta-delta calculation: The delta-delta calculation helps determine if there is more than one type of metabolic acidosis occurring in a patient. For example, if you dissolve 1 unit of metabolic acid (H^+A^-) into the blood, the acid dissociates to an H^+ and an unmeasured anion A^-. The H^+ decreases the serum HCO_3 by 1 point, while the unmeasured anion increases the anion gap by 1 point, yielding a delta-delta value of 1.0, a pure anion gap acidosis. Alternatively, when the fall in the serum HCO_3 is more than expected from the change in anion gap, this may be due to a non-anion gap acidosis. In this situation, the additional fall in HCO_3 is due to further buffering of an acid that does not contribute to the anion gap (such as HCl from stomach acid, where the anion Cl^- is measured).

Remember to Use the Corrected AG Based on Albumin Here:

$$(\text{Measured AG} - \text{Normal AG})/(\text{Normal HCO}_3 - \text{Measured HCO}_3)$$
$$(26 - 7)/(24 - 7) = \textbf{19/17, which is } > 1 \textbf{ but} < 2.$$

Delta-Delta interpretation.	
Delta-Delta Value	Condition Present
< 0.4	Non-anion gap only
0.4–1.0	Anion gap *and* non-anion gap acidosis
1.0–2.0	**Anion gap acidosis only**
> 2.0	Anion gap acidosis and metabolic alkalosis

This indicates that the change in serum HCO_3 for this patient is what we would expect from the change in the anion gap. If we had not corrected the "normal" anion gap for this patient, we would have determined that an anion gap and a non-anion gap acidosis were contributing.

Q3-5: A
This is the appropriate evaluation for a patient with an anion gap acidosis.

Rationale: This is the laboratory evaluation that is performed when patients have a pure anion gap acidosis (see table). This will help identify some of the more common causes of an anion gap acidosis including lactic acidosis, ketoacidosis, organic alcohol ingestion, aspirin toxicity, and acetaminophen toxicity. Option B is a laboratory evaluation for renal failure, and option C would be appropriate if the patient were suspected or known to have adrenal insufficiency.

Causes of anion gap metabolic acidosis.	
Common	Less Common
Lactic acidosis (including transient)	Cyanide poisoning
Renal failure ("uremia")	Carbon monoxide poisoning
Diabetic ketoacidosis	Aminoglycosides
Alcohol ketoacidosis	Phenformin use
Starvation ketoacidosis	D-Lactic acidosis
Salicylate poisoning (ASA)	Paraldehyde
Acetaminophen poisoning (paracetamol)	Iron use
Organic alcohol poisoning (ethylene glycol, methanol, propylene glycol)	Isoniazid use
Toluene poisoning ("glue-sniffing")	Inborn errors of metabolism

Q3-6: D
59.

Rationale: The serum osmolal gap is the difference between the laboratory measured ("true") serum osmolality, and a "calculated" osmolality based on commonly measured compounds that are known to contribute to the serum osmolality. Therefore, similar to the serum anion gap, the serum osmolal gap represents the "unmeasured" compounds also contributing to the serum osmolality. The serum osmolal gap can be helpful in determining if an organic alcohol ingestion has occurred recently. The following are potential causes of an elevated serum osmolality:

With an elevated serum anion gap:

1. Ethanol ingestion with alcohol ketoacidosis (acetone is an unmeasured osmole, in addition to ethanol)—the osmolality is usually elevated more so by the increased ethanol concentration, so the osmolal "gap" depends on whether the term for ethanol is included in the osmolality calculation.*

---

*A mildly elevated osmolal gap has been reported in the literature in patients with lactic acidosis in critical illness, particularly severe distributive shock. The pathology is not quite clear, although it is likely related to multiorgan failure—particularly of the liver and kidneys—and the release of cellular components known to contribute to the osmolal gap. The serum osmolal gap in this situation is typically around 10, although it may be as high as 20 to 25 mOsm/L.

2. Organic alcohol ingestions (methanol, ethylene glycol, diethylene glycol, propylene glycol).
3. Diabetic ketoacidosis—similar to ethanol ingestion above, glucose and acetone contribute to the osmolality since the glucose term is always included in the calculation.
4. Salicylate toxicity.
5. Renal failure—the BUN is nearly always included in the osmolality.

Without an elevated serum anion gap:

1. Hyperosmolar therapy (mannitol, glycerol)
2. Other organic solvent ingestion (eg, acetone)
3. Isopropyl alcohol ingestion (produces only acetone rather than an organic acid, so no anion gap is seen)
4. Hypertriglyceridemia
5. Hyperproteinemia

Similar to the serum anion gap, the serum osmolal gap is determined by the difference between the "calculated" serum osmolality and the true, measured serum osmolality. The equation for the serum osmolal gap typically includes factors for sodium, glucose, BUN, and ethanol, as these are readily measurable in most laboratories. Therefore, the serum osmolal gap will represent the osmolality of those "unmeasured" osmoles, including organic alcohols and acetone. The most common form is shown as follows.

$$\text{Calculated Serum Osmolality} = 2*[\text{Na}^+] + \frac{[\text{Glucose}]}{18} + \frac{[\text{BUN}]}{2.8} + \frac{[\text{EtOH}]}{3.7},$$

In which the units are as follows: Na, mEq/L; glucose, mg/dL; BUN, mg/dL; EtOH, mg/dL. The conversion factors are provided in the equation as well. A normal serum osmolal gap is around -10 to $+10$ mOsm/L (or mOsm/kg).

Therefore, for this patient:

$$\begin{aligned}
\text{Calculated Serum Osmolality} &= [2*\text{Na}] + [\text{Glucose}/18] + [\text{BUN}/2,8] + [\text{EtOH}/3.7] \\
&= (2*131) + (80/18) + (68/2.8) + (0.37) \\
&= 291.
\end{aligned}$$

$$\begin{aligned}
\text{Serum Osmolal Gap} &= \text{Measured Serum Osmolality} - \text{Calculated Osmolality} \\
&= (350 - 291) = 59 > 10 \rightarrow \text{positive serum osmolal gap.}
\end{aligned}$$

A normal serum osmolal gap is less than 10. There are four primary causes of an elevated osmolal gap:

1. Alcohol ingestion (ethanol, methanol, ethylene glycol, isopropyl alcohol)
2. Carbohydrate/sugars, namely mannitol
3. Hypertriglyceridemia
4. Hypergammaglobulinemia

In this patient, we would primarily worry about the first etiology, particularly methanol or ethylene glycol ingestion.

Q3-7: C
No, a concomitant respiratory acidosis is present.

Rationale: Using the Winter formula, one can calculate what the expected arterial $Paco_2$ should be for a given serum HCO_3 if the patient were completely compensated.

Respiratory Compensation for Acute Metabolic Acidosis (Winter Formula):

$$\text{Expected } Paco_2 = 15 * [\text{Actual } HCO_3] + 8 \pm 2 \text{ (in mm Hg).}$$

Therefore,

$$\text{Expected } Paco_2 = 15 * (\text{Actual } HCO_3) + 8 \, (+/-2)$$
$$= (15 * 7) + 8 = 10.5 + 8 = 18.5 +/-2 = (17 - 21) \text{ mm Hg.}$$

Since the patient's $Paco_2$ on presentation (**30 mm Hg**) was higher than the expected **17 to 21 mm Hg**, the patient also has a relative respiratory acidosis on top of the anion gap metabolic acidosis.

Q3-8: J
Both D and F would be the next appropriate steps in management.

Rationale: Treatment should never be delayed in a case of suspected methanol or ethylene glycol ingestion while awaiting confirmation. The elevated osmolar gap with suspicion of ingestion based on the blurred vision is sufficient evidence in this case. The severe morbidity associated with untreated methanol (blindness) or ethylene glycol (renal failure) necessitates immediate action, so fomepizole (preferred, if available) and intermittent dialysis are essential. Fomepizole prevents the conversion of the organic alcohols to the more toxic organic acids, while allowing intermittent hemodialysis to remove the remaining unmetabolized alcohols.

CASE 4

A 33-year-old man with unknown medical history and altered mental status is brought to the emergency department by EMS. He is wearing a medical bracelet that states he is a diabetic patient. No family or friends are present. He is moaning and complaining of abdominal pain but is otherwise not interacting meaningfully. Vital signs are T 37.4°C, RR 32, HR 133, BP 110/70, and SaO_2 100% on 2 L NC. WBC count is $11.2 \times 10^3/\mu L$ with a mild left shift. The lipase level is normal. The patient has had several episodes of emesis since arrival, but overall is protecting his airway. On examination, the patient has a benign abdomen and a normal cardiopulmonary examination, with the exception of sinus tachycardia. The patient's mucous membranes are quite dry.

Laboratory data.			
ABGs		Basic Metabolic Panel	
pH	7.08	Na	128 mEq/L
$Paco_2$	17 mm Hg	K	5.9 mEq/L
Pao_2	81 mm Hg	Cl	72 mEq/L
HCO_3	5 mEq/L	CO_2	5 mEq/L
		BUN	45 mg/dL
		Cr	1.1 mg/dL
		Glucose	845 mg/dL
		Albumin	4.0 g/dL
		EtOH	0 mg/dL

QUESTIONS

Q4-1: Define the patient's baseline acid-base status: Does this patient have an underlying chronic acid-base disorder that we need to account for in order to appropriately interpret the acute acid-base disorders?

A. There is no evidence for an underlying chronic respiratory or metabolic acid-base disorder in this patient, so we would assume a baseline $Paco_2$ of 40 mm Hg and an HCO_3 of 24 mEq/L.

B. While the patient has a condition predisposing him to a chronic acid-base disorder, there is insufficient information to estimate the patient's baseline $Paco_2$ and HCO_3 values; therefore, we will assume a baseline $Paco_2$ of 40 mm Hg and a baseline HCO_3 of 24 mEq/L.

C. The patient has an underlying acid-base condition, and we have sufficient information to estimate the patient's baseline $Paco_2$ and HCO_3 values.

Q4-2: What is/are the primary acid-base disturbance(s) occurring in this case?

A. Metabolic acidosis only
B. Respiratory acidosis only
C. Metabolic alkalosis only
D. Respiratory alkalosis only
E. Metabolic acidosis and a respiratory acidosis
F. Metabolic alkalosis and a respiratory alkalosis

Q4-3: How would the metabolic acidosis component be classified in this case?

A. Anion gap acidosis
B. Non-anion gap acidosis
C. Anion and non-anion gap acidosis
D. Anion gap acidosis and a metabolic alkalosis

Q4-4: Your laboratory testing returns the following values:

Serum EtOH	0 mg/dL
Serum acetaminophen level	< 3 mg/dL (ULN for therapeutic use 20 mg/dL)
Serum salicylates level	< 5 mg/dL (ULN for therapeutic use 30 mg/dL)
Serum osmolality	332 mOsm/kg
Serum L-lactate	2.1 mmol/L (ULN 2.0 mmol/L venous)
Beta-hydroxybutyrate (acetone)	4.5 mmol/L (ULN 0.18 mmol/L)
Serum glucose	845 mg/dL

Does the patient have a serum osmolal gap?

A. Yes, there is a serum osmolal gap and we should obtain laboratory results for organic alcohol ingestion.

B. No, there is no serum osmolal gap.

C. Yes, there is a serum osmolal gap but this is not due to organic alcohol ingestion.

Q4-5: Does the patient in this case demonstrate appropriate respiratory or metabolic compensation?

A. Yes, the respiratory compensation is appropriate.
B. No, a concomitant respiratory alkalosis is present.
C. No, a concomitant respiratory acidosis is present.
D. Yes, the metabolic compensation is appropriate.
E. No, a concomitant metabolic acidosis is present.
F. No, a concomitant metabolic alkalosis is present.

Q4-6: The patient's urine studies are as follows:

Urine Na	13 mEq/L
Urine K	9 mEq/L
Urine Cl	6 mEq/L
Urine urea	450 mg/dL
Urine glucose	151 mg/dL
Urine osmolality	840 mOsm/L
Urine pH	4.9
Urine RBCs	None
Urine WBCs	None
Urine protein	Minimal
Urine microscopic	None

What is the most likely cause of the patient's concomitant metabolic alkalosis?

A. Emesis
B. Current thiazide diuretic use
C. Hypoaldosteronism
D. Hyperaldosteronism
E. Laxative abuse

ANSWERS

Q4-1: A

There is no evidence for an underlying chronic respiratory or metabolic acid-base disorder in this patient, so we would assume a baseline $Paco_2$ of 40 mm Hg and an HCO_3 of 24 mEq/L.

Rationale: Ignoring these underlying chronic acid-base disorders can significantly alter the interpretation of a patient's acute acid-base status. This was demonstrated in the first case of the series. However, often we do not have the necessary information (eg, prior ABG or VBG, or prior serum chemistry with an HCO_3) and are forced to assume the ongoing processes are all acute in nature. We are primarily concerned about chronic respiratory acid-base disorders, as these can significantly alter the patient's baseline or expected values for the serum HCO_3 and $Paco_2$, and we have reliable equations to predict the expected baseline values. The respiratory compensation for both chronic metabolic acidosis and alkalosis is generally poor, so there are no equations or rules to predict what the $Paco_2$ should be in these cases. While the baseline serum HCO_3 may be significantly off from our standard value of 24 mEq/L in these patients, we would assume a baseline $Paco_2$ of 40 mm Hg in patients with chronic metabolic processes. Once we identify the patient's baseline $Paco_2$ and HCO_3 values, we will need to use these values in the appropriate equations to identify the ongoing acute processes.

Q4-2: A

Metabolic acidosis only.

Rationale:

1. The pH is 7.08; therefore, the primary disorder is an **acidosis.**
2. The $Paco_2$ of 17 mm Hg is less than 40 mm Hg, so this is not the cause of acidosis.
3. The HCO_3 of 5 mEq/L is less than 24 mEq/L, so there is a **primary metabolic acidosis.**

Q4-3: D

Anion gap acidosis and a metabolic alkalosis.

Rationale:

1. Is there evidence for a chronic respiratory acid-base disorder that requires adjustment of the patient's "normal" HCO_3? No, there is no evidence for a chronic respiratory acid-base disorder, so we would assume a baseline $Paco_2$ of 40 mm Hg and an HCO_3 of 24 mEq/L.
2. Expected anion gap:

$$\text{Expected Anion Gap} = 12 - (2.5) * \left[4.0 \frac{g}{dL} - \text{Actual Serum Albumin} \right]$$

$$= 12 - (2.5 * [4.0 - 4.0])$$

$$= 12 - (2.5 * [0]) = \mathbf{12 \ mEq/L.}$$

3. Anion gap calculation:

Serum Anion Gap = $[Na^+] - [HCO_3^-] - [Cl^-]$

    128 – (72 + 5) = 51 mEq/L, which is > 12 mEq/L → **anion gap acidosis is present.**

4. Delta-delta calculation:

$$\Delta\Delta = \frac{(\text{Actual Anion Gap} - \text{Expected Anion Gap})}{(\text{Baseline HCO}_3 - \text{Actual HCO}_3)}$$

    (50 – 12)/(24 – 5) = **39/19, which is ~2.1.**

Delta-Delta interpretation.	
Delta-Delta Value	Condition Present
< 0.4	Non-anion gap only
0.4–0.9	Anion gap *and* non-anion gap acidosis
1.0–2.0	Anion gap acidosis only
> 2.0	**Anion gap acidosis and metabolic alkalosis**

Q4-4: C
Yes, there is a serum osmolal gap, but this is not due to organic alcohol ingestion.

Rationale: The serum osmolal gap is the difference between the laboratory measured ("true") serum osmolality and a "calculated" osmolality based on commonly measured compounds that are known to contribute to the serum osmolality. Therefore, similar to the serum anion gap, the serum osmolal gap represents the "unmeasured" compounds also contributing to the serum osmolality. The serum osmolal gap can be helpful in determining whether an organic alcohol ingestion has occurred recently.

Similar to the serum anion gap, the serum osmolal gap is determined by the difference between the "calculated" serum osmolality and the true, measured serum osmolality. The equation for the serum osmolal gap typically includes factors for sodium, glucose, BUN, and ethanol, as these are readily measurable in most laboratories. Therefore, the serum osmolal gap will represent the osmolality of those "unmeasured" osmoles, including organic alcohols and acetone. The most common form is shown as the following:

$$\text{Calculated Serum Osmolality} = 2*[Na^+] + \frac{[\text{Glucose}]}{18} + \frac{[\text{BUN}]}{2.8} + \frac{[\text{EtOH}]}{3.7},$$

In which the units of measure are as follows: Na, mEq/L; glucose, mg/dL; BUN, mg/dL; EtOH, mg/dL. The conversion factors (for values in mg/dL) are provided in the previous table. One can include additional factors if the concentrations of other osmoles are known. No correction factor is needed if units are in mmol/L; the following corrections are for values in mg/dL: methanol, 3.2; isopropyl alcohol, 6.0; ethylene glycol, 6.2; and acetone, 5.8. The osmolal gap is generally between −10 and +10; anything greater than +15 mOsm/L is considered a critical value.

Calculated Serum Osmolality = [2 * Na] + [Glucose/18] + [BUN/2.8] + [EtOH/3.7]
$$= (2 * 128) + (845/18) + (45/2.8) + (0/3.7)$$
$$= 319.$$

Serum Osmolal Gap = Measured Serum Osmolality – Calculated Osmolality
$$= (332 - 319) = 13 > 10 \rightarrow positive \text{ serum osmolal gap.}$$

While the serum anion gap is elevated, the patient has a positive ketone study. The unit of measure of the ketone study is mmol/L. Since this is unit of measure for serum osmolality, we do not need a conversion factor, and we can subtract it from the current serum osmolal gap and see if the result is still abnormal—after we account for the elevated beta-hydroxybutyrate (BHB), keeping in mind that acetone is the breakdown product of BHB and acetoacetate:

Serum Osmolal Gap – BHB = 13 – 4.5 = 8.5 mOsm/L.

Therefore, after we account for the elevated ketone bodies, the serum osmolal gap is normal and we should not be concerned about an organic alcohol ingestion. This patient has a classic presentation of DKA, with a mildly elevated serum osmolal gap due to the presence of ketone bodies.

Q4-5: A
Yes, the respiratory compensation is appropriate.

Rationale: Using the Winter formula, one can calculate what the expected arterial $Paco_2$ should be for a given serum HCO_3 if the patient were completely compensated.

Respiratory Compensation for Acute Metabolic Acidosis (Winter Formula):

Expected $Paco_2$ = 1.5 * (Actual HCO_3) + 8 ± 2 (in mm Hg).

Therefore, for this patient,

Expected $Paco_2$ = 1.5 * (Actual HCO_3) + 8 (± 2)
$$= (1.5 * 5) + 8 = 7.5 + 8 = 15.5 \pm 2 = (13.5 - 17.5).$$

Accordingly, this patient has an appropriate compensatory response to the metabolic acidosis.

Q4-6: A
Emesis.

Rationale: This patient presented with emesis in the setting of DKA, likely due to reduced gastric peristalsis associated with hyperglycemia and possibly gastritis. The patient has a metabolic alkalosis, with a low urine chloride level, and therefore a chloride-responsive process is most likely. Hyperemesis is the only cause in this scenario that generally meets these criteria. Current thiazide diuretic use and hyperaldosteronism as associated with chloride-resistant alkalosis, while hypoaldosteronisms is associated with a type 4 RTA. Laxative abuse is complicated, as it can cause either a metabolic alkalosis or a metabolic acidosis. However, when it does cause a metabolic

Causes of metabolic alkalosis.
History: Rule Out the Following as Causes
• Alkali load ("milk-alkali" or calcium-alkali syndrome, oral sodium bicarbonate, IV sodium bicarbonate) • Genetic causes (cystic fibrosis [CF]) • Presence of hypercalcemia • IV β-lactam antibiotics • Laxative abuse (may also cause a metabolic acidosis depending on diarrheal HCO_3 losses)
If None of the Above, Then. . .
Urine Chloride < 20 mEq/L • Loss of gastric acid (hyperemesis, NGT suctioning) • Prior diuretic use (in hours to days following discontinuation) • Post-hypercapnia • Villous adenoma • Congenital chloridorrhea • Chronic laxative abuse (may also cause a metabolic acidosis depending on diarrheal HCO_3 losses) • CF **OR: Urine Chloride > 20 mEq/L**
Urine Chloride > 20 mEq/L, Lack of Hypertension (HTN), Urine Potassium < 30 mEq/L
• Hypokalemia or hypomagnesemia • Laxative abuse (if dominated by hypokalemia) • Bartter syndrome • Gitelman syndrome
Urine Chloride > 20 mEq/L, Lack of HTN, Urine Potassium > 30 mEq/L
• Current diuretic use
Urine Chloride > 20 mEq/L, Presence of HTN, Urine Potassium Variable but Usually > 30 mEq/L
Elevated plasma renin level: • Renal artery stenosis • Renin-secreting tumor • Renovascular disease
Low plasma renin, low plasma aldosterone: • Cushing syndrome • Exogenous mineralocorticoid • Genetic disorder (11-hydoxylase or 17-hydrolyase deficiency, 11β-HSD deficiency) • Liddle syndrome • Licorice toxicity
Low plasma renin, high plasma aldosterone: • Primary hyperaldosteronism • Adrenal adenoma • Bilateral adrenal hyperplasia

alkalosis, this is usually associated with hypokalemia and is not responsive to simple fluid resuscitation alone.

References

Abreo K, Adlakha A, Kilpatrick S, et al. The milk-alkali syndrome. A reversible form of acute renal failure. Arch Intern Med. 1993;153:1005.

Arroliga AC, Shehab N, McCarthy K, Gonzales JP. Relationship of continuous infusion lorazepam to serum propylene glycol concentration in critically ill adults. Crit Care Med. 2004;32:1709.

Barton CH, Vaziri ND, Ness RL, et al. Cimetidine in the management of metabolic alkalosis induced by nasogastric drainage. Arch Surg. 1979;114:70.

Bear R, Goldstein M, Phillipson E, et al. Effect of metabolic alkalosis on respiratory function in patients with chronic obstructive lung disease. Can Med Assoc J. 1977;117:900.

Braden GL, Strayhorn CH, Germain MJ, et al. Increased osmolal gap in alcoholic acidosis. Arch Intern Med. 1993;153:2377.

Cámara-Lemarroy CR, Gónzalez-Moreno EI, Rodriguez-Gutierrez R, González-González JG. Clinical presentation and management in acute toluene intoxication: a case series. Inhal Toxicol. 2012;24:434.

DeFronzo RA, Matzuda M, Barret E. Diabetic ketoacidosis: a combined metabolic-nephrologic approach to therapy. Diabetes Rev. 1994;2:209.

Fulop M, Murthy V, Michilli A, et al. Serum beta-hydroxybutyrate measurement in patients with uncontrolled diabetes mellitus. Arch Intern Med. 1999;159:381.

Gabow PA. Ethylene glycol intoxication. Am J Kidney Dis. 1988;11:277.

Galla JH, Gifford JD, Luke RG, Rome L. Adaptations to chloride-depletion alkalosis. Am J Physiol. 1991;261:R771.

Garella S, Chang BS, Kahn SI. Dilution acidosis and contraction alkalosis: review of a concept. Kidney Int. 1975;8:279.

Gennari FJ. Current concepts. Serum osmolality. Uses and limitations. N Engl J Med. 1984;310:102.

Gennari FJ, Weise WJ. Acid-base disturbances in gastrointestinal disease. Clin J Am Soc Nephrol. 2008;3:1861.

Glasser L, et. al. Serum osmolality and its applicability to drug overdose. Am J Clin Pathol. 1973;60:695.

Hamm LL, Nakhoul N, Hering-Smith KS. Acid-base homeostasis. Clin J Am Soc Nephrol. 2015;10:2232.

Hulter HN, Sebastian A, Toto RD, et al. Renal and systemic acid-base effects of the chronic administration of hypercalcemia-producing agents: calcitriol, PTH, and intravenous calcium. Kidney Int. 1982;21:445.

Khanna A, Kurtzman NA. Metabolic alkalosis. J Nephrol. 2006;19(suppl 9):S86.

Kraut JA, Kurtz I. Toxic alcohol ingestions: clinical features, diagnosis, and management. Clin J Am Soc Nephrol. 2008;3:208.

Kraut JA, Nagami GT. The serum anion gap in the evaluation of acid-base disorders: what are its limitations and can its effectiveness be improved? Clin J Am Soc Nephrol. 2013;8:2018.

Kraut JA, Xing SX. Approach to the evaluation of a patient with an increased serum osmolal gap and high-anion-gap metabolic acidosis. Am J Kidney Dis. 2011;58:480.

Laski ME, Sabatini S. Metabolic alkalosis, bedside and bench. Semin Nephrol. 2006;26:404.

Luke RG, Galla JH. It is chloride depletion alkalosis, not contraction alkalosis. J Am Soc Nephrol. 2012;23:204.

Lynd LD, Richardson KJ, Purssell RA, et al. An evaluation of the osmole gap as a screening test for toxic alcohol poisoning. BMC Emerg Med. 2008;8:5.

Marraffa JM, Holland MG, Stork CM, et al. Diethylene glycol: widely used solvent presents serious poisoning potential. J Emerg Med. 2008;35:401.

Miller PD, Berns AS. Acute metabolic alkalosis perpetuating hypercarbia. A role for acetazolamide in chronic obstructive pulmonary disease. JAMA. 1977;238:2400.

Oster JR, Materson BJ, Rogers AI. Laxative abuse syndrome. Am J Gastroenterol. 1980;74:451.

Patel AM, Goldfarb S. Got calcium? Welcome to the calcium-alkali syndrome. J Am Soc Nephrol. 2010;21:1440.

Porter WH, Yao HH, Karounos DG. Laboratory and clinical evaluation of assays for beta-hydroxybutyrate. Am J Clin Pathol. 1997;107:353.

Purssell RA, Pudek M, Brubacher J, Abu-Laban RB. Derivation and validation of a formula to calculate the contribution of ethanol to the osmolal gap. Ann Emerg Med. 2001;38:653.

Robinson AG, Loeb JN. Ethanol ingestion—commonest cause of elevated plasma osmolality? N Engl J Med. 1971;284:1253.

Rose BD, Post TW. Clinical Physiology of Acid-Base and Electrolyte Disorders. 5e. New York, NY: McGraw Hill; 2001:559, 809-815.

Schelling JR, Howard RL, Winter SD, Linas SL. Increased osmolal gap in alcoholic ketoacidosis and lactic acidosis. Ann Intern Med. 1990;113:580.

Schwartz WB, Van Ypersele de Strihou, Kassirer JP. Role of anions in metabolic alkalosis and potassium deficiency. N Engl J Med. 1968;279:630.

Shen T, Braude S. Changes in serum phosphate during treatment of diabetic ketoacidosis: predictive significance of severity of acidosis on presentation. Intern Med J. 2012;42:1347.

Streicher HZ, Gabow PA, Moss AH, et al. Syndromes of toluene sniffing in adults. Ann Intern Med. 1981;94:758.

Sweetser LJ, Douglas JA, Riha RL, Bell SC. Clinical presentation of metabolic alkalosis in an adult patient with cystic fibrosis. Respirology. 2005;10:254.

Taher SM, Anderson RJ, McCartney R, et al. Renal tubular acidosis associated with toluene "sniffing". N Engl J Med. 1974;290:765.

Taki K, Mizuno K, Takahashi N, Wakusawa R. Disturbance of CO_2 elimination in the lungs by carbonic anhydrase inhibition. Jpn J Physiol. 1986;36:523.

Turban S, Beutler KT, Morris RG, et al. Long-term regulation of proximal tubule acid-base transporter abundance by angiotensin II. Kidney Int. 2006;70:660.

Wachtel TJ, Tetu-Mouradjian LM, Goldman DL, et al. Hyperosmolarity and acidosis in diabetes mellitus: a three-year experience in Rhode Island. J Gen Intern Med. 1991;6:495.

Yücel M, Takagi M, Walterfang M, Lubman DI. Toluene misuse and long-term harms: a systematic review of the neuropsychological and neuroimaging literature. Neurosci Biobehav Rev. 2008;32:910.

CASE 5

A 56-year-old man with ESRD presents after several days of profuse diarrhea and associated weakness. His medical history includes *Clostridium difficile* infection last month, and he just finished a course of antibiotics for an associated Permac-ath infection. He is somewhat delirious and unable to answer questions. He takes calcitriol, amlodipine, nicardipine, sodium bicarbonate tablets, and revlamer. His vital signs on arrival are T 37.9°C, HR 110, RR 28, BP 90/40, and Sao_2 99% on RA. According to the patient's caretaker, he missed dialysis 2 days ago due to weakness. Laboratory values are as follows:

Laboratory data.			
ABGs		Basic Metabolic Panel	
pH	7.21	Na	131 mEq/L
$Paco_2$	23 mm Hg	K	5.9 mEq/L
Pao_2	77 mm Hg	Cl	88 mEq/L
HCO_3	9 mEq/L	CO_2	9 mEq/L
		BUN	184 mg/dL
		Cr	11.9 mg/dL
		Glucose	110 mg/dL
		Albumin	3.0 g/dL
		EtOH	0 mg/dL

QUESTIONS

Q5-1: Define the patient's baseline acid-base status: Does this patient have an underlying chronic acid-base disorder that we need to account for in order to appropriately interpret the acute acid-base disorders?

A. There is no evidence of an underlying chronic respiratory or metabolic acid-base disorder in this patient, so we would assume a baseline $Paco_2$ of 40 mm Hg and an HCO_3 of 24 mEq/L.

B. While the patient has a condition that predisposing him to a chronic acid-base disorder, there is insufficient information to estimate the patient's baseline $Paco_2$ and HCO_3 values; therefore, we will assume a baseline $Paco_2$ of 40 mm Hg and a baseline HCO_3 of 24 mEq/L.

C. The patient has an underlying acid-base condition, and we have sufficient information to estimate the patient's baseline $Paco_2$ and HCO_3 values.

Q5-2: What is/are the primary acid-base disturbance(s) occurring in this case?

A. Metabolic acidosis only
B. Respiratory acidosis only
C. Metabolic alkalosis only
D. Respiratory alkalosis only
E. Metabolic acidosis and a respiratory acidosis
F. Metabolic alkalosis and a respiratory alkalosis

Q5-3: For a perfectly healthy patient, a normal anion gap is assumed to be 12. What should be considered a normal anion gap in this patient?

A. 12 mEq/L
B. 9.5 mEq/L
C. 7.5 mEq/L
D. 4 mEq/L

Q5-4: How would the metabolic acidosis component be classified in this case?

A. Anion gap acidosis
B. Non-anion gap acidosis
C. Anion and non-anion gap acidosis
D. Anion gap acidosis and a metabolic alkalosis

Q5-5: Your laboratory testing returns the following values:

Serum EtOH	0 mg/dL
Serum acetaminophen level	< 3 mg/dL (ULN for therapeutic use 20 mg/dL)
Serum salicylates level	< 5 mg/dL (ULN for therapeutic use 30 mg/dL)
Serum osmolality	341 mOsm/kg
Serum L-lactate	4.3 mmol/L (ULN 2.0 mmol/L venous)
Beta-hydroxybutyrate (acetone)	< 0.18 mmol/L (ULN 0.18 mmol/L)
Serum glucose	110 mg/dL

Which of the following is/are likely contributing to the patient's anion gap acidosis?

A. Lactic acidosis secondary to distributive shock
B. Methanol intoxication
C. Renal failure
D. Acetaminophen toxicity
E. Hypoaldosteronism
F. A and B
G. B and C
H. A and C
I. C and D
J. A, B, and E.

Q5-6: Does the patient in this case demonstrate appropriate respiratory or metabolic compensation?

A. Yes, the respiratory compensation is appropriate.
B. No, a concomitant respiratory alkalosis is present.
C. No, a concomitant respiratory acidosis is present.
D. Yes, the metabolic compensation is appropriate.
E. No, a concomitant metabolic acidosis is present.
F. No, a concomitant metabolic alkalosis is present.

ANSWERS

Q5-1: B

This patient has a condition, ESRD that is typically associated with a chronic metabolic acidosis. However, we don't have enough information regarding the patient's baseline HCO_3; therefore, we will use a baseline value of 24 mEq/L.

Rationale: Ignoring these underlying chronic acid-base disorders can significantly alter the interpretation of a patient's acute acid-base status. This was demonstrated in the first case of the series. However, often, we do not have the necessary information (eg, prior ABG or VBG, or prior serum chemistry with an HCO_3) and are forced to assume the ongoing processes are all acute in nature. We are primarily concerned about chronic respiratory acid-base disorders, as this can significantly alter the patient's baseline or expected values for the serum HCO_3 and $Paco_2$, and we have reliable equations to predict the expected baseline values. The respiratory compensation for both chronic metabolic acidosis and alkalosis is generally poor, so there are no equations or rules to predict what the $Paco_2$ should be in these cases. While the baseline serum HCO_3 may be significantly off from our standard value of 24 mEq/L in these patients, we would assume a baseline $Paco_2$ of 40 mm Hg in patients with chronic metabolic processes. Once we identify the patient's baseline $Paco_2$ and HCO_3 values, we will need to use these values in the appropriate equations to identify the ongoing acute processes.

Q5-2: A

Metabolic acidosis only.

Rationale:

1. The pH is 7.21; therefore, the primary disorder is an **acidosis.**
2. The $Paco_2$ of 23 mm Hg is less than 40 mm Hg, so this is not the cause of acidosis.
3. The HCO_3 of 9 mEq/L is less than 24 mEq/L, so there is a **metabolic acidosis.**

Q5-3: B

9.5 mEq/L.

Rationale: The normal anion gap is 12 mEq/L. The term *anion gap* refers to those ions (negatively charged molecules) in the bloodstream that we do not routinely measure, including phosphates, sulfates, organic acids, and negatively charged plasma proteins. One of the most abundant negatively charged ions in the blood is serum albumin. A normal serum albumin is 4.0 g/dL. For patients with hypoalbuminemia (low serum albumin), the normal or expected anion gap is smaller.

Expected Anion Gap (AG):

$$\text{Expected AG} = 12 - (2.5) * \left[4.0\frac{g}{dL} - \text{Actual Serum Albumin} \right].$$

So for this patient,

$$\text{Expected AG} = 12 - [2.5 * (4 - 3)] = 12 - (2.5 * 1) = 9.5 \text{ mEq/L}.$$

This is an important concept as patients with hypoalbuminemia may "hide" an anion gap acidosis if this correction is not performed.

Q5-4: C
Anion and non-anion gap acidosis.

Rationale:

1. Does the patient have an underlying, chronic acid-base disorder (is there information provided to suggest the patient's baseline acid-base values)? No, although the patient likely has very poor renal function, we do not have any data regarding an underlying chronic metabolic acidosis. Therefore, we will assume the ongoing processes are acute.
2. Expected anion gap: We calculated this in the prior question, and the expected anion gap is 9.5.
3. Anion gap calculation:

$$\text{Serum AG} = [Na^+] - [HCO_3^-] - [Cl^-]$$
$$131 - (88 + 9) = 34 \text{ mEq/L, which is} > 9.5 \text{ mEq/L}$$
$$\rightarrow \textbf{anion gap acidosis is present.}$$

4. Delta-delta calculation:

$$\Delta\Delta = \frac{(\text{Actual AG} - \text{Expected AG})}{(\text{Baseline HCO}_3 - \text{Actual HCO}_3)}$$

$(34 - 9.5)/(24 - 9) = \textbf{23.5/15, which is ~1.6.}$

Delta-Delta interpretation.	
Delta-Delta Value	Condition Present
< 0.4	Non-anion gap only
0.4–0.9	Anion gap *and* non-anion gap acidosis
1.0–2.0	**Anion gap acidosis only**
> 2.0	Anion gap acidosis and metabolic alkalosis

Q5-5: H
Both option A (lactic acidosis secondary to distributive shock) and option C (renal failure) are correct.

Rationale: The patient presents with hypotension in the setting of volume depletion from several days of severe diarrhea. He has an elevated serum lactate. Additionally, the patient has a significantly elevated BUN in the setting of his ESRD and recently missed dialysis session, indicating that his chronic renal failure is likely also contributing to the acidosis. There is no evidence of acetaminophen toxicity based on the laboratory data above, and hypoaldosteronism is associated with a non-anion gap acidosis. The final remaining answer to rule out is an organic alcohol intoxication.

The serum osmolal gap is calculated as the difference between the patient's measured serum osmolarity (or osmolality) and the calculated serum osmolality based on laboratory data. The calculated osmolality equation is:

Calculated Serum Osmolality:

$$2*[Na^+] + \frac{[Glucose]}{18} + \frac{[BUN]}{2.8} + \frac{[EtOH]}{3.7}$$

Calculated Serum Osmolality = [2 * Na] + [Glucose/18] + [BUN/2.8] + [EtOH/3.7]
$$- (2 * 131) + (110/18) + (184/2.8) + (0/3.7)$$
$$= 334.$$

Serum Osmolal Gap = Measured Serum Osmolality – Calculated Osmolality
$$= (341 - 334) = 8, \text{ which is} < 10 \rightarrow \textbf{\textit{no}} \text{ serum osmolal gap is present.}$$

The lack of an elevated serum osmolar gap effectively rules out organic alcohol poisoning.

Causes of anion gap metabolic acidosis.	
Common	Less Common
Lactic acidosis (including transient)	Cyanide poisoning
Renal failure ("uremia")	Carbon monoxide poisoning
Diabetic ketoacidosis	Aminoglycosides
Alcohol ketoacidosis	Phenformin use
Starvation ketoacidosis	D-Lactic acidosis
Salicylate poisoning (ASA)	Paraldehyde
Acetaminophen poisoning (paracetamol)	Iron
Organic alcohol poisoning (ethylene glycol, methanol, propylene glycol)	Isoniazid
Toluene poisoning ("glue-sniffing")	Inborn errors of metabolism

Q5-6: A
Yes, the respiratory compensation is appropriate.

Rationale: Using the Winter formula, one can calculate what the expected arterial $Paco_2$ should be for a given serum HCO_3 if the patient were completely compensated.

Respiratory Compensation for Acute Metabolic Acidosis (Winter Formula):

Expected $Paco_2$ = 1.5 * [Actual HCO_3] + 8 ± 2 (in mm Hg)
Expected $Paco_2$ = 1.5 * (Actual HCO_3) + 8 (± 2)
$$= (1.5 * 9) + 8 = 13.5 + 8 = 21.5 \pm 2 = (19.5 - 23.5 \text{ mm Hg}).$$

Therefore, this patient has an appropriate compensatory response to the metabolic acidosis.

References

Adeva-Andany M, López-Ojén M, Funcasta-Calderón R, et al. Comprehensive review on lactate metabolism in human health. Mitochondrion. 2014;17:76.

Bailey JL. Metabolic acidosis: an unrecognized cause of morbidity in the patient with chronic kidney disease. Kidney Int Suppl. 2005;S15.

Batlle D, Grupp M, Gaviria M, Kurtzman NA. Distal renal tubular acidosis with intact capacity to lower urinary pH. Am J Med. 1982;72:751.

Batlle D, Haque SK. Genetic causes and mechanisms of distal renal tubular acidosis. Nephrol Dial Transplant. 2012;27:3691.

Batlle DC, Hizon M, Cohen E, et al. The use of the urinary anion gap in the diagnosis of hyperchloremic metabolic acidosis. N Engl J Med. 1988;318:594.

Batlle DC, von Riotte A, Schlueter W. Urinary sodium in the evaluation of hyperchloremic metabolic acidosis. N Engl J Med. 1987;316:140.

Bern M. Clinically significant pseudohyponatremia. Am J Hematol. 2006;81:558.

Buckalew VM Jr, McCurdy DK, Ludwig GD, et al. Incomplete renal tubular acidosis. Physiologic studies in three patients with a defect in lowering urine pH. Am J Med. 1968;45:32.

Corey HE. Stewart and beyond: new models of acid-base balance. Kidney Int. 2003;64:777.

Feldman M, Soni N, Dickson B. Influence of hypoalbuminemia or hyperalbuminemia on the serum anion gap. J Lab Clin Med. 2005;146:317.

Fenves AZ, Kirkpatrick HM 3rd, Patel VV, et al. Increased anion gap metabolic acidosis as a result of 5-oxoproline (pyroglutamic acid): a role for acetaminophen. Clin J Am Soc Nephrol. 2006;1:441.

Fernandez PC, Cohen RM, Feldman GM. The concept of bicarbonate distribution space: the crucial role of body buffers. Kidney Int. 1989;36:747.

Forni LG, McKinnon W, Lord GA, et al. Circulating anions usually associated with the Krebs cycle in patients with metabolic acidosis. Crit Care. 2005;9:R591.

Halperin ML, Ethier JH, Kamel KS. Ammonium excretion in chronic metabolic acidosis: benefits and risks. Am J Kidney Dis. 1989;14:267.

Karet FE. Mechanisms in hyperkalemic renal tubular acidosis. J Am Soc Nephrol. 2009;20:251.

Komaru Y, Inokuchi R, Ueda Y, et al. Use of the anion gap and intermittent hemodialysis following continuous hemodiafiltration in extremely high dose acute-on-chronic lithium poisoning: a case report. Hemodial Int. 2018;22:E15.

Kraut JA, Kurtz I. Metabolic acidosis of CKD: diagnosis, clinical characteristics, and treatment. Am J Kidney Dis. 2005;45:978.

Kraut JA, Kurtz I. Toxic alcohol ingestions: clinical features, diagnosis, and management. Clin J Am Soc Nephrol. 2008;3:208.

Kraut JA, Nagami GT. The serum anion gap in the evaluation of acid-base disorders: what are its limitations and can its effectiveness be improved? Clin J Am Soc Nephrol. 2013;8:2018.

Kraut JA, Xing SX. Approach to the evaluation of a patient with an increased serum osmolal gap and high-anion-gap metabolic acidosis. Am J Kidney Dis. 2011;58:480.

Krieger NS, Frick KK, Bushinsky DA. Mechanism of acid-induced bone resorption. Curr Opin Nephrol Hypertens. 2004;13:423.

Levy B. Lactate and shock state: the metabolic view. Curr Opin Crit Care. 2006;12:315.

Lu J, Zello GA, Randell E, et al. Closing the anion gap: contribution of D-lactate to diabetic ketoacidosis. Clin Chim Acta. 2011;412:286.

Madias NE. Lactic acidosis. Kidney Int. 1986;29:752.

Madias NE, Ayus JC, Adrogué HJ. Increased anion gap in metabolic alkalosis: the role of plasma-protein equivalency. N Engl J Med. 1979;300:1421.

Mikkelsen ME, Miltiades AN, Gaieski DF, et al. Serum lactate is associated with mortality in severe sepsis independent of organ failure and shock. Crit Care Med. 2009;37:1670.

Murray T, Long W, Narins RG. Multiple myeloma and the anion gap. N Engl J Med. 1975;292:574.

Pierce NF, Fedson DS, Brigham KL, et al. The ventilatory response to acute base deficit in humans. Time course during development and correction of metabolic acidosis. Ann Intern Med. 1970;72:633.

Relman AS. What are acids and bases? Am J Med. 1954;17:435.

Rodríguez Soriano J. Renal tubular acidosis: the clinical entity. J Am Soc Nephrol. 2002;13:2160.

Schwartz WB, Relman AS. A critique of the parameters used in the evaluation of acid-base disorders. "Whole-blood buffer base" and "standard bicarbonate" compared with blood pH and plasma bicarbonate concentration. N Engl J Med. 1963;268:1382.

Warnock DG. Uremic acidosis. Kidney Int. 1988;34:278.

Widmer B, Gerhardt RE, Harrington JT, Cohen JJ. Serum electrolyte and acid base composition. The influence of graded degrees of chronic renal failure. Arch Intern Med. 1979;139:1099.

Zimmer BW, Marcus RJ, Sawyer K, Harchelroad F. Salicylate intoxication as a cause of pseudohyperchloremia. Am J Kidney Dis. 2008;51:346.

CASE 6

A 23-year-old man with history of alcohol abuse is brought to the emergency department by EMS. The patient is unresponsive with agonal breathing. He has shown some improvement with naloxone but has evidence of recent aspiration and emesis. He is intubated for airway protection. EMS reports finding the patient face down in an alley in the middle of a nearby city. No identification is found and the patient has no medical bracelets or medications on his person. Vital signs on arrival were RR 4 and agonal, HR 40, BP 90/60, and Sao$_2$ 63% on RA. He is hypothermic to 35.3°C. Initial laboratory values are shown as follows:

Laboratory data.			
ABGs		Basic Metabolic Panel	
pH	6.95	Na	133 mEq/L
Paco$_2$	79 mm Hg	K	5.6 mEq/L
Pao$_2$	109 mm Hg	Cl	89 mEq/L
HCO$_3$	17 mEq/L	CO$_2$	17 mEq/L
		BUN	12 mg/dL
		Cr	1.1 mg/dL
		Glucose	187 mg/dL
		Albumin	4 g/dL
		EtOH	33 mg/dL

QUESTIONS

Q6-1: Define the patient's baseline acid-base status: Does this patient have an underlying chronic acid-base disorder that we need to account for in order to appropriately interpret the acute acid-base disorders?

A. There is no evidence of an underlying chronic respiratory or metabolic acid-base disorder in this patient, so we would assume a baseline $Paco_2$ of 40 mm Hg and an HCO_3 of 24 mEq/L.

B. While the patient has a condition that predisposing him to a chronic acid-base disorder, there is insufficient information to estimate the patient's baseline $Paco_2$ and HCO_3 values; therefore, we will assume a baseline $Paco_2$ of 40 mm Hg and a baseline HCO_3 of 24 mEq/L.

C. The patient has an underlying acid-base condition, and we have sufficient information to estimate the patient's baseline $Paco_2$ and HCO_3 values.

Q6-2: What is/are the primary acid-base disturbance(s) occurring in this case?

A. Metabolic acidosis only
B. Respiratory acidosis only
C. Metabolic alkalosis only
D. Respiratory alkalosis only
E. Metabolic acidosis and a respiratory acidosis
F. Metabolic alkalosis and a respiratory alkalosis

Q6-3: How would the metabolic acidosis component be classified in this case?

A. Anion gap acidosis
B. Non-anion gap acidosis
C. Anion and non-anion gap acidosis
D. Anion gap acidosis and a metabolic alkalosis

Q6-4: Your laboratory testing returns the following values:

Serum EtOH	33 mg/dL
Serum acetaminophen level	< 5 mg/dL (ULN for therapeutic use 20 mg/dL)
Serum salicylates level	< 5 mg/dL (ULN for therapeutic use 30 mg/dL)
Serum osmolality	333 mOsm/kg
Serum L-lactate	2.3 mmol/L (ULN 2.0 mmol/L venous)
Beta-hydroxybutyrate (acetone)	< 0.18 mmol/L (ULN 0.18 mmol/L)
Serum glucose	187 mg/dL
Urine drug screen	+++ Positive for opioids, THC, benzodiazepines

Which of the following is the likely cause of the patient's respiratory acidosis?

A. Benzodiazepine overdose
B. Ethylene glycol intoxication
C. Opioid intoxication
D. Progesterone overdose
E. Aspirin overdose

Q6-5. Referring to the laboratory values listed for Q6-4, which of the following is the likely cause of the patient's metabolic acidosis?

A. Lactic acidosis
B. Alcoholic ketoacidosis
C. Ethylene glycol intoxication
D. Acute renal failure
E. Adrenal crisis

Q6-6: The patient's urine chloride is less than 10, with a urine anion gap of −10 and urine osmolal gap of 150 mOsm/L. What is the most likely cause of the patient's concomitant metabolic alkalosis?

A. Emesis
B. Current thiazide diuretic use
C. Current high-dose corticosteroid use
D. Laxative abuse

ANSWERS

Q6-1: A

There is no evidence of an underlying chronic respiratory or metabolic acid-base disorder in this patient, so we would assume a baseline $Paco_2$ of 40 mm Hg and an HCO_3 of 24 mEq/L.

Rationale: Ignoring these underlying chronic acid-base disorders can significantly alter the interpretation of a patient's acute acid-base status. This was demonstrated in the first case of the series. However, often, we do not have the necessary information (eg, prior ABG or VBG or prior serum chemistry with an HCO_3) and are forced to assume the ongoing processes are all acute in nature. We are primarily concerned about chronic respiratory acid-base disorders, as this can significantly alter the patient's baseline or expected values for the serum HCO_3 and $Paco_2$, and we have reliable equations to predict the expected baseline values. The respiratory compensation for both chronic metabolic acidosis and alkalosis is generally poor, so there are no equations or rules to predict what the $Paco_2$ should be in these cases. While the baseline serum HCO_3 may be significantly off from our standard value of 24 mEq/L in these patients, we would assume a baseline $Paco_2$ of 40 mm Hg in patients with chronic metabolic processes. Once we identify the patient's baseline $Paco_2$ and HCO_3 values, we will need to use these values in the appropriate equations to identify the ongoing acute processes.

Q6-2: E

Metabolic acidosis and a respiratory acidosis.

Rationale:

1. The pH is 6.95; therefore, the primary disorder is an **acidosis.**
2. The $Paco_2$ of 79 mm Hg is less than 40 mm Hg, so there is a **respiratory acidosis.**
3. The HCO_3 of 17 mEq/L is less than 24 mEq/L, so there is a **metabolic acidosis.**

Therefore, there appears to be both a metabolic and respiratory acidosis.

Q6-3: C

Anion and non-anion gap acidosis.

Rationale:

1. Does the patient have an underlying chronic acid-base disorder (is there information provided to suggest the patient's baseline acid-base values)? No, there does not appear to be any underlying chronic acid-base disorder.
2. Expected anion gap:

$$\text{Expected Anion Gap} = 12 - (2.5) * \left[4.0\frac{g}{dL} - \text{Actual Serum Albumin} \right]$$

$$= 12 - (2.5 * [4.0 - 4.0])$$
$$= 12 - (2.5 * [0]) = \textbf{12 mEq/L.}$$

3. Anion gap calculation:

Serum Anion Gap = [Na⁺] − [HCO₂⁻] − [Cl⁻]

$$\text{Serum Anion Gap} = [Na^+] - [HCO_2^-] - [Cl^-]$$

133 − (89 + 17) = 27 mEq/L, which is > 12 mEq/L → **anion gap acidosis is present.**

4. Delta-delta calculation:

$$\Delta\Delta = \frac{(\text{Actual Anion Gap} - \text{Expected Anion Gap})}{(\text{Baseline HCO}_3 - \text{Actual HCO}_3)}$$

ΔΔ = (27 − 12)/(24 − 17) = **15/7, which is ~2.2.**

Delta-delta interpretation.	
Delta-Delta Value	Condition Present
< 0.4	Non-anion gap only
0.4–0.9	Anion gap *and* non-anion gap acidosis
1.0–2.0	Anion gap acidosis only
> 2.0	**Anion gap acidosis and metabolic alkalosis**

Q6-4: C
Opioid intoxication.

Rationale: See discussion that follows for Q6-5.

Q6-5: C
Ethylene glycol intoxication.

Rationale: The patient's respiratory acidosis is most likely due to opioid intoxication, as determined by the response to naloxone and the positive urine drug screen. There is no evidence of benzodiazepine use. While alcohol intoxication can cause respiratory suppression, the patient's current ethyl alcohol blood level is not significantly elevated. Aspirin and progesterone are more likely to cause a respiratory alkalosis than an acidosis. To determine the etiology of the anion gap acidosis, we need to consider a possible co-ingestion with another organic alcohol. The serum osmolal gap is calculated as the difference between the patient's measured serum osmolarity (or osmolality) and the calculated serum osmolality based on laboratory data. The calculated osmolality equation is as follows:

Calculated Serum Osmolality:

$$\text{Calculated Serum Osmolality} = 2 * [Na^+] + \frac{[\text{Glucose}]}{18} + \frac{[\text{BUN}]}{2.8} + \frac{[\text{EtOH}]}{3.7}$$

Therefore, for this patient,

Calculated Serum Osmolality = [2 * Na] + [Glucose/18] + [BUN/2.8] + [EtOH/3.7]
= (2 * 133) + (187/18) + (12/2.8) + (33/3.7)
= 290 mOsm/L.

Serum Osmolal Gap = Measured Serum Osmolality − Calculated Osmolality
= (333 − 290) = 43 mOsm/L, which is
> 10 mOsm/L → **serum osmolal gap is present.**

The presence of an elevated serum anion gap and an elevated serum osmolar gap helps to narrow the differential for this patient's underlying condition.

Conditions associated with or without an elevated serum osmolal gap.
With an Elevated Serum Anion Gap
1. Ethanol ingestion with alcoholic ketoacidosis (acetone is an unmeasured osmole, in addition to ethanol)—the osmolality is usually elevated more so by the increased ethanol concentration, so the osmolal "gap" depends on whether the term for ethanol is included in the osmolality calculation*
2. Organic alcohol ingestions (methanol, ethylene glycol, diethylene glycol, propylene glycol)
3. DKA—similar to ethanol ingestion, earlier, glucose and acetone contribute to the osmolality. Since the glucose terms is always included in the calculation
4. Salicylate toxicity
5. Renal failure—the BUN is nearly always included in the osmolality.
Without an Elevated Serum Anion Gap
1. Hyperosmolar therapy (mannitol, glycerol)
2. Other organic solvent ingestion (eg, acetone)
3. Isopropyl alcohol ingestion (produces only acetone rather than an organic acid, so no anion gap is seen).
4. Hypertriglyceridemia
5. Hyperproteinemia
A mildly elevated osmolal gap has been reported in the literature in patients with lactic acidosis in critical illness, particularly severe distributive shock. The pathology is not quite clear, although it likely is related to multiorgan failure—particularly involving the liver and kidneys—and the release of cellular components known to contribute to the osmolal gap. This is typically around 10 mOsm/L, although it may be as high as 20–25 mOsm/L.

In this patient, we would be primarily worried about the first etiology, particularly methanol or ethylene glycol ingestion. Ethylene glycol or methanol ingestion can cause an elevated serum osmolal gap and an elevated serum anion gap. Additionally, metabolites of both organic alcohol can interfere with the serum lactate assay and cause elevated levels. The patient's lactate is mildly elevated, but not to the point it would account for the anion gap present. While the patient has been drinking ethyl alcohol (EtOH), there are no ketones present to suggest a ketoacidosis. The patient does not appear to have renal failure.

Q6-6: A
Emesis.

Rationale: The patient has a metabolic alkalosis, with a urine chloride less than 10. This is consistent with chloride-responsive process such as hyperemesis or prior diuretic use. Given the clinical scenario of ethanol, ethylene glycol, and opioid use described in this case, hyperemesis seems the most likely cause. Recall that the urine osmolal gap is useful in non-anion gap metabolic acidosis, not metabolic alkalosis.

Causes of metabolic alkalosis.
History: Rule Out the Following as Causes:
• Alkali load ("milk-alkali" or calcium-alkali syndrome, oral sodium bicarbonate, IV sodium bicarbonate) • Genetic causes (CF) • Presence of hypercalcemia • IV β-lactam antibiotics • Laxative abuse (may also cause a metabolic acidosis depending on diarrheal HCO_3 losses)
If None of the Above, Then…
Urine Chloride < 20 mEq/L • Loss of gastric acid (hyperemesis, NGT suctioning) • Prior diuretic use (in hours to days following discontinuation) • Post-hypercapnia • Villous adenoma • Congenital chloridorrhea • Chronic laxative abuse (may also cause a metabolic acidosis depending on diarrheal HCO_3 losses) • CF **OR: Urine Chloride > 20 mEq/L**
Urine Chloride > 20 mEq/L, Lack of HTN, Urine Potassium < 30 mEq/L
• Hypokalemia or hypomagnesemia • Laxative abuse (if dominated by hypokalemia) • Bartter syndrome • Gitelman syndrome
Urine Chloride > 20 mEq/L, Lack of HTN, Urine Potassium > 30 mEq/L
• Current diuretic use
Urine Chloride > 20 mEq/L, Presence of HTN, Urine Potassium Variable but Usually > 30 mEq/L
Elevated plasma renin level: • Renal artery stenosis • Renin-secreting tumor • Renovascular disease
Low plasma renin, low plasma aldosterone: • Cushing syndrome • Exogenous mineralocorticoid use • Genetic disorder (11-hydoxylase or 17-hydrolyase deficiency, 11β-HSD deficiency) • Liddle syndrome • Licorice toxicity
Low plasma renin, high plasma aldosterone: • Primary hyperaldosteronism • Adrenal adenoma • Bilateral adrenal hyperplasia

References

Abreo K, Adlakha A, Kilpatrick S, et al. The milk-alkali syndrome. A reversible form of acute renal failure. Arch Intern Med. 1993;153:1005.

Barton CH, Vaziri ND, Ness RL, et al. Cimetidine in the management of metabolic alkalosis induced by nasogastric drainage. Arch Surg. 1979;114:70.

Bear R, Goldstein M, Phillipson E, et al. Effect of metabolic alkalosis on respiratory function in patients with chronic obstructive lung disease. Can Med Assoc J. 1977;117:900.

Carlisle EJ, Donnelly SM, Vasuvattakul S, et al. Glue-sniffing and distal renal tubular acidosis: sticking to the facts. J Am Soc Nephrol. 1991;1:1019.

Church AS, Witting MD. Laboratory testing in ethanol, methanol, ethylene glycol, and isopropanol toxicities. J Emerg Med. 1997;15:687.

Eder AF, Dowdy YG, Gardiner JA, et al. Serum lactate and lactate dehydrogenase in high concentrations interfere in enzymatic assay of ethylene glycol. Clin Chem. 1996;42:1489.

Galla JH, Gifford JD, Luke RG, Rome L. Adaptations to chloride-depletion alkalosis. Am J Physiol. 1991;261:R771.

Garella S, Chang BS, Kahn SI. Dilution acidosis and contraction alkalosis: review of a concept. Kidney Int. 1975;8:279.

Gennari FJ, Weise WJ. Acid-base disturbances in gastrointestinal disease. Clin J Am Soc Nephrol. 2008;3:1861.

Hamm LL, Nakhoul N, Hering-Smith KS. Acid-base homeostasis. Clin J Am Soc Nephrol. 2015;10:2232.

Hoffman RS, Smilkstein MJ, Howland MA, Goldfrank LR. Osmol gaps revisited: normal values and limitations. J Toxicol Clin Toxicol. 1993;31:81.

Höjer J. Severe metabolic acidosis in the alcoholic: differential diagnosis and management. Hum Exp Toxicol. 1996;15:482.

Hulter HN, Sebastian A, Toto RD, et al. Renal and systemic acid-base effects of the chronic administration of hypercalcemia-producing agents: calcitriol, PTH, and intravenous calcium. Kidney Int. 1982;21:445.

Khanna A, Kurtzman NA. Metabolic alkalosis. J Nephrol. 2006;19(suppl 9):S86.

Laski ME, Sabatini S. Metabolic alkalosis, bedside and bench. Semin Nephrol. 2006;26:404.

Liesivuori J, Savolainen H. Methanol and formic acid toxicity: biochemical mechanisms. Pharmacol Toxicol. 1991;69:157.

Luke RG, Galla JH. It is chloride depletion alkalosis, not contraction alkalosis. J Am Soc Nephrol. 2012;23:204.

Lynd LD, Richardson KJ, Purssell RA, et al. An evaluation of the osmole gap as a screening test for toxic alcohol poisoning. BMC Emerg Med. 2008;8:5.

Malandain H, Cano Y. Interferences of glycerol, propylene glycol, and other diols in the enzymatic assay of ethylene glycol. Eur J Clin Chem Clin Biochem 1996; 34:651.

Miller PD, Berns AS. Acute metabolic alkalosis perpetuating hypercarbia. A role for acetazolamide in chronic obstructive pulmonary disease. JAMA. 1977;238:2400.

Oster JR, Materson BJ, Rogers AI. Laxative abuse syndrome. Am J Gastroenterol. 1980;74:451.

Patel AM, Goldfarb S. Got calcium? Welcome to the calcium-alkali syndrome. J Am Soc Nephrol. 2010;21:1440.

Purssell RA, Pudek M, Brubacher J, Abu-Laban RB. Derivation and validation of a formula to calculate the contribution of ethanol to the osmolal gap. Ann Emerg Med. 2001;38:653.

Rose BD, Post TW. Clinical Physiology of Acid-Base and Electrolyte Disorders. 5e, New York, NY: McGraw Hill; 2001:559.

Schwartz WB, Van Ypersele de Strihou, Kassirer JP. Role of anions in metabolic alkalosis and potassium deficiency. N Engl J Med. 1968;279:630.

Shirey T, Sivilotti M. Reaction of lactate electrodes to glycolate. Crit Care Med. 1999;27:2305.

Sivilotti ML. Methanol intoxication. Ann Emerg Med. 2000;35:313.

Streicher HZ, Gabow PA, Moss AH, et al. Syndromes of toluene sniffing in adults. Ann Intern Med. 1981;94:758.

Sweetser LJ, Douglas JA, Riha RL, Bell SC. Clinical presentation of metabolic alkalosis in an adult patient with cystic fibrosis. Respirology. 2005;10:254.

Taher SM, Anderson RJ, McCartney R, et al. Renal tubular acidosis associated with toluene "sniffing". N Engl J Med. 1974;290:765.

Taki K, Mizuno K, Takahashi N, Wakusawa R. Disturbance of CO_2 elimination in the lungs by carbonic anhydrase inhibition. Jpn J Physiol. 1986;36:523.

Turban S, Beutler KT, Morris RG, et al. Long-term regulation of proximal tubule acid-base transporter abundance by angiotensin II. Kidney Int. 2006;70:660.

CASE 7

A female patient presents to urgent care with complaints of dizziness, nausea, emesis, confusion, and headaches that have been rapidly progressive over the past few days. She reports the onset of headaches about 3 months ago. At first they progressed slowly, but beginning this week they developed more rapidly and were associated with the reported symptoms. She is an otherwise healthy 33-year-old woman. She is having trouble providing any additional history. Vital signs are RR 23, HR 110, BP 80/40, and Sao_2 100% on RA. She is afebrile. She appears flush with excessive sweating and is complaining of joint pain and flank pain, although there is no apparent abnormality on examination. She reports a 10-lb weight loss over the past 2 weeks.

Laboratory data.			
ABGs		Basic Metabolic Panel	
pH	7.31	Na	124 mEq/L
$Paco_2$	34 mm Hg	K	6.1 mEq/L
Pao_2	109 mm Hg	Cl	89 mEq/L
HCO_3	17 mEq/L	CO_2	17 mEq/L
		BUN	12 mg/dL
		Cr	0.9 mg/dL
		Glucose	65 mg/dL
		Albumin	4.0 g/dL
		EtOH	0 mg/dL

QUESTIONS

Q7-1: **Define the patient's baseline acid-base status: Does this patient have an underlying chronic acid-base disorder that we need to account for in order to appropriately interpret the acute acid-base disorders?**

A. There is no evidence of an underlying chronic respiratory or metabolic acid-base disorder in this patient, so we would assume a baseline $Paco_2$ of 40 mm Hg and an HCO_3 of 24 mEq/L.

B. While the patient has a condition predisposing her to a chronic acid-base disorder, there is insufficient information to estimate the patient's baseline $Paco_2$ and HCO_3 values; therefore, we will assume a baseline $Paco_2$ of 40 mm Hg and a baseline HCO_3 of 24 mEq/L.

C. The patient has an underlying acid-base condition, and we have sufficient information to estimate the patient's baseline $Paco_2$ and HCO_3 values.

Q7-2: **What is/are the primary acid-base disturbance(s) occurring in this case?**

A. Metabolic acidosis only
B. Respiratory acidosis only
C. Metabolic alkalosis only
D. Respiratory alkalosis only
E. Metabolic acidosis and a respiratory acidosis
F. Metabolic alkalosis and a respiratory alkalosis

Q7-3: **Does the patient in this case demonstrate appropriate respiratory or metabolic compensation?**

A. Yes, the respiratory compensation is appropriate.
B. No, a concomitant respiratory alkalosis is present.
C. No, a concomitant respiratory acidosis is present.
D. Yes, the metabolic compensation is appropriate.
E. No, a concomitant metabolic acidosis is present.
F. No, a concomitant metabolic alkalosis is present.

Q7-4: **How would the metabolic acidosis component be classified in this case?**

A. Anion gap acidosis
B. Non-anion gap acidosis
C. Anion and non-anion gap acidosis
D. Anion gap acidosis and a metabolic alkalosis

Q7-5: **Your laboratory testing returns the following values:**

Serum EtOH	< 3 mg/dL
Serum acetaminophen level	< 5 mg/dL (ULN for therapeutic use 20 mg/dL)
Serum salicylates level	< 5 mg/dL (ULN for therapeutic use 30 mg/dL)
Serum osmolality	264 mOsm/kg
Serum L-lactate	4.3 mmol/L (ULN 2.0 mmol/L venous)
Beta-hydroxybutyrate (acetone)	< 0.18 mmol/L (ULN 0.18 mmol/L)
Serum glucose	65 mg/dL

Is there a serum osmolal gap?

A. No
B. Yes

Q7-6: You decide to further investigate the patient's metabolic acidosis. The patient's other studies are as follows:

Urine Na	45 mEq/L
Urine K	10 mEq/L
Urine Cl	22 mEq/L
Urine urea	145 mg/dL
Urine glucose	0 mg/dL
Urine osmolality	255 mOsm/L
Urine pH	5.0
Urine RBCs	None
Urine WBCs	None
Urine protein	None
Urine microscopic	None

What is the likely cause of the patient's anion gap acidosis?

A. Lactic acidosis
B. Diabetic ketoacidosis
C. Alcoholic ketoacidosis
D. Methanol ingestion
E. Toluene ingestion
F. Acetaminophen ingestion

Q7-7. What is the cause of the patient's non-anion gap acidosis?

A. Type 1 (distal) RTA
B. Type 2 (proximal) RTA
C. GI losses of HCO_3
D. Type 4 RTA

Q7-8: Additional laboratory studies show that the patient has mild anemia and mild peripheral eosinophilia. Blood cultures and a urine culture are pending. A procalcitonin test returns negative results. Which of the following would you order next to determine the underlying cause of the patient's presentation?

A. Serum parathyroid hormone level
B. Serum vitamin D (25-OH) level
C. Plasma renin and aldosterone levels
D. Serum cortisol stimulation test
E. Urine metanephrine study
F. 24-Hour urine collection for electrophoresis

Q7-9: What is the most important step in management of this patient?

A. Epinephrine infusion
B. Sodium bicarbonate infusion
C. Oral prednisone therapy
D. IV hydrocortisone therapy
E. IV levothyroxine therapy

ANSWERS

Q7-1: B

While the patient has a condition predisposing her to a chronic acid-base disorder, there is insufficient information to estimate the patient's baseline $Paco_2$ and HCO_3 values; therefore, we will assume a baseline $Paco_2$ of 40 mm Hg and a baseline HCO_3 of 24 mEq/L. The vignette suggests the patient's constellation of symptoms is subacute (ie, evolving over weeks), so there is a chance that whatever is ongoing is a chronic issue. However, there is no concrete evidence at this point. For the time being, we will assume this is an acute process.

Rationale: Ignoring these underlying chronic acid-base disorders can significantly alter the interpretation of a patient's acute acid-base status. This was demonstrated in the first case of the series. However, oftentimes, we do not have the necessary information (eg, prior ABG or VBG or prior serum chemistry with an HCO_3) and are forced to assume the ongoing processes are all acute in nature. We are primarily concerned about chronic respiratory acid-base disorders, as this can significantly alter the patient's baseline or expected values for the serum HCO_3 and $Paco_2$, and we have reliable equations to predict the expected baseline values. The respiratory compensation for both chronic metabolic acidosis and alkalosis is generally poor, so there are no equations or rules to predict what the $Paco_2$ should be in these cases. While the baseline serum HCO_3 may be significantly off from our standard value 24 mEq/L in these patients, we would assume a baseline $Paco_2$ of 40 mm Hg in patients with chronic metabolic processes. Once we identify the patient's baseline $Paco_2$ and HCO_3 values, we will need to use these values in the appropriate equations to identify the ongoing acute processes.

Q7-2: A

Metabolic acidosis only.

Rationale:

1. The pH is 7.31; therefore, the primary disorder is an **acidosis.**
2. The $Paco_2$ of 34 mm Hg is less than 40 mm Hg, so this is not the cause of acidosis.
3. The HCO_3 of 17 mEq/L is less than 24 mEq/L, so there is a **metabolic acidosis.**

Therefore, the patient has a primary metabolic acidosis.

Q7-3: A

Yes, the respiratory compensation is appropriate.

Rationale: While the patient's vignette suggests a subacute or chronic process, the primary process appears to be metabolic. However, we lack any useful information to make a reliable inference. Therefore, for primary metabolic acidosis, we assume an acute process. Using the Winter formula, we can calculate what the expected arterial $Paco_2$ should be for a given serum HCO_3 if the patient were completely compensated.

Respiratory Compensation for Acute Metabolic Acidosis (Winter Formula):

$$\text{Expected Paco}_2 = 1.5 * [\text{Actual HCO}_3] + 8 \pm (\text{in mm Hg}).$$

Therefore, for this patient,

$$\text{Expected Paco}_2 = 1.5 * (\text{Actual HCO}_3) + 8 \,(\pm 2)$$
$$= (1.5 * 17) + 8 = 25.5 + 8 = 33.5 \pm 2 = (31.5\text{-}35.5) \text{ mm Hg.}$$

As this patient's Paco$_2$ falls in this range, the patient has an appropriate compensatory response to the metabolic acidosis. Therefore, there does not appear to be a primary respiratory acidosis or alkalosis.

Q7-4: C
Anion and non-anion gap acidosis.

Rationale:

1. Is there evidence for a chronic acid-base disorder that requires adjustment of the patient's "normal" HCO$_3$? No, in this case, there is no evidence of a chronic respiratory process.
2. Expected anion gap:

$$\text{Expected Anion Gap} = 12 - (2.5) * \left[4.0\frac{\text{g}}{\text{dL}} - \text{Actual Serum Albumin} \right]$$

$$= 12 - (2.5 * [4.0 - 4.0])$$
$$= 12 - (2.5 * [0]) = \mathbf{12 \text{ mEq/L.}}$$

3. Anion gap calculation:

$\text{Serum Anion Gap} = [\text{Na}^+] - [\text{HCO}_3^-] - [\text{Cl}^-]$
$124 - (89 + 17) = 18 \text{ mEq/L}$, which is $> 12 \text{ mEq/L} \rightarrow$ **anion gap acidosis is present.**

4. Delta-delta calculation:

$$\Delta\Delta = \frac{(\text{Actual Anion Gap} - \text{Expected Anion Gap})}{(\text{Baseline HCO}_3 - \text{Actual HCO}_3)}$$

$$= (18 - 12)/(24 - 17) = \mathbf{6/7,} \text{ which is } \mathbf{\sim 0.85.}$$

Delta-Delta interpretation.	
Delta-Delta Value	Condition Present
< 0.4	Non-anion gap only
0.4–0.9	**Anion gap *and* non-anion gap acidosis**
1.0–2.0	Anion gap acidosis only
> 2.0	Anion gap acidosis and metabolic alkalosis

The delta-delta value is 0.85, which indicates this patient has a concomitant anion gap and non-anion gap metabolic acidosis.

Q7-5: A
No.

Rationale: Given the patient has an anion gap acidosis, we should consider whether the patient has a serum osmolal gap. The serum osmolal gap is calculated as the difference between the patient's measured serum osmolarity (or osmolality) and the calculated serum osmolality based on laboratory data. The calculated osmolality equation is as follows:

Calculated Serum Osmolality:

$$\text{Calculated Serum Osmolality} = 2*[Na^+] + \frac{[\text{Glucose}]}{18} + \frac{[\text{BUN}]}{2.8} + \frac{[\text{EtOH}]}{3.7}.$$

Therefore, for this patient,

$$\begin{aligned}
\text{Calculated Serum Osmolality} &= [2 * Na] + [\text{Glucose}/18] + [\text{BUN}/2.8] + [\text{EtOH}/3.7] \\
&= (2 * 124) + (65/18) + (12/2.8) + (0/3.7) \\
&= 256 \text{ mOsm/L.}
\end{aligned}$$

$$\begin{aligned}
\text{Serum Osmolar Gap} &= \text{Measured Serum Osmolality} - \text{Calculated Osmolality} \\
&= (264 - 256) = 8, \text{ which is} < 10 \text{ mOsm/L} \\
&\rightarrow \textbf{there is } \textit{no} \textbf{ serum osmolal gap.}
\end{aligned}$$

Therefore, there is no osmolal (osmolar) gap.

Q7-6: A
Lactic acidosis.

Rationale: See Q 7-7 below for discussion.

Q7-7: D
Type 4 RTA.

Rationale: For the etiology of the high anion gap acidosis, there is no evidence of acetaminophen ingestion, methanol ingestion, or a ketoacidosis. Therefore, the primary difference would be between toluene ingestion and lactic acidosis. Toluene ingestion is not associated with a lactic acidosis but can be associated with a mixed anion gap and non-anion gap acidosis. Since the patient presented with hypotension and an elevated lactate level, a lactic acidosis is the more likely answer. Additionally, as we will see further, the patient has a type 4 RTA, rather than a type 1 RTA usually associated with toluene toxicity.

Urine Anion Gap:

$$\text{Urine Anion Gap (UAG)} = [U_{Na}] + [U_K] - [U_{Cl}].$$

The patient's UAG is:

$$UAG = U_{Na} + U_K - U_{Cl}$$
$$= (45 + 10) - 22 = (+33) \text{ mEq/L.}$$

Interpretation:

- A UAG > ~20 → reduced renal acid excretion (RTA).
- A UAG of −20 → GI loss of bicarbonate (eg, diarrhea), although type 2 RTA is possible.
- A UAG between −20 and +10 is generally considered inconclusive.

Limitation:

- The UAG can be inappropriately elevated in anion gap acidosis, a situation in which multiple unmeasured anions may be present in the urine (beta-hydroxybutyrate/acetoacetate [ketoacidosis], hippurate [toluene], bicarbonate [proximal RTA], D-lactate [D-lactic acidosis], L-lactate, 5-oxoproline [acetaminophen toxicity]).
- Therefore, in patients with a significant anion gap, the urine osmolar gap (UOG) is typically more useful.

Calculated Urine Osmolality:

$$\text{Calculated Urine Osmolality} = 2 * [U_{Na} + U_K] + \frac{[U_{BUN}]}{2.8} + \frac{[U_{glucose}]}{18}.$$

For this patient, the UOG is:

Calculated Urine Osmolarity = $2 * ([U_{Na}] + [U_K]) + (U_{Urea} \text{ (mg/dL)}/2.8) + [U_{glucose} \text{ (mg/dL)}/18]$
Calculated Urine Osmolarity = $2 * [45 + 10] + [145/2.8] + [0/18] = 161 \text{ mOsm/L}$

$$UOG = \text{Measured Urine Osmolality} - \text{Calculated Serum Osmolality}$$
$$UOG = 255 - 161 \text{ mOsm/L} = 93 \text{ mOsm.}$$

Similar to the UAG, the UOG is used as a surrogate for the urine ammonium concentration. Therefore, a larger gap indicates increased urinary NH_4 excretion. In normal acid-base conditions, the UOG is between 10 and 100 mOsm/L. During a significant metabolic acidosis, patients with impaired renal tubular acidification (type 1 and type 4 RTA) are unable to excrete additional acid (NH_4), and therefore the osmolar gap does not change. Patients with an intact renal response to acidemia (ie, GI losses) should have a significant urine osmolar gap (~ > 300 to 400 mOsm/L) as a result of increased NH_4 excretion.

Interpretation (in Setting of a Metabolic Acidosis):

- UOG > 400 mOsm/L (or kg) → appropriate urinary acidification, consistent with a GI source and normal renal acidification.
- UOG < 100 to 150 mOsm/L (of kg) → inappropriately low urinary acidification, most consistent with a type 1 or 4 RTA.
- Again, this is not particularly useful for the diagnosis of a type 2 (proximal) RTA, where other serum or urine lab abnormalities are more helpful.

Limitations:

- The primary limitation is its use in conditions with a high osmolar gap, where non-ammonium solutes not included in the calculation may be present in the urine (particularly mannitol).
- The presence of these unmeasured solutes will increase the osmolal gap inappropriately.
- Also, the UOG should not be used in patients with a urinary tract infection caused by a urease-producing organism, as urea is metabolized to HCO_3 bicarbonate and ammonium in urine.

To determine the type of RTA, one can look at the urine pH, serum potassium, and for evidence of kidney stones.

RTA classifications.			
	Type I RTA	Type 2 RTA	Type 4 RTA
Severity of metabolic acidosis, [HCO$_3$]	Severe (< 10–12 mEq/L typically)	Intermediate (12–20 mEq/L)	Mild (15–20 mEq/L)
Associated urine abnormalities	Urinary phosphate, calcium increased; bone disease often present	Urine glucose, amino acids, phosphate, calcium may be elevated	
Urine pH	HIGH (> 5.5)	Low (acidic), until serum HCO$_3$ level exceeds resorptive ability of proximal tubule; then becomes alkalotic once reab-sorptive threshold is crossed	Low (acidic)
Serum K$^+$	Low to normal; should correct with oral HCO$_3$ therapy	Classically low, although may be nor-mal or even high with rare genetic defects; worsens with oral HCO$_3$ therapy	HIGH
Renal stones	Often	No	No
Renal tubular defect	Reduced NH$_4$ secretion in distal tubule	Reduced HCO$_3$ resorption in proximal tubule	Reduced H$^+$/K$^+$ exchange in distal and collecting tubules due to decreased aldosterone or aldosterone resistance
Urine anion gap	> 10	Negative	> 10
Urine osmolal gap	Reduced during acute acidosis		Reduced during acute acidosis

The patient's urine pH is low and she has hyperkalemia. This is most consistent with type 4 RTA.

Q7-8: D
Serum cortisol stimulation test.

Rationale: The next most appropriate study in this patient would be to examine the patient's ACTH-cortisol axis. This patient presents with symptoms concerning for acute adrenal crisis, with hypotension, hyponatremia, hyperkalemia, metabolic acidosis, and hypoglycemia, all associated with adrenal insufficiency. In a patient with known adrenal insufficiency, adrenal crisis can be brought on by any stressful situation, including infection or trauma, or medication noncompliance. Patients who have been on high-dose steroids (usually > 20 mg/d of prednisone-equivalents for several weeks) and are then abruptly withdrawn from these drugs are also at risk. Adrenal insufficiency may arise from either a direct issue with production of cortisol in the adrenal gland or from lack of stimulation of the adrenal gland from ACTH produced in the pituitary gland. This patient has been complaining of headaches and vision changes, and this is concerning for a mass causing damage to the pituitary gland. The cortisol stimulation test will help differentiate between primary (adrenal) and secondary (pituitary or ACTH-related) causes, and a brain MRI would be most useful to investigate this possibility. Immediate initiation of therapy for adrenal insufficiency (eg, IV corticosteroids) can be lifesaving. Additionally, studies should be performed to examine the patient's thyroid function as this may need to be supplemented as well.

Q7-9: D
IV hydrocortisone therapy.

Rationale: The most appropriate therapy for this patient with adrenal crisis would be to start IV hydrocortisone therapy, along with appropriate fluid resuscitation and electrolyte repletion. Oral therapy would be appropriate at this point. While it is appropriate to test for hypothyroidism, levothyroxine should not be initiated without confirming an elevated TSH. A sodium bicarbonate infusion is not appropriate, and an epinephrine infusion would not solve the underlying condition. If adrenal insufficiency testing has not been completed, a dexamethasone infusion would be appropriate as it does not interfere with testing; however, as it lacks mineralocorticoid efficacy, aggressive fluid and electrolyte resuscitation is essential when dexamethasone is used alone.

References

Arlt W. The approach to the adult with newly diagnosed adrenal insufficiency. J Clin Endocrinol Metab. 2009;94:1059.

Arlt W, Society for Endocrinology Clinical Committee. Society for Endocrinology Endocrine Emergency Guidance: Emergency management of acute adrenal insufficiency (adrenal crisis) in adult patients. Endocr Connect. 2016;5:G1.

Hahner S, Allolio B. Therapeutic management of adrenal insufficiency. Best Pract Res Clin Endocrinol Metab. 2009;23:167.

Iwasaku M, Shinzawa M, Tanaka S, et al. Clinical characteristics of adrenal crisis in adult population with and without predisposing chronic adrenal insufficiency: a retrospective cohort study. BMC Endocr Disord. 2017;17:58.

Loriaux DL, Fleseriu M. "Relative" adrenal insufficiency in critical illness. Curr Opin Endocrinol Diabetes Obes. 2009;15:632.

Ono Y, Ono S, Yasunaga H, et al. Clinical features and practice patterns of treatment for adrenal crisis: a nationwide cross-sectional study in Japan. Eur J Endocrinol. 2017;176:329.

Weant KA, Sasaki-Adams D, Dziedzic K, et al. Acute relative adrenal insufficiency after aneurysmal subarachnoid hemorrhage. Neurosurgery. 2008; 63:645; discussion 649.

CASE 8

A 76-year-old man is brought to the hospital with altered mental status and hypoxemia. His daughter reports that she had difficulty contacting him for several days. When she arrived at his home, he was very confused and appeared to be hyperventilating. She called EMS, and the patient was brought to the emergency department. The daughter states that her father told her he fell at home 4 days ago and strained his lower back, but did not want to ask his children for help. He had been taking OTC medications since then to help with the pain. His vital signs on arrival are T 37.5°C, RR 25, HR 110, BP 140/80, and Sao$_2$ 86% on RA, which improves to 92% on 2L NC. His examination is unremarkable except for delirium. The daughter states that her father had also reported having nausea, and there was some non-bloody, non-bilious emesis in the house.

Laboratory data.			
ABGs		Basic Metabolic Panel	
pH	7.67	Na	146 mEq/L
Paco$_2$	15 mm Hg	K	3.8 mEq/L
Pao$_2$	64 mm Hg	Cl	100 mEq/L
HCO$_3$	17 mEq/L	CO$_2$	17 mEq/L
		BUN	12 mg/dL
		Cr	0.9 mg/dL
		Glucose	89 mg/dL
		Albumin	4.0 g/dL
		EtOH	0 mg/dL

QUESTIONS

Q8-1: Define the patient's baseline acid-base status: Does this patient have an underlying chronic acid-base disorder that we need to account for in order to appropriately interpret the acute acid-base disorders?

A. There is no evidence of an underlying chronic respiratory or metabolic acid-base disorder in this patient, so we would assume a baseline $PaCO_2$ of 40 mm Hg and an HCO_3 of 24 mEq/L.

B. While the patient has a condition predisposing him to a chronic acid-base disorder, there is insufficient information to estimate the patient's baseline $PaCO_2$ and HCO_3 values; therefore, we will assume a baseline $PaCO_2$ of 40 mm Hg and a baseline HCO_3 of 24 mEq/L.

C. The patient has an underlying acid-base condition and we have sufficient information to estimate the patient's baseline $PaCO_2$ and HCO_3 values.

Q8-2: What is/are the primary acid-base disturbance(s) occurring in this case?

A. Metabolic acidosis only

B. Respiratory acidosis only

C. Metabolic alkalosis only

D. Respiratory alkalosis only

E. Metabolic acidosis and a respiratory acidosis

F. Metabolic alkalosis and a respiratory alkalosis

Q8-3: Is the reduction in the patient's serum HCO_3 a result of a primary metabolic acidosis or is it representative of an appropriate compensation for the patient's respiratory alkalosis?

A. It is a primary metabolic acidosis.

B. It is appropriate renal compensation for an acute respiratory alkalosis.

Q8-4: How would the metabolic acidosis component be classified in this case?

A. Anion gap acidosis

B. Non-anion gap acidosis

C. Anion and non-anion gap acidosis

D. Anion gap acidosis and a metabolic alkalosis

Q8-5: In patient with a primary anion gap metabolic acidosis *and* an overlying respiratory alkalosis, what is the most appropriate test to order next?

A. Serum drug screen (EtOH, ASA, salicylates)

B. Serum lactate

C. Serum beta-hydroxybutyrate

D. Serum osmolality

Q8-6: The patient's urine studies are as follows:

Urine Na	12 mEq/L
Urine K	6 mEq/L
Urine Cl	8 mEq/L
Urine urea	300 mg/dL
Urine glucose	0 mg/dL
Urine osmolality	567 mOsm/L
Urine pH	5.0
Urine RBCs	None
Urine WBCs	None
Urine protein	None
Urine microscopic	None

What is the likely cause of the patient's metabolic alkalosis?

A. Diarrhea
B. Hyperemesis
C. Current diuretic use
D. Laxative abuse

Q8-7: The patient's daughter reports that her father purchased several "powder packets" from a local gas station 2 days ago as "pain relievers" for his back issues. What other intoxication should you be concerned for?

A. Nicotine
B. Opioids
C. THC
D. Acetaminophen
E. Barbiturates

Q8-8: Aside from the previously mentioned acid-base abnormalities, which of the following is *not* a potential complication of aspirin toxicity?

A. Tinnitus.
B. Nausea/emesis.
C. Pulmonary edema.
D. Cardiac arrhythmia.
E. Thrombocytopenia.
F. Encephalopathy.
G. All of the above are potential complications of aspirin toxicity.

Q8-9: The patient is not in respiratory distress and therefore there is no need for intubation. His airway, breathing, and circulation have been examined and are stable. Due to the patient's altered mental status, he is not a candidate for activated charcoal at this point. Emergent dialysis is planned, but it will take some time to organize the appropriate staff. The Poison Control Center informs you that the next step in management is to alkalinize the urine to increase the excretion of salicylate and reduce CNS effects. How should this be accomplished?

A. Acetazolamide or another carbonic anhydrase inhibitor

B. IV sodium bicarbonate infusion

ANSWERS

Q8-1: A

There is no evidence of an underlying chronic respiratory or metabolic acid-base disorder in this patient, so we would assume a baseline $Paco_2$ of 40 mm Hg and an HCO_3 of 24 mEq/L. Based on the vignette, this process appears to be entirely acute in nature.

Rationale: Ignoring these underlying chronic acid-base disorders can significantly alter the interpretation of a patient's acute acid-base status. This was demonstrated in the first case of the series. However, often, we do not have the necessary information (eg, prior ABG or VBG or prior serum chemistry with an HCO_3) and are forced to assume the ongoing processes are all acute in nature. We are primarily concerned about chronic respiratory acid-base disorders, as these can significantly alter the patient's baseline or expected values for the serum HCO_3 and $Paco_2$, and we have reliable equations to predict the expected baseline values. The respiratory compensation for both chronic metabolic acidosis and alkalosis is generally poor, so there are no equations or rules to predict what the $Paco_2$ should be in these cases. While the baseline serum HCO_3 may be significantly off from our standard value of 24 mEq/L in these patients, we would assume a baseline $Paco_2$ of 40 mm Hg in patients with chronic metabolic processes. Once we identify the patient's baseline $Paco_2$ and HCO_3 values, we will need to use these values in the appropriate equations to identify the ongoing acute processes.

Q8-2: D

Respiratory alkalosis only.

Rationale:

1. The pH is 7.67; therefore, the primary disorder is an **alkalosis.**
2. The $Paco_2$ of 15 mm Hg is less than 40 mm Hg, so there is a **respiratory alkalosis.**
3. The HCO_3 of 17 mEq/L is less than 24 mEq/L, so this is not the primary cause of the alkalosis, but there appears to be a metabolic acidosis present.

Therefore, the primary acid-base disorder appears to be a respiratory alkalosis.

Q8-3: A

It is a primary metabolic acidosis.

Rationale: There are two factors that support that this is a primary process, and not simply a compensatory response by the kidney with an appropriate drop in the serum HCO_3. First, we can calculate what the expected serum HCO_3 would be if this were simply compensation for an acute respiratory alkalosis.

Metabolic Compensation for Acute Respiratory Alkalosis:

$$\text{Expected } HCO_3 = \text{Baseline } HCO_3 - (0.20) [\text{Actual } Paco_2 - \text{Baseline } Paco_2].$$

Metabolic Compensation for Chronic Respiratory Alkalosis:

Expected HCO_3 = Baseline HCO_3 − (0.40) [Actual $Paco_2$ − Baseline $Paco_2$].

For an acute respiratory alkalosis, the HCO_3 would be:

Expected HCO_3 = 24 + [0.20 * (Actual $Paco_2$ − Expected $Paco_2$)]

Expected HCO_3 = 24 + [0.20 * (15 − 40 mm Hg)] = 24 + (0.2) * (−25) ~ **19 mEq/L.**

Since the actual serum HCO_3 of 17 mEq/L is less than the expected 19 mEq/L, there is also a concomitant metabolic acidosis present. Second, there is an anion gap present (anion gap is 29). Compensation for a respiratory acidosis would yield a non-anion gap process rather than an anion gap process.

Q8-4: D
Anion gap acidosis and a metabolic alkalosis.

Rationale:

1. Is there evidence for a chronic acid-base disorder that requires adjustment of the patient's "normal" HCO_3? Here, given the vignette, we would assume this to be an acute disorder. Recall that it takes up to a week for appropriate renal compensation to a chronic respiratory process.

2. Expected anion gap: Since the patient's serum albumin is 4 g/dL, the expected anion gap is 12 mEq/L.

$$\text{Expected Anion Gap} = 12 - (2.5) * \left[4.0 \frac{g}{dL} - \text{Actual Serum Albumin} \right]$$

3. Anion gap calculation:

Serum Anion Gap = $[Na^+] - [HCO_3^-] - [Cl^-]$

146 − (100 + 17) = 29 mEq/L, which is > 12 mEq/L → **anion gap acidosis is present.**

4. Delta-delta calculation: The delta-delta calculation helps determine if there is more than one type of metabolic acidosis occurring in a patient. For example, if you dissolve one unit of metabolic acid (H^+A^-) into the blood, the acid dissociates to an H^+ and an unmeasured anion A^-. The H^+ decreases the serum HCO_3 by 1 point, while the unmeasured anion increases the anion gap by 1 point, yielding a delta-delta value of 1.0, a pure anion gap acidosis. Alternatively, when the fall in the serum HCO_3 is more than expected from the change in anion gap, this may be due to a non-anion gap acidosis. In this situation, the additional decrease in HCO_3 is due to further buffering of an acid that does not contribute to the anion gap (such as HCl from stomach acid, where the anion Cl^- is measured). Here, we will assume the patient's baseline HCO_3 is 24 mEq/L.

$$\Delta\Delta = \frac{(\text{Actual Anion Gap} - \text{Expected Anion Gap})}{(\text{Baseline } HCO_3 - \text{Actual } HCO_3)}$$

$$= (29 - 12)/(24 - 17) = \textbf{17/7, which is} = \textbf{~2.4.}$$

Delta-Delta interpretation.	
Delta-Delta Value	Condition Present
< 0.4	Non-anion gap only
0.4–1.0	Anion gap *and* non-anion gap acidosis
1.0–2.0	Anion gap acidosis only
> 2.0	**Anion gap acidosis and metabolic alkalosis**

As the patient's delta-delta value is 2.4, the patient has a concomitant anion gap acidosis and metabolic alkalosis.

Q8-5: A
Serum drug screen for ASA.

Rationale: All of the listed tests are appropriate for a patient with an anion gap metabolic acidosis. However, when patients present with a primary respiratory alkalosis that is otherwise unexplained, or a primary respiratory alkalosis with a concomitant metabolic acidosis, aspirin toxicity should always be considered in the differential diagnosis. Patients rarely present with a solitary anion gap metabolic acidosis, with the exception being children presenting early after ingestion.

Acute salicylate toxicity is associated with abnormalities in both cellular metabolism and the control of ventilator centers. Salicylate causes stimulation of the medulla centers responsible for controlling ventilation as well as chemoreceptors zones controlling nausea and emesis. Patients often present with hyperventilation, nausea, and emesis. Additionally, salicylates interfere with cellular metabolism pathways including oxidative phosphorylation and the citric acid cycle, leading to anaerobic metabolism and a resultant lactic acidosis. While we would expect the lactate level to be elevated in this setting, the patient's blood pressure is normal and distributive shock does not appear to be the leading cause for this patient's acid-base disorder. Therefore, checking the patient's serum salicylate level would more directly identify the underlying etiology.

The prompt indicated that the patient was taking OTC medications, and likely took an accidental overdose of aspirin.

Q8-6: B
Hyperemesis.

Rationale: The patient has a metabolic alkalosis and is relatively normotensive. He is likely dehydrated and has a recent history of emesis. The urine chloride is low, indicating that the metabolic alkalosis is likely a chloride-responsive process. Of the options listed, the most likely cause would be hyperemesis. Diarrhea is associated with a non-anion gap metabolic acidosis, while current diuretic use is generally associated with a chloride-resistant metabolic alkalosis. Laxative abuse generally causes a metabolic alkalosis as a result of hypokalemia, although significant abuse can also lead to severe diarrhea and a non-anion gap metabolic acidosis. The urine chloride is not usually diagnostic in laxative abuse (which usually occurs in combination with other body image or eating disorders, such as bulimia), and there is no indication from the prompt that this is the cause.

Causes of metabolic alkalosis.
History: Rule Out the Following as Causes
• Alkali load ("milk-alkali" or calcium-alkali syndrome, oral sodium bicarbonate, IV sodium bicarbonate);   • Genetic causes (CF)   • Presence of hypercalcemia   • IV β-lactam antibiotics   • Laxative abuse (may also cause a metabolic acidosis depending on diarrheal HCO_3 losses)
If None of the Above, Then. . .
Urine Chloride < 20 mEq/L   • Loss of gastric acid (hyperemesis, NGT suctioning)   • Prior diuretic use (in hours to days following discontinuation)   • Post-hypercapnia   • Villous adenoma   • Congenital chloridorrhea   • Chronic laxative abuse (may also cause a metabolic acidosis depending on diarrheal HCO_3 losses)   • CF   **OR: Urine Chloride > 20 mEq/L**
Urine Chloride > 20 mEq/L, Lack of HTN, Urine Potassium < 30 mEq/L
• Hypokalemia or hypomagnesemia   • Laxative abuse (if dominated by hypokalemia)   • Bartter syndrome   • Gitelman syndrome
Urine Chloride > 20 mEq/L, Lack of HTN, Urine Potassium > 30 mEq/L
• Current diuretic use
Urine Chloride > 20 mEq/L, Presence of HTN, Urine Potassium Variable but Usually > 30 mEq/L
Elevated plasma renin level: • Renal artery stenosis   • Renin-secreting tumor   • Renovascular disease
Low plasma renin, low plasma aldosterone: • Cushing syndrome   • Exogenous mineralocorticoid use   • Genetic disorder (11-hydoxylase or 17-hydrolyase deficiency, 11β-HSD deficiency)   • Liddle syndrome   • Licorice toxicity
Low plasma renin, high plasma aldosterone: • Primary hyperaldosteronism   • Adrenal adenoma   • Bilateral adrenal hyperplasia

Q8-7: D

Acetaminophen.

Rationale: A number of OTC anti-inflammatory medications are available in powder form, including Goody's Powder or BC Powder. These medications most commonly contain acetaminophen, aspirin, and caffeine. Therefore, it would also be prudent to test for acetaminophen toxicity in this patient, as untreated acetaminophen toxicity could lead to liver failure.

Q8-8: G
All of the above are potential complications of aspirin toxicity.

Rationale: Aspirin, or salicylate toxicity may be either acute or chronic. Common symptoms of aspirin toxicity include tinnitus, nausea, emesis, tachypnea, and abdominal pain, and occasionally fever. More severe complications may include pulmonary edema, hypoglycemia, hypokalemia, encephalopathy, seizures (secondary to cerebral edema and increased ICP), thrombocytopenia, cardiac arrhythmias, and cardiopulmonary arrest (most commonly due to severe hypoxemia in setting of pulmonary edema).

Q8-9: B
IV sodium bicarbonate infusion.

Rationale: While acetazolamide will in effect alkalinize the urine, this is accomplished through renal sodium bicarbonate wasting, which will further lower the patient's serum HCO_3 and worsen the metabolic acidosis overall. The lowering of the patient's pH will actually worsen the CNS effects of salicylate by driving salicylate across the blood-brain barrier. Providing exogenous sodium bicarbonate via an infusion will alkalinize the urine appropriately, and the rate should be adjusted to obtain a urine pH greater than 7.5. It is important to treat any hypokalemia present as this will result in appropriate alkalinization.

Intermittent hemodialysis is indicated for patients who have encephalopathy, pulmonary edema, cerebral edema, volume overload, or a general medication condition that prevents the use of large-volume sodium bicarbonate infusion; acute or chronic renal failure that will prevent salicylate excretion; severe acidemia (pH 7.20 or less); extremely high salicylate levels (typically greater than 70 to 80 mg/dL); and those whose conditions are deteriorating despite appropriate medical care.

References

Fertel BS, Nelson LS, Goldfarb DS. The underutilization of hemodialysis in patients with salicylate poisoning. Kidney Int. 2009;75:1349.

Greenberg MI, Hendrickson RG, Hofman M. Deleterious effects of endotracheal intubation in salicylate poisoning. Ann Emerg Med. 2003;41:583.

Hill JB. Salicylate intoxication. N Engl J Med. 1973;288:1110

Kent K, Ganetsky M, Cohen J, Bird S. Non-fatal ventricular dysrhythmias associated with severe salicylate toxicity. Clin Toxicol (Phila). 2008;46:297.

O'Malley GF. Emergency department management of the salicylate-poisoned patient. Emerg Med Clin North Am. 2007;25:333.

Prescott LF, Balali-Mood M, Critchley JA, et al. Diuresis or urinary alkalinisation for salicylate poisoning? Br Med J (Clin Res Ed). 1982;285:1383.

Proudfoot AT, Krenzelok EP, Vale JA. Position paper on urine alkalinization. J Toxicol Clin Toxicol. 2004;42:1.

Walters JS, Woodring JH, Stelling CB, Rosenbaum HD. Salicylate-induced pulmonary edema. Radiology. 1983;146:289.

Winters RW, White JS, Hughes MC, Ordway NK. Disturbances of acid-base equilibrium in salicylate intoxication. Pediatrics. 1959;23:260.

CASE 9

A 31-year-old man with myasthenia gravis presents to the pulmonary clinic for routine follow-up care. The patient has had intermittent flares requiring hospitalization and invasive ventilation in the past but has never required a tracheostomy. His ABGs (when healthy) demonstrate no chronic hypercarbia. Home medications include baclofen for intermittent muscle spasms as well as oxycodone for chronic pain. He has a history of aspiration pneumonia. He is being seen in clinic for follow-up for a recent pneumonia that required intubation. On triage, the nurse calls you to see the patient for abnormal vital signs, as follows: T 39.5°C, RR 22, HR 125, BP 85/55, and Sao_2 91% on RA. The physical examination is notable for a chronically ill–appearing young man in no distress with temporal wasting, contractures, and limited chest excursion with each breath. The patient is transferred to the emergency department next door for continued management. Laboratory results are as follows:

Laboratory data.			
ABGs		Basic Metabolic Panel	
pH	7.19	Na	130 mEq/L
$Paco_2$	32 mm Hg	K	2.9 mEq/L
Pao_2	64 mm Hg	Cl	100 mEq/L
HCO_3	12 mEq/L	HCO_3	12 mEq/L
		BUN	38 mg/dL
		Cr	1.7 mg/dL
		Lactate	4.5 mmol/L
		Albumin	4.0

QUESTIONS

Q9-1: Define the patient's baseline acid-base status: Does this patient have an underlying chronic acid-base disorder that we need to account for in order to appropriately interpret the acute acid-base disorders?

A. There is no evidence of an underlying chronic respiratory or metabolic acid-base disorder in this patient, so we would assume a baseline $Paco_2$ of 40 mm Hg and an HCO_3 of 24 mEq/L.

B. While the patient has a condition predisposing him to a chronic acid-base disorder, there is insufficient information to estimate the patient's baseline $Paco_2$ and HCO_3 values; therefore, we will assume a baseline $Paco_2$ of 40 mm Hg and a baseline HCO_3 of 24 mEq/L.

C. The patient has an underlying acid-base condition and we have sufficient information to estimate the patient's baseline $Paco_2$ and HCO_3 values.

Q9-2: What is/are the primary acid-base disturbance(s) occurring in this case?

A. Metabolic acidosis only
B. Respiratory acidosis only
C. Metabolic acidosis and a respiratory acidosis
D. Metabolic alkalosis and a respiratory alkalosis
E. Metabolic alkalosis
F. Respiratory alkalosis

Q9-3: How would the metabolic acidosis component be classified in this case?

A. Anion gap acidosis
B. Non-anion gap acidosis
C. Anion and non-anion gap acidosis
D. Anion gap acidosis and a metabolic alkalosis

Q9-4: Does the patient in this case demonstrate appropriate respiratory or metabolic compensation?

A. Yes, the respiratory compensation is appropriate.
B. No, a concomitant respiratory alkalosis is present.
C. No, a concomitant respiratory acidosis is present.
D. Yes, the metabolic compensation is appropriate.
E. No, a concomitant metabolic acidosis is present.
F. No, a concomitant metabolic alkalosis is present.

Q9-5: The patient's urine is negative for ketones and the serum drug screen is also negative. The patient's serum osmolal gap is 8. What is the likely cause of his anion gap acidosis?

A. Aspirin toxicity
B. Lactic acidosis
C. Opioid overdose
D. Acetaminophen overdose
E. Diabetic ketoacidosis
F. Alcoholic ketoacidosis

Q9-6: Additional laboratory results are obtained as follows: Urine anion gap, 10; urine osmolal gap, 80 mOsm/L; urine chloride, < 10 mEq/L; urine pH, 6.8; urine microscopic examination, negative. Which of the following medications would you suspect the patient received recently?

A. Amphotericin B
B. Prednisone
C. Acetazolamide
D. Atorvastatin
E. Spironolactone

Q9-7: The patient is diagnosed with aspiration pneumonia and severe sepsis in the setting of a flare of his myasthenia gravis. After several days, his condition stabilizes and his acid-base status returns to a new baseline. An ABG on transfer to the medicine service shows pH of 7.35, $Paco_2$ of 55, Pao_2 of 66, and HCO_3 30 mEq/L. After several days, the patient develops some volume overload and the decision is made to administer a diuretic. The patient receives the medication and several hours later is noted to be altered and somewhat hypotensive. An ABG now shows a new acidosis with a pH of 7.22, $Paco_2$ 55, Pao_2 79, and HCO_3 22. The patient's anion gap is 6. The urine anion gap is −6. Which of the following diuretics did the patient most likely receive?

A. Furosemide
B. Spironolactone
C. Acetazolamide
D. Amiloride

ANSWERS

Q9-1: A

There is no evidence of an underlying chronic respiratory or metabolic acid-base disorder in this patient, so we would assume a baseline $Paco_2$ of 40 mm Hg and an HCO_3 of 24 mEq/L. While this patient does have a predisposing condition for chronic respiratory acidosis (myasthenia gravis), the vignette states that the patient has no evidence of a chronic respiratory acidosis at baseline.

Rationale: Ignoring these underlying chronic acid-base disorders can significantly alter the interpretation of a patient's acute acid-base status. This was demonstrated in the first case of the series. However, often, we do not have the necessary information (eg, prior ABG or VBG or prior serum chemistry with an HCO_3) and are forced to assume the ongoing processes are all acute in nature. We are primarily concerned about chronic respiratory acid-base disorders, as these can significantly alter the patient's baseline or expected values for the serum HCO_3 and $Paco_2$, and we have reliable equations to predict the expected baseline values. The respiratory compensation for both chronic metabolic acidosis and alkalosis is generally poor, so there are no equations or rules to predict what the $Paco_2$ should be in these cases. While the baseline serum HCO_3 may be significantly off from our standard value of 24 mEq/L in these patients, we would assume a baseline $Paco_2$ of 40 mm Hg in patients with chronic metabolic processes. Once we identify the patient's baseline $Paco_2$ and HCO_3 values, we will need to use these values in the appropriate equations to identify the ongoing acute processes.

Q9-2: A

Metabolic acidosis only.

Rationale:

1. The pH is 7.25; therefore, the primary disorder is an **acidosis.**
2. The $Paco_2$ of 28 mm Hg is less than 40 mm Hg, so this is **not a primary respiratory acidosis.**
3. The HCO_3 of 12 mEq/L is less than 24 mEq/L, so there is a **metabolic acidosis.**

Therefore, the patient has an acute metabolic acidosis.

Q9-3: C

Anion and non-anion gap acidosis.

Rationale:

1. Is there evidence for a chronic respiratory acid-base disorder that requires adjustment of the patient's "normal" HCO_3? This is a case where we might be particularly concerned about a chronic respiratory acidosis, as the patient has a neuromuscular disorder. However, we have no evidence for a chronic respiratory acidosis at this point, and no information has been provided regarding an elevated serum

HCO_3 at baseline. Therefore, for the sake of the case, we would have to assume a normal baseline ($Paco_2$ 40 mm Hg, HCO_3 24 mEq/L).

2. Expected anion gap:

$$\text{Expected Anion Gap} = 12 - (2.5) * \left[4.0 \frac{g}{dL} - \text{Actual Serum Albumin} \right]$$

$$= 12 - (2.5 * [4.0 - 4.0])$$
$$= 12 - (2.5 * [0]) = \textbf{12 mEq/L.}$$

3. Anion gap calculation:

$$\text{Serum Anion Gap} = [Na^+] - [HCO_3^-] - [Cl^-]$$
$$= 130 - (110 + 12) = 18 \text{ mEq/L, which is} > 12 \text{ mEq/L}$$
$$\rightarrow \textbf{anion gap acidosis is present.}$$

4. Delta-delta calculation:

$$\Delta\Delta = \frac{(\text{Actual Anion Gap} - \text{Expected Anion Gap})}{(\text{Baseline HCO}_3 - \text{Actual HCO}_3)}$$

$$= (18 - 12)/(24 - 12) = \textbf{6/12, which is ~0.5.}$$

Delta-Delta Interpretation.	
Delta-Delta Value	Condition Present
< 0.4	Non-anion gap only
0.4–0.9	**Anion gap *and* non-anion gap acidosis**
1.0–2.0	Anion gap acidosis only
> 2.0	Anion gap acidosis and metabolic alkalosis

The delta-delta value is 0.5, therefore this patient has a concomitant anion gap and non-anion gap metabolic acidosis.

Q9-4: C
No, a concomitant respiratory acidosis is present.

Rationale: Using the Winter formula, one can calculate what the expected arterial $Paco_2$ should be for a given serum HCO_3 if the patient were completely compensated.

$$\text{Expected Paco}_2 = 1.5 * (\text{Actual HCO}_3) + 8 \,(\pm 2)$$
$$= (1.5 * 12) + 8 = 18 + 8 = 26 \pm 2 = (24 \text{ to } 28) \text{ mm Hg.}$$

This patient has a $Paco_2$ of 32 mm Hg, which is elevated compared with the expected value of 24 to 28 mm Hg. Therefore, the patient has a concomitant respiratory acidosis. This is likely due to the patient's underlying neuromuscular disorder, which can be associated with reduced pulmonary function/reserve. When these patients develop a metabolic acidosis, they may lack the reserve to compensate appropriately and are prone to developing respiratory muscle fatigue much faster than patients with intact neuromuscular function.

Q9-5: B
Lactic acidosis.

Rationale: The patient presented with symptoms prompting concern for infection, with hypotension, tachycardia, and fever. He has a history of aspiration pneumonia. He presents with an elevated serum lactate. His other laboratory findings suggest that the patient does not have a ketoacidosis, organic acid ingestion, acetaminophen toxicity, or salicylate toxicity. Opioid overdose is associated with a respiratory rather than a metabolic acidosis. Therefore, lactic acidosis is the most appropriate answer here.

Causes of anion gap metabolic acidosis.	
Common	Less Common
Lactic acidosis (including transient)	Cyanide poisoning
Renal failure ("uremia")	Carbon monoxide poisoning
Diabetic ketoacidosis	Aminoglycosides
Alcohol ketoacidosis	Phenformin use
Starvation ketoacidosis	D-Lactic acidosis
Salicylate poisoning (ASA)	Paraldehyde
Acetaminophen poisoning (paracetamol)	Iron
Organic alcohol poisoning (ethylene glycol, methanol, propylene glycol)	Isoniazid

Q9-6: A
Amphotericin B.

Rationale: The patient's laboratory studies point toward a type 1 (distal) RTA (high urine pH, indeterminant urine anion gap but a low urine osmolar gap, low serum K^+). Medications associated with a type 1 RTA include amphotericin B, lithium, toluene, and cisplatin. High-dose prednisone and spironolactone can both be associated with a type 4 RTA, while acetazolamide is associated with a type 2 RTA.

Causes of RTA.
Causes of Type 1 (Distal) RTA
Primary • Idiopathic or familial (may be recessive or dominant)
Secondary • Medications: Lithium, amphotericin, ifosfamide, NSAIDs • Rheumatologic disorders: Sjögren syndrome, SLE, RA • Hypercalciuria (idiopathic) or associated with vitamin D deficiency or hyperparathyroidism • Sarcoidosis • Obstructive uropathy • Wilson disease • Rejection of renal transplant allograft

(Continued)

Causes of RTA. (*continued*)
Causes of Type 2 (Proximal) RTA
Primary • Idiopathic • Familial (primarily recessive disorders) • Genetic: Fanconi syndrome, cystinosis, glycogen storage disease (type 1), Wilson disease, galactosemia
Secondary • Medications: Acetazolamide, topiramate, aminoglycoside antibiotics, ifosfamide, reverse transcriptase inhibitors (tenofovir) • Heavy metal poisoning: Lead, mercury, copper • Multiple myeloma or amyloidosis (secondary to light chain toxicity) • Sjögren syndrome • Vitamin D deficiency • Rejection of renal transplant allograft
Causes of Type 4 RTA (Hypoaldosteronism or Aldosterone Resistance)
Primary • Primary adrenal insufficiency • Inherited disorders associated with hypoaldosteronism • Pseudohypoaldosteronism (types 1 and 2)
Secondary • Causes of hyporeninemic hypoaldosteronism such as renal disease (diabetic nephropathy), NSAID use, calcineurin inhibitors, volume expansion/volume overload • Causes of distal tubule voltage defects such as sickle cell disease, obstructive uropathy, SLE • Severe illness/septic shock • Angiotensin II-associated medications: ACE inhibitors, ARBs, direct renin inhibitors • Potassium-sparing diuretics: Spironolactone, amiloride, triamterene • Antibiotics: Trimethoprim, pentamidine

Q9-7: C
Acetazolamide.

Rationale: Compared with the patient's prior ABG (which represents the patient's new baseline), the patient has a new normal anion gap acidosis. Notably, the patient's initial ABG after the resolution of his acute issues showed a chronic respiratory acidosis with appropriate renal compensation (HCO_3 30 mEq/L). However, his serum HCO_3 has dropped from 30 to 22 mEq/L quickly, and it appears he is not able to compensate from a respiratory standpoint for the new metabolic acidosis. The urine anion gap is not particularly helpful here as it is indeterminate. This scenario is most consistent with a type 2 RTA (proximal kidney), most likely caused by administration of acetazolamide. A carbonic anhydrase inhibitor, acetazolamide works at the proximal convoluted tubule in the kidney, preventing reabsorption of HCO_3 and stimulating a metabolic acidosis. The metabolic acidosis will stimulate the body to increase minute ventilation to compensate, largely through tachypnea. This patient with significant muscle weakness was unable to compensate and became significantly acidemic. He has a chronic respiratory acidemia with compensatory metabolic alkalosis, but once the acetazolamide was administered, the compensatory mechanism was lost.

References

Adamson R, Swenson ER. Acetazolamide use in severe chronic obstructive pulmonary disease. Pros and cons. Ann Am Thorac Soc. 2017;14:1086.

Batlle D, Grupp M, Gaviria M, Kurtzman NA. Distal renal tubular acidosis with intact capacity to lower urinary pH. Am J Med. 1982;72:751.

Batlle D, Haque SK. Genetic causes and mechanisms of distal renal tubular acidosis. Nephrol Dial Transplant. 2012;27:3691.

Batlle DC, Hizon M, Cohen E, et al. The use of the urinary anion gap in the diagnosis of hyperchloremic metabolic acidosis. N Engl J Med. 1988;318:594.

Batlle DC, von Riotte A, Schlueter W. Urinary sodium in the evaluation of hyperchloremic metabolic acidosis. N Engl J Med. 1987;316:140.

Buckalew VM Jr, McCurdy DK, Ludwig GD, et al. Incomplete renal tubular acidosis. Physiologic studies in three patients with a defect in lowering urine pH. Am J Med. 1968;45:32.

Karet FE. Mechanisms in hyperkalemic renal tubular acidosis. J Am Soc Nephrol. 2009;20:251.

Rodríguez Soriano J. Renal tubular acidosis: the clinical entity. J Am Soc Nephrol. 2002;13:2160.

CASE 10

A 77-year-old man with a history of obesity (BMI 33), hypertension, diabetes mellitus (non-insulin dependent), and hyperlipidemia presents to the emergency department with shortness of breath and nonproductive cough. The patient returned yesterday from an overseas trip with his wife. He noticed some mild left lower leg discomfort after arriving home, but thought nothing of it. He takes valsartan, amlodipine, glipizide, and atorvastatin. He denies any fevers, chills, sweats, chest pain (pleuritic or crushing in nature), weight loss, or abdominal pain. The patient's vital signs are T 99.1 F, RR 29, HR 122, BP 90/60, and Sao_2 92% on 6 L NC. He reports the sudden onset of shortness of breath this morning after taking a shower. There was no associated diaphoresis, but he has been feeling lightheaded for the past few hours. An ECG shows an S1-Q3-T3 pattern. His D-dimer is grossly elevated. A serum BNP is significantly elevated and the patient's CXR is clear. His cardiopulmonary examination is unremarkable. His left lower extremity has asymmetric edema with some mild tenderness to palpation in the left thigh and mild redness. A V/Q scan is performed and is very high probability.

Laboratory data.			
ABGs		Basic Metabolic Panel	
pH	7.45	Na	134 mEq/L
$Paco_2$	25 mm Hg	K	5.6 mEq/L
Pao_2	64 (6 L NC) mm Hg	Cl	100 mEq/L
HCO_3	17 mEq/L	CO_2	17 mEq/L
		BUN	40 mg/dL
		Cr	3.2 mg/dL
		Glucose	100 mg/dL
		Albumin	4.0 g/dL
		EtOH	0 mg/dL

QUESTIONS

Q10-1: Define the patient's baseline acid-base status: Does this patient have an underlying chronic acid-base disorder that we need to account for in order to appropriately interpret the acute acid-base disorders?

A. There is no evidence of an underlying chronic respiratory or metabolic acid-base disorder in this patient, so we would assume a baseline $Paco_2$ of 40 mm Hg and an HCO_3 of 24 mEq/L.

B. While the patient has a condition predisposing him to a chronic acid-base disorder, there is insufficient information to estimate the patient's baseline $Paco_2$ and HCO_3 values; therefore, we will assume a baseline $Paco_2$ of 40 mm Hg and a baseline HCO_3 of 24 mEq/L.

C. The patient has an underlying acid-base condition, and we have sufficient information to estimate the patient's baseline $Paco_2$ and HCO_3 values.

Q10-2: What is/are the primary acid-base disturbance(s) occurring in this case?

A. Metabolic acidosis only
B. Respiratory acidosis only
C. Metabolic alkalosis only
D. Respiratory alkalosis only
E. Metabolic acidosis and a respiratory acidosis
F. Metabolic alkalosis and a respiratory alkalosis

Q10-3: What is the likely cause of the patient's respiratory alkalosis?

A. Aspirin overdose
B. Pulmonary edema
C. Pulmonary embolism
D. Pulmonary effusion
E. Pericardial effusion
F. Opioid overdose

Q10-4: How would the reduction in the patient's serum HCO_3 be classified in this case?

A. Anion gap acidosis.
B. Non-anion gap acidosis.
C. Anion and non-anion gap acidosis.
D. Anion gap acidosis and a metabolic alkalosis.
E. There is no concomitant metabolic acidosis; the reduction in HCO_3 represents an appropriate metabolic compensation for the respiratory alkalosis present.

Q10-5: The patient's urine is negative for ketones and the serum drug screen is also negative. What factors may be contributing to the patient's anion gap acidosis?

A. Aspirin toxicity
B. Lactic acidosis secondary to sepsis
C. Acetaminophen overdose
D. Lactic acidosis secondary to heart failure
E. Diabetic ketoacidosis
F. Acute renal failure
G. A and C
H. B and F
I. D and F
J. E and F
K. B and C

Q10-6: The patient's urine anion gap is +22 mEq/L. A urine pH is 5.3. Which of the patient's medications is most likely to be associated with his non-anion gap acidosis?

A. Valsartan
B. Amlodipine
C. Glipizide
D. Atorvastatin

ANSWERS

Q10-1: A

There is no evidence of an underlying chronic respiratory or metabolic acid-base disorder in this patient, so we would assume a baseline $Paco_2$ of 40 mm Hg and an HCO_3 of 24 mEq/L.

Rationale: Ignoring these underlying chronic acid-base disorders can significantly alter the interpretation of a patient's acute acid-base status. This was demonstrated in the first case of the series. However, often, we do not have the necessary information (eg, prior ABG or VBG, or prior serum chemistry with an HCO_3) and are forced to assume the ongoing processes are all acute in nature. We are primarily concerned about chronic respiratory acid-base disorders, as these can significantly alter the patient's baseline or expected values for the serum HCO_3 and $Paco_2$, and we have reliable equations to predict the expected baseline values. The respiratory compensation for both chronic metabolic acidosis and alkalosis is generally poor, so there are no equations or rules to predict what the $Paco_2$ should be in these cases. While the baseline serum HCO_3 may be significantly off from our standard value of 24 mEq/L in these patients, we would assume a baseline $Paco_2$ of 40 mm Hg in patients with chronic metabolic processes. Once we identify the patient's baseline $Paco_2$ and HCO_3 values, we will need to use these values in the appropriate equations to identify the ongoing acute processes.

Q10-2: D

Respiratory alkalosis only.

Rationale:

1. The pH is 7.45; therefore, the primary disorder is an **alkalosis.**
2. The $Paco_2$ of 25 mm Hg is less than 40 mm Hg, so this is a **respiratory alkalosis.**
3. The HCO_3 of 17 mEq/L is less than 24 mEq/L, so there is **not a primary metabolic alkalosis.**

Therefore, the primary disorder is a respiratory alkalosis.

Q10-3: C

Pulmonary embolism.

Rationale: The patient presented with signs and symptoms that are most concerning for a massive or submassive pulmonary embolism with cor pulmonale. He has a clear chest radiograph, asymmetric swelling of the left lower extremity, a clear inciting event (prolonged plane ride), an S1-Q3-T3 right heart strain pattern on ECG, a positive D-dimer, and a positive V/Q scan. The elevated BNP is common in massive or submassive pulmonary embolism, indicative of evolving right-sided heart failure. Aspirin overdose can cause a respiratory alkalosis, but there is no clear indication for that at this point in the case. The CXR shows no evidence of pulmonary edema or a pleural effusion. While a pericardial effusion is possible and could be associated with pain and hypotension, again, a pulmonary embolism seems more likely. Opioid overdose is most commonly associated with a respiratory acidosis.

Pulmonary embolism can often result in a respiratory alkalosis. Gas exchange in pulmonary embolism is characterized by a shift to areas of high ventilation-to-perfusion ratio (increased V/Q), as the areas with embolism are receiving reduced or no blood flow but may still have some degree of ventilation. Overall, this yields some degree of increased physiologic dead space, the severity of which is dependent on the size or territory affected by the pulmonary emboli. Pulmonary blood flow through the unaffected portions of the lung increases proportionally to the severity of the embolism, requiring an overall increase in minute ventilation to match the ventilation in these areas. This increase is accomplished through multiple mechanisms that include local reductions in Pao_2 and increases in $Paco_2$, causing a reflex stimulation of irritant (pain) and juxtacapillary sensors in the lung parenchyma. This mechanism leads to hyperventilation and an increase in the total minute ventilation. In rare circumstances, a patient with a pulmonary embolism may experience respiratory acidosis. These circumstances include a patient who cannot increase minute ventilation sufficiently as a result of being intubated and being delivered a fixed minute ventilation, paralysis, or receiving ample narcotic pain medications. Some reports indicate that hypercapnia may occur in scenarios where the extent of clot burden leads to massive dead space ventilation, although this is rare.

Q10-4: C
Anion and non-anion gap acidosis.

Rationale:

1. Is there evidence for a chronic respiratory acid-base disorder that requires adjustment of the patient's "normal" HCO_3? No, in this patient there is no evidence of a chronic disorder and the respiratory alkalosis is likely acute in nature. We will therefore assume the patient's baseline $Paco_2$ and HCO_3 are 40 mm Hg and 24 mEq/L, respectively.
2. Does the reduction in the patient's HCO_3 represent an appropriate acute compensation to a respiratory alkalosis? Here, we use the following equation to determine if the patient's reduced bicarbonate is due to the respiratory alkalosis.
Metabolic Compensation for Acute Respiratory Acidosis:

$$\text{Expected } HCO_3 - \text{Baseline } HCO_3 + (0.10)\,[\text{Actual } Paco_2 - \text{Baseline } Paco_2].$$

For this patient, the expected HCO_3 would be:

$$\text{Expected } HCO_3 = 24 + (0.10) * [25 \text{ mm Hg} - 40 \text{ mm Hg}] = 24 - 1.5 = 22.5 \text{ mEq/L}.$$

Since the HCO_3 is lower (17 mEq/L) than the expected 22.5 mEq/L, we would diagnosis a concomitant metabolic acidosis as well.

3. Expected anion gap:

$$\text{Expected Anion Gap} = 12 - (2.5) * \left[4.0\,\frac{g}{dL} - \text{Actual Serum Albumin} \right]$$

$$= 12 - (2.5 * [4.0 - 4.0])$$
$$= 12 - (2.5 * [0]) = \mathbf{12.}$$

4. Anion gap calculation:

$$\text{Serum Anion Gap} = [Na^+] - [HCO_3^-] - [Cl^-]$$
$134 - (100 + 17) = 17$, which is $> 12 \rightarrow$ **anion gap acidosis is present.**

5. Delta-delta calculation:

$$\Delta\Delta = \frac{(\text{Actual Anion Gap} - \text{Expected Anion Gap})}{(\text{Baseline HCO}_3 - \text{Actual HCO}_3)}$$

$$= (17 - 12)/(24 - 17) = \mathbf{5/7, \ which \ is \sim 0.7,}$$
so there is a non-anion gap acidosis as well.

Delta-Delta interpretation.	
Delta-Delta Value	**Condition Present**
< 0.4	Non-anion gap only
0.4–0.9	**Anion gap *and* non-anion gap acidosis**
1.0–2.0	Anion gap acidosis only
> 2.0	Anion gap acidosis and metabolic alkalosis

The delta-delta value is 0.7, therefore this patient has a concomitant anion gap and non-anion gap metabolic acidosis.

Q10-5: I
Options D (lactic acidosis secondary to heart failure) and F (acute renal failure) are both likely contributing to the patient's high anion gap acidosis.

Rationale: The patient has an acute pulmonary embolus causing acute right-sided heart failure and poor forward flow, leading to a lactic acidosis from poor oxygen delivery to the tissues of the body. Additionally, this process has resulted in acute renal failure that can also be associated with the accumulation of organic acids usually cleared by the kidney.

Q10-6: A
Valsartan.

Rationale: The patient's urine anion gap is suggestive of a renal cause for the non-anion gap acidosis portion, and with a low urine pH and an elevated serum potassium, a type 4 RTA is most likely. Although the acute renal failure alone could account for the non-anion gap acidosis present, the patient does take an angiotensin receptor blocker, valsartan, that is associated with the development of a type 4 RTA. The remaining medications are generally not associated with a type 4 RTA. Other medications associated with the development of a type 4 RTA include ACE inhibitors (eg, lisinopril), ARBs, renin inhibitors (eg, aliskerin), aldosterone antagonists (eg, spironolactone, eplerenone), and ENaC inhibitors (eg, amiloride, cimetidine, pentamidine, trimethoprim).

Diagnosis of RTA.			
	Type 1 RTA	Type 2 RTA	Type 4 RTA
Severity of metabolic acidosis, [HCO_3]	Severe (< 10–12 mEq/L typically)	Intermediate (12–20 mEq/L)	Mild (15–20 mEq/L)
Associated urine abnormalities	Urinary phosphate, calcium are increased; bone disease often present	Urine glucose, amino acids, phosphate, calcium may be elevated	
Urine pH	HIGH (> 5.5)	Low (acidic), until serum HCO_3 level exceeds the resorptive ability of the proximal tubule; then becomes alkalotic once reabsorptive threshold is crossed	Low (acidic)
Serum K^+	Low to normal; should correct with oral HCO_3 therapy	Classically low, although may be normal or even high with rare genetic defects; worsens with oral HCO_3 therapy	HIGH
Renal stones	Often	No	No
Renal tubular defect	Reduced NH_4 secretion in distal tubule	Reduced HCO_3 resorption in proximal tubule	Reduced H^+/K^+ exchange in distal and collecting tubule due to decreased aldosterone or aldosterone resistance
Urine anion gap	> 10	Negative	> 10
Urine osmolal gap	Reduced during acute acidosis		Reduced during acute acidosis

Causes of RTA.
Causes of Type 1 (Distal) RTA
Primary   • Idiopathic or familial (may be recessive or dominant)
Secondary   • Medications: Lithium, amphotericin, ifosfamide, NSAIDs   • Rheumatologic disorders: Sjögren syndrome, SLE, RA   • Hypercalciuria (idiopathic) or associated with vitamin D deficiency or hyperparathyroidism   • Sarcoidosis   • Obstructive uropathy   • Wilson disease   • Rejection of renal transplant allograft

(Continued)

Causes of RTA. (*continued*)
Causes of Type 2 (Proximal) RTA
Primary • Idiopathic • Familial (primarily recessive disorders) • Genetic: Fanconi syndrome, cystinosis, glycogen storage disease (type 1), Wilson disease, galactosemia
Secondary • Medications: Acetazolamide, topiramate, aminoglycoside antibiotics, ifosfamide, reverse transcriptase inhibitors (tenofovir) • Heavy metal poisoning: Lead, mercury, copper • Multiple myeloma or amyloidosis (secondary to light chain toxicity) • Sjögren syndrome • Vitamin D deficiency • Rejection of renal transplant allograft
Causes of Type 4 RTA (Hypoaldosteronism or Aldosterone Resistance)
Primary • Primary adrenal insufficiency • Inherited disorders associated with hypoaldosteronism • Pseudohypoaldosteronism (types 1 and 2)
Secondary • Causes of hyporeninemic hypoaldosteronism such as renal disease (diabetic nephropathy), NSAID use, calcineurin inhibitors, volume expansion/volume overload • Causes of distal tubule voltage defects such as sickle cell disease, obstructive uropathy, SLE • Severe illness/septic shock • Angiotensin II-associated medications: ACE inhibitors, ARBs, direct renin inhibitors • Potassium-sparing diuretics: Spironolactone, amiloride, triamterene • Antibiotics: Trimethoprim, pentamidine

References

Batlle D, Grupp M, Gaviria M, Kurtzman NA. Distal renal tubular acidosis with intact capacity to lower urinary pH. Am J Med. 1982;72:751.

Batlle D, Haque SK. Genetic causes and mechanisms of distal renal tubular acidosis. Nephrol Dial Transplant. 2012;27:3691.

Batlle DC, Hizon M, Cohen E, et al. The use of the urinary anion gap in the diagnosis of hyperchloremic metabolic acidosis. N Engl J Med. 1988;318:594.

Batlle DC, von Riotte A, Schlueter W. Urinary sodium in the evaluation of hyperchloremic metabolic acidosis. N Engl J Med. 1987;316:140.

Buckalew VM Jr, McCurdy DK, Ludwig GD, et al. Incomplete renal tubular acidosis. Physiologic studies in three patients with a defect in lowering urine pH. Am J Med. 1968;45:32.

Karet FE. Mechanisms in hyperkalemic renal tubular acidosis. J Am Soc Nephrol. 2009;20:251.

Mélot C, Naeije R. Pulmonary vascular diseases. Compr Physiol. 2011,1:593.

Rodríguez Soriano J. Renal tubular acidosis: the clinical entity. J Am Soc Nephrol. 2002;13:2160.

Santolicandro A, Prediletto R, Fornai E, et al. Mechanisms of hypoxemia and hypocapnia in pulmonary embolism. Am J Respir Crit Care Med. 1995;152:336.

CASE 11

You are called for an ICU consult of a patient on the general medicine service. The patient is a 44-year-old man who is a marathon runner with no chronic medical issues except bipolar disorder, for which he takes lithium. He initially presented to his primary care physician for general malaise and weakness; his vital signs at that time were T 36.5°C RR 20, HR 97, BP 105/60, and Sao₂ 95% on RA. He was directly admitted to the general medicine service for an expedited cardiac evaluation because a murmur was heard on examination, and the patient was noted to have frequent PVCs when undergoing an in-office ECG. He was admitted to the hospital where he was noted to be somewhat tachypneic and mildly tachycardic. His vital signs were T 37.2°C, RR 22, HR 105, BP 97/55, and Sao₂ 97% on RA. A CXR was normal and a CT scan with contrast revealed no evidence of a pulmonary embolism. An ECG and rhythm strip demonstrated intermittent PACs and PVCs, with sinus tachycardia. He had recently been training for a marathon. His initial laboratory results are as follows:

Laboratory data.			
ABGs		**Basic Metabolic Panel**	
pH	7.31	Na	149 mEq/L
$Paco_2$	24 mm Hg	K	5.9 mEq/L
Pao_2	104 mm Hg	Cl	116 mEq/L
HCO_3	12 mEq/L	CO_2	12 mEq/L
		BUN	118 mg/dL
		Cr	3.8 mg/dL
		Glucose	70 mg/dL
		Albumin	4.0 g/dL
		EtOH	0 mg/dL

QUESTIONS

Q11-1: Define the patient's baseline acid-base status: Does this patient have an underlying chronic acid-base disorder that we need to account for in order to appropriately interpret the acute acid-base disorders?

A. There is no evidence of an underlying chronic respiratory or metabolic acid-base disorder in this patient, so we would assume a baseline $Paco_2$ of 40 mm Hg and an HCO_3 of 24 mEq/L.

B. While the patient has a condition predisposing him to a chronic acid-base disorder, there is insufficient information to estimate the patient's baseline $Paco_2$ and HCO_3 values; therefore, we will assume a baseline $Paco_2$ of 40 mm Hg and a baseline HCO_3 of 24 mEq/L.

C. The patient has an underlying acid-base condition and we have sufficient information to estimate the patient's baseline $Paco_2$ and HCO_3 values.

Q11-2: What is/are the primary acid-base disturbance(s) occurring in this case?

A. Metabolic acidosis only
B. Respiratory acidosis only
C. Metabolic alkalosis only
D. Respiratory alkalosis only
E. Metabolic acidosis and a respiratory acidosis
F. Metabolic alkalosis and a respiratory alkalosis

Q11-3: How would the metabolic acidosis component be classified in this case?

A. Anion gap acidosis
B. Non-anion gap acidosis
C. Anion and non-anion gap acidosis
D. Anion gap acidosis and a metabolic alkalosis

Q11-4: The patient's serum osmolality is 350 mOsm/L as measured by the lab. The resident on the general medicine team is concerned about possible ethylene glycol poisoning because the serum osmolality seems quite high, the patient has some confusion, and he is also oliguric. The resident suggests initiating treatment with a fomepizole infusion and intermittent hemodialysis. Should you follow this recommendation?

A. No
B. Yes

Q11-5: The laboratory analysis returns the following results:

Serum EtOH	< 3 mg/dL
Serum acetaminophen level	< 5 mg/dL (ULN for therapeutic use 20 mg/dL)
Serum salicylates level	< 5 mg/dL (ULN for therapeutic use 30 mg/dL)
Serum osmolality	350 mOsm/kg
Serum L-lactate	0.9 mmol/L (ULN 2.0 mmol/L venous)
Beta-hydroxybutyrate (acetone)	< 0.18 mmol/L (ULN 0.18 mmol/L)
Serum glucose	70 mg/dL
Serum creatinine kinase (CK)	1300 IU/L (ULN 198 IU/L

What is the most likely cause of the patient's anion gap acidosis?

A. Starvation ketoacidosis
B. Diabetic ketoacidosis
C. Alcohol ketoacidosis
D. Lactic acidosis
E. Renal failure

Q11-6: You decide to investigate the patient's non-anion gap acidosis. The urine studies return the following results:

Urine Na	33 mEq/L
Urine K	15 mEq/L
Urine Cl	13 mEq/L
Urine urea	123 mg/dL
Urine glucose	0 mg/dL
Urine osmolality	140 mOsm/L
Urine pH	6.5
Urine RBCs	Few present
Urine WBCs	None
Urine protein	Mild
Urine microscopic	None

What is the cause of the patient's non-anion gap acidosis?

A. Lithium toxicity
B. Acetazolamide toxicity
C. Laxative abuse
D. Hyperaldosteronism

Q11-7. Does the patient in this case demonstrate appropriate respiratory or metabolic compensation?

A. Yes, the respiratory compensation is appropriate.

B. No, a concomitant respiratory alkalosis is present.

C. No, a concomitant respiratory acidosis is present.

D. Yes, the metabolic compensation is appropriate.

E. No, a concomitant metabolic acidosis is present.

F. No, a concomitant metabolic alkalosis is present.

ANSWERS

Q11-1: A
There is no evidence of an underlying chronic respiratory or metabolic acid-base disorder in this patient, so we would assume a baseline $Paco_2$ of 40 mm Hg and an HCO_3 of 24 mEq/L.

Rationale: Ignoring these underlying chronic acid-base disorders can significantly alter the interpretation of a patient's acute acid-base status. This was demonstrated in the first case of the series. However, often, we do not have the necessary information (eg, prior ABG or VBG, or prior serum chemistry with an HCO_3) and are forced to assume the ongoing processes are all acute in nature. We are primarily concerned about chronic respiratory acid-base disorders, as these can significantly alter the patient's baseline or expected values for the serum HCO_3 and $Paco_2$, and we have reliable equations to predict the expected baseline values. The respiratory compensation for both chronic metabolic acidosis and alkalosis is generally poor, so there are no equations or rules to predict what the $Paco_2$ should be in these cases. While the baseline serum HCO_3 may be significantly off from our standard value of 24 mEq/L in these patients, we would assume a baseline $Paco_2$ of 40 mm Hg in patients with chronic metabolic processes. Once we identify the patient's baseline $Paco_2$ and HCO_3 values, we will need to use these values in the appropriate equations to identify the ongoing acute processes.

Q11-2: A
Metabolic acidosis only.

Rationale:

1. The pH is 7.31; therefore, the primary disorder is an **acidosis.**
2. The $Paco_2$ of 24 mm Hg is less than 40 mm Hg, so this is not the cause of **acidosis.**
3. The HCO_3 of 12 mEq/L is less than 24 mEq/L, so there is a **metabolic acidosis.**

Therefore, this patient has a primary metabolic acidosis.

Q11-3: C
Anion and non-anion gap acidosis

Rationale:

1. Is there evidence for a chronic respiratory acid-base disorder that requires adjustment of the patient's "normal" HCO_3? No, in this case, there is no evidence of a chronic respiratory acid-base disorder; therefore, the baseline serum HCO_3 is presumed to be 24 mEq/L.
2. Expected anion gap:

$$\text{Expected Anion Gap} = 12 - (2.5) * \left[4.0 \frac{g}{dL} - \text{Actual Serum Albumin} \right]$$

$$= 12 - (2.5 * [4.0 - 4.0])$$
$$= 12 - (2.5 * [0]) = \textbf{12 mEq/L.}$$

3. Anion gap calculation:

$$\text{Serum Anion Gap} = [Na^+] - [HCO_3^-] - [Cl^-]$$
$$149 - (116 + 12) = 21 \text{ mEq/L, which is} > 12 \text{ mEq/L}$$
$$\rightarrow \textbf{anion gap acidosis is present.}$$

4. Delta-delta calculation:

$$\Delta\Delta = \frac{(\text{Actual Anion Gap} - \text{Expected Anion Gap})}{(\text{Baseline HCO}_3 - \text{Actual HCO}_3)}$$

$(21 - 12)/(24 - 12) = \textbf{9/12, which is} \sim\textbf{0.75.}$

Delta-delta interpretation.	
Delta-Delta Value	Condition Present
< 0.4	Non-anion gap only
0.4–0.9	**Anion gap *and* non-anion gap acidosis**
1.0–2.0	Anion gap acidosis only
> 2.0	Anion gap acidosis and metabolic alkalosis

Therefore, this patient has both an anion gap as well as a non-anion gap metabolic acidosis.

Q11-4: A
No.

Rationale: While it is always important to consider ethylene glycol (or other organic alcohol ingestion) in the differential diagnosis of an anion gap acidosis, the patient has no overt risk factors (known suicidal ideation, alcohol abuse disorder, etc) to suggest this as the etiology. The only way to formally rule out this possibility is to send blood samples for analysis of ethylene glycol/methanol and their metabolites. However, this study is often sent to other facilities for analysis, which can take more than 24 hours to return results—far too long to allow for appropriate intervention.

The serum osmolal gap is the difference between the laboratory-measured ("true") serum osmolality and a "calculated" osmolality based on commonly measured compounds that are known to contribute to the serum osmolality. Therefore, similar to the serum anion gap, the serum osmolal gap represents the "unmeasured" compounds also contributing to the serum osmolality. The serum osmolal gap can be helpful in determining whether an organic alcohol ingestion has occurred recently. The following are potential causes of an elevated serum osmolality.

Conditions associated with elevated serum osmolality.
With an Elevated Serum Anion Gap
1. Ethanol ingestion with alcohol ketoacidosis (acetone is an unmeasured osmole, in addition to ethanol)—the osmolality is usually elevated more so by the increased ethanol concentration, so the osmolal "gap" depends on whether the term for ethanol is included in the osmolality calculation*
2. Organic alcohol ingestions (methanol, ethylene glycol, diethylene glycol, propylene glycol)
3. Diabetic ketoacidosis—similar to ethanol ingestion, earlier, glucose and acetone contribute to the osmolality, since the glucose term is always included in the calculation
4. Salicylate toxicity
5. Renal failure—the BUN is nearly always included in the osmolality
Without an Elevated Serum Anion Gap
1. Hyperosmolar therapy (mannitol, glycerol)
2. Other organic solvent ingestion (eg, acetone)
3. Isopropyl alcohol ingestion (produces only acetone rather than an organic acid, so no anion gap is seen)
4. Hypertriglyceridemia
5. Hyperproteinemia
*A mildly elevated osmolal gap has been reported in the literature in patients with lactic acidosis in critical illness, particularly severe distributive shock. The pathology is not quite clear, although it likely is related to multiorgan failure—particularly involving the liver and kidneys—and the release of cellular components known to contribute to the osmolal gap. This is typically around 10 mOsm/L, although it may be as high as 20–25 mOsm/L.

Similar to the serum anion gap, the serum osmolal gap is determined by the difference between the "calculated" serum osmolality and the true, measured serum osmolality. The equation for the serum osmolal gap typically includes factors for sodium, glucose, BUN, and ethanol, as these are readily measurable in most laboratories. Therefore, the serum osmolal gap will represent the osmolality of those "unmeasured" osmoles, including organic alcohols and acetone. The most common form is shown as follows:

$$\text{Calculated Serum Osmolality} = 2*[Na^+] + \frac{[Glucose]}{18} + \frac{[BUN]}{2.8} + \frac{[EtOH]}{3.7};$$

In which the units of measure are as follows: Na, mEq/L; glucose, mg/dL; BUN, mg/dL; and EtOH, mg/dL. The conversion factors are shown in the preceding equation as well. A normal serum osmolal gap is around −10 to +10 mOsm/L (or mOsm/kg).

Patients with ethylene glycol or methanol ingestion will have an elevated osmolal gap, an elevated anion gap, or both. The outcome is dependent on the time from ingestion, metabolism, and renal function. This is because both ethylene glycol and methanol increase the osmolality of blood, but they are not anions and do not contribute to the anion gap. As the alcohols are metabolized, they produce organic acids (which cause the more significant toxicities); these acids dissociate to H^+ and an organic anion, thus increasing the anion gap while reducing the osmolar gap. Therefore, initially after ingestion, the osmolal gap is very elevated while the anion gap may be normal. As the alcohols are metabolized, the osmolal gap will decrease while the anion gap will increase accordingly. The serum osmolal gap alone is not 100% sensitive for organic alcohol ingestion, as patients may have completely metabolized the alcohols and only have an anion gap. However, the important factor is that the treatment of toxic organic alcohol ingestions (eg, fomepizole or ethanol infusion, hemodialysis) is most useful in patients with an osmolal gap as it is focused on removing the alcohol prior to metabolism to the more harmful organic acids/anions. Studies have shown that the serum osmolal gap is about 90% sensitive for any toxic alcohol ingestion, but nearly 100% sensitive in identifying patients in whom advanced therapies and ICU-level care (ie, dialysis) are needed.

In this case, we can calculate the serum osmolality as follows:

Calculated Serum Osmolality = [2 * Na] + [Glucose/18] + [BUN/2.8] + [EtOH/3.7]
$$= (2 * 149) + (70/18) + (118/2.8) + (0/3.7)$$
$$= 344 \text{ mOsm/L.}$$

Serum Osmolar Gap = Measured Serum Osmolality – Calculated Osmolality
$$= (350 – 344) = 6, \text{ which is} < 10 \text{ mOsm/L}$$
→ **negative serum osmolar gap**.

Therefore, this patient does not have an elevated serum osmolal gap. The patient's actual serum osmolality is increased overall from a normal value (usually around 285 mOsm/kg), but this increase is accounted for by "measured" compounds, namely the elevated BUN. Hence, there is no elevation in the serum osmolal gap. Fomepizole is a compound that prevents the metabolism of methanol and ethylene glycol by the rate-limiting alcohol dehydrogenase (which eventually leads to the generation of the toxic metabolites formic acid and glycolic acid, respectively). This allows time for dialysis to remove the organic alcohols, and also allows time for the liver to process the toxic metabolites before they accumulate in tissues and cause permanent end-organ damage.

Q11-5: E
Renal failure.

Rationale: The patient presented with a metabolic acidosis, an elevated BUN, hyperkalemia, and elevated serum Cr. He was noted to be oliguric as well. We would assume, from the prompt, that this is an acute process. The patient is in acute renal failure without evidence of another cause for an elevated anion gap acidosis. He has an elevated serum CK and is an elite athlete, so rhabdomyolysis may be the primary etiology for the renal failure. Additionally, he received contrast during the admission process and this may have further contributed to the process.

Acute renal failure may present as an anion gap, a non-anion gap, or a mixed acidosis, depending on how the kidney is affected. Anion filtration and excretion occurs primarily at the glomerulus and in the proximal tubules, while urine acidification occurs primarily in distal tubules/collecting ducts. Uremia develops when the kidney is unable to process and excrete the end products of amino acid and protein metabolism.

Causes of anion gap metabolic acidosis.	
Common	Less Common
Lactic acidosis (including transient)	Cyanide poisoning
Renal failure ("uremia")	Carbon monoxide poisoning
Diabetic ketoacidosis	Aminoglycosides
Alcohol ketoacidosis	Phenformin use
Starvation ketoacidosis	D-Lactic acidosis
Salicylate poisoning (ASA)	Paraldehyde
Acetaminophen poisoning (paracetamol)	Iron
Organic alcohol poisoning (ethylene glycol, methanol, propylene glycol)	Isoniazid
Toluene poisoning ("glue-sniffing")	Inborn errors of metabolism

Q11-6: A
Lithium toxicity associated with a type 1 RTA (distal).

Rationale: The urine anion gap and the urine osmolal gap are both useful here.

Urine Anion Gap:

$$\text{Urine Anion Gap} = [U_{Na}] + [U_K] - [U_{Cl}].$$

Therefore, for this patient:

$$\text{Urine Anion Gap} = U_{Na} + U_K - U_{Cl} = (33 + 15) - 13 = (+35).$$

Interpretation:

- A urine anion gap that is greater than ~20 → reduced renal acid excretion (RTA).
- A urine anion gap that is −20 → GI loss of bicarbonate (eg, diarrhea), although type 2 RTA is possible.
- A urine anion gap between −20 and +10 is generally considered inconclusive.

An alternative approach is to consider the urine osmolar gap. This is particularly useful in patients with a high anion gap. Here the urine osmolar gap is:

Calculated Urine Osmolality:

$$\text{Urine Osmolality} = 2 * [U_{Na} + U_K] + \frac{[U_{BUN}]}{2.8} + \frac{[U_{glucose}]}{18}.$$

Therefore, for this patient:

Calculated Urine Osmolarity = $2 * [33 + 15] + [123/2.8] + [0/18] = 123$ mOsm/L;

And the urine osmolar gap is therefore:

$$\text{Urine Osmolar Gap (UOG)} = \text{Measured Urine Osmolality} \\ - \text{Calculated Serum Osmolality} \\ \text{UOG} = 140 - 123 \text{ Osm/L} = 17 \text{ mOsm/L}.$$

Similar to the urine anion gap, the urine osmolar gap is used as a surrogate for the urine ammonium concentration. Therefore, a larger gap indicates increased urinary NH_4 excretion. In normal acid-base conditions, the urine osmolar gap is between 10 and 100 mOsm/L. During a significant metabolic acidosis, patients with impaired renal tubular acidification (type 1 and type 4 RTA) are unable to excrete additional acid (NH_4), and therefore the osmolar gap does not change. Patients with an intact renal response to acidemia (ie, GI losses) should have a significant urine osmolar gap ($\sim$ >300 to 400 mOsm/L) as a result of increased NH_4 excretion. Therefore, this patient has a reduced ability to acidify the urine and has either a type 1 or a type 4 RTA. Recall that the urine anion gap and urine osmolar gap are not as useful in patients with a type 2 RTA (proximal). The diagnosis of a type 2 RTA is usually guided by additional information (eg, toxic drug exposure or specific metabolic disorder).

Diagnosis of RTA.			
	Type 1 RTA	**Type 2 RTA**	**Type 4 RTA**
Severity of metabolic acidosis, [HCO_3]	Severe (< 10–12 mEq/L typically)	Intermediate (12–20 mEq/L)	Mild acidosis (15–20 mEq/L)
Associated urine abnormalities	Urinary phosphate, calcium are increased; bone disease often present	Urine glucose, amino acids, phosphate, calcium may be elevated	
Urine pH	HIGH (> 5.5)	Low (acidic), until serum HCO_3 level exceeds the resorptive ability of the proximal tubule; then becomes alkalotic once reabsorptive threshold is crossed	Low (acidic)
Serum K^+	Low to normal; should correct with oral HCO_3 therapy	Classically low, although may be normal or even high with rare genetic defects; worsens with oral HCO_3 therapy	HIGH
Renal stones	Often	No	No
Renal tubular defect	Reduced NH_4 secretion in distal tubule	Reduced HCO_3 resorption in proximal tubule	Reduced H^+/K^+ exchange in distal and collecting tubule due to decreased aldosterone or aldosterone resistance
Urine anion gap	> 10	Negative	> 10
Urine osmolal gap	Reduced during acute acidosis		Reduced during acute acidosis

The patient's urine pH is 6.0 despite the acidosis. This is consistent with a type 1 RTA (distal), which affects the ability of the kidney to acidify the urine. Although patients often have a low to normal serum K^+ when a distal RTA is present in isolation, this patient also has acute renal failure, which is associated with hyperkalemia. If the distal RTA is chronic, kidney stones are often present.

In this patient, the acute renal failure may have led to lithium toxicity, manifested by hypernatremia and a distal RTA. Acetazolamide causes a type 2 (proximal RTA), whereas laxative abuse and hyperaldosteronism are associated with a metabolic alkalosis.

Causes of RTA.
Causes of Type 1 (Distal) RTA
Primary   • Idiopathic or familial (may be recessive or dominant)
Secondary   • Medications: Lithium, amphotericin, ifosfamide, NSAIDs   • Rheumatologic disorders: Sjögren syndrome, SLE, RA   • Hypercalciuria (idiopathic) or associated with vitamin D deficiency or hyperparathyroidism   • Sarcoidosis   • Obstructive uropathy   • Wilson disease   • Rejection of renal transplant allograft
Causes of Type 2 (Proximal) RTA
Primary   • Idiopathic   • Familial (primarily recessive disorders)   • Genetic: Fanconi syndrome, cystinosis, glycogen storage disease (type 1), Wilson disease, galactosemia
Secondary   • Medications: Acetazolamide, topiramate, aminoglycoside antibiotics, ifosfamide, reverse transcriptase inhibitors (tenofovir)   • Heavy metal poisoning: Lead, mercury, copper   • Multiple myeloma or amyloidosis (secondary to light chain toxicity)   • Sjögren syndrome   • Vitamin D deficiency   • Rejection of renal transplant allograft
Causes of Type 4 RTA (Hypoaldosteronism or Aldosterone Resistance)
Primary   • Primary adrenal insufficiency   • Inherited disorders associated with hypoaldosteronism   • Pseudohypoaldosteronism (types 1 and 2)
Secondary   • Causes of hyporeninemic hypoaldosteronism such as renal disease (diabetic nephropathy), NSAID use, calcineurin inhibitors, volume expansion/volume overload   • Causes of distal tubule voltage defects such as sickle cell disease, obstructive uropathy, SLE   • Severe illness/septic shock   • Angiotensin II-associated medications: ACE inhibitors, ARBs, direct renin inhibitors   • Potassium-sparing diuretics: Spironolactone, amiloride, triamterene   • Antibiotics: Trimethoprim, pentamidine

Q11-7: A
Yes, the respiratory compensation is appropriate.

Rationale: Using the Winter formula one can calculate what the expected arterial $Paco_2$ should be for a given serum HCO_3 if the patient were completely compensated.

Respiratory Compensation for Acute Metabolic Acidosis (Winter formula):

$$\text{Expected Paco}_2 = 1.5 * [\text{Actual HCO}_3] + 8 \pm 2 \text{ (in mm Hg)}.$$

Therefore, for this patient,

$$
\begin{aligned}
\text{Expected Paco}_2 &= 1.5 * (\text{Actual HCO}_3) + 8 \ (\pm 2) \\
&= (1.5 * 12) + 8 = 18 + 8 = 26 \pm 2 = (24 \text{ to } 28) \text{ mm Hg}.
\end{aligned}
$$

This patient has an appropriate compensatory response to the metabolic acidosis.

References

Krasowski MD, Wilcoxon RM, Miron J. A retrospective analysis of glycol and toxic alcohol inges-tion: utility of anion and osmolal gaps. BMC Clin Pathol. 2012;12:1.

Kraut JA, Kurtz I. Metabolic acidosis of CKD: diagnosis, clinical characteristics, and treatment. Am J Kidney Dis. 2005;45:978.

Kraut JA, Xing SX. Approach to the evaluation of a patient with an increased serum osmolal gap and high-anion-gap metabolic acidosis. Am J Kidney Dis. 2011;58:480.

Lynd LD. An evaluation of the osmole gap as a screening test for toxic alcohol poisoning. BMC Emerg Med. 2008;8:5.

Petejova N, Martinek A. Acute kidney injury due to rhabdomyolysis and renal replacement therapy: a critical review. Crit Care. 2014;18:224.

Sood MM, Richardson R. Lactate and the osmolar gap. CMAJ. 2007;177:489.

CASE 12

A 58-year-old man is admitted to the emergency department with nausea and vomiting. His medical history includes hypertension, for which he takes amlodipine, and prior sports hernia repair. He is found on CT scan of the abdomen to have a small bowel obstruction. An NGT that is placed and attached to continuous wall suction produces copious output. Over the next day, the patient becomes hypotensive. On examination, his abdomen is tense and diffusely tender to palpation. His T 37.9°C RR is 33, HR 120, BP 80/40, and Sao$_2$ 94% on RA. Laboratory results are as follows:

Laboratory data.			
ABGs		Basic Metabolic Panel	
pH	7.31	Na	139 mEq/L
Paco$_2$	37 mm Hg	K	2.3 mEq/L
Pao$_2$	98 mm Hg	Cl	95 mEq/L
HCO$_3$	18 mEq/L	CO$_2$	18 mEq/L
		BUN	44 mg/dL
		Cr	1.3 mg/dL
		Glucose	103 mg/dL
		Albumin	4.0 g/dL
		EtOH	0 mg/dL

QUESTIONS

Q12-1: Define the patient's baseline acid-base status: Does this patient have an underlying chronic acid-base disorder that we need to account for in order to appropriately interpret the acute acid-base disorders?

A. There is no evidence of an underlying chronic respiratory or metabolic acid-base disorder in this patient, so we would assume a baseline $Paco_2$ of 40 mm Hg and an HCO_3 of 24 mEq/L.

B. While the patient has a condition predisposing him to a chronic acid-base disorder, there is insufficient information to estimate the patient's baseline $Paco_2$ and HCO_3 values; therefore, we will assume a baseline $Paco_2$ of 40 mm Hg and a baseline HCO_3 of 24 mEq/L.

C. The patient has an underlying acid-base condition and we have sufficient information to estimate the patient's baseline $Paco_2$ and HCO_3 values.

Q12-2: What is/are the primary acid-base disturbance(s) occurring in this case?

A. Metabolic acidosis only
B. Respiratory acidosis only
C. Metabolic alkalosis only
D. Respiratory alkalosis only
E. Metabolic acidosis and a respiratory acidosis
F. Metabolic alkalosis and a respiratory alkalosis

Q12-3: How would the metabolic acidosis component be classified in this case?

A. Anion gap acidosis
B. Non-anion gap acidosis
C. Anion and non-anion gap acidosis
D. Anion gap acidosis and a metabolic alkalosis

Q12-4: The patient's measured serum osmolality is 306. Does the patient have a serum osmolal gap?

A. No
B. Yes

Q12-5: Does the patient in this case demonstrate appropriate respiratory or metabolic compensation?

A. Yes, the respiratory compensation is appropriate.
B. No, a concomitant respiratory alkalosis is present.
C. No, a concomitant respiratory acidosis is present.
D. Yes, the metabolic compensation is appropriate.
E. No, a concomitant metabolic acidosis is present.
F. No, a concomitant metabolic alkalosis is present.

Q12-6: Which of the following laboratory tests is most likely to reveal the source of the patient's anion gap metabolic acidosis?

A. Serum acetone
B. Serum drug screen
C. Urine anion gap
D. Urine chloride
E. Serum osmolality
F. Urine osmolality
G. Serum lactate

Q12-7: The urine electrolytes are as follows:

Urine Na	23	mEq/L
Urine K	10	mEq/L
Urine Cl	< 10	mEq/L
Urine urea	NA	mg/dL
Urine glucose	0	mg/dL
Urine osmolality	NA	mOsm/L
Urine pH	5.5	
Urine RBCs	None	
Urine WBCs	None	
Urine protein	None	
Urine microscopic	None	

What is most likely cause of the patient's metabolic alkalosis?

A. Bicarbonate infusion
B. Addison disease
C. Milk-alkali ingestion
D. Cystic fibrosis
E. Hyperemesis/NGT suctioning
F. Diarrhea
G. Bactrim use
H. Acetazolamide use
I. Aminoglycoside use
J. Ifosfamide chemotherapy

ANSWERS

Q12-1: A

There is no evidence of an underlying chronic respiratory or metabolic acid-base disorder in this patient, so we would assume a baseline $Paco_2$ of 40 mm Hg and an HCO_3 of 24 mEq/L.

Rationale: Ignoring these underlying chronic acid-base disorders can significantly alter the interpretation of a patient's acute acid-base status. This was demonstrated in the first case of the series. However, often, we do not have the necessary information (eg, prior ABG or VBG, or prior serum chemistry with an HCO_3) and are forced to assume the ongoing processes are all acute in nature. We are primarily concerned about chronic respiratory acid-base disorders, as these can significantly alter the patient's baseline or expected values for the serum HCO_3 and $Paco_2$, and we have reliable equations to predict the expected baseline values. The respiratory compensation for both chronic metabolic acidosis and alkalosis is generally poor, so there are no equations or rules to predict what the $Paco_2$ should be in these cases. While the baseline serum HCO_3 may be significantly off from our standard value of 24 mEq/L in these patients, we would assume a baseline $Paco_2$ of 40 mm Hg in patients with chronic metabolic processes. Once we identify the patient's baseline $Paco_2$ and HCO_3 values, we will need to use these values in the appropriate equations to identify the ongoing acute processes.

Q12-2: A

Metabolic acidosis only.

Rationale:

1. The pH is 7.31; therefore, the primary disorder is an acidosis.
2. The $Paco_2$ of 37 mm Hg is less than 40 mm Hg, so this is not the cause of acidosis.
3. The HCO_3 of 18 mEq/L is less than 24, so there is a **metabolic acidosis.**

Q12-3: D

Anion gap acidosis and a metabolic alkalosis.

Rationale:

1. Is there evidence of a chronic respiratory acid-base disorder that requires adjustment of the patient's "normal" HCO_3? No, in this vignette, there is no information or evidence of a chronic respiratory acid-base disorder; therefore we would assume the patient's baseline serum HCO_3 is 24 mEq/L.
2. Expected anion gap:

$$\text{Expected Anion Gap} = 12 - (2.5) * \left[4.0\,\frac{g}{dL} - \text{Actual Serum Albumin} \right]$$

$$= 12 - (2.5 * [4.0 - 4.0])$$
$$= 12 - (2.5 * [0]) = 12 \text{ mEq/L.}$$

3. Anion gap calculation:

$$\text{Serum Anion Gap} = [Na^+] - [HCO_3^-] - [Cl^-]$$
$$139 - (95 + 18) = 26 \text{ mEq/L, which is} > 12 \text{ mEq/L}$$

→ **anion gap acidosis is present.**

4. Delta-delta calculation:

$$\Delta\Delta = \frac{(\text{Actual Anion Gap} - \text{Expected Anion Gap})}{(\text{Baseline HCO}_3 - \text{Actual HCO}_3)}$$

$$= (26 - 12)/(24 - 19) = \textbf{14/5, which is} \sim\textbf{2.3.}$$

Delta-Delta interpretation.	
Delta-Delta Value	**Condition Present**
< 0.4	Non-anion gap only
0.4–0.9	Anion gap *and* non-anion gap acidosis
1.0–2.0	Anion gap acidosis only
> 2.0	**Anion gap acidosis and metabolic alkalosis**

Therefore, both an anion gap metabolic acidosis and a metabolic alkalosis are present.

Q12-4: A
No.

Rationale: Similar to the serum anion gap, the serum osmolal gap is determined by the difference between the "calculated" serum osmolality and the true measured serum osmolality. The equation for the serum osmolal gap typically includes factors for sodium, glucose, BUN, and ethanol, as these are readily measurable in most laboratories. Therefore, the serum osmolal gap will represent the osmolality of those "unmeasured" osmoles, including organic alcohols and acetone. The most common form is shown as follows:

$$\text{Calculated Serum Osmolality} = 2 * [Na^+] + \frac{[\text{Glucose}]}{18} + \frac{[\text{BUN}]}{2.8} + \frac{[\text{EtOH}]}{3.7};$$

In which the units of measure are as follows: Na, mEq/L; glucose, mg/dL; BUN, mg/dL; and EtOH, mg/dL. The conversion factors are shown in the preceding equation as well. A normal serum osmolal gap is around −10 to +10 mOsm/L (or mOsm/kg).

Therefore, for this patient,

$$\text{Calculated Serum Osmolality} = [2 * Na] + [\text{Glucose}/18] + [\text{BUN}/2.8] + [\text{EtOH}/3.7]$$
$$= (2 * 139) + (103/18) + (44/2.8) + (0/3.7)$$
$$= 299 \text{ mOsm/L.}$$

Serum Osmolal Gap = Measured Serum Osmolality – Calculated Osmolality
$$= (306 - 299) = 7, \text{ which is } < 10 \text{ mOsm/L}$$
→ *no* **serum osmolal gap is present.**

Therefore, this patient does not have a serum osmolal gap.

Q12-5: A
Yes, the respiratory compensation is appropriate.

Rationale: Using the Winter formula, one can calculate what the expected arterial $Paco_2$ should be for a given serum HCO_3 if the patient were completely compensated.

Respiratory Compensation for Acute Metabolic Acidosis (Winter formula):

$$\text{Expected } Paco_2 = 1.5 * [\text{Actual } HCO_3] + 8 \pm 2 \text{ (in mm Hg)}.$$

Therefore, for this patient,

$$\text{Expected } Paco_2 = 1.5 * (\text{Actual } HCO_3) + 8 (\pm 2)$$
$$= (1.5 * 18) + 8 = 27 + 8 = 35 \pm 2 = (33 \text{ to } 37) \text{ mm Hg}.$$

As the patient's $Paco_2$ falls within this range, he has an appropriate compensatory response to the metabolic acidosis.

Q12-6: G
Serum lactate.

Rationale: The patient is hypotensive with signs of an acute abdomen and a lactic acidosis is the most likely cause of the patient's anion acidosis. A serum acetone level is useful for identifying ketoacidosis, whereas a serum drug screen would be useful for acetaminophen, alcohol, and ASA toxicity. A urine anion gap is helpful in determining non-anion gap acidosis and the urine chloride alone is helpful in metabolic alkalosis. A serum osmolality is helpful if an organic acid is the probable cause of an anion gap metabolic acidosis. A urine osmolality can be helpful in differentiating certain types of RTAs.

Q12-7: E
Hyperemesis.

Rationale: According to the vignette, the patient had hyperemesis and then had an NGT inserted to remove gastric fluid. This suctioning essentially eliminates acid from the body along with fluid and results in a net metabolic alkalosis. The urine chloride is less than 10 mEq/L, indicating this is likely a chloride-responsive process. The differential diagnosis is shown as follows:

Differential diagnosis of metabolic alkalosis.
History: Rule Out the Following as Causes
• Alkali load ("milk-alkali" or calcium-alkali syndrome, oral sodium bicarbonate, IV sodium bicarbonate); • Genetic causes (CF) • Presence of hypercalcemia • IV β-lactam antibiotics • Laxative abuse (may also cause a metabolic acidosis depending on diarrheal HCO_3 losses)
If None of the Above, Then…
Chloride-Responsive
Urine Chloride < 20 mEq/L
• Loss of gastric acid (hyperemesis, NGT suctioning) • Prior diuretic use (in hours to days following discontinuation) • Post-hypercapnia • Villous adenoma • Congenital chloridorrhea • Chronic laxative abuse (may also cause a metabolic acidosis depending on diarrheal HCO_3 losses) • Cystic fibrosis
OR
Chloride-Resistant
Urine Chloride > 20 mEq/L, Lack of HTN, Urine Potassium < 30 mEq/L
• Hypokalemia or hypomagnesemia • Laxative abuse (if dominated by hypokalemia) • Bartter syndrome • Gitelman syndrome
Urine Chloride > 20 mEq/L, Lack of HTN, Urine Potassium > 30 mEq/L
• Current diuretic use
Urine Chloride > 20 mEq/L, Presence of HTN, Urine Potassium Variable but Usually > 30 mEq/L
Elevated plasma renin level: • Renal artery stenosis • Renin-secreting tumor • Renovascular disease
Low plasma renin, low plasma aldosterone: • Cushing syndrome • Exogenous mineralocorticoid use • Genetic disorder (11-hydoxylase or 17-hydrolyase deficiency, 11β-HSD deficiency) • Liddle syndrome • Licorice toxicity
Low plasma renin, high plasma aldosterone: • Primary hyperaldosteronism • Adrenal adenoma • Bilateral adrenal hyperplasia

Given the differential for chloride-responsive metabolic alkalosis, and the clinical vignette, the most likely etiology is loss of gastric acid via emesis and NGT suctioning.

References

Adrogué HJ, Madias NE. Secondary responses to altered acid-base status: the rules of engagement. J Am Soc Nephrol. 2010;21:920.

Berend K, de Vries AP, Gans RO. Physiological approach to assessment of acid-base disturbances. N Engl J Med. 2014;371:1434.

Feldman M, Soni N, Dickson B. Influence of hypoalbuminemia or hyperalbuminemia on the serum anion gap. J Lab Clin Med. 2005;146:317.

Gennari FJ, Weise WJ. Acid-base disturbances in gastrointestinal disease. Clin J Am Soc Nephrol. 2008;3:1861.

Kraut JA, Nagami GT. The serum anion gap in the evaluation of acid-base disorders: what are its limitations and can its effectiveness be improved? Clin J Am Soc Nephrol. 2013;8:2018.

Luke RG, Galla JH. It is chloride depletion alkalosis, not contraction alkalosis. J Am Soc Nephrol. 2012;23:204.

Rastegar A. Use of the deltaAG/deltaHCO$_3^-$ ratio in the diagnosis of mixed acid-base disorders. J Am Soc Nephrol. 2007;18:2429.

Rose BD, Post TW. Clinical Physiology of Acid-Base and Electrolyte Disorders, 5e. New York, NY: McGraw-Hill; 2001:583.

Schwartz WB, Van Ypersele de Strihou, Kassirer JP. Role of anions in metabolic alkalosis and potassium deficiency. N Engl J Med. 1968;279:630.

Turban S, Beutler KT, Morris RG, et al. Long-term regulation of proximal tubule acid-base transporter abundance by angiotensin II. Kidney Int. 2006;70:660.

CASE 13

A 56-year-old man with a history of gastroesophageal reflux disease, alcohol abuse, and gout, presents with bloody emesis and hypotension. He is in extremis on presentation with T of 36.6°C, RR 38, HR 144, Sao$_2$ 88% and BP 60/40. He was found lying on the floor of his apartment after the downstairs neighbor reported hearing a loud noise consistent with a possible fall. The patient is intubated emergently for airway protection and an NGT is inserted, resulting in rapid return of copious bright red blood. A central line is placed and he is started on vasopressors while volume resuscitation and blood transfusion are undertaken. A head CT is negative for an acute process and CT scans of the face, neck, chest, and abdomen are all negative for significant trauma or other obvious pathology. His laboratory studies are as follows:

Laboratory data.			
ABGs		Basic Metabolic Panel	
pH	7.29	Na	129 mEq/L
Paco$_2$	21 mm Hg	K	2.1 mEq/L
Pao$_2$	55 mm Hg	Cl	75 mEq/L
HCO$_3$	10 mEq/L	CO$_2$	10 mEq/L
		BUN	55 mg/dL
		Cr	0.9 mg/dL
		Glucose	133 mg/dL
		Albumin	2.8 g/dL
		EtOH	125 mg/dL

QUESTIONS

Q13-1: Define the patient's baseline acid-base status: Does this patient have an underlying chronic acid-base disorder that we need to account for in order to appropriately interpret the acute acid-base disorders?

A. There is no evidence of an underlying chronic respiratory or metabolic acid-base disorder in this patient, so we would assume a baseline $Paco_2$ of 40 mm Hg and an HCO_3 of 24 mEq/L.

B. While the patient has a condition predisposing him to a chronic acid-base disorder, there is insufficient information to estimate the patient's baseline $Paco_2$ and HCO_3 values; therefore, we will assume a baseline $Paco_2$ of 40 mm Hg and a baseline HCO_3 of 24 mEq/L.

C. The patient has an underlying acid-base condition and we have sufficient information to estimate the patient's baseline $Paco_2$ and HCO_3 values.

Q13-2: What is/are the primary acid-base disturbance(s) occurring in this case?

A. Metabolic acidosis only
B. Respiratory acidosis only
C. Metabolic alkalosis only
D. Respiratory alkalosis only
E. Metabolic acidosis and a respiratory acidosis
F. Metabolic alkalosis and a respiratory alkalosis

Q13-3: For a perfectly healthy patient, a normal anion gap is assumed to be 12 mEq/L. What should be considered a normal anion gap in this patient?

A. 12 mEq/L
B. 10 mEq/L
C. 9 mEq/L
D. 4 mEq/L

Q13-4: How would the metabolic acidosis component be classified in this case?

A. Anion gap acidosis
B. Non-anion gap acidosis
C. Anion and non-anion gap acidosis
D. Anion gap acidosis and a metabolic alkalosis

Q13-5: What is the patient's calculated serum osmolality?

A. 288 mOsm/L
B. 301 mOsm/L
C. 319 mOsm/L
D. 355 mOsm/L

Q13-6: The following laboratory findings are also reported for the patient:

Serum EtOH	125 mg/dL
Serum acetaminophen level	< 5 mg/dL (ULN for therapeutic use 20 mg/dL)
Serum salicylates level	< 5 mg/dL (ULN for therapeutic use 30 mg/dL)
Serum osmolality	323 mOsm/kg
Serum L-lactate	5.6 mmol/L (ULN 2.0 mmol/L venous)
Beta-hydroxybutyrate (BHB; acetone)	1.81 mmol/L (ULN 0.18 mmol/L)
Serum glucose	133 mg/dL
WBCs	4.1 ($\times$ 10^3/μL) – NOTE: 66% PMNs
Hemoglobin	5.8 g/dL (LLN 13.5 g/dL)
Platelets	101 ($\times$ 10^3/μL)
Lipase	Elevated

What is/are the likely cause(s) of the patient's anion gap acidosis?

A. Ethylene glycol ingestion
B. Distributive shock secondary to intra-abdominal sepsis
C. Distributive shock secondary to acute blood loss anemia
D. Diabetic ketoacidosis
E. Alcoholic ketoacidosis
F. A and B
G. B and D
H. B and E
I. A and C
J. C and D
K. C and E

Q13-7: The patient's urine chloride is 8 mEq/L. The urine anion gap is –10 mEq/L. What is the most likely cause of the patient's concomitant metabolic alkalosis?

A. Hyperemesis.
B. Ongoing thiazide diuretic use
C. Primary hyperaldosteronism
D. Liddle syndrome

Q13-8: Does the patient in this case demonstrate appropriate respiratory or metabolic compensation?

A. Yes, the respiratory compensation is appropriate.
B. No, a concomitant respiratory alkalosis is present.
C. No, a concomitant respiratory acidosis is present.
D. Yes, the metabolic compensation is appropriate.
E. No, a concomitant metabolic acidosis is present.
F. No, a concomitant metabolic alkalosis is present.

ANSWERS

Q13-1: A

There is no evidence of an underlying chronic respiratory or metabolic acid-base disorder in this patient, so we would assume a baseline $Paco_2$ of 40 mm Hg and an HCO_3 of 24 mEq/L. We would assume from the vignette that the acid-base issues are acute in this case.

Rationale: Ignoring these underlying chronic acid-base disorders can significantly alter the interpretation of a patient's acute acid-base status. This was demonstrated in the first case of the series. However, often, we do not have the necessary information (eg, prior ABG or VBG, or prior serum chemistry with an HCO_3) and are forced to assume the ongoing processes are all acute in nature. We are primarily concerned about chronic respiratory acid-base disorders, as these can significantly alter the patient's baseline or expected values for the serum HCO_3 and $Paco_2$, and we have reliable equations to predict the expected baseline values. The respiratory compensation for both chronic metabolic acidosis and alkalosis is generally poor, so there are no equations or rules to predict what the $Paco_2$ should be in these cases. While the baseline serum HCO_3 may be significantly off from our standard value of 24 mEq/L in these patients, we would assume a baseline $Paco_2$ of 40 mm Hg in patients with chronic metabolic processes. Once we identify the patient's baseline $Paco_2$ and HCO_3 values, we will need to use these values in the appropriate equations to identify the ongoing acute processes.

Q13-2: A

Metabolic acidosis only.

Rationale:

1. The pH is 7.29; therefore, the primary disorder is an **acidosis.**
2. The $Paco_2$ of 21 mm Hg is less than 40 mm Hg, so this is not the cause of acidosis.
3. The HCO_3 of 10 mEq/L is less than 24 mEq/L, so there is a **metabolic acidosis.**

Q13-3: C

9 mEq/L.

Rationale: The normal anion gap is 12 mEq/L. The term *anion gap* refers to those ions (negatively charged molecules) in the bloodstream that we do not routinely measure, including phosphates, sulfates, organic acids, and negatively charged plasma proteins. One of the most abundant negatively charged ions in the blood is serum albumin. A normal serum albumin is 4.0 g/dL. For patients with hypoalbuminemia (low serum albumin), the normal or expected anion gap is smaller:

$$\text{Expected Anion Gap} = 12 - (2.5) * \left[4.0\,\frac{g}{dL} - \text{Actual Serum Albumin} \right].$$

So for this patient,

Expected Anion Gap = 12 − [2.5 ∗ (4 mg/dL − 2.8 mg/dL)] = 12 − (2.5 ∗ 1.2) = 9 mEq/L.

This is an important concept as patients with hypoalbuminemia may "hide" an anion gap acidosis if this correction is not performed.

Q13-4: C
Anion and non-anion gap acidosis.

Rationale:

1. Is there evidence for a chronic respiratory acid-base disorder that requires adjustment of the patient's "normal" HCO_3? No, there is no information or evidence to suggest the patient has a chronic respiratory acid-base disorder, so we would anticipate a baseline serum HCO_3 of 24 mEq/L and a $Paco_2$ of 40 mm Hg.
2. Expected anion gap:

$$\text{Expected Anion Gap} = 12 - (2.5) * \left[4.0 \frac{g}{dL} - \text{Actual Serum Albumin} \right]$$
$$= 12 - (2.5 * [4.0 - 2.8])$$
$$= 12 - (2.5 * [1.2]) = \textbf{9 mEq/L.}$$

3. Anion gap calculation:

$$\text{Serum Anion Gap} = [Na^+] - [HCO_3^-] - [Cl^-]$$

129 − (75 + 10) = 44 mEq/L, which is > 12 mEq/L → **anion gap acidosis is present.**

4. Delta-delta calculation:

$$\Delta\Delta = \frac{(\text{Actual Anion Gap} - \text{Expected Anion Gap})}{(\text{Baseline HCO}_3 - \text{Actual HCO}_3)}$$
$$= (44 - 9)/(24 - 10) = \textbf{35/14, which is ~2.5.}$$

Delta-Delta interpretation.	
Delta-Delta Value	Condition Present
< 0.4	Non-anion gap only
0.4–0.9	Anion gap *and* non-anion gap acidosis
1.0–2.0	Anion gap acidosis only
> 2.0	**Anion gap acidosis and metabolic alkalosis**

The delta-delta value is 2.5, therefore this patient has a concomitant anion gap acidosis and a metabolic alkalosis.

Q13-5: C
319 mOsm/L.

Rationale: The calculated serum osmolality is determined as follows:

$$\text{Calculated Serum Osmolality} = 2*[Na^+] + \frac{[\text{Glucose}]}{18} + \frac{[\text{BUN}]}{2.8} + \frac{[\text{EtOH}]}{3.7}.$$

$$
\begin{aligned}
\text{Calculated Serum Osmolality} &= [2*Na] + [\text{Glucose}/18] + [\text{BUN}/2.8] + [\text{EtOH}/3.7] \\
&= (2*129) + (133/18) + (55/2.8) + (125/3.7) \\
&= 319 \text{ mOsm/L (or kg; 1 kg of water} = 1 \text{ L).}
\end{aligned}
$$

Q13-6: K
Options C and E are both likely correct.

Rationale: This patient presented with acute blood loss anemia, with an Hbg of 5.8 g/dL (no known history of anemia), and hypotension, raising concern for likely distributive shock secondary to acute blood loss anemia. Although sepsis is possible in this patient, from either an intra-abdominal process or aspiration, he does not have a left shift, elevated WBCs, or a fever, and there is no clear source for infection, given the imaging described in the case vignette. Additionally, while this patient does meet the former criteria for the systemic inflammatory response syndrome (SIRS), recall that the SIRS criteria are longer used to determine sepsis given their poor sensitivity and specificity. The patient's BUN is elevated, but his Cr indicates that the GFR is likely preserved (although the patient may in fact have some degree of acute kidney injury depending on the baseline Cr). In fact, an elevated BUN is associated with upper GI bleeding, as blood is a good source of urea, which is resorbed through the GI system. The positive BHB and acetone in a patient without hyperglycemia, a concomitant history of alcoholism, and a positive EtOH level, should point to an alcoholic ketoacidosis as opposed to a diabetic ketoacidosis. The elevated lactate is likely associated with both conditions as well. There is no serum osmolal gap (323 – 319 = 4 mOsm/L), so ethylene glycol poisoning is unlikely.

Q13-7: A
Hyperemesis.

Rationale: In this patient, the likely cause of the concomitant metabolic alkalosis is hyperemesis. The reduced urine chloride points to a chloride-responsive process, and he presents with a history of recent emesis. It is likely he developed alcoholic gastritis sometime in the recent past and with continued emesis has suffered an arterial bleed. The urine anion gap is not particularly useful in metabolic alkalosis. Low serum potassium is also common in chronic alcoholism, further supporting this diagnosis. The remaining causes are associated with an elevated urine chloride.

Q13-8: A
Yes, the respiratory compensation is appropriate.

Rationale: Using the Winter formula, one can calculate what the expected arterial $Paco_2$ should be for a given serum HCO_3 if the patient were completely compensated.

Respiratory Compensation for Acute Metabolic Acidosis (Winter formula):

$$\text{Expected } Paco_2 = 1.5 * [\text{Actual } HCO_3] + 8 \pm 2 \text{ (in mm Hg)}.$$

So, for this patient,

$$\text{Expected } Paco_2 = 1.5 * (\text{Actual } HCO_3) + 8 \ (\pm 2)$$
$$= (1.5 * 10) + 8 = 15 + 8 = 23 \pm 2 = (21 \text{ to } 25) \text{ mm Hg}.$$

The patient's $Paco_2$ falls within this range. Therefore, this patient has an appropriate compensatory response to the metabolic acidosis.

References

Cecconi M, Evans L, Levy M, Rhodes A. Sepsis and septic shock. Lancet. 2018;392:75.

Chandrasekara H, Fernando P, Danjuma M, Jayawarna C. Ketoacidosis is not always due to diabetes. BMJ Case Rep. 2014;2014. pii: bcr2013203263.

Gerrity RS, Pizon AF, King AM, et al. A patient with alcoholic ketoacidosis and profound lactemia. J Emerg Med. 2016;51:447.

Jenkins DW, Eckle RE, Craig JW. Alcoholic ketoacidosis. JAMA. 1971;217:177.

Levy LJ, Duga J, Girgis M, Gordon EE. Ketoacidosis associated with alcoholism in nondiabetic subjects. Ann Intern Med. 1973;78:213.

Noor NM, Basavaraju K, Sharpstone D. Alcoholic ketoacidosis: a case report and review of the literature. Oxf Med Case Rep. 2016;2016:31.

Palmer BF, Clegg DJ. Electrolyte disturbances in patients with chronic alcohol-use disorder. N Engl J Med. 2017;377:1368.

Reichard GA Jr, Owen OE, Haff AC, et al. Ketone-body production and oxidation in fasting obese humans. J Clin Invest. 1974;53:508.

Schelling JR, Howard RL, Winter SD, Linas SL. Increased osmolal gap in alcoholic ketoacidosis and lactic acidosis. Ann Intern Med. 1990;113:580.

Srygley FD, Gerardo CJ, Tran T, Fisher DA. Does this patient have a severe upper gastrointestinal bleed? JAMA. 2012;307:1072.

Toth HL, Greenbaum LA. Severe acidosis caused by starvation and stress. Am J Kidney Dis. 2003;42:E16.

Umpierrez GE, DiGirolamo M, Tuvlin JA, et al. Differences in metabolic and hormonal milieu in diabetic- and alcohol-induced ketoacidosis. J Crit Care. 2000;15:52.

CASE 14

A 24-year-old man with a history of type 1 diabetes mellitus, hyperlipidemia, and diabetic nephropathy (baseline Cr 1.5) presents with lethargy and abdominal tenderness. He is unable to provide a history. An abdominal plain film series shows no free air under the diaphragm. A CT scan of the abdomen is concerning for acute appendicitis. The patient's vital signs are T 39.1°C, RR 26, HR 133, BP 90/70, and Sao_2 99% on 2 L NC. He has copious urine output. The laboratory studies are as follows:

Laboratory data.			
ABGs		Basic Metabolic Panel	
pH	6.99	Na	124 mEq/L
$Paco_2$	21 mm Hg	K	5.9 mEq/L
Pao_2	213 mm Hg	Cl	85 mEq/L
HCO_3	5 mEq/L	CO_2	5 mEq/L
		BUN	60 mg/dL
		Cr	1.8 mg/dL
		Glucose	560 mg/dL
		Albumin	4.8 g/dL
		EtOH	45 mg/dL

QUESTIONS

Q14-1: Define the patient's baseline acid-base status: Does this patient have an underlying chronic acid-base disorder that we need to account for in order to appropriately interpret the acute acid-base disorders?

A. There is no evidence of an underlying chronic respiratory or metabolic acid-base disorder in this patient, so we would assume a baseline $Paco_2$ of 40 mm Hg and an HCO_3 of 24 mEq/L.

B. While the patient has a condition predisposing him to a chronic acid-base disorder, there is insufficient information to estimate the patient's baseline $Paco_2$ and HCO_3 values; therefore, we will assume a baseline $Paco_2$ of 40 mm Hg and a baseline HCO_3 of 24 mEq/L.

C. The patient has an underlying acid-base condition and we have sufficient information to estimate the patient's baseline $Paco_2$ and HCO_3 values.

Q14-2: What is/are the primary acid-base disturbance(s) occurring in this case?

A. Metabolic acidosis only
B. Respiratory acidosis only
C. Metabolic alkalosis only
D. Respiratory alkalosis only
E. Metabolic acidosis and a respiratory acidosis
F. Metabolic alkalosis and a respiratory alkalosis

Q14-3: For a perfectly healthy patient, a normal anion gap is assumed to be 12 mEq/L. What should be considered a normal anion gap in this patient?

A. 12 mEq/L
B. 14 mEq/L
C. 7 mEq/L
D. 4 mEq/L

Q14-4: How would the metabolic acidosis component be classified in this case?

A. Anion gap acidosis
B. Non-anion gap acidosis
C. Anion and non-anion gap acidosis
D. Anion gap acidosis and a metabolic alkalosis

Q14-5: Your laboratory testing returns the following values:

Serum EtOH	45 mg/dL
Serum acetaminophen level	< 5 mg/dL (ULN for therapeutic use 20 mg/dL)
Serum salicylates level	< 5 mg/dL (ULN for therapeutic use 30 mg/dL)
Serum osmolality	320 mOsm/kg
Serum L-lactate	2.3 mmol/L (ULN 2.0 mmol/L venous)
Beta-hydroxybutyrate (acetone)	1.18 mmol/L (ULN 0.18 mmol/L)
Serum glucose	560 mg/dL

What is the serum osmolal gap?

A. −7
B. 7
C. 14
D. 44

Q14-6: Does the patient in this case demonstrate appropriate respiratory or metabolic compensation?

A. Yes, the respiratory compensation is appropriate.
B. No, a concomitant respiratory alkalosis is present.
C. No, a concomitant respiratory acidosis is present.
D. Yes, the metabolic compensation is appropriate.
E. No, a concomitant metabolic acidosis is present.
F. No, a concomitant metabolic alkalosis is present.

Q14-7: What is the likely primary cause of the patient's metabolic acidosis?

A. Distributive shock with lactic acidosis
B. Diabetic ketoacidosis
C. Renal failure
D. Neurogenic shock
E. Methanol ingestion

Q14-8: The patient is managed appropriately in the ICU, and his follow-up laboratory studies are as follows:

Laboratory data.					
ABGs			Basic Metabolic Panel		
pH	7.35		Na	135 mEq/L	
Paco$_2$	24 mm Hg		K	3.8 mEq/L	
Pao$_2$	100 mm Hg		Cl	111 mEq/L	
HCO$_3$	13 mEq/L		CO$_2$	13 mEq/L	
			BUN	60 mg/dL	
			Cr	1.8 mg/dL	
			Glucose	230 mg/dL	
			Albumin	3.6 g/dL	
			EtOH	0 mg/dL	

What is the primary acid-base disorder present now?

A. Respiratory acidosis
B. Anion gap metabolic acidosis
C. Non-anion gap metabolic acidosis
D. Anion and non-anion gap metabolic acidosis
E. Metabolic alkalosis

Q14-9: What is the likely cause of the patient's non-anion gap metabolic acidosis?

A. Volume resuscitation with normal saline
B. Diuretic use
C. Antibiotic administration
D. Intra-abdominal sepsis and associated shock
E. NGT suctioning

ANSWERS

Q14-1: B

While the patient has a condition predisposing him to a chronic acid-base disorder, there is insufficient information to estimate the patient's baseline $Paco_2$ and HCO_3 values; therefore, we will assume a baseline $Paco_2$ of 40 mm Hg and a baseline HCO_3 of 24 mEq/L. The patient's diagnosis of diabetic nephropathy is a risk factor for a chronic metabolic acidosis; however, we have insufficient evidence from the vignette to make a reasonable assumption regarding this fact.

Rationale: Ignoring these underlying chronic acid-base disorders can significantly alter the interpretation of a patient's acute acid-base status. This was demonstrated in the first case of the series. However, often, we do not have the necessary information (eg, prior ABG or VBG, or prior serum chemistry with an HCO_3) and are forced to assume the ongoing processes are all acute in nature. We are primarily concerned about chronic respiratory acid-base disorders, as these can significantly alter the patient's baseline or expected values for the serum HCO_3 and $Paco_2$, and we have reliable equations to predict the expected baseline values. The respiratory compensation for both chronic metabolic acidosis and alkalosis is generally poor, so there are no equations or rules to predict what the $Paco_2$ should be in these cases. While the baseline serum HCO_3 may be significantly off from our standard value of 24 mEq/L in these patients, we would assume a baseline $Paco_2$ of 40 mm Hg in patients with chronic metabolic processes. Once we identify the patient's baseline $Paco_2$ and HCO_3 values, we will need to use these values in the appropriate equations to identify the ongoing acute processes.

Q14-2: A

Metabolic acidosis only.

Rationale:

1. The pH is 6.99, therefore the primary disorder is an **acidosis.**
2. The $Paco_2$ of 21 mm Hg is less than 40 mm Hg, so this is not the cause of acidosis.
3. The HCO_3 of 5 mEq/L is less than 24 mEq/L, so there is a **metabolic acidosis**.

Q14-3: B

14 mEq/L.

Rationale: The normal anion gap is 12 mEq/L. The term *anion gap* refers to those ions (negatively charged molecules) in the bloodstream that we do not routinely measure, including phosphates, sulfates, organic acids, and negatively charged plasma proteins. One of the most abundant negatively charged ions in the blood is serum albumin. A normal serum albumin is 4.0 g/dL. For patients with hypoalbuminemia (low serum albumin), the normal or expected anion gap is smaller:

$$\text{Expected Anion Gap} = 12 - (2.5) * \left[4.0 \frac{\text{g}}{\text{dL}} - \text{Actual Serum Albumin} \right].$$

So for this patient,

Expected Anion Gap $= 12 - [2.5 * (4 - 4.8)] = 12 - [(2.5) * (-0.8)] = 12 - (-2) = 14$ mEq/L.

Q14-4: A
Anion gap acidosis.

Rationale:

1. Is there evidence of a chronic respiratory acid-base disorder that requires adjustment of the patient's "normal" HCO_3? No, the ongoing process appears acute based on the clinical vignette and associated information. Therefore, we would assume a baseline serum HCO_3 of 24 mEq/L and a $Paco_2$ of 40 mm Hg.
2. Expected anion gap:

$$\text{Expected Anion Gap} = 12 - (2.5) * \left[4.0 \frac{g}{dL} - \text{Actual Serum Albumin} \right]$$

$$= 12 - (2.5 * [4.0 - 4.8])$$
$$= 12 - (2.5 * [-0.8]) = \textbf{14 mEq/L.}$$

3. Anion gap calculation:

$$\text{Serum Anion Gap} = [Na^+] - [HCO_3^-] - [Cl^-]$$
$$124 - (85 + 5) = 34 \text{ mEq/L, which is} > 14 \text{ mEq/L}$$
$$\rightarrow \textbf{anion gap acidosis is present.}$$

Note: If we did not correct for the reduced albumin we would have missed the anion gap acidosis.

4. Delta-delta calculation:

$$\Delta\Delta = \frac{(\text{Actual Anion Gap} - \text{Expected Anion Gap})}{(\text{Baseline } HCO_3 - \text{Actual } HCO_3)}$$

$$= (34 - 14)/(24 - 5) = \textbf{20/19, which is ~1.}$$

Delta-delta interpretation.	
Delta-Delta Value	Condition Present
< 0.4	Non-anion gap only
0.4–0.9	Anion gap *and* non-anion gap acidosis
1.0–2.0	**Anion gap acidosis only**
> 2.0	Anion gap acidosis and metabolic alkalosis

The delta-delta value is 1, therefore the patient has an isolated anion gap metabolic acidosis.

Q14-5: B
7.

Rationale: Similar to the serum anion gap, the serum osmolal gap is determined by the difference between the "calculated" serum osmolality and the true measured serum osmolality. The equation for the serum osmolal gap typically includes factors for sodium, glucose, BUN, and ethanol, as these are readily measurable in most laboratories. Therefore, the serum osmolal gap will represent the osmolality of those "unmeasured" osmoles, including organic alcohols and acetone. The most common form is shown as follows:

$$\text{Calculated Serum Osmolality} = 2*[Na^+] + \frac{[\text{Glucose}]}{18} + \frac{[\text{BUN}]}{2.8} + \frac{[\text{EtOH}]}{3.7}.$$

In which the units of measure are as follows: Na, mEq/L; glucose, mg/dL; BUN, mg/dL; and EtOH, mg/dL. The conversion factors are shown in the preceding equation as well. A normal serum osmolal gap is around −10 to +10 mOsm/L (or mOsm/kg). A serum osmolal gap more than 10 to 15 mOsm/L is considered a critical finding.

Therefore, in this patient,

$$\begin{aligned}\text{Calculated Serum Osmolality} &= [2*Na] + [\text{Glucose}/18] + [\text{BUN}/2.8] + [\text{EtOH}/3.7]\\ &= (2*124) + (560/18) + (60/2.8) + (45/3.7)\\ &= 313 \text{ mOsm/L.}\end{aligned}$$

$$\begin{aligned}\text{Serum Osmolal Gap} &= \text{Measured Serum Osmolality} - \text{Calculated Osmolality}\\ &= (320 - 313) = 7, \text{ which is} < 10 \text{ mOsm/L}\\ &\rightarrow \textbf{no serum osmolal gap is present.}\end{aligned}$$

Note that in this patient, if we had not included the extra term for the contribution of ethyl alcohol to the osmolar gap, we would have a different result:

$$\begin{aligned}\text{Calculated Serum Osmolality (without EtOH term)} &= [2*Na] + [\text{Glucose}/18] + [\text{BUN}/2.8]\\ &= (2*124) + (560/18) + (60/2.8)\\ &= 300 \text{ mOsm/L;}\end{aligned}$$

and the osmolal gap would be 20 mOsm/L, which would be positive and potentially concerning for a toxic ingestion of another organic alcohol in addition to alcohol. Including the term provides some additional clarity of the clinical situation.

Q14-6: C
No, a concomitant respiratory acidosis is present.

Rationale: Here, we would assume the metabolic acidosis is an acute process. Using the Winter formula, one can calculate what the expected arterial $Paco_2$ should be for a given serum HCO_3 if the patient were completely compensated.

Respiratory Compensation for Acute Metabolic Acidosis (Winters formula):

$$\text{Expected Paco}_2 = 1.5 * [\text{Actual HCO}_3] + 8 \pm 2 \text{ (in mm Hg)}.$$

Therefore, in this patient,

$$\text{Expected Paco}_2 = 1.5 * (\text{actual HCO}_3) + 8 (+/-2)$$
$$= (1.5 * 5) + 8 = 7.5 + 8 = 15.5 +/-2 = (13 \text{ to } 17) \text{ mm Hg}.$$

This patient has a concomitant respiratory acidosis possibly due to splinting from abdominal pain or related to encephalopathy from the severe acidosis.

Q14-7: B
Diabetic ketoacidosis.

Rationale: The patient is a known diabetic with insulin dependence, presenting with an acute illness (likely appendicitis), without evidence of septic shock at this point. The patient's blood glucose is very elevated and his beta-hydroxybutyrate is elevated as well, consistent with DKA (although alcoholic and/or starvation ketoacidosis may also be contributing). Renal failure may be contributing to some degree, although the patient's Cr is not far from baseline and he is still making urine. There is no evidence of neurogenic shock. The serum osmolal gap is normal, making methanol ingestion much less likely.

Q14-8: C
Non-anion gap metabolic acidosis.

Rationale: The patient continues to have an acidosis as the primary problem and the HCO_3 is reduced at 13 mEq/L while the $Paco_2$ is also reduced at 24 mm Hg. Therefore, there is no primary respiratory disorder, but there is a primary metabolic acidosis. The patient's albumin is now 3.6 g/dL, so the expected anion gap is 11 mEq/L. The patient's anion gap now is 11, so there is no anion gap acidosis present. Therefore, the primary problem is a non-anion gap acidosis.

Q14-9: A
Volume resuscitation with normal saline.

Rationale: The most likely reason for the patient's non-anion gap acidosis is volume resuscitation with a hyperchloremic fluid such as a normal saline. This is a common complication during the recovery phase of DKA and the severity can be reduced—to some degree—by the use of other fluids that are closer to physiologic, such as PlasmaLyte. This remains an active area of research. Recall that DKA is a generally a volume-depletion disorder. As the primary anion in normal saline is chloride, chloride is rapidly resorbed with sodium, rather than HCO_3 (which is not present in sufficient quantity to appropriately balance anion resorption). This can, at least initially during resuscitation, actually lead to a further drop in HCO_3 levels, although over time the anion gap will be closed by increases in both chloride and HCO_3.

References

Basnet S, Venepalli PK, Andoh J, et al. Effect of normal saline and half normal saline on serum electrolytes during recovery phase of diabetic ketoacidosis. J Intensive Care Med. 2014;29:38.

DeFronzo RA, Matzuda M, Barret E. Diabetic ketoacidosis: a combined metabolic-nephrologic approach to therapy. Diabetes Rev. 1994;2:209.

Dhatariya K. Diabetic ketoacidosis. BMJ. 2007;334:1284.

Dymot JA, McKay GA. Type 1 (distal) renal tubular acidosis in a patient with type 1 diabetes mellitus—not all cases of metabolic acidosis in type 1 diabetes mellitus are due to diabetic ketoacidosis. Diabet Med. 2008;25:114.

Fulop M, Murthy V, Michilli A, et al. Serum beta-hydroxybutyrate measurement in patients with uncontrolled diabetes mellitus. Arch Intern Med. 1999;159:381.

Mahler SA, Conrad SA, Wang H, Arnold TC. Resuscitation with balanced electrolyte solution prevents hyperchloremic metabolic acidosis in patients with diabetic ketoacidosis. Am J Emerg Med. 2011;29:670.

Oh MS, Banerji MA, Carroll HJ. The mechanism of hyperchloremic acidosis during the recovery phase of diabetic ketoacidosis. Diabetes. 1981;30:310.

Porter WH, Yao HH, Karounos DG. Laboratory and clinical evaluation of assays for beta-hydroxybutyrate. Am J Clin Pathol. 1997;107:353.

Rose BD, Post TW. Clinical Physiology of Acid-Base and Electrolyte Disorders. 5e. New York, NY: McGraw-Hill; 2001:809.

Shen T, Braude S. Changes in serum phosphate during treatment of diabetic ketoacidosis: predictive significance of severity of acidosis on presentation. Intern Med J. 2012;42:1347.

Van Zyl DG, Rheeder P, Delport E. Fluid management in diabetic-acidosis– Ringer's lactate versus normal saline: a randomized controlled trial. QJM. 2012;105:337.

Wachtel TJ, Tetu-Mouradjian LM, Goldman DL, et al. Hyperosmolarity and acidosis in diabetes mellitus: a three-year experience in Rhode Island. J Gen Intern Med. 1991;6:495.

CASE 15

An 88-year-old woman is transferred from the general medicine service to the medical ICU unit with worsening encephalopathy and hypotension. She had initially presented to the hospital 6 hours earlier with weakness, fatigue, poor PO intake, and mild confusion. She has a history of COPD (FEV_1 33% predicted), hypertension, diastolic heart failure, and hyperlipidemia. Her current medications include aspirin, amlodipine, furosemide (taken PRN), hydrochlorothiazide, tiotropium, and albuterol PRN. She has had similar episodes in the past when she has had urinary tract infections. Initiation of antibiotics was delayed on admission as the patient was unable to provide a urine sample and was unwilling to allow catheterization. On transfer to the ICU, her vital signs are T 38.7°C, RR 25, HR 92, BP 75/50, and Sao_2 90% on 2 L NC. On examination, the patient is delirious. She has mild expiratory wheezing on pulmonary examination. Her mucous membranes appear dry. She has no lower extremity (LE) edema, rashes, or bruising. On abdominal examination, she does have right-sided flank tenderness. A Foley catheter is inserted and a urinalysis shows many WBCs, with positive nitrates and leukocyte esterase. Laboratory results are as follows:

Laboratory data.			
ABGs		Basic Metabolic Panel	
pH	7.10	Na	132 mEq/L
$Paco_2$	49 mm Hg	K	2.3 mEq/L
Pao_2	213 mm Hg	Cl	82 mEq/L
HCO_3	15 mEq/L	CO_2	15 mEq/L
		BUN	40 mg/dL
		Cr	1.2 mg/dL
		Glucose	100 mg/dL
		Albumin	3.6 g/dL
		EtOH	0 mg/dL

QUESTIONS

Q15-1: Define the patient's baseline acid-base status: Does this patient have an underlying chronic acid-base disorder that we need to account for in order to appropriately interpret the acute acid-base disorders?

A. There is no evidence of an underlying chronic respiratory or metabolic acid-base disorder in this patient, so we would assume a baseline $Paco_2$ of 40 mm Hg and an HCO_3 of 24 mEq/L.

B. While the patient has a condition predisposing her to a chronic acid-base disorder, there is insufficient information to estimate the patient's baseline $Paco_2$ and HCO_3 values; therefore, we will assume a baseline $Paco_2$ of 40 mm Hg and a baseline HCO_3 of 24 mEq/L.

C. The patient has an underlying acid-base condition and we have sufficient information to estimate the patient's baseline $Paco_2$ and HCO_3 values.

Q15-2: What is/are the primary acid-base disturbance(s) occurring in this case?

A. Metabolic acidosis only
B. Respiratory acidosis only
C. Metabolic alkalosis only
D. Respiratory alkalosis only
E. Metabolic acidosis and a respiratory acidosis
F. Metabolic alkalosis and a respiratory alkalosis

Q15-3: For a perfectly healthy patient, a normal anion gap is assumed to be 12 mEq/L. What should be considered a normal anion gap in this patient?

A. 12 mEq/L
B. 11 mEq/L
C. 10 mEq/L
D. 9 mEq/L

Q15-4: How would the metabolic acidosis component be classified in this case?

A. Anion gap acidosis
B. Non-anion gap acidosis
C. Anion and non-anion gap acidosis
D. Anion gap acidosis and a metabolic alkalosis

Q15-5: Your laboratory testing returns the following values:

Serum EtOH	< 3 mg/dL
Serum acetaminophen level	< 5 mg/dL (ULN for therapeutic use 20 mg/dL)
Serum salicylates level	< 5 mg/dL (ULN for therapeutic use 30 mg/dL)
Serum osmolality	290 mOsm/kg
Serum L-lactate	5.0 mmol/L (ULN 2.0 mmol/L venous)
Beta-hydroxybutyrate (acetone)	< 0.18 mmol/L (ULN 0.18 mmol/L)
Serum glucose	80 mg/dL

What is the serum osmolal gap?

A. −4 mOsm/L
B. 0 mOsm/L
C. 6 mOsm/L
D. 12 mOsm/L

Q15-6: The following additional laboratory findings are obtained:

Urine Na	22 mEq/L
Urine K	41 mEq/L
Urine Cl	39 mEq/L
Urine urea	569 mg/dL
Urine glucose	0 mg/dL
Urine osmolality	600 mOsm/L
Urine pH	5.5
Urine RBCs	None
Urine WBCs	None
Urine protein	None
Urine microscopic	None
Serum phosphorus	2.8 mEq/L

Choose the primary etiologies for each acid-base disorder present from the list below (choose only one answer per disorder):

A. Diabetic ketoacidosis
B. Liver failure
C. Lactic acidosis
D. Hyperemesis
E. Underlying pulmonary disease (COPD)
F. Pulmonary embolism
G. Neuromuscular disease
H. Type 4 RTA
I. Type I RTA
J. Acetaminophen overdose
K. Methanol poisoning
L. Chronic diarrhea
M. Current diuretic use
N. Prior diuretic use
___Anion gap metabolic acidosis
___Respiratory acidosis
___Metabolic alkalosis

Q15-7: What would you expect the patient's arterial partial pressure of carbon dioxide ($Paco_2$) and arterial pH to be if she was compensating appropriately for the metabolic acidosis present?

A. $Paco_2$ 22 mm Hg, pH 7.45

B. $Paco_2$ 25 mm Hg, pH 7.39

C. $Paco_2$ 19 mm Hg, pH 7.51

D. $Paco_2$ 30 mm Hg, pH 7.31

E. $Paco_2$ 36 mm Hg, pH 7.23

F. $Paco_2$ 40 mm Hg, pH 7.19

Q15-8: Now, assume this patient has a respiratory acidosis alone, with no metabolic acidosis present. What would you expect the patient's pH and serum HCO_3 to be if the respiratory acidosis was acute (assume that sufficient time has passed for the acute compensation to be complete)?

A. pH 7.20, HCO_3 30 mEq/L

B. pH 7.29, HCO_3 24 mEq/L

C. pH 7.32, HCO_3 25 mEq/L

D. pH 7.17, HCO_3 21 mEq/L

ANSWERS

Q15-1: B

While the patient has a condition predisposing her to a chronic acid-base disorder, there is insufficient information to estimate the patient's baseline $Paco_2$ and HCO_3 values; therefore, we will assume a baseline $Paco_2$ of 40 mm Hg and a baseline HCO_3 of 24 mEq/L. She does have COPD, which is a risk factor for chronic hypercarbic respiratory failure and chronic respiratory acidosis, but we do not have sufficient evidence to support this, let alone estimate the patient's baseline acid-base status. Therefore, we will assume the "normal" values above.

Rationale: Ignoring these underlying chronic acid-base disorders can significantly alter the interpretation of a patient's acute acid-base status. This was demonstrated in the first case of the series. However, often, we do not have the necessary information (eg, prior ABG or VBG, or prior serum chemistry with an HCO_3) and are forced to assume the ongoing processes are all acute in nature. We are primarily concerned about chronic respiratory acid-base disorders, as these can significantly alter the patient's baseline or expected values for the serum HCO_3 and $Paco_2$, and we have reliable equations to predict the expected baseline values. The respiratory compensation for both chronic metabolic acidosis and alkalosis is generally poor, so there are no equations or rules to predict what the $Paco_2$ should be in these cases. While the baseline serum HCO_3 may be significantly off from our standard value of 24 mEq/L in these patients, we would assume a baseline $Paco_2$ of 40 mm Hg in patients with chronic metabolic processes. Once we identify the patient's baseline $Paco_2$ and HCO_3 values, we will need to use these values in the appropriate equations to identify the ongoing acute processes.

Q15-2: E

Metabolic acidosis and a respiratory acidosis.

Rationale:

1. The pH is 7.10; therefore, the primary disorder is an **acidosis**.
2. The $Paco_2$ of 49 mm Hg is less than 40 mm Hg, so there is a **respiratory acidosis**.
3. The HCO_3 of 15 mEq/L is less than 24 mEq/L, so there is a **metabolic acidosis**.

Q15-3: B

11 mEq/L.

Rationale: The normal anion gap is 12 mEq/L. The term *anion gap* refers to those ions (negatively charged molecules) in the bloodstream that we do not routinely measure, including phosphates, sulfates, organic acids, and negatively charged plasma proteins. One of the most abundant negatively charged ions in the blood is serum albumin. A normal serum albumin is 4.0 g/dL. For patients with hypoalbuminemia (low serum albumin), the normal or expected anion gap is smaller:

$$\text{Expected Anion Gap} = 12 - (2.5) * \left[4.0 \frac{g}{dL} - \text{Actual Serum Albumin} \right].$$

So for this patient,

Expected Anion Gap = 12 − [2.5 * (4 − 3.6)] = 12 − (2.5 * 0.4) = **11 mEq/L.**

Q15-4: C
Anion and non-anion gap acidosis.

Rationale:

1. Is there evidence of a chronic respiratory acid-base disorder that requires adjustment of the patient's "normal" HCO_3? While the patient does carry a diagnosis of COPD, there is not enough information in the vignette to make the assumption of chronic hypercarbic respiratory failure, and therefore we would assume a serum HCO_3 of 24 mEq/L and a serum $PaCO_2$ of 40 mm Hg.

2. Expected anion gap:

$$\text{Expected Anion Gap} = 12 - (2.5) * \left[4.0\, \frac{g}{dL} - \text{Actual Serum Albumin} \right]$$

$$= 12 - (2.5 * [4.0 - 3.6])$$
$$= 12 - (2.5 * [0.4]) = \mathbf{11\ mEq/L.}$$

3. Anion gap calculation:

$$\text{Serum Anion Gap} = [Na^+] - [HCO_3^-] - [Cl^-]$$
$$132 - (82 + 15) = 35\ \text{mEq/L, which is} > 11\ \text{mEq/L}$$
$$\rightarrow \textbf{anion gap acidosis is present.}$$

4. Delta-delta calculation:

$$\Delta\Delta = \frac{(\text{Actual Anion Gap} - \text{Expected Anion Gap})}{(\text{Baseline } HCO_3 - \text{Actual } HCO_3)}$$

(35 − 11)/(24 − 15) = **24/9, which is ~2.7.**

Delta-delta interpretation.	
Delta-Delta Value	Condition Present
< 0.4	Non-anion gap only
0.4–0.9	Anion gap *and* non-anion gap acidosis
1.0–2.0	Anion gap acidosis only
> 2.0	**Anion gap acidosis and metabolic alkalosis**

The delta-delta value is 2.7, therefore the patient has a concomitant anion gap metabolic acidosis and a metabolic alkalosis.

Q15-5: C
6 mOsm/L.

Rationale: Similar to the serum anion gap, the serum osmolal gap is determined by the difference between the "calculated" serum osmolality and the true measured serum osmolality. The equation for the serum osmolal gap typically includes factors for sodium, glucose, BUN, and ethanol, as these are readily measurable in most laboratories. Therefore, the serum osmolal gap will represent the osmolality of those "unmeasured" osmoles, including organic alcohols and acetone. The most common form is shown as follows:

$$\text{Calculated Serum Osmolality} = 2*[\text{Na}^+] + \frac{[\text{Glucose}]}{18} + \frac{[\text{BUN}]}{2.8} + \frac{[\text{EtOH}]}{3.7};$$

In which the units of measure are as follows: Na, mEq/L; glucose, mg/dL; BUN, mg/dL; and EtOH, mg/dL. The conversion factors are shown in the preceding equation as well. A normal serum osmolal gap is around −10 to +10 mOsm/L (or mOsm/kg).

Therefore, in this patient,

$$\begin{aligned}
\text{Calculated Serum Osmolality} &= [2*\text{Na}] + [\text{Glucose}/18] + [\text{BUN}/2.8] + [\text{EtOH}/3.7] \\
&= (2*132) + (100/18) + (40/2.8) + (0/3.7) \\
&= 284 \text{ mOsm/L}.
\end{aligned}$$

$$\begin{aligned}
\text{Serum Osmolar Gap} &= \text{Measured Serum Osmolality} - \text{Calculated Osmolality} \\
&= (290 - 284) = 6, \text{ which is} < 10 \text{ mOsm/L}
\end{aligned}$$
→ **no serum osmolal gap is present**.

In this patient, there is no evidence of a serum osmolal gap.

Q15-6: C; E; M
Lactic acidosis; Underlying pulmonary disease (COPD); Current diuretic use.

Rationale: The patient's laboratory values are most consistent with a lactic acidosis as the primary cause of the anion gap acidosis. The patient presents with hypotension in the setting of a likely urinary tract infection and an elevated serum lactate. While the patient may have some mild renal failure, this is unlikely the primary cause.

The patient's history of COPD with severe airflow obstruction and associated underlying lung disease is the likely cause of the patient's respiratory acidosis. Patients with reduced pulmonary reserve (eg, COPD, interstitial lung disease, cystic fibrosis) are often unable to adequately compensate for a significant metabolic acidosis, or they tire more quickly from the increased energy expenditure necessary to adequately compensate. Patients with COPD, in particular, can develop significant problems with hyperinflation/air-trapping resulting from the increased respiratory rate. Therefore, in this patient, her underlying lung disease is likely the reason that she developed a respiratory acidosis.

The patient has a concomitant metabolic alkalosis. The urine chloride is the first step in classifying the cause of a patient's metabolic alkalosis. The urine chloride is elevated (> 20 mEq/L) indicating that a chloride-resistant process is ongoing. Recall that active or current diuretic use results in a chloride-resistant metabolic alkalosis, and as the diuretics are metabolized and cleared (eg, "prior" diuretic use), the metabolic alkalosis can shift to a chloride-responsive process. As this patient presented within the past 24 hours, the diuretics she has been taking are likely still active.

Q15-7: D
$Paco_2$ of 30 mm Hg, pH 7.31.

Rationale: First, we need to determine what the patient's $Paco_2$ should be if the patient was compensating appropriately for the acute metabolic acidosis. Using the Winter formula, we can calculate what the expected arterial $Paco_2$ should be for a given serum HCO_3 if the patient was completely compensated (assume the metabolic acidosis is an acute process).

Respiratory Compensation for Acute Metabolic Acidosis (Winters formula):

Expected $Paco_2$ = 1.5 = * [Actual HCO_3] + 8 ± 2 (in mm Hg)
Expected $Paco_2$ = (1.5 * 15) + 8 = 22.5 + 8 = 30.5 ± 2 = ~(28 to 32) mm Hg.

Therefore, we would expect the patient's $Paco_2$ to be between 28 and 32 (approximately). Next, we can use the Henderson-Hasselbach equation to determine the predicted pH (assuming a value of 30 mm Hg for the $Paco_2$ and the HCO_3 of 15 mEq/L:

Henderson-Hasselbalch Equation:

$$pH = 6.10 + \log\left(\frac{[HCO_3]}{0.03 * PCO_2}\right),$$

or,

$$pH = 7.61 + \log_{10}\left(\frac{[HCO_3]}{Paco_2}\right).$$

Therefore, the pH would be 7.31 (between 7.28 and 7.34), with a $Paco_2$ of approximately 30 mm Hg.

Q15-8: C
pH 7.32, HCO_3 25 mEq/L.

Rationale: To determine the serum HCO_3 level if the patient has appropriate compensation for an *acute* process, you need the following equation:

Metabolic Compensation for Acute Respiratory Acidosis:

Expected = HCO_3 = Baseline HCO_3 + (0.10) [Actual $Paco_2$ – Baseline $Paco_2$]
Expected HCO_3 = 24 + [0.10 * 9] ~ **25 mEq/L.**

Then, applying the following Henderson-Hasselbach equation from the prior question, you would obtain a pH of approximately 7.32.

$$pH = 6.10 + \log\left(\frac{[HCO_3]}{0.03 * P_{CO_2}}\right),$$

or,

$$pH = 7.61 + \log_{10}\left(\frac{[HCO_3]}{Pa_{CO_2}}\right).$$

References

Adrogué HJ, Madias NE. Secondary responses to altered acid-base status: the rules of engagement. J Am Soc Nephrol. 2010;21:920.

Berend K, de Vries AP, Gans RO. Physiological approach to assessment of acid-base disturbances. N Engl J Med. 2014;371:1434.

Feldman M, Soni N, Dickson B. Influence of hypoalbuminemia or hyperalbuminemia on the serum anion gap. J Lab Clin Med. 2005;146:317.

Gennari FJ, Weise WJ. Acid-base disturbances in gastrointestinal disease. Clin J Am Soc Nephrol. 2008;3:1861.

Kraut JA, Nagami GT. The serum anion gap in the evaluation of acid-base disorders: what are its limitations and can its effectiveness be improved? Clin J Am Soc Nephrol. 2013;8:2018.

Luke RG, Galla JH. It is chloride depletion alkalosis, not contraction alkalosis. J Am Soc Nephrol. 2012;23:204.

Rastegar A. Use of the deltaAG/deltaHCO$_3^-$ ratio in the diagnosis of mixed acid-base disorders. J Am Soc Nephrol. 2007;18:2429.

Rose BD, Post TW. Clinical Physiology of Acid-Base and Electrolyte Disorders, 5e. New York, NY: McGraw-Hill; 2001:583.

Schwartz WB, Van Ypersele de Strihou, Kassirer JP. Role of anions in metabolic alkalosis and potassium deficiency. N Engl J Med. 1968;279:630.

Turban S, Beutler KT, Morris RG, et al. Long-term regulation of proximal tubule acid-base transporter abundance by angiotensin II. Kidney Int. 2006;70:660.

CASE 16

A 66-year-old white man with longstanding, poorly controlled diabetes mellitus, resultant diabetic nephropathy (stage IV, Cr 2.6 baseline), diabetic neuropathy, hyperlipidemia, hypertension, coronary artery disease, gout, and chronic back pain presents with sudden cardiopulmonary arrest in the waiting room of the emergency department (ED). He had come to the ED for issues with chronic back pain. He takes gabapentin for this condition. He reported worsening back pain over the past few days. His vital signs at triage were within normal limits. An ECG showed evidence of prior inferior and anterior myocardial infarctions, but no acute changes. According to the patient's caretaker, who accompanied him to the ER, the patient had noted some mild dizziness and shortness of breath 5 minutes before the code event, and appeared diaphoretic. He was transferred to a trauma bay immediately while CPR was underway. The initial rhythm was ventricular fibrillation. He received a 200 J cardioversion, which was successful. He obtained ROSC about 5 minutes after the initial code. He received 1 mg epinephrine, 1 amp of calcium chloride, and a 300-mg amiodarone bolus during the code event. He was minimally responsive following recovery and was intubated for airway protection following the code. His laboratory values immediately post code are as follows:

Laboratory data.			
ABGs		Basic Metabolic Panel	
pH	7.01	Na	140 mEq/L
$Paco_2$	76 mm Hg	K	6.1 mEq/L
Pao_2	213 mm Hg	Cl	109 mEq/L
HCO_3	19 mEq/L	CO_2	19 mEq/L
		BUN	27 mg/dL
		Cr	3.3 mg/dL
		Glucose	154 mg/dL
		Albumin	3 g/dL
		EtOH	0 mg/dL

QUESTIONS

Q16-1: Define the patient's baseline acid-base status: Does this patient have an underlying chronic acid-base disorder that we need to account for in order to appropriately interpret the acute acid-base disorders?

A. There is no evidence for an underlying chronic respiratory or metabolic acid-base disorder in this patient, so we would assume a baseline $Paco_2$ of 40 mm Hg and an HCO_3 of 24 mEq/L.

B. While the patient has a condition predisposing him to a chronic acid-base disorder, there is insufficient information to estimate the patient's baseline $Paco_2$ and HCO_3 values; therefore, we will assume a baseline $Paco_2$ of 40 mm Hg and a baseline HCO_3 of 24 mEq/L.

C. The patient has an underlying acid-base condition, and we have sufficient information to estimate the patient's baseline $Paco_2$ and HCO_3 values.

Q16-2: What is/are the primary acid-base disturbance(s) occurring in this case?

A. Metabolic acidosis only
B. Respiratory acidosis only
C. Metabolic alkalosis only
D. Respiratory alkalosis only
E. Metabolic acidosis and a respiratory acidosis
F. Metabolic alkalosis and a respiratory alkalosis

Q16-3: For a perfectly healthy patient, a normal anion gap is assumed to be 12 mEq/L. What should be considered a normal anion gap in this patient?

A. 12 mEq/L
B. 9.5 mEq/L
C. 8 mEq/L
D. 7 mEq/L

Q16-4: How would the metabolic acidosis component be classified in this case?

A. Anion gap acidosis
B. Non-anion gap acidosis
C. Anion and non-anion gap acidosis
D. Anion gap acidosis and a metabolic alkalosis

Q16-5: Laboratory testing returns the following results:

Serum EtOH	< 3 mg/dL
Serum acetaminophen level	< 5 mg/dL (ULN for therapeutic use 20 mg/dL)
Serum salicylates level	< 5 mg/dL (ULN for therapeutic use 30 mg/dL)
Serum osmolality	306 mOsm/kg
Serum L-lactate	3.8 mmol/L (ULN 2.0 mmol/L venous)
Beta-hydroxybutyrate (acetone)	< 0.18 mmol/L (ULN 0.18 mmol/L)
Serum glucose	154 mg/dL
Urine drug screen	Negative

What is the serum osmolal gap?

A. −4 mOsm/L
B. 4 mOsm/L
C. 8 mOsm/L
D. 12 mOsm/L

Q16-6: **What is the likely cause of the patient's anion gap acidosis?**

A. Diabetic ketoacidosis
B. Alcoholic ketoacidosis
C. Lactic acidosis
D. Organic alcohol ingestion
E. Chronic diarrhea

Q16-7: **What is the likely cause of the patient's respiratory acidosis?**

A. Acetaminophen toxicity
B. Opioid overdose
C. Benzodiazepine overdose
D. Cardiac arrest
E. Aspirin toxicity

Q16-8: **You decide to investigate the patient's non-anion gap acidosis. The patient's urine studies are as follows:**

Urine Na	15 mEq/L
Urine K	18 mEq/L
Urine Cl	24 mEq/L
Urine urea	89 mg/dL
Urine glucose	0 mg/dL
Urine osmolality	198 mOsm/L
Urine pH	5.3
Urine RBCs	None
Urine WBCs	None
Urine protein	None
Urine microscopic	None

What is the cause of the patient's non-anion gap acidosis?

A. Type 1 (distal) RTA
B. Type 2 (proximal) RTA
C. GI losses of bicarbonate
D. Type 4 RTA

ANSWERS

Q16-1: B

While the patient has a condition predisposing him to a chronic acid-base disorder, there is insufficient information to estimate the patient's baseline $Paco_2$ and HCO_3 values; therefore, we will assume a baseline $Paco_2$ of 40 mm Hg and a baseline HCO_3 of 24 mEq/L. The patient has a diabetic nephropathy, which predisposes to a chronic metabolic acidosis, but we lack any additional information to determine if his baseline HCO_3 is different from our presumed "normal" value of 24 mEq/L.

Rationale: Ignoring these underlying chronic acid-base disorders can significantly alter the interpretation of a patient's acute acid-base status. This was demonstrated in the first case of the series. However, often, we do not have the necessary information (eg, prior ABG or VBG, or prior serum chemistry with an HCO_3) and are forced to assume the ongoing processes are all acute in nature. We are primarily concerned about chronic respiratory acid-base disorders, as these can significantly alter the patient's baseline or expected values for the serum HCO_3 and $Paco_2$, and we have reliable equations to predict the expected baseline values. The respiratory compensation for both chronic metabolic acidosis and alkalosis is generally poor, so there are no equations or rules to predict what the $Paco_2$ should be in these cases. While the baseline serum HCO_3 may be significantly off from our standard value of 24 mEq/L in these patients, we would assume a baseline $Paco_2$ of 40 mm Hg in patients with chronic metabolic processes. Once we identify the patient's baseline $Paco_2$ and HCO_3 values, we will need to use these values in the appropriate equations to identify the ongoing acute processes.

Q16-2: E

Metabolic acidosis and a respiratory acidosis.

Rationale:

1. The pH is 7.01; therefore, the primary disorder is an **acidosis.**
2. The $Paco_2$ of 76 mm Hg is greater than 40 mm Hg, so there is a **respiratory acidosis.**
3. The HCO_3 of 19 mEq/L is less than 24 mEq/L, so there is a **metabolic acidosis.**

Q16-3: B

9.5 mEq/L.

Rationale: The normal anion gap is 12 mEq/L. The term *anion gap* refers to those ions (negatively charged molecules) in the bloodstream that we do not routinely measure, including phosphates, sulfates, organic acids, and negatively charged plasma proteins. One of the most abundant negatively charged ions in the blood is serum albumin. A normal serum albumin is 4.0 g/dL. For patients with hypoalbuminemia (low serum albumin), the normal or expected anion gap is smaller:

$$\text{Expected Anion Gap} = 12 - (2.5) * \left[4.0\,\frac{g}{dL} - \text{Actual Serum Albumin} \right].$$

So for this patient,

$$\text{Expected Anion Gap} = 12 - [2.5 * (4 - 3)] = 12 - (2.5 * 1) = 9.5 \text{ mEq/L.}$$

This is an important concept as patients with hypoalbuminemia may "hide" an anion gap acidosis if this correction is not performed.

Q16-4: C
Anion and non-anion gap acidosis.

Rationale:

1. Is there evidence for a chronic respiratory acid-base disorder that requires adjustment of the patient's "normal" HCO_3? While the patient does have risk factors for a chronic metabolic acidosis (diabetic nephropathy), we lack sufficient information to confirm this. Given the lack of information, we will assume a "normal" baseline acid-base status.

2. Expected anion gap:

$$\text{Expected Anion Gap} = 12 - (2.5) * \left[4.0 \frac{g}{dL} - \text{Actual Serum Albumin} \right]$$
$$= 12 - (2.5 * [4.0 - 3.0])$$
$$= 12 - (2.5 * [0]) = \textbf{9.5 mEq/L.}$$

3. Anion gap calculation:

$$\text{Serum Anion Gap} = [Na^+] - [HCO_3^-] - [Cl^-]$$
$$140 - (109 + 19) = 12 \text{ mEq/L, which is} > 9.5 \text{ mEq/L}$$
$$\rightarrow \textbf{anion gap acidosis is present.}$$

Note: If we did not correct for the reduced albumin we would have missed the anion gap acidosis.

4. Delta-delta calculation:

$$\Delta\Delta = \frac{(\text{Actual Anion Gap} - \text{Expected Anion Gap})}{(\text{Baseline HCO}_3 - \text{Actual HCO}_3)}$$
$$= (12 - 9.5)/(24 - 19) = 2.5/5, \textbf{ which is ~0.5.}$$

Delta-delta interpretation.	
Delta-Delta Value	**Condition Present**
< 0.4	Non-anion gap only
0.4–0.9	**Anion gap *and* non-anion gap acidosis**
1.0–2.0	Anion gap acidosis only
> 2.0	Anion gap acidosis and metabolic alkalosis

Again, note here that we would have missed the patient's anion gap acidosis if we had ignored the hypoalbuminemia.

Q16-5: C
8 mOsm/L.

Rationale: Similar to the serum anion gap, the serum osmolal gap is determined by the difference between the "calculated" serum osmolality and the true laboratory -measured serum osmolality. The equation for the serum osmolal gap typically includes factors for sodium, glucose, BUN, and ethanol, as these are readily measurable in most laboratories. Therefore, the serum osmolal gap will represent the osmolality of those "unmeasured" osmoles, including organic alcohols and acetone. The most common form is as follows:

$$\text{Calculated Serum Osmolality} = 2 * [Na^+] + \frac{[Glucose]}{18} + \frac{[BUN]}{2.8} + \frac{[EtOH]}{3.7};$$

In which the units of measure are as follows: Na, mEq/L; glucose, mg/dL; BUN, mg/dL; and EtOH, mg/dL. The conversion factors are shown in the preceding equation as well. A normal serum osmolal gap is around −10 to +10 mOsm/L (or mOsm/kg).

For this patient,

$$\begin{aligned}
\text{Calculated Serum Osmolality} &= [2 * Na] + [Glucose/18] + [BUN/2.8] + [EtOH/3.7] \\
&= (2 * 140) + (154/18) + (27/2.8) + (0/3.7) \\
&= 298 \text{ mOsm/kg.}
\end{aligned}$$

$$\begin{aligned}
\text{Serum Osmolal Gap} &= \text{Measured Serum Osmolality} - \text{Calculated Osmolality} \\
&= (306 - 298) = 8 \text{ mOsm/L, which is} < 10 \text{ mOsm/L} \\
&\rightarrow \textit{no} \textbf{ serum osmolal gap is present.}
\end{aligned}$$

Q16-6: C
Lactic acidosis.

Rationale: During a cardiac arrest, even with CPR, the cardiac output is significantly lower than would be expected during normal cardiac function. A lactic acidosis is a very common finding in the post-code period. The patient's lactate is mildly elevated, consistent with the mild elevation in the anion gap. The laboratory testing indicates no evidence of a ketoacidosis or organic alcohol ingestion. Additionally, a chronic diarrhea usually leads to a non-anion gap acidosis (unless hypovolemia and distributive shock are involved). Another consideration in this patient would be renal failure.

Q16-7: D
Cardiac arrest.

Rationale: It is always critical to rule out potential drug toxicity as a cause of a sudden cardiopulmonary arrest, particularly in patients with a history of substance abuse, issues with chronic pain, or new-onset renal failure. The patient's laboratory testing did not show use of acetaminophen, aspirin, narcotics, or benzodiazepines on the initial screen. Although the rapid urine drug screens are not 100% sensitive for low-level use of some illicit substances (or in the acute setting of a massive ingestion), the patient did not present in a comatose or confused state that would suggest an acute intoxication, and there is no mention in the prompt regarding use of narcotics. Another concern would be for gabapentin toxicity. Gabapentin is cleared primarily by the kidney and accumulation of gabapentin in patients with acute or chronic renal failure can lead to confusion, drowsiness, encephalopathy, and coma. Narcotics, benzodiazepines, and gabapentin toxicity are more commonly associated with an arrest due to pulmonary issues.

Overall, the prompt is more concerning for a cardiac then a pulmonary cause of the arrest. The patient's initial presenting symptoms are concerning for acute coronary syndrome (ACS), particularly in a patient with a history of coronary artery disease. Additionally, the initial rhythm was ventricular fibrillation, raising concern for a primary cardiac arrest from ACS, prior structural heart disease, or an electrolyte abnormality. During cardiac arrest, the patient is dependent on ventilation from advanced cardiac life support and a respiratory acidosis is very common in the immediate post-arrest period.

Q16-8: D
Type 4 RTA.

Rationale: Recall that we can use either the urine anion gap (UAG) or urine osmolar gap (UOG) to qualitatively estimate urinary ammonium excretion. This is a case where the UAG alone is inconclusive. The patient's UAG is as follows:

$$UAG = [U_{Na}] + [U_K] - [U_{Cl}].$$

So for this patient,

$$UAG = U_{Na} + U_K - U_{Cl} = (15 + 18) - 24 = (+9) \text{ mEq/L}.$$

Interpretation:

- A UAG that is greater than ~20 → reduced renal acid excretion (RTA).
- A UAG that is −20 → GI loss of HCO_3 (eg, diarrhea), although type 2 RTA is possible.
- A UAG between −20 and +10 is generally considered inconclusive.

Limitations:

The UAG can be inappropriately elevated in anion gap acidosis, a situation in which multiple unmeasured anions may be present in the urine (beta-hydroxybutyrate/acetoacetate [ketoacidosis], hippurate [toluene], HCO_3 [proximal RTA], D-lactate

[D-lactic acidosis], L-lactate, 5-oxoproline [acetaminophen toxicity]). Therefore, in patients with a significant anion gap, the UOG is typically more useful.

Here the UOG is:

$$\text{Calculated Urine Osmolality} = 2*([Na^+]+[K^+]) + \frac{[Urea]}{2.8} + \frac{[Glucose]}{18}$$

$$\text{UOG} = \text{Measured Urine Osmolality}$$
$$- \text{Measured Urine Osmolality}.$$

So for this patient,

$$\text{Calculated Urine Osmolarity} = 2*[15+18]+[89/2.8]+[0/18] = 98 \text{ mOsm/L}$$
$$\text{UOG} = \text{Measured Urine Osmolality}$$
$$- \text{Calculated Serum Osmolality}$$
$$\text{UOG} = 198 - 98 \text{ Osm/L} = \textbf{100 mOsm.}$$

Interpretation (in setting of a metabolic acidosis):

- UOG greater than 400 mOsm/L (or kg): Appropriate urinary acidification, consistent with a GI source and normal renal acidification.
- UOG less than 100 to 150 mOsm/L (of kg): Inappropriately low urinary acidification, most consistent with a type 1 or 4 RTA.
- Again, this is not particularly useful for the diagnosis of a type 2 (proximal) RTA, where other serum or urine lab abnormalities are more helpful.

Limitations:

The primary limitation is the use of the UOG in conditions with a high osmolar gap, where non-ammonium solutes not included in the calculation may be present in the urine (particularly mannitol). The presence of these unmeasured solutes will increase the osmolal gap inappropriately. Also, the UOG should not be used in patients with a urinary tract infection caused by a urease-producing organism as urea is metabolized to HCO_3 and ammonium in urine.

Similar to the UAG, the UOG is used as a surrogate for the urine ammonium concentration. Therefore, a larger gap indicates increased urinary NH_4 excretion. In normal acid-base conditions, the urine osmolar gap is between **10** and **100 mOsm/L**. During a significant metabolic acidosis, patients with impaired renal tubular acidification (type 1 and type 4 RTA) are unable to excrete additional acid (NH_4), and therefore the osmolar gap does not change. Patients with an intact renal response to acidemia (ie, GI losses) should have a significant urine osmolar gap (~ **> 300** to **400 mOsm/L**) as a result of increased NH_4 excretion. Therefore, this patient has reduced urinary acidification consistent with a type 1 or type 4 RTA.

To determine the type of RTA, one can look at the urine pH, serum potassium, and for evidence of kidney stones.

Diagnosis of RTA.			
	Type 1 RTA	Type 2 RTA	Type 4 RTA
Severity of metabolic acidosis, (HCO_3)	Severe (< 10–12 mEq/L typically)	Intermediate (12–20 mEq/L)	Mild (15–20 mEq/L)
Associated urine abnormalities	Urinary phosphate, calcium are increased; bone disease often present	Urine glucose, amino acids, phosphate, calcium may be elevated	
Urine pH	HIGH (> 5.5)	Low (acidic), until serum HCO_3 level exceeds the resorptive ability of the proximal tubule; then becomes alkalotic once reabsorptive threshold is crossed	Low (acidic)
Serum K^+	Low to normal; should correct with oral HCO_3 therapy	Classically low, although may be normal or even high with rare genetic defects; worsens with oral HCO_3 therapy	HIGH
Renal stones	Often	No	No
Renal tubular defect	Reduced NH_4 secretion in distal tubule	Reduced HCO_3 resorption in proximal tubule	Reduced H^+/K^+ exchange in distal and collecting tubule due to decreased aldosterone or aldosterone resistance
Urine anion gap	> 10	Negative	> 10
Urine osmolal gap	Reduced during acute acidosis		Reduced during acute acidosis

The patient here has an elevated potassium and a low-normal urine pH, most consistent with a type 4 RTA. Diabetic nephropathy is commonly associated with development of a type 4 RTA.

The causes of renal tubular acidoses are summarized in the following table:

Causes of renal tubular acidosis.
Causes of Type 1 (Distal) RTA
Primary • Idiopathic or familial (may be recessive or dominant)
Secondary • Medications: Lithium, amphotericin, ifosfamide, NSAIDs • Rheumatologic disorders: Sjögren syndrome, SLE, RA • Hypercalciuria (idiopathic) or associated with vitamin D deficiency or hyperparathyroidism • Sarcoidosis • Obstructive uropathy • Wilson disease • Rejection of renal transplant allograft

(Continued)

Causes of renal tubular acidosis. (*continued*)
Causes of Type 2 (Proximal) RTA
Primary   • Idiopathic   • Familial (primarily recessive disorders)   • Genetic: Fanconi syndrome, cystinosis, glycogen storage disease (type 1), Wilson disease, galactosemia
Secondary   • Medications: Acetazolamide, topiramate, aminoglycoside antibiotics, ifosfamide, reverse transcriptase inhibitors (tenofovir)   • Heavy metal poisoning: Lead, mercury, copper   • Multiple myeloma or amyloidosis (secondary to light chain toxicity)   • Sjögren syndrome   • Vitamin D deficiency   • Rejection of renal transplant allograft
Causes of Type 4 RTA (Hypoaldosteronism or Aldosterone Resistance)
Primary   • Primary adrenal insufficiency   • Inherited disorders associated with hypoaldosteronism   • Pseudohypoaldosteronism (types 1 and 2)
Secondary   • Causes of hyporeninemic hypoaldosteronism such as renal disease (diabetic nephropathy), NSAID use, calcineurin inhibitors, volume expansion/volume overload   • Causes of distal tubule voltage defects such as sickle cell disease, obstructive uropathy, SLE   • Severe illness/septic shock   • Angiotensin II-associated medications: ACE inhibitors, ARBs, direct renin inhibitors   • Potassium-sparing diuretics: Spironolactone, amiloride, triamterene   • Antibiotics: Trimethoprim, pentamidine

References

Adrogué HJ, Madias NE. Secondary responses to altered acid-base status: the rules of engagement. J Am Soc Nephrol. 2010;21:920.

Batlle D, Chin-Theodorou J, Tucker BM. Metabolic acidosis or respiratory alkalosis? Evaluation of a low plasma bicarbonate using the urine anion gap. Am J Kidney Dis. 2017;70:440.

Batlle D, Grupp M, Gaviria M, Kurtzman NA. Distal renal tubular acidosis with intact capacity to lower urinary pH. Am J Med. 1982;72:751.

Batlle D, Haque SK. Genetic causes and mechanisms of distal renal tubular acidosis. Nephrol Dial Transplant. 2012;27:3691.

Batlle DC, Hizon M, Cohen E, et al. The use of the urinary anion gap in the diagnosis of hyperchloremic metabolic acidosis. N Engl J Med. 1988;318:594.

Batlle DC, von Riotte A, Schlueter W. Urinary sodium in the evaluation of hyperchloremic metabolic acidosis. N Engl J Med. 1987;316:140.

Berend K, de Vries AP, Gans RO. Physiological approach to assessment of acid-base disturbances. N Engl J Med. 2014;371:1434.

Buckalew VM Jr, McCurdy DK, Ludwig GD, et al. Incomplete renal tubular acidosis. Physiologic studies in three patients with a defect in lowering urine pH. Am J Med. 1968;45:32.

Feldman M, Soni N, Dickson B. Influence of hypoalbuminemia or hyperalbuminemia on the serum anion gap. J Lab Clin Med. 2005;146:317.

Karet FE. Mechanisms in hyperkalemic renal tubular acidosis. J Am Soc Nephrol. 2009;20:251.

Kraut JA, Madias NE. Differential diagnosis of nongap metabolic acidosis: value of a systematic approach. Clin J Am Soc Nephrol. 2012;7:671.

Kraut JA, Nagami GT. The serum anion gap in the evaluation of acid-base disorders: what are its limitations and can its effectiveness be improved? Clin J Am Soc Nephrol. 2013;8:2018.

Rastegar A. Use of the deltaAG/deltaHCO$_3^-$ ratio in the diagnosis of mixed acid-base disorders. J Am Soc Nephrol. 2007;18:2429.

Rodríguez Soriano J. Renal tubular acidosis: the clinical entity. J Am Soc Nephrol. 2002;13:2160.

Rose BD, Post TW. Clinical Physiology of Acid-Base and Electrolyte Disorders, 5e. New York, NY: McGraw-Hill; 2001:583.

CASE 17

A 33-year-old man with non-ischemic cardiomyopathy secondary to chronic amphetamine and cocaine abuse (EF 15%) presents with reduced exercise tolerance, paroxysmal nocturnal dyspnea, weight gain, and lower extremity edema. The patient is oriented to person and place, but is not oriented to time, date, or the current situation. He is in extremis on presentation and is placed on BiPAP on arrival for work-of-breathing. On examination, his lower extremities are mottled and cool to the touch, with 2+ pitting edema and faint pulses. He has crackles at the bases on inspiration. His abdomen is soft, but there is a positive fluid-wave present on examination. His vital signs are HR 110, BP 80/40, Sao_2 87% on 4 L/min bleed-in to the BiPAP. He is afebrile. His home medications include lisinopril, carvedilol, furosemide, and metolazone. He denies any recent drug use, alcohol use, or smoking. A CXR shows diffuse linear interstitial opacities.

Laboratory data.			
ABGs		Basic Metabolic Panel	
pH	7.35	Na	128 mEq/L
$Paco_2$	25 mm Hg	K	5.3 mEq/L
Pco_2	56 mm Hg	Cl	84 mEq/L
HCO_3	14 mEq/L	CO_2	14 mEq/L
		BUN	44 mg/dL
		Cr	2.2 mg/dL
		Glucose	104 mg/dL
		Albumin	2.6 g/dL
		EtOH	0 mg/dL

QUESTIONS

Q17-1: Define the patient's baseline acid-base status: Does this patient have an underlying chronic acid-base disorder that we need to account for in order to appropriately interpret the acute acid-base disorders?

A. There is no evidence for an underlying chronic respiratory or metabolic acid-base disorder in this patient, so we would assume a baseline $Paco_2$ of 40 mm Hg and an HCO_3 of 24 mEq/L.

B. While the patient has a condition predisposing him to a chronic acid-base disorder, there is insufficient information to estimate the patient's baseline $Paco_2$ and HCO_3 values; therefore, we will assume a baseline $Paco_2$ of 40 mm Hg and a baseline HCO_3 of 24 mEq/L.

C. The patient has an underlying acid-base condition, and we have sufficient information to estimate the patient's baseline $Paco_2$ and HCO_3 values.

Q17-2: What is/are the primary acid-base disturbance(s) occurring in this case?

A. Metabolic acidosis only
B. Respiratory acidosis only
C. Metabolic alkalosis only
D. Respiratory alkalosis only
E. Metabolic acidosis and a respiratory acidosis
F. Metabolic alkalosis and a respiratory alkalosis

Q17-3: For a perfectly healthy patient, a normal anion gap is assumed to be 12 mEq/L. What should be considered a normal anion gap in this patient?

A. 12 mEq/L
B. 10 mEq/L
C. 8.5 mEq/L
D. 6 mEq/L

Q17-4: How would the metabolic acidosis component be classified in this case?

A. Anion gap acidosis
B. Non-anion gap acidosis
C. Anion and non-anion gap acidosis
D. Anion gap acidosis and a metabolic alkalosis

Q17-5: Laboratory testing returns the following results:

Serum EtOH	< 3 mg/dL
Serum acetaminophen level	< 5 mg/dL (ULN for therapeutic use 20 mg/dL)
Serum salicylates level	< 5 mg/dL (ULN for therapeutic use 30 mg/dL)
Serum osmolality	284 mOsm/kg
Beta-hydroxybutyrate (acetone)	< 0.18 mmol/L (ULN 0.18 mmol/L)
Serum glucose	80 mg/dL

What is the serum osmolal gap?

A. 0
B. −7
C. 7
D. 17

Q17-6: The patient's Hgb is 15 g/dL and WBCs are 5.5 × 10³/microliter, with no evidence of a neutrophilia or bands. What is the next most appropriate test to order to determine the etiology of the anion gap acidosis present in this patient?

A. Brain natriuretic peptide (BNP)
B. Serum lactate
C. Serum procalcitonin
D. Urine chloride
E. Diagnostic paracentesis
F. Urine anion gap

Q17-7: The results of the patient's other serum and urine studies are as follows:

Urine Na	10 mEq/L
Urine K	13 mEq/L
Urine Cl	33 mEq/L
Urine urea	234 mg/dL
Urine glucose	0 mg/dL
Urine osmolality	231 mOsm/L
Urine pH	5.1

Which of the following is likely the cause of the patient's metabolic alkalosis?

A. Acetazolamide use
B. Thiazide/loop diuretic use
C. Hyperemesis
D. Primary hyperaldosteronism

Q17-8: Which lab test can help distinguish between primary and secondary hyperaldosteronism in a patient with a chloride-resistant metabolic alkalosis?

A. Urine urea
B. Urine osmolar gap
C. Urine anion gap
D. Plasma aldosterone-to-renin ratio
E. Urine catecholamines

Q17-9: Does the patient in this case demonstrate appropriate respiratory or metabolic compensation?

A. Yes, the respiratory compensation is appropriate.
B. No, a concomitant respiratory alkalosis is present.
C. No, a concomitant respiratory acidosis is present.
D. Yes, the metabolic compensation is appropriate.
E. No, a concomitant metabolic acidosis is present.
F. No, a concomitant metabolic alkalosis is present.

Q17-10: Which of the following is the most likely cause of the patient's respiratory alkalosis?

A. Liver failure/cirrhosis
B. Pulmonary edema
C. Pulmonary embolism
D. Cushing syndrome
E. Liddle syndrome
F. Milk-alkali syndrome

ANSWERS

Q17-1: B

While the patient has a condition predisposing him to a chronic acid-base disorder, there is insufficient information to estimate the patient's baseline $Paco_2$ and HCO_3 values; therefore, we will assume a baseline $Paco_2$ of 40 mm Hg and a baseline HCO_3 of 24 mEq/L. The patient has chronic congestive heart failure that can be associated with a chronic metabolic alkalosis (secondary to diuretic use or hypoaldosteronism) as well as with chronic metabolic acidosis in the setting of resultant CKD from poor forward flow. However, the vignette does not provide any evidence for a chronic acid-base disorder, so we will assume the standard baseline values as listed earlier.

Rationale: Ignoring these underlying chronic acid-base disorders can significantly alter the interpretation of a patient's acute acid-base status. This was demonstrated in the first case of the series. However, often, we do not have the necessary information (eg, prior ABG or VBG, or prior serum chemistry with an HCO_3) and are forced to assume the ongoing processes are all acute in nature. We are primarily concerned about chronic respiratory acid-base disorders, as these can significantly alter the patient's baseline or expected values for the serum HCO_3 and $Paco_2$, and we have reliable equations to predict the expected baseline values. The respiratory compensation for both chronic metabolic acidosis and alkalosis is generally poor, so there are no equations or rules to predict what the $Paco_2$ should be in these cases. While the baseline serum HCO_3 may be significantly off from our standard value of 24 mEq/L in these patients, we would assume a baseline $Paco_2$ of 40 mm Hg in patients with chronic metabolic processes. Once we identify the patient's baseline $Paco_2$ and HCO_3 values, we will need to use these values in the appropriate equations to identify the ongoing acute processes.

Q17-2: A

Metabolic acidosis only.

Rationale:

1. The pH is 7.35; therefore, the primary disorder is an **acidosis.**
2. The $Paco_2$ of 25 mm Hg is less than 40 mm Hg, so this is not the cause of acidosis.
3. The HCO_3 of 14 mEq/L is less than 24 mEq/L, so there is a **primary metabolic acidosis.**

Q17-3: C

8.5 mEq/L.

Rationale: The normal anion gap is 12 mEq/L. The term *anion gap* refers to those ions (negatively charged molecules) in the bloodstream that we do not routinely measure, including phosphates, sulfates, organic acids, and negatively charged plasma proteins. One of the most abundant negatively charged ions in the blood is serum albumin. A normal serum albumin is 4.0 g/dL. For patients with hypoalbuminemia (low serum albumin) the normal or expected anion gap is smaller.

$$\text{Expected Anion Gap} = 12 - (2.5) * \left[4.0 \frac{g}{dL} - \text{Actual Serum Albumin} \right].$$

So for this patient,

$$\text{Expected Anion Gap} = 12 - [2.5 * (4 - 2.6)] = 12 - (2.5 * 1.4) = 12\text{-}3.5 = 8.5 \text{ mEq/L}.$$

Q17-4: D
Anion gap acidosis and a metabolic alkalosis.

Rationale:

1. Is there evidence for a chronic respiratory acid-base disorder that requires adjustment of the patient's "normal" HCO_3? While the patient does have chronic congestive heart failure, which can be associated with various respiratory acid-base disorders, there is not enough information from the vignette to confirm that this patient has a chronic process, and therefore we will assume a serum HCO_3 of 24 mEq/L and a $Paco_2$ of 40 mm Hg.

2. Expected anion gap:

$$\text{Expected Anion Gap} = 12 - (2.5) * \left[4.0 \frac{g}{dL} - \text{Actual Serum Albumin} \right]$$

$$= 12 - (2.5 * [4.0 - 2.6])$$
$$= 12 - (2.5 * [1.4]) = \textbf{8.5 mEq/L.}$$

3. Anion gap calculation:

$$\text{Serum Anion Gap} = [Na^+] - [HCO_3^-] - [Cl^-]$$
$$128 - (84 + 14) = 30 \text{ mEq/L, which is} > 8.5 \text{ mEq/L}$$
$$\rightarrow \textbf{anion gap acidosis is present.}$$

4. Delta-delta calculation:

$$\Delta\Delta = \frac{(\text{Actual Anion Gap} - \text{Expected Anion Gap})}{(\text{Baseline } HCO_3 - \text{Actual } HCO_3)}$$

$$= (30 - 8.5)/(24 - 14) = \textbf{22.5/10, which is} \sim\textbf{2.25.}$$

Delta-delta interpretation.	
Delta-Delta Value	Condition Present
< 0.4	Non-anion gap only
0.4–0.9	Anion gap *and* non-anion gap acidosis
1.0–2.0	Anion gap acidosis only
> 2.0	**Anion gap acidosis and metabolic alkalosis**

The delta-delta value is 2.25, therefore this patient has an anion gap acidosis and a concomitant metabolic alkalosis.

Q17-5: C
7.

Rationale: Similar to the serum anion gap, the serum osmolal gap is determined by the difference between the "calculated" serum osmolality and the true measured serum osmolality. The equation for the serum osmolal gap typically includes factors for sodium, glucose, BUN, and ethanol, as these are readily measurable in most laboratories. Therefore, the serum osmolal gap will represent the osmolality of those "unmeasured" osmoles, including organic alcohols and acetone. The most common form is shown as follows:

$$\text{Calculated Serum Osmolality} = 2*[Na^+] + \frac{[\text{Glucose}]}{18} + \frac{[\text{BUN}]}{2.8} + \frac{[\text{EtOH}]}{3.7};$$

In which the units of measure are as follows: Na, mEq/L; glucose, mg/dL; BUN, mg/dL; and EtOH, mg/dL. The conversion factors are shown in the preceding equation as well. A normal serum osmolal gap is around −10 to +10 mOsm/L (or mOsm/kg).

Therefore, this patient,

$$\begin{aligned}\text{Calculated Serum Osmolality} &= [2*Na] + [\text{Glucose}/18] + [\text{BUN}/2.8] + [\text{EtOH}/3.7] \\ &= (2*128) + (104/18) + (44/2.8) + (0/3.7) \\ &= 277 \text{ mOsm/L.}\end{aligned}$$

$$\begin{aligned}\text{Serum Osmolal Gap} &= \text{Measured Serum Osmolality} - \text{Calculated Osmolality} \\ &= (284 - 277) = 7 \text{ mOsm/L, which is} < 10 \text{ mOsm/L}\end{aligned}$$

→ *no* **serum osmolal gap is present.**

Q17-6: B
Serum lactate.

Rationale: The patient's presentation with cool, wet extremities, hypotension, and evidence of pulmonary edema with a known history of severe systolic LV dysfunction should raise the concern for cardiogenic shock; therefore a lactic acidosis would be most likely. The next most likely causes would be PE leading to cardiogenic shock, septic shock, or hemorrhagic shock, all of which would manifest as a lactic acidosis as well. The most appropriate test to order next would be the serum lactate, which we would anticipate is significantly elevated. A serum BNP, while potentially helpful, can also be elevated in conditions such as pneumonia or pulmonary embolism. A serum procalcitonin could be helpful to rule out a bacterial infection; however, its utility in patients with renal dysfunction is unclear, and the patient has no other history suggestive of infection. A diagnostic paracentesis may help identify the cause of the ascites as portal hypertension, but this again does not get to the underlying cause of the non-anion gap acidosis.

Q17-7: B
Thiazide/loop diuretic use.

Rationale: The patient's urine chloride is elevated (> 20 mEq/L), indicating that a chloride-resistant process is present. Loop and thiazide diuretics, when in active use, cause a chloride-resistant metabolic alkalosis, as the drug is actively interfere with the resorption of sodium and chloride in the loop of Henle and distal tubule. When these drugs are metabolized and/or excreted, the alkalosis can shift from a chloride-resistant to a chloride-responsive process. This patient presented with daily use of furosemide, a loop diuretic, in addition to metolazone (a thiazide-like diuretic), which is the most likely cause of the patient's metabolic alkalosis. Acetazolamide use is associated with a non-anion gap metabolic acidosis/renal tubular acidosis. Hyperemesis is associated with a low urine chloride, typically, and the patient has no history of hyperemesis (however, note that a patient with hyperemesis who is also taking loop and/or thiazide diuretic could potentially have an elevated urine chloride). Primary aldosteronism is associated with a metabolic alkalosis with a high urinary chloride. However, this is typically also associated with hypertension and is unlikely in this patient. In cases of congestive heart failure, a metabolic alkalosis due to secondary hyperaldosteronism is possible, and this would be a reasonable answer to this question as well. Secondary hyperaldosteronism can develop from reduced blood flow to the kidneys, most commonly seen in renovascular disease (renal artery stenosis) and in edematous conditions such as congestive heart failure or cirrhosis.

Differential diagnosis of metabolic alkalosis.
History: Rule Out the Following as Causes
• Alkali load ("milk-alkali" or calcium-alkali syndrome, oral sodium bicarbonate, IV sodium bicarbonate)   • Genetic causes (CF)   • Presence of hypercalcemia   • IV β-lactam antibiotics   • Laxative abuse (may also cause a metabolic acidosis depending on diarrheal HCO_3 losses)
If None of the Above, Then…
Urine Chloride < 20 mEq/L (Chloride-Responsive Causes)
• Loss of gastric acid (hyperemesis, NGT suctioning)   • Prior diuretic use (in hours to days following discontinuation)   • Post-hypercapnia   • Villous adenoma   • Congenital chloridorrhea   • Chronic laxative abuse (may also cause a metabolic acidosis depending on diarrheal HCO_3 losses)   • Cystic fibrosis
OR
Urine Chloride > 20 mEq/L (Chloride-Resistant Causes)
Urine Chloride > 20 mEq/L, Lack of HTN, Urine Potassium < 30 mEq/L
• Hypokalemia or hypomagnesemia   • Laxative abuse (if dominated by hypokalemia)   • Bartter syndrome   • Gitelman syndrome

(Continued)

Differential diagnosis of metabolic alkalosis. (*continued*)
Urine Chloride > 20 mEq/L, Lack of HTN, Urine Potassium > 30 mEq/L
• Current diuretic use
Urine Chloride > 20 mEq/L, Presence of HTN, Urine Potassium Variable but Usually > 30 mEq/L
Elevated plasma renin level: • Renal artery stenosis • Renin-secreting tumor • Renovascular disease
Low plasma renin, low plasma aldosterone: • Cushing syndrome • Exogenous mineralocorticoid use • Genetic disorder (11-hydoxylase or 17-hydrolyase deficiency, 11β-HSD deficiency) • Liddle syndrome • Licorice toxicity
Low plasma renin, high plasma aldosterone: • Primary hyperaldosteronism • Adrenal adenoma • Bilateral adrenal hyperplasia

Q17-8: D
Plasma aldosterone-to-renin ratio.

Rationale: In chloride-resistant metabolic alkalosis, the patient's BP, physical examination, serum and urine potassium, plasma renin, and serum aldosterone levels can be used to differentiate these conditions. However, of note, the use of diuretics, including loop, thiazide, and potassium-sparing diuretics such as spironolactone (which directly impacts aldosterone effects in the kidney), as well as ACE inhibitors, can alter all of these results, so it is generally recommended that patients have a washout period of several days if not weeks before testing.

In primary hyperaldosteronism, as might occur with an adrenal adenoma or hyperplasia, patients are typically hypertensive, with low serum potassium, elevated urinary potassium, normal or mildly elevated serum sodium, markedly reduced plasma renin, and elevated serum aldosterone. Given that the plasma renin level is quite low and the aldosterone level is elevated, the ratio of aldosterone to renin is therefore elevated. Edema is rarely present in these conditions.

In secondary hyperaldosteronism resulting from renovascular disease, patients typically present with refractory hypertension, low serum potassium and elevated urinary potassium, normal serum sodium level, elevated plasma renin, and elevated serum aldosterone. Therefore, the aldosterone-to-renin ratio is lower than in primary hyperaldosteronism. Edema is rarely present in this condition.

In secondary hyperaldosteronism resulting from congestive heart failure, patients are typically normotensive, with low serum potassium, elevated urinary potassium, low serum sodium, elevated renin, and elevated aldosterone. The key factor that can differentiate this condition from other causes is the significant edema that is usually present. The pathogenesis is likely multifactorial, including reduced renal blood flow from poor forward flow, yielding activation of the hypovolemic response of the renin-angiotensin-aldosterone axis; reduced hepatic blood flow and/or congestion, leading to reduced aldosterone metabolism; and intravascular volume depletion from diuresis despite total body volume overload. Spironolactone is highly effective in the treatment of secondary hyperaldosteronism. More recent evidence also suggests a possible role of parathyroid hormone and calcium balance in the pathogenesis of secondary hyperaldosteronism.

Q17-9: B
No, a concomitant respiratory alkalosis is present.

Rationale: Using the Winter formula, one can calculate what the expected arterial $Paco_2$ should be for a given serum HCO_3 if the patient were completely compensated.

$$Expected\ Paco_2 = 1.5 * (Actual\ HCO_3) + 8\ (\pm 2)$$
$$= (1.5 * 14) + 8 = 21 + 8 = 29 \pm 2 = (27\ to\ 31)\ mm\ Hg.$$

This patient's $Paco_2$ is slightly below the expected level of 27 to 31 mm Hg so a respiratory alkalosis is also present.

Q17-10: B
Pulmonary edema.

Rationale: The patient presented with signs and symptoms of decompensated congestive heart failure, with both right- and left-sided symptoms. Pulmonary edema is therefore the most likely cause of the respiratory alkalosis. Although the patient has evidence of ascites, this may be due to portal hypertension secondary to elevated filling pressures in the heart and pulmonary hypertension, all due to congestive heart failure. Pulmonary edema generally leads to tachypnea and a respiratory alkalosis, as it is associated with reduced oxygenation more than reduced ventilation. However, patients with predisposing lung conditions, or those who are tiring from the work of breathing, may also develop a respiratory acidosis. A pulmonary embolism is another reasonable cause to consider, particularly in a patient presenting with hypotension and hypoxemia. However, the chest radiograph and the history are more consistent with pulmonary edema as the most likely cause. The remaining choices are all causes of metabolic alkalosis rather than respiratory alkalosis.

References

Byrd JB, Turcu AF, Auchus RJ. Primary aldosteronism. Circulation. 2018;138:823.

Chhokar VS, Sun Y, Bhattacharya SK, et al. Hyperparathyroidism and the calcium paradox of aldosteronism. Circulation. 2005;111:87.

Corry DB, Tuck ML. Secondary aldosteronism. Endocrinol Metab Clin North Am. 1995;24:511.

Frangiosa A, De Santo LS, Anastasio P, De Santo NG. Acid-base balance in heart failure. J Nephrol. 2006;19(suppl 9):S115-20.

Khanna A, Kurtzman NA. Metabolic alkalosis. J Nephrol. 2006;19(suppl 9):S86-96.

Urso C, Brucculeri S, Caimi G. Acid-base and electrolyte abnormalities in heart failure: pathophysiology and implications. Heart Fail Rev. 2015;20:493.

Oster JR, Preston RA, Materson BJ. Fluid and electrolyte disorders in congestive heart failure. Semin Nephrol. 1994;14:485.

Radó JP, Marosi J, Takó J. High doses of spironolactone (Aldactone, SC-14266, Verospirone) alone and in combination with triamterene and-or diuretics in the treatment of refractory edema associated with secondary hyperaldosteronism. Endokrinologie. 1970;57:46.

Romani JD. The secondary hyperaldosteronism of cardiac insufficiency. Pathogenic study and physiopathological implications. Presse Med. 1960;68:441.

Seller RH, Ramirez O, Brest AN. Secondary aldosteronism in refractory edema. GP. 1967;35:104.

Soifer JT, Kim HT. Approach to metabolic alkalosis. Emerg Med Clin North Am. 2014;32:453.

Weber KT, Villarreal D. Aldosterone and antialdosterone therapy in congestive heart failure. Am J Cardiol. 1993;71:3A.

CASE 18

A 44-year-old male veteran with a history of major depressive disorder (MDD), PTSD, anxiety and associated panic disorder, possible schizophrenia, and alcoholism presents to the emergency department with confusion, lightheadedness, and dyspnea. He reports a 2-week history of binge drinking, with 12 to 24 alcoholic beverages consumed daily during that time period. Approximately 2 to 3 days ago, he developed sharp, nonradiating epigastric pain, exacerbated by PO intake, and has had several episodes of emesis over the past 24 to 48 hours. He has had poor PO intake over the past week and cannot recall his last proper meal. He takes no medications regularly, although he was prescribed prazosin for PTSD and citalopram for depression. He reports his last drink was approximately 40 hours ago, primarily due to pain and emesis. He reports a desire to quit consuming alcohol. He denies any illicit drug use or other ingestions. He appears tremulous, is pacing around the room, and states that "people are out to get him." On examination, he is tachypneic, with RR of 32, HR 131, BP 166/76, and Sao_2 100% on RA. His cardiopulmonary examination is unremarkable. The patient has diffuse mild tenderness to palpation throughout the abdomen. In addition to the findings listed below, his lab tests reveal elevated lipase and amylase levels.

Laboratory data.

ABGs		Basic Metabolic Panel	
pH	7.53	Na	138 mEq/L
$Paco_2$	11 mm Hg	K	4.8 mEq/L
Pao_2	111 mm Hg	Cl	81 mEq/L
HCO_3	9 mEq/L	CO_2	9 mEq/L
		BUN	5 mg/dL
		Cr	1.8 mg/dL
		Glucose	266 mg/dL
		Albumin	5.9 g/dL
		EtOH	0 mg/dL

QUESTIONS

Q18-1: Define the patient's baseline acid-base status: Does this patient have an underlying chronic acid-base disorder that we need to account for in order to appropriately interpret the acute acid-base disorders?

A. There is no evidence for an underlying chronic respiratory or metabolic acid-base disorder in this patient, so we would assume a baseline $Paco_2$ of 40 mm Hg and an HCO_3 of 24 mEq/L.

B. While the patient has a condition predisposing him to a chronic acid-base disorder, there is insufficient information to estimate the patient's baseline $Paco_2$ and HCO_3 values; therefore, we will assume a baseline $Paco_2$ of 40 mm Hg and a baseline HCO_3 of 24 mEq/L.

C. The patient has an underlying acid-base condition, and we have sufficient information to estimate the patient's baseline $Paco_2$ and HCO_3 values.

Q18-2: What is/are the primary acid-base disturbance(s) occurring in this case?

A. Metabolic acidosis only
B. Respiratory acidosis only
C. Metabolic alkalosis only
D. Respiratory alkalosis only
E. Metabolic acidosis and a respiratory acidosis
F. Metabolic alkalosis and a respiratory alkalosis

Q18-3: For a perfectly healthy patient, a normal anion gap is assumed to be 12 mEq/L. What should be considered a normal anion gap in this patient?

A. 12 mEq/L
B. 10 mEq/L
C. 17 mEq/L
D. 9 mEq/L

Q18-4: Is a metabolic acidosis present, and, if so, how would the metabolic acid-base derangements be classified?

A. Anion gap acidosis.
B. Non-anion gap acidosis.
C. Anion and non-anion gap acidosis.
D. Anion gap acidosis and a metabolic alkalosis.
E. The reduction in the serum HCO_3 represents a complete metabolic compensation for the patient's respiratory alkalosis.

Q18-5: Laboratory testing returns the following results:

Serum EtOH	< 3 mg/dL
Serum acetaminophen level	< 5 mg/dL (ULN for therapeutic use 20 mg/dL)
Serum salicylates level	< 5 mg/dL (ULN for therapeutic use 30 mg/dL)

(Continued)

Serum osmolality	303 mOsm/kg
Serum L-lactate	2.8 mmol/L (ULN 2.0 mmol/L venous)
Beta-hydroxybutyrate (acetone)	2.77 mmol/L (ULN 0.18 mmol/L)
Serum glucose	266 mg/dL

What is the serum osmolal gap?

A. 0 mOsm/L
B. 9 mOsm/L
C. 22 mOsm/L
D. 59 mOsm/L

Q18-6: Additional laboratory values have resulted for the patient. The updated laboratory values are provided below. What is the likely primary cause of the patient's anion gap acidosis?

Serum EtOH	< 3 mg/dL
Serum acetaminophen level	< 5 mg/dL (ULN for therapeutic use 20 mg/dL)
Serum salicylates level	< 5 mg/dL (ULN for therapeutic use 30 mg/dL)
Serum osmolality	303 mOsm/kg
Serum L-lactate	2.8 mmol/L (ULN 2.0 mmol/L venous)
Beta-hydroxybutyrate (acetone)	2.77 mmol/L (ULN 0.18 mmol/L)
Serum glucose	266 mg/dL
Serum triglycerides	485 mg/dL

A. Alcoholic ketoacidosis
B. Diabetic ketoacidosis
C. Lactic acidosis
D. Renal failure
E. Metformin use
F. Hypoaldosteronism

Q18-7: Which of the following is not a common cause of respiratory alkalosis?

A. Aspirin overdose
B. Panic disorder
C. Pain
D. Hyperaldosteronism
E. Progesterone toxicity

Q18-8: You suspect the patient's metabolic acidosis is due to hyperemesis and volume depletion based on the preceding analyses. Your colleague believes it is due to primary hyperaldosteronism. What would you expect the patient's urine electrolyte panel to be if you are correct?

A. Urine Cl < 20 mEq/L
B. Urine Cl > 20 mEq/L
C. Urine Cl > 20 mEq/L and urine K < 30 mEq/L
D. Urine Cl > 20 mEq/L and urine K < 30 mEq/L

ANSWERS

Q18-1: B

While the patient has a condition predisposing him to a chronic acid-base disorder, there is insufficient information to estimate the patient's baseline $Paco_2$ and HCO_3 values; therefore, we will assume a baseline $Paco_2$ of 40 mm Hg and a baseline HCO_3 of 24 mEq/L. The patient has a several-week history of alcohol consumption, which can be associated with an acute or chronic metabolic acidosis. However, given the information provided, we will assume the process is acute.

Rationale: Ignoring these underlying chronic acid-base disorders can significantly alter the interpretation of a patient's acute acid-base status. This was demonstrated in the first case of the series. However, often, we do not have the necessary information (eg, prior ABG or VBG, or prior serum chemistry with an HCO_3) and are forced to assume the ongoing processes are all acute in nature. We are primarily concerned about chronic respiratory acid-base disorders, as these can significantly alter the patient's baseline or expected values for the serum HCO_3 and $Paco_2$, and we have reliable equations to predict the expected baseline values. The respiratory compensation for both chronic metabolic acidosis and alkalosis is generally poor, so there are no equations or rules to predict what the $Paco_2$ should be in these cases. While the baseline serum HCO_3 may be significantly off from our standard value 24 mEq/L in these patients, we would assume a baseline $Paco_2$ of 40 mm Hg in patients with chronic metabolic processes. Once we identify the patient's baseline $Paco_2$ and HCO_3 values, we will need to use these values in the appropriate equations to identify the ongoing acute processes.

Q18-2: D

Respiratory alkalosis only.

Rationale:

1. The pH is 7.06; therefore, the primary disorder is an **alkalosis.**
2. The $Paco_2$ of 11 mm Hg is less than 40 mm Hg, so there is a **primary respiratory alkalosis.**
3. The HCO_3 of 9 mEq/L is less than 24 mEq/L, so a primary metabolic alkalosis is not present.

Q18-3: C

17 mEq/L.

Rationale: The normal anion gap is 12 mEq/L. The term *anion gap* refers to those ions (negatively charged molecules) in the bloodstream that we do not routinely measure, including phosphates, sulfates, organic acids, and negatively charged plasma proteins. One of the most abundant negatively charged ions in the blood is serum albumin. A normal serum albumin is 4.0 g/dL. For patients with hypoalbuminemia (low serum albumin), the normal or expected anion gap is smaller.

$$\text{Expected Anion Gap} = 12 - (2.5) * \left[4.0 \frac{g}{dL} - \text{Actual Serum Albumin} \right].$$

So for this patient,

$$\text{Expected Anion Gap} = 12 - [2.5 * (4 - 5.9)] = 12 - (2.5 * -1.9)$$
$$= 12 - (-4.75) = 12 + 4.75 = \sim 17 \text{ mEq/L.}$$

Q18-4: D
Anion gap acidosis and a metabolic alkalosis.

Rationale:

1. Is there a metabolic acidosis? Yes, a respiratory alkalosis is present, so first we should determine whether the reduction in the patient's serum HCO_3 is expected as a compensatory mechanism. If the patient's respiratory alkalosis was acute respiratory alkalosis (as we have assumed), we would expect the patient's serum HCO_3 to be as follows:

Metabolic Compensation for Acute Respiratory Alkalosis:

$$\text{Expected } HCO_3 = \text{Baseline } HCO_3 - (0.20) [\text{Actual } Paco_2 - \text{Baseline } Paco_2]$$

$$\text{Expected Serum } HCO_3 = \text{Normal Serum } HCO_3$$
$$- [(\text{Normal } Paco_2 - \text{Actual } Paco_2) * 0.2]$$
$$= 24 - [(40\text{-}11) * 0.20] = 24 - [29 * 0.2] = 24 - 5.8 = 18.2 \text{ mEq/L.}$$

Since the serum HCO_3 is lower than 18.2 mEq/L, a concomitant metabolic acidosis appears to be present as well, which we will explore further. For a chronic respiratory alkalosis, the compensatory response of the kidney is more significant, and we would expect a serum HCO_3 of approximately 12.4 mEq/L. Even if the patient's serum HCO_3 was as expected for complete compensation in chronic respiratory alkalosis, it would be dangerous to assume that the patient has a chronic respiratory alkalosis without a supporting collateral history (a definite diagnosis of cirrhosis, etc), as the clinician might be missing another ongoing critical process. It would be safer to assume that an acute process is ongoing.

2. Expected anion gap (AG):

$$\text{Expected AG} = 12 - (2.5 * [4.0 - \text{Actual Albumin}])$$
$$= 12 - (2.5 * [4.0 - 5.9])$$
$$= 12 - (2.5 * [-1.9]) = \textbf{17 mEq/L.}$$

3. Anion gap calculation:

$$AG = Na - (Cl + HCO_3)$$
$$138 - (81 + 9) = 48 \text{ mEq/L, which is} > 17 \text{ mEq/L}$$
$$\rightarrow \textbf{anion gap acidosis is present.}$$

4. Delta-delta calculation:

$$(\text{Measured AG} - \text{Normal AG})/(\text{Normal } HCO_3 - \text{Measured } HCO_3)$$
$$(48 - 17)/(24 - 9) = \textbf{31/15, which is} \sim \textbf{2.1.}$$

Delta-delta interpretation.	
Delta-Delta Value	Condition Present
< 0.4	Non-anion gap only
0.4–0.9	Anion gap *and* non-anion gap acidosis
1.0–2.0	Anion gap acidosis only
> 2.0	**Anion gap acidosis and metabolic alkalosis**

The delta-delta value is 2.1, therefore this patient has an anion gap acidosis and a concomitant metabolic alkalosis.

Q18-5: B

9 mOsm/L.

Rationale: Similar to the serum anion gap, the serum osmolal gap is determined by the difference between the "calculated" serum osmolality and the true, measured serum osmolality. The equation for the serum osmolal gap typically includes factors for sodium, glucose, BUN, and ethanol, as these are readily measurable in most laboratories. Therefore, the serum osmolal gap will represent the osmolality of those "unmeasured" osmoles, including organic alcohols and acetone. The most common form is shown as follows:

$$\text{Calculated Serum Osmolality} = 2 * [Na^+] + \frac{[Glucose]}{18} + \frac{[BUN]}{2.8} + \frac{[EtOH]}{3.7};$$

In which the units of measure are as follows: Na, mEq/L; glucose, mg/dL; BUN, mg/dL; and EtOH, mg/dL. The conversion factors are shown in the preceding equation as well. A normal serum osmolal gap is around −10 to +10 mOsm/L (or mOsm/kg).

Therefore, for this patient,

$$\text{Calculated Serum Osmolality} = [2 * Na] + [Glucose/18] + [BUN/2.8] + [EtOH/3.7]$$
$$= (2 * 138) + (266/18) + (5/2.8) + (0/3.7)$$
$$= 293 \text{ mOsm/L.}$$

$$\text{Serum Osmolal Gap} = \text{Measured Serum Osmolality} - \text{Calculated Osmolality}$$
$$= (302 - 293) = 9 \text{ mOsm/L, which is} < 10 \text{ mOsm/L}$$
$$\rightarrow \textbf{no serum osmolal gap.}$$

Q18-6: A

Alcoholic ketoacidosis.

Rationale: The patient's laboratory studies are most consistent with a ketoacidosis as the primary cause of the anion gap acidosis. The patient's studies show a very mildly elevated lactate, positive serum BHB and urinary ketones, and some evidence of renal failure. Given the clinical scenario, the patient's renal failure is likely the result of volume depletion from the ketoacidosis, and while this is possibly contributing to the anion gap acidosis, it likely is not the primary cause given the lack of uremia. The patient does not have a history of metformin use or diabetes mellitus to suggest either of these conditions as the cause (we will come back to the elevated blood glucose in a moment). Additionally, the patient has no evidence of hypoaldosteronism (which is associated with a non-anion gap rather than an anion gap acidosis). The elevation in the lactate is, again, very mild, and unlikely to account for the presence of such a significant anion gap.

Alcoholic ketoacidosis typically occurs after periods of binge drinking associated with poor PO carbohydrate intake. In addition to the diuretic effects of alcohol (osmolar diuretic), patients will often develop gastritis or pancreatitis (as in this case) which leads to further volume depletion. This leads to a sympathetic response, resulting in reduced insulin secretion (and increased peripheral insulin resistance), increased glucagon release, and increased catecholamines. Metabolism shifts from glucose utilization to gluconeogenesis to protein catabolism and ketogenesis as fuel sources are consumed and insulin resistance increases. This leads to hyperglycemia and increased fatty release into the bloodstream to provide a fuel source for lipolysis. The metabolism of fatty acids to glycerol also further contributes to volume depletion through increasing the osmolar gap. The metabolism of alcohol, by stripping the body of reduced NAD (NADH), also prevents appropriate functioning of the Kreb cycle, leading to production of lactate through anaerobic metabolism and ketogenesis.

Alcoholic ketoacidosis should be considered in patients presenting with an anion gap acidosis and an appropriate history. It can have a very similar presentation to diabetic ketoacidosis, except that there is usually no prior history of diabetes. Glucose levels can vary from hypoglycemia to hyperglycemia, and an osmolar gap may be present depending on the time from last ethanol intake and the severity of lipolysis.

Q18-7: D
Hyperaldosteronism.

Rationale: Hyperaldosteronism is associated with a metabolic alkalosis rather than a respiratory acidosis. Both panic disorders and pain may be associated with acute respiratory alkalosis but are uncommon causes of chronic respiratory alkalosis. Aspirin is also a stimulant of the respiratory center and is associated with respiratory alkalosis. Pulmonary embolism is another common cause of a respiratory alkalosis. In this instance, the patient's panic disorder, PTSD, and schizophrenia are more likely causes of the respiratory alkalosis. Additionally, the abrupt discontinuation of alcohol may further contribute to anxiety and panic.

Q18-8: A
Urine Cl < 20 mEq/L.

Rationale: The urine chloride is a helpful tool in differentiating chloride-responsive versus chloride-resistant causes of metabolic alkalosis. The term *chloride responsive* indicates that the metabolic alkalosis improves or corrects with administration of an isotonic, chloride-containing fluid such as normal saline or lactated Ringer solution. Chloride-responsive causes of metabolic alkalosis include GI loss of acid (hyperemesis, villous adenoma, congenital hyperchloridorrhea), contraction alkalosis (including from diuretic use—*only* when the diuretics are discontinued does this convert to chloride-responsive etiology), sweat loss in cystic fibrosis, laxative abuse, ingestion of HCO_3, and in the post-hypercapnic period as the kidney is excreting retained HCO_3. Chloride-resistant causes include mechanisms that result in inappropriate renal loss of acid, including those with hypertension—primary hyperaldosteronism, congenital adrenal hyperplasia, secondary hyperaldosteronism, exogenous or congenital causes of increased mineralocorticoid or glucocorticoid, in some cases diuretics (particularly loop and thiazides) for the treatment of hypertension (not causing volume depletion), renovascular hypertension, and Liddle syndrome; those without hypertension—glycyrrhizin-containing products (eg, black licorice), Bartter or Gitelman syndrome, profound hypokalemia/hypomagnesemia; and diuretic use. Other causes of metabolic alkalosis where the urine chloride is less helpful include certain antibiotics (penicillins typically), milk-alkali syndrome, ingestion of large quantities of HCO_3, hypercalcemia, carbohydrate refeeding after a prolonged fast, massive transfusion, and possibly hypoproteinemia.

In chloride-responsive cases, the urine chloride is generally less than 10 to 20 mEq/L, as the kidney is attempting to retain all possible chloride and water. In chloride-resistance cases, the urine chloride is generally greater than 20 mEq/L. Additionally, the urine potassium can provide further information regarding the etiology of a chloride-resistant cause when coupled with the patient's BP.

Causes of metabolic alkalosis.
History: Rule Out the Following as Causes
• Alkali load ("milk-alkali" or calcium-alkali syndrome, oral sodium bicarbonate, IV sodium bicarbonate); • Genetic causes (CF) • Presence of hypercalcemia • IV β-lactam antibiotics • Laxative abuse (may also cause a metabolic acidosis depending on diarrheal HCO_3 losses)
If None of the Above, Then…
Urine Chloride < 20 mEq/L (Chloride-Responsive Causes)
• Loss of gastric acid (hyperemesis, NGT suctioning) • Prior diuretic use (in hours to days following discontinuation) • Post-hypercapnia • Villous adenoma • Congenital chloridorrhea • Chronic laxative abuse (may also cause a metabolic acidosis depending on diarrheal HCO_3 losses) • Cystic fibrosis
OR
Urine Chloride > 20 mEq/L (Chloride-Resistant Causes)
Urine Chloride > 20 mEq/L, Lack of HTN, Urine Potassium < 30 mEq/L
• Hypokalemia or hypomagnesemia • Laxative abuse (if dominated by hypokalemia) • Bartter syndrome • Gitelman syndrome

(Continued)

Causes of metabolic alkalosis. (*continued*)
Urine Chloride > 20 mEq/L, Lack of HTN, Urine Potassium > 30 mEq/L
• Current diuretic use
Urine Chloride > 20 mEq/L, Presence of HTN, Urine Potassium Variable but Usually > 30 mEq/L
Elevated plasma renin level: • Renal artery stenosis • Renin-secreting tumor • Renovascular disease
Low plasma renin, low plasma aldosterone: • Cushing syndrome • Exogenous mineralocorticoid use • Genetic disorder (11-hydoxylase or 17-hydrolyase deficiency, 11β-HSD deficiency) • Liddle syndrome • Licorice toxicity
Low plasma renin, high plasma aldosterone: • Primary hyperaldosteronism • Adrenal adenoma • Bilateral adrenal hyperplasia

Alternatively, measurements of the serum renin and aldosterone levels can provide additional information. The urine sodium is rarely helpful in this setting.

References

Allison MG, McCurdy MT. Alcoholic metabolic emergencies. Emerg Med Clin North Am. 2014;32:293.

Fulop M. Alcoholic ketoacidosis. Endocrinol Metab Clin North Am. 1993;22:209.

Gennari FJ. Pathophysiology of metabolic alkalosis: a new classification based on the centrality of stimulated collecting duct ion transport. Am J Kidney Dis. 2011;58:626.

Gennari FJ, Weise WJ. Acid-base disturbances in gastrointestinal disease. Clin J Am Soc Nephrol. 2008;3:1861.

Gillion V, Jadoul M, Devuyst O, Pochet JM. The patient with metabolic alkalosis. Acta Clin Belg. 2019;74:34.

Kraut JA, Madias NE. Serum anion gap: its uses and limitations in clinical medicine. Clin J Am Soc Nephrol. 2007;2:162.

McGuire L, Cruickshank A, Munro P. Alcoholic ketoacidosis. Emerg Med J. 2006;23:417.

Tanaka M, Myyazaki Y, Ishikawa S, Matsuyama K. Alcoholic ketoacidosis associated with multiple complications: report of 3 cases. Intern Med. 2004;43:955.

CASE 19

A 45-year-old man presents to your clinic with moderate confusion, having had multiple similar recent episodes at home recently. Approximately 1 year ago, the patient had a prolonged critical illness secondary to influenza A infection. He developed ARDS requiring ECMO support, which was further complicated by a secondary bacterial pneumonia, septic shock, and resultant ischemic bowel requiring resection of a significant amount of small bowel. He also suffered from *Clostridium difficile* infection during the hospitalization. Since, returning home, the patient had two additional bouts of *C difficile* infection requiring treatment. His wife reports that he intermittently has episodes of confusion, echolalia, and slurred speech. He has not been experiencing significant diarrhea recently. He does not drink alcohol or use illicit drugs, but his wife characterizes these episodes as the patient being in a "drunk-like" state. His medications include citalopram, pantoprazole, and *Lactobacillus*. On examination, the patient has some mild ataxia and slurred speech. He is disoriented. His mucous membranes are normal. His vital signs are all within normal limits: T 37.1°C, RR 20, HR 85, and BP 120/70.

Laboratory data.			
ABGs		Basic Metabolic Panel	
pH	7.24	Na	145 mEq/L
$Paco_2$	35 mm Hg	K	2.9 mEq/L
Pao_2	93 mm Hg	Cl	115 mEq/L
HCO_3	15 mEq/L	CO_2	15 mEq/L
		BUN	34 mg/dL
		Cr	0.6 mg/dL
		Glucose	103 mg/dL
		Albumin	3.6 g/dL
		EtOH	0 mg/dL

QUESTIONS

Q19-1: Define the patient's baseline acid-base status: Does this patient have an underlying chronic acid-base disorder that we need to account for in order to appropriately interpret the acute acid-base disorders?

A. There is no evidence for an underlying chronic respiratory or metabolic acid-base disorder in this patient, so we would assume a baseline $Paco_2$ of 40 mm Hg and an HCO_3 of 24 mEq/L.

B. While the patient has a condition predisposing him to a chronic acid-base disorder, there is insufficient information to estimate the patient's baseline $Paco_2$ and HCO_3 values; therefore, we will assume a baseline $Paco_2$ of 40 mm Hg and a baseline HCO_3 of 24 mEq/L.

C. The patient has an underlying acid-base condition, and we have sufficient information to estimate the patient's baseline $Paco_2$ and HCO_3 values.

Q19-2: What is/are the primary acid-base disturbance(s) occurring in this case?

A. Metabolic acidosis only
B. Respiratory acidosis only
C. Metabolic alkalosis only
D. Respiratory alkalosis only
E. Metabolic acidosis and a respiratory acidosis
F. Metabolic alkalosis and a respiratory alkalosis

Q19-3: How would the metabolic acidosis component be classified in this case?

A. Anion gap acidosis
B. Non-anion gap acidosis
C. Anion and non-anion gap acidosis
D. Anion gap acidosis and a metabolic alkalosis

Q19-4: Does the patient in this case demonstrate appropriate respiratory or metabolic compensation?

A. Yes, the respiratory compensation is appropriate.
B. No, a concomitant respiratory alkalosis is present.
C. No, a concomitant respiratory acidosis is present.
D. Yes, the metabolic compensation is appropriate.
E. No, a concomitant metabolic acidosis is present.
F. No, a concomitant metabolic alkalosis is present.

Q19-5: You begin to evaluate the patient's anion gap metabolic acidosis. Below are some additional laboratory results:

Serum EtOH	< 3 mg/dL
Serum acetaminophen level	< 5 mg/dL (ULN for therapeutic use 20 mg/dL)
Serum salicylates level	< 5 mg/dL (ULN for therapeutic use 30 mg/dL)
Serum osmolality	311 mOsm/kg
Serum L-lactate	1.1 mmol/L (ULN 2.0 mmol/L venous)
Beta-hydroxybutyrate (acetone)	< 0.18 mmol/L (ULN 0.18 mmol/L)
Serum glucose	103 mg/dL

What is the serum osmolal gap?

A. −8
B. 3
C. 11
D. 109

Q19-6. You decide to investigate the patient's non-anion gap acidosis. The results of the patient's urine studies are as follows:

Urine Na	33 mEq/L
Urine K	26 mEq/L
Urine Cl	27 mEq/L
Urine urea	215 mg/dL
Urine glucose	0 mg/dL
Urine osmolality	678 mOsm/L
Urine pH	5.1
Urine RBCs	None
Urine WBCs	None
Urine protein	None
Urine microscopic	None

What is the cause of the patient's non-anion gap acidosis?

A. Type 1 (distal) RTA
B. Type 4 RTA
C. GI losses of bicarbonate
D. Other disorder

Q19-7. What is the most likely unifying diagnosis in this patient?

A. Toluene ingestion
B. D-Lactic acidosis
C. Hypoaldosteronism
D. Diuretic abuse
E. Milk-alkali syndrome

ANSWERS

Q19-1: A

There is no evidence for an underlying chronic respiratory or metabolic acid-base disorder in this patient, so we would assume a baseline $Paco_2$ of 40 mm Hg and an HCO_3 of 24 mEq/L. While the patient had a significant illness the year before, there is no indication that he has an ongoing chronic acid-base disorder.

Rationale: Ignoring these underlying chronic acid-base disorders can significantly alter the interpretation of a patient's acute acid-base status. This was demonstrated in the first case of the series. However, often, we do not have the necessary information (eg, prior ABG or VBG, or prior serum chemistry with an HCO_3) and are forced to assume the ongoing processes are all acute in nature. We are primarily concerned about chronic respiratory acid-base disorders, as these can significantly alter the patient's baseline or expected values for the serum HCO_3 and $Paco_2$, and we have reliable equations to predict the expected baseline values. The respiratory compensation for both chronic metabolic acidosis and alkalosis is generally poor, so there are no equations or rules to predict what the $Paco_2$ should be in these cases. While the baseline serum HCO_3 may be significantly off from our standard value of 24 mEq/L in these patients, we would assume a baseline $Paco_2$ of 40 mm Hg in patients with chronic metabolic processes. Once we identify the patient's baseline $Paco_2$ and HCO_3 values, we will need to use these values in the appropriate equations to identify the ongoing acute processes.

Q19-2: A

Metabolic acidosis only.

Rationale:

1. The pH is 7.24; therefore, the primary disorder is an **acidosis.**
2. The $Paco_2$ of 35 mm Hg is less than 40 mm Hg, so this is not the cause of acidosis.
3. The HCO_3 of 15 mEq/L is less than 24 mEq/L, so there is a **metabolic acidosis.**

Q19-3: C

Anion and non-anion gap acidosis.

Rationale:

1. Is there evidence for a chronic respiratory acid-base disorder that requires adjustment of the patient's "normal" HCO_3? No, there is no evidence for an underlying chronic respiratory acid-base disorder, so we would assume a baseline $Paco_2$ of 40 mm Hg and an HCO_3 of 24 mEq/L.
2. Expected anion gap:

$$\text{Expected Anion Gap} = 12 - (2.5) * \left[4.0 \frac{g}{dL} - \text{Actual Serum Albumin} \right]$$

$$= 12 - (2.5 * [4.0 - 3.6])$$
$$= 12 - (2.5 * [0.4]) = \textbf{11 mEq/L.}$$

3. Anion gap calculation:

$$\text{Serum Anion Gap} = [Na^+] - [HCO_3^-] - [Cl^-]$$
$$145 - (115 + 15) = 15 \text{ mEq/L, which is} > 11 \text{ mEq/L}$$
$$\rightarrow \textbf{anion gap acidosis is present.}$$

4. Delta-delta calculation:

$$\Delta\Delta = \frac{(\text{Actual Anion Gap} - \text{Expected Anion Gap})}{(\text{Baseline HCO}_3 - \text{Actual HCO}_3)}$$

Therefore, for this patient,

$$\text{Delta-Delta} = (15 - 11)/(24 - 15) = \textbf{4/9, which is ~0.44.}$$

Delta-delta interpretation.	
Delta-Delta Value	Condition Present
< 0.4	Non-anion gap only
0.4–0.9	**Anion gap *and* non-anion gap acidosis**
1.0–2.0	Anion gap acidosis only
> 2.0	Anion gap acidosis and metabolic alkalosis

Therefore, this patient appears to have both an anion gap acidosis as well as a non-anion gap acidosis.

Q19-4: C
No, a concomitant respiratory acidosis is present.

Rationale: Using the Winter formula, one can calculate what the expected arterial $Paco_2$ should be for a given serum HCO_3 if the patient were completely compensated.

Respiratory Compensation for Acute Metabolic Acidosis (Winter Formula):

$$\text{Expected Paco}_2 = 1.5 * [\text{Actual HCO}_3] + 8 \pm 2 \text{ (in mm Hg).}$$

So for this patient,

$$\text{Expected Paco}_2 = 1.5 * (\text{Actual HCO}_3) + 8 (\pm 2)$$
$$= (1.5 * 15) + 8 = 22.5 + 8 = 30.5 \pm 2 = (28.5 \text{ to } 32.5) \text{ mm Hg.}$$

This patient's $Paco_2$ is 35 mm Hg, which is higher than the expected range for appropriate compensation. Therefore, in this patient a concomitant respiratory acidosis is present, as well as an anion gap and non-anion gap metabolic acidosis. This may be due to residual lung scarring from his prior bout of ARDS.

Q19-5: B
3.

Rationale: Similar to the serum anion gap, the serum osmolal gap is determined by the difference between the "calculated" serum osmolality and the true, measured serum osmolality. The equation for the serum osmolal gap typically includes factors for sodium, glucose, BUN, and ethanol, as these are readily measurable in most laboratories. Therefore, the serum osmolal gap will represent the osmolality of those "unmeasured" osmoles, including organic alcohols and acetone. The most common form is shown as follows:

$$\text{Calculated Serum Osmolality} = 2*[Na^+] + \frac{[Glucose]}{18} + \frac{[BUN]}{2.8} + \frac{[EtOH]}{3.7};$$

In which the units of measure are as follows: Na, mEq/L; glucose, mg/dL; BUN, mg/dL; and EtOH, mg/dL. The conversion factors are shown in the preceding equation as well. A normal serum osmolal gap is around −10 to +10 mOsm/L (or mOsm/kg).

Therefore, for this patient,

$$\begin{aligned}
\text{Calculated Serum Osmolality} &= [2*Na] + [Glucose/18] + [BUN/2.8] + [EtOH/3.7] \\
&= (2*145) + (103/18) + (34/2.8) + (0/3.7) \\
&= 308 \text{ mOsm/L.}
\end{aligned}$$

$$\begin{aligned}
\text{Serum Osmolal Gap} &= \text{Measured Serum Osmolality} - \text{Calculated Osmolality} \\
&= (311 - 308) = 3 \text{ mOsm/L, which is} < 10 \text{ mOsm/L} \\
&\rightarrow no \text{ serum osmolal gap.}
\end{aligned}$$

Given the earlier information, the cause of the patient's anion gap acidosis remains unclear. The cause does not appear to be a ketoacidosis, L-lactic acidosis, organic alcohol ingestion, salicylate ingestion, or acetaminophen ingestion. Additionally, the patient does not have acute renal failure.

Q19-6: D
Other disorder.

Rationale: This is an important case in which the urine anion gap can be misleading, and the urine osmolar gap is more helpful. Recall the limitations of the urine anion gap.

The urine anion gap can be inappropriately elevated in **severe anion gap acidosis**, a situation in which multiple unmeasured anions may be present in the urine (beta-hydroxybutyrate/acetoacetate [ketoacidosis], hippurate [toluene], bicarbonate [proximal RTA], D-lactate [D-lactic acidosis], L-lactate, 5-oxoproline [acetaminophen toxicity]). Therefore, in patients with a significant anion gap, the urine osmolar gap is typically more useful.

First, we will look at the urine anion gap:

$$\text{Urine Anion Gap} = [N_{Na}] + [U_K] - [U_{Cl}]$$
$$\text{UAG} = U_{Na} + U_K - U_{Cl} = (33 + 26) - 27 = (+32).$$

Interpretation:

- A UAG that is greater than ~20 → reduced renal acid excretion (RTA).
- A UAG that is −20 → GI loss of bicarbonate (eg, diarrhea), although type 2 RTA is possible.
- A UAG between −20 and +10 is generally considered inconclusive.

Based on this information alone, one would assume that the patient's non-anion gap acidosis is due to a reduced ability of the kidney to acidify the urine, consistent with a potential RTA. We may be tempted to make a diagnosis of distal RTA. However, the urine pH is quite low for a type 1 RTA, and the serum potassium is quite low for a type 4 RTA.

Diagnosis of RTA.			
	Type 1 RTA	Type 2 RTA	Type 4 RTA
Severity of metabolic acidosis, (HCO$_3$)	Severe (< 10–12 mEq/L typically)	Intermediate (12–20 mEq/L)	Mild (15–20 mEq/L)
Associated urine abnormalities	Urinary phosphate, calcium are increased; bone disease often present	Urine glucose, amino acids, phosphate, calcium may be elevated	
Urine pH	HIGH (> 5.5)	Low (acidic), until serum HCO$_3$ level exceeds the resorptive ability of the proximal tubule; then becomes alkalotic once reabsorptive threshold is crossed	Low (acidic)
Serum K$^+$	Low to normal; should correct with oral HCO$_3$ therapy	Classically low, although may be normal or even high with rare genetic defects; worsens with oral HCO$_3$ therapy	HIGH
Renal stones	Often	No	No
Renal tubular defect	Reduced NH$_4$ secretion in distal tubule	Reduced HCO$_3$ resorption in proximal tubule	Reduced H$^+$/K$^+$ exchange in distal and collecting tubule due to decreased aldosterone or aldosterone resistance
Urine anion gap	> 10	Negative	> 10
Urine osmolal gap	Reduced during acute acidosis		Reduced during acute acidosis

As we noted earlier, in patients with a high anion gap acidosis, the UAG can be misleading as the unmeasured anions in the bloodstream are excreted with sodium and potassium, leading to a falsely elevated UAG. In this situation, the urine osmolar gap is more useful.

Here the urine osmolar gap is:

$$\text{Calculated Urine Osmolality} = 2 * ([Na^+] + [K^+]) + \frac{[Urea]}{2.8} + \frac{[Glucose]}{18}$$

Urine Osmolal Gap (UOG) = Measured Urine Osmolality − Measured Urine Osmolality.

Therefore, for this patient,

Calculated Urine Osmolarity = 2 * ([U_{Na}] + [U_K]) + (U_{Urea} (mg/dL)/2.8]
  + [$U_{glucose}$ (mg/dL)/18]

Calculated Urine Osmolarity = 2 * [33 + 26] + [215/2.8] + [0/18] = 195 mOsm/L

UOG = Measured Urine Osmolality
  − Calculated Serum Osmolality

UOG = 678 − 195 Osm/L = 483 mOsm/L.

The UOG is more reliable than the UAG in patients with a high anion gap acidosis, whereas the UAG is generally more appropriate in patients with a serum osmolal gap. Similar to the UAG, the UOG is used as a surrogate for the urine ammonium concentration. Therefore, a larger gap indicates increased urinary NH_4 excretion. In normal acid-base conditions, the UOG is between 10 and 100 mOsm/L. During a significant metabolic acidosis, patients with impaired renal tubular acidification (type 1 and type 4 RTA) are unable to excrete additional acid (NH_4), and therefore the osmolar gap does not change/increase appropriately. Patients with an intact renal response to acidemia (ie, GI losses) should have a significant urine osmolar gap ($\sim$ >300 to 400 mOsm/L) as a result of increased NH_4 excretion.

The elevated UOG indicates that the patient has a preserved ability to acidify the urine. Therefore, options A and B are not correct. There is no indication of significant diarrhea noted in the history, and typically the UAG will be negative in cases of chronic diarrhea. Therefore, it seems that some alternative diagnosis is responsible for the patient's anion gap acidosis.

Q19-7: B
D-Lactic acidosis.

Rationale: This is a classic presentation of D-lactic acidosis. This is a disorder that occurs most commonly in patients with malabsorption disorders or short gut syndrome, although it may also be associated with large-volume ingestions of infusion or propylene glycol or severe diabetic ketoacidosis. The presenting symptoms are typically neurologic in nature including confusion, encephalopathy, ataxia, and slurred speech. In humans, L-lactate is produced from anaerobic metabolism and is largely utilized by the liver to generate pyruvate (although it also is excreted in the urine). D-lactate, on the other hand, is not normally produced during metabolism in humans (with the two exceptions noted below) and cannot be converted to pyruvate by lactate dehydrogenase (a stereospecific enzyme). D-Lactic acid can be produced by gram-positive anaerobes, such as *Lactobacillus* in colon. In normal subjects, the vast majority of carbohydrates are absorbed or metabolized in the small intestine, but in patients with malabsorption syndromes, significant carbohydrate loads can be delivered to the large intestine, leading to generation of D-lactic acid. D-lactate can also be produced during metabolism of propylene glycol and acetone/dihydroxyacetone (produced during ketoacidosis). Importantly, the enzymatic assay used in most laboratories for determination of lactate concentration is stereospecific and will not detect D-lactate. A chromatographic assay or a stereospecific enzyme assay is required to detect D-lactate in the urine or serum.

D-Lactic acid is converted into a hydrogen ion and D-lactate. The hydrogen ion reacts with HCO_3 to yield CO_2 and water, leading to the reduction in serum HCO_3. The increased D-lactate anion concentration accounts for the increased anion gap. However, D-lactate is not well absorbed in the kidney (again due to stereospecificity of the L-lactate transporter). As a result, the anion can be excreted quickly through the urine. When it is excreted, it is generally excreted with Na^+ or K^+ in addition to NH_4^+. As a result of the increased Na^+ and K^+ excretion, patients may also have hypokalemia and hypovolemia. This also leads to retention of chloride as NH_4 is excreted with alternate anions. Overall, this has the effect of increasing the urine anion gap despite the fact that the kidney is able to appropriately acidify the urine.

Patients with D-lactic acidosis in short bowel syndrome often experience transient symptoms after large carbohydrate loads. This can be further exacerbated by antibiotics that modify the colonic flora or increase the concentration of D-lactic acid-producing bacteria in the colon. The predominant symptoms are likely due to other toxins produced in concert with D-lactate, as D-lactate has not been shown to induce such change alone.

References

Coronado BE, Opal SM, Yoburn DC. Antibiotic-induced D-lactic acidosis. Ann Intern Med 1995;122:839.

Halperin ML, Kamel KS. D-lactic acidosis: turning sugar into acids in the gastrointestinal tract. Kidney Int 1996;49:1.

Jorens PG, Demey HE, Schepens PJ, et al. Unusual D-lactic acid acidosis from propylene glycol metabolism in overdose. J Toxicol Clin Toxicol 2004;42:163.

Lu J, Zello GA, Randell E, et al. Closing the anion gap: contribution of D-lactate to diabetic ketoacidosis. Clin Chim Acta 2011;412:286.

Stolberg L, Rolfe R, Gitlin N, et al. d-Lactic acidosis due to abnormal gut flora: diagnosis and treatment of two cases. N Engl J Med 1982;306:1344.

Uribarri J, Oh MS, Carroll HJ. D-lactic acidosis. A review of clinical presentation, biochemical features, and pathophysiologic mechanisms. Medicine (Baltimore) 1998;77:73.

Yilmaz B, Schibli S, Macpherson AJ, Sokollik C. D-lactic Acidosis: successful suppression of D-lactate-producing *Lactobacillus* by probiotics. Pediatrics. 2018 Sep;142(3): e20180337. doi: 10.1542/peds.2018-0337. Epub 2018 Aug 8.

CASE 20

A 55-year-old man with alcoholic cirrhosis complicated by hepatic encephalopathy, large-volume ascites, and varices presents to the hospital with complaints of lightheadedness and dizziness several days after a transjugular intrahepatic portosystemic shunt (TIPS) procedure. After the procedure, his gastroenterologist increased his lactulose dose considerably to prevent the development of encephalopathy post-procedure. Since then the patient has been experiencing high-volume, frequent bowel movements. He has also continued to take his diuretic regimen, including furosemide and spironolactone. His CXR is clear, and the patient's ECG shows only sinus tachycardia. His vital signs are as follows: T 37.2°C, RR 24, HR 109, and BP 85/35. On examination, he has large-volume ascites with a nontender abdomen. The patient is mildly jaundiced. Referring back to his laboratory results at the time of the TIPS procedure, he has a normal serum HCO_3 (24 mEq/L) and a normal $Paco_2$ (40 mm Hg) on an ABG.

Laboratory data.			
ABGs		Basic Metabolic Panel	
pH	7.49	Na	124 mEq/L
$Paco_2$	21 mm Hg	K	3.1 mEq/L
Pao_2	70 mm Hg	Cl	104 mEq/L
HCO_3	16 mEq/L	CO_2	16 mEq/L
		BUN	5 mg/dL
		Cr	0.3 mg/dL
		Glucose	144 mg/dL
		Albumin	2.0 g/dL
		EtOH	0 mg/dL

QUESTIONS

Q20-1: What is/are the primary acid-base disturbance(s) occurring in this case?

A. Metabolic acidosis only
B. Metabolic alkalosis only
C. Respiratory alkalosis only
D. Respiratory acidosis only
E. Metabolic acidosis and a respiratory acidosis
F. Metabolic alkalosis and a respiratory alkalosis

Q20-2: For a perfectly healthy patient, a normal anion gap is assumed to be 12 mEq/L. What should be considered a normal anion gap in this patient?

A. 12 mEq/L
B. 10 mEq/L
C. 7 mEq/L
D. 4 mEq/L

Q20-3: Which of the following is the most likely cause of the patient's respiratory alkalosis?

A. Aspirin overdose
B. Liver failure
C. Pulmonary embolism
D. Neuromuscular disorder (eg, ALS)

Q20-4: If we assume the respiratory alkalosis is *acute*, is there a concomitant metabolic acidosis, and if so, how would the metabolic acidosis component be classified in this case?

A. Anion gap acidosis.
B. Non-anion gap acidosis.
C. Anion and non-anion gap acidosis.
D. Anion gap acidosis and a metabolic alkalosis.
E. No metabolic acidosis; the reduction in serum HCO_3 represents appropriate metabolic compensation.

Q20-5: You decide to investigate the patient's non-anion gap acidosis. The results of the patient's urine studies are as follows:

Urine Na	10 mEq/L
Urine K	8 mEq/L
Urine Cl	NA
Urine urea	75 mg/dL
Urine glucose	0 mg/dL
Urine osmolality	545 mOsm/L
Urine pH	7.7
Urine RBCs	None
Urine WBCs	None
Urine protein	None
Urine microscopic	None

What is the cause of the patient's non-anion gap acidosis?

A. Type 1 (distal) RTA
B. Type 2 (proximal) RTA
C. GI losses of bicarbonate
D. Type 4 RTA

ANSWERS

Q20-1: C
Respiratory alkalosis only.

Rationale:

1. The pH is 7.49; therefore, the primary disorder is an **alkalosis.**
2. The $Paco_2$ of 21 mm Hg is less than 40 mm Hg, so there is a **respiratory alkalosis.**
3. The HCO_3 of 18 mEq/L is less than 24 mEq/L, so there is **no metabolic alkalosis.**

Q20-2: C
7 mEq/L.

Rationale: The normal anion gap is 12 mEq/L. The term *anion gap* refers to those ions (negatively charged molecules) in the bloodstream that we do not routinely measure, including phosphates, sulfates, organic acids, and negatively charged plasma proteins. One of the most abundant negatively charged ions in the blood is serum albumin. A normal serum albumin is 4.0 g/dL. For patients with hypoalbuminemia (low serum albumin), the normal or expected anion gap is smaller.

$$\text{Expected Anion Gap} = 12 - (2.5) * \left[4.0 \, \frac{\text{g}}{\text{dL}} - \text{Actual Serum Albumin} \right].$$

So for this patient,

$$\text{Expected Anion Gap} = 12 - [2.5 * (4 - 2)] = 12 - (2.5 * 2) = 7 \, \text{mEq/L}.$$

This is an important concept, as patients with hypoalbuminemia may "hide" an anion gap acidosis if this correction is not performed. This is particularly important for patients with cirrhosis or other malnutrition states.

Q20-2: B
Liver failure.

Rationale: Liver failure is associated with respiratory alkalosis due to an inability to clear or metabolize hormones and other compounds (eg, progesterone), which can stimulate the respiratory centers. Aspirin is also a stimulant of the respiratory center. Pulmonary embolism is another common cause of a respiratory alkalosis, and this patient's vignette is most consistent with an acute pulmonary embolism. Neuromuscular disorders are more commonly associated with a respiratory acidosis, although intracranial pathology can also produce a respiratory alkalosis. In this patient, the most likely cause of the respiratory alkalosis is cirrhosis.

Q20-4: B
Non-anion gap acidosis.

Rationale: While cirrhosis can cause a chronic respiratory alkalosis, we will assume that the patient developed an acute respiratory alkalosis as a result of the recent TIPS procedure. This is supported by the fact that the patient had a normal acid-base status at the time of the TIPS procedure. We can estimate the HCO_3 for an appropriate metabolic compensation to a respiratory alkalosis (acute) as follows:

Metabolic Compensation for Acute Respiratory Alkalosis:

$$\text{Expected } HCO_3 = \text{Baseline } HCO_3 - (0.20)\, [\text{Actual } Paco_2 - \text{Baseline } Paco_2]$$
$$= 24 - [0.2 * (40 - 21)] = 24 - [0.2 * 19] = 24 - 4 = 20 \text{ mEq/L}.$$

As the patient's current serum HCO_3 is 16, which is less than the expected 20 mEq/L, we would assume a concomitant metabolic acidosis is present.

Next, we calculate the anion gap:

$$\text{Expected Anion Gap} = 7 \text{ mEq/L}$$
$$\text{Actual Anion Gap} = (124 - 104 - 16)$$
$$= 4 \text{ mEq/L; therefore } \textbf{no anion gap is present.}$$

We would therefore assume the metabolic acidosis is due to a **non-anion gap acidosis**.

Note, again how important it is to identify the chronicity of a process. If we had assumed the respiratory alkalosis as *chronic* rather than acute, we would have missed the concomitant metabolic acidosis.

Metabolic Compensation for Chronic Respiratory Alkalosis:

$$\text{Expected } HCO_3 = \text{Baseline } HCO_3 - (0.40)\, [\text{Actual } Paco_2 - \text{Baseline } Paco_2]$$
$$= 24 - [0.4 * (40 - 21)] = 24 - [0.4 * 19] = 24 - 8 = 16 \text{ mEq/L}.$$

Therefore, the HCO_3 of 16 mEq/L would have represented an appropriate metabolic compensation for a *chronic* respiratory alkalosis, and we would assume there was no additional metabolic acidosis.

Q20-5: C
GI losses of bicarbonate.

Rationale: We were not provided with a urine chloride level, but we have enough information to calculate the urine osmolar gap (UOG):

$$\text{Calculated Urine Osmolality} = 2 * ([Na^+] + [K^+]) + \frac{[\text{Urea}]}{2.8} + \frac{[\text{Glucose}]}{18}$$

$$\text{UOG} = \text{Measured Urine Osmolality}$$
$$- \text{Measured Urine Osmolality}.$$

Therefore, for this patient,

$$\text{Calculated Urine Osmolarity} = 2 * [10 + 8] + [75/2.8] + [0/18] = 63 \text{ mOsm/L}$$
$$\text{UOG} = 545 - 63 \text{ Osm/L} = 482 \text{ mOsm/L}.$$

Similar to the urine anion gap, the UOG is used as a surrogate for the urine ammonium concentration. Therefore, a larger gap indicates increased urinary NH_4 excretion. In normal acid-base conditions, the UOG is between 10 and 100 mOsm/L. During a significant metabolic acidosis, patients with impaired renal tubular acidification (type 1 and type 4 RTA) are unable to excrete additional acid (NH_4), and therefore the osmolar gap does not change. Patients with an intact renal response to acidemia (ie, GI losses) should have a significant UOG (~ > 400 mOsm/L) as a result of increased NH_4 excretion. Therefore, we would assume this patient's non-anion gap acidosis is due to HCO_3 losses in the GI tract, likely secondary to the diarrhea described by the patient on presentation.

References

Adrogué HJ, Madias NE. Secondary responses to altered acid-base status: the rules of engagement. J Am Soc Nephrol 2010; 21:920.

Batlle D, Chin-Theodorou J, Tucker BM. Metabolic Acidosis or Respiratory Alkalosis? Evaluation of a Low Plasma Bicarbonate Using the Urine Anion Gap. Am J Kidney Dis. 2017 Sep;70(3):440-444. doi: 10.1053/j.ajkd.2017.04.017. Epub 2017 Jun 7.

Batlle D, Grupp M, Gaviria M, Kurtzman NA. Distal renal tubular acidosis with intact capacity to lower urinary pH. Am J Med 1982; 72:751.

Batlle D, Haque SK. Genetic causes and mechanisms of distal renal tubular acidosis. Nephrol Dial Transplant 2012; 27:3691.

Batlle DC, Hizon M, Cohen E, Gutterman C, Gupta R. The use of the urinary anion gap in the diagnosis of hyperchloremic metabolic acidosis. N Engl J Med. 1988 Mar 10;318(10):594-9.

Batlle DC, von Riotte A, Schlueter W. Urinary sodium in the evaluation of hyperchloremic metabolic acidosis. N Engl J Med 1987; 316:140.

Berend K, de Vries AP, Gans RO. Physiological approach to assessment of acid-base disturbances. N Engl J Med. 2014 Oct 9;371(15):1434-45. doi: 10.1056/NEJMra1003327.

Buckalew VM Jr, McCurdy DK, Ludwig GD, et al. Incomplete renal tubular acidosis. Physiologic studies in three patients with a defect in lowering urine pH. Am J Med 1968; 45:32.

Dyck RF, Asthana S, Kalra J, et al. A modification of the urine osmolal gap: an improved method for estimating urine ammonium. Am J Nephrol 1990; 10:359.

Farwell WR, Taylor EN. Serum anion gap, bicarbonate and biomarkers of inflammation in healthy individuals in a national survey. CMAJ 2010; 182:137.

Feldman M, Soni N, Dickson B. Influence of hypoalbuminemia or hyperalbuminemia on the serum anion gap. J Lab Clin Med 2005; 146:317.

Gardner WN. The pathophysiology of hyperventilation disorders. Chest 1996; 109:516.

Karet FE. Mechanisms in hyperkalemic renal tubular acidosis. J Am Soc Nephrol 2009; 20:251.

Kim GH, Han JS, Kim YS, et al. Evaluation of urine acidification by urine anion gap and urine osmolal gap in chronic metabolic acidosis. Am J Kidney Dis 1996; 27:42.

Kraut JA, Madias NE. Differential diagnosis of nongap metabolic acidosis: value of a systematic approach. Clin J Am Soc Nephrol. 2012 Apr;7(4):671-9. doi: 10.2215/CJN.09450911. Epub 2012 Mar 8.

Kraut JA, Nagami GT. The serum anion gap in the evaluation of acid-base disorders: what are its limitations and can its effectiveness be improved? Clin J Am Soc Nephrol 2013; 8:2018.

Meregalli P, Lüthy C, Oetliker OH, Bianchetti MG. Modified urine osmolal gap: an accurate method for estimating the urinary ammonium concentration? Nephron 1995; 69:98.

Rastegar A. Use of the DeltaAG/DeltaHCO3- ratio in the diagnosis of mixed acid-base disorders. J Am Soc Nephrol 2007; 18:2429.

Rastegar M, Nagami GT. Non-Anion Gap Metabolic Acidosis: A Clinical Approach to Evaluation. Am J Kidney Dis. 2017 Feb;69(2):296-301. doi: 10.1053/j.ajkd.2016.09.013. Epub 2016 Oct 28.

Rodríguez Soriano J. Renal tubular acidosis: the clinical entity. J Am Soc Nephrol 2002; 13:2160.

Rose BD, Post TW. Clinical Physiology of Acid-Base and Electrolyte Disorders, 5th ed, McGraw-Hill, New York 2001. p.583.

Wang F, Butler T, Rabbani GH, Jones PK. The acidosis of cholera. Contributions of hyperproteinemia, lactic acidemia, and hyperphosphatemia to an increased serum anion gap. N Engl J Med 1986; 315:1591.

CASE 21

A 66-year-old woman presents to the emergency department (ED) with fevers and generalized weakness. The patient underwent lung transplantation 22 years ago and has a diagnosis of chronic rejection. She also has a diagnosis of osteoporosis. Her medications include hydrochlorothiazide (HCTZ), lisinopril, mycophenolate, tacrolimus, prednisone, pantoprazole, and atovaquone. Twelve years ago, she developed bladder cancer, requiring a radical cystectomy and the creation of an ileal conduit for urinary diversion. The stoma has been well-healed. Unfortunately, she had had frequent complications with recurrent pyelonephritis. Her vital signs are T 39.6°C, RR 38, HR 133, BP 70/40, and Sao$_2$ 94% on 2 L NC. On examination, she has considerable right flank tenderness. A CXR is clear. An ECG reveals sinus tachycardia. Her daughter, who accompanied her to the ED, notes that the patient has had significantly reduced urine output over the past 24 hours. The patient's laboratory values are as follows:

Laboratory data.			
ABGs		Basic Metabolic Panel	
pH	7.06	Na	132 mEq/L
Paco$_2$	46 mm Hg	K	3.3 mEq/L
Pao$_2$	70 mm Hg	Cl	101 mEq/L
HCO$_3$	13 mEq/L	CO$_2$	13 mEq/L
		BUN	55 mg/dL
		Cr	1.2 mg/dL
		Glucose	104 mg/dL
		Albumin	3.3 g/dL
		EtOH	0 mg/dL

QUESTIONS

Q21-1: Define the patient's baseline acid-base status: Does this patient have an underlying chronic acid-base disorder that we need to account for in order to appropriately interpret the acute acid-base disorders?

A. There is no evidence for an underlying chronic respiratory or metabolic acid-base disorder in this patient, so we would assume a baseline $Paco_2$ of 40 mm Hg and an HCO_3 of 24 mEq/L.

B. While the patient has a condition predisposing her to a chronic acid-base disorder, there is insufficient information to estimate the patient's baseline $Paco_2$ and HCO_3 values; therefore, we will assume a baseline $Paco_2$ of 40 mm Hg and a baseline HCO_3 of 24 mEq/L.

C. The patient has an underlying acid-base condition, and we have sufficient information to estimate the patient's baseline $Paco_2$ and HCO_3 values.

Q21-2: What is/are the primary acid-base disturbance(s) occurring in this case?

A. Metabolic acidosis only
B. Respiratory acidosis only
C. Metabolic alkalosis only
D. Respiratory alkalosis only
E. Metabolic acidosis and a respiratory acidosis
F. Metabolic alkalosis and a respiratory alkalosis

Q21-3: For a perfectly healthy patient, a normal anion gap is assumed to be 12 mEq/L. What should be considered a normal anion gap in this patient?

A. 12 mEq/L
B. 10 mEq/L
C. 7 mEq/L
D. 4 mEq/L

Q21-4: How would the metabolic acidosis component be classified in this case?

A. Anion gap acidosis
B. Non-anion gap acidosis
C. Anion and non-anion gap acidosis
D. Anion gap acidosis and a metabolic alkalosis

Q21-4: Additional laboratory testing returns the following results:

Serum EtOH	< 3 mg/dL
Serum acetaminophen level	< 5 mg/dL (ULN for therapeutic use 20 mg/dL)
Serum salicylates level	< 5 mg/dL (ULN for therapeutic use 30 mg/dL)
Serum osmolality	290 mOsm/kg
Serum L-lactate	6.7 mmol/L (ULN 2.0 mmol/L venous)
Beta-hydroxybutyrate (acetone)	< 0.18 mmol/L (ULN 0.18 mmol/L)
Serum glucose	66 mg/dL

What is the likely etiology of the patient's anion gap acidosis?

A. Methanol intoxication
B. Urinary diversion
C. Renal failure
D. Lactic acidosis
E. Salicylate intoxication

Q21-5: This patient has a concomitant respiratory acidosis with an elevated $Paco_2$ of 46 mm Hg. If the patient were compensating appropriately for the metabolic acidosis, what would be the patient's expected $Paco_2$?

A. 20 mm Hg
B. 22 mm Hg
C. 27 mm Hg
D. 32 mm Hg
E. 36 mm Hg

Q21-6: Assuming the patient's HCO_3 is 13 mEq/L and the $Paco_2$ is 27 mm Hg, as expected with appropriate compensation, what would be the expected value of the patient's arterial pH?

A. 7.10
B. 7.18
C. 7.30
D. 7.40
E. 7.35

Q21-7: You decide to investigate the patient's non-anion gap acidosis. The patient's urine studies are as follows:

Urine Na	20 mEq/L
Urine K	10 mEq/L
Urine Cl	53 mEq/L
Urine urea	122 mg/dL
Urine glucose	0 mg/dL
Urine osmolality	450 mOsm/L
Urine pH	5.3
Urine RBCs	Too numerous to count
Urine WBCs	Too numerous to count
Urine protein	Moderate
Urine microscopic:	No stones present

What is the cause of the patient's non-anion gap acidosis?

A. Type 1 (distal) RTA due to diuretic use
B. Type 2 (proximal) RTA due to acetazolamide use
C. GI losses of bicarbonate secondary to ileal conduit
D. Type 4 RTA due to calcineurin inhibitor use

ANSWERS

Q21-1: B

While the patient has a condition predisposing her to a chronic acid-base disorder, there is insufficient information to estimate the patient's baseline $Paco_2$ and HCO_3 values; therefore, we will assume a baseline $Paco_2$ of 40 mm Hg and a baseline HCO_3 of 24 mEq/L. Patients with an ileal conduit are at increased risk for certain types of acidosis when complications arise. However, in this case, it appears to be an acute process.

Rationale: Ignoring these underlying chronic acid-base disorders can significantly alter the interpretation of a patient's acute acid-base status. This was demonstrated in the first case of the series. However, often, we do not have the necessary information (eg, prior ABG or VBG, or prior serum chemistry with an HCO_3) and are forced to assume the ongoing processes are all acute in nature. We are primarily concerned about chronic respiratory acid-base disorders, as these can significantly alter the patient's baseline or expected values for the serum HCO_3 and $Paco_2$, and we have reliable equations to predict the expected baseline values. The respiratory compensation for both chronic metabolic acidosis and alkalosis is generally poor, so there are no equations or rules to predict what the $Paco_2$ should be in these cases. While the baseline serum HCO_3 may be significantly off from our standard value of 24 mEq/L in these patients, we would assume a baseline $Paco_2$ of 40 mm Hg in patients with chronic metabolic processes. Once we identify the patient's baseline $Paco_2$ and HCO_3 values, we will need to use these values in the appropriate equations to identify the ongoing acute processes.

Q21-2: E

Metabolic acidosis and respiratory acidosis.

Rationale:

1. The pH is 7.21; therefore, the primary disorder is an **acidosis.**
2. The $Paco_2$ of 46 mm Hg is greater than 40 mm Hg, so there is a **respiratory acidosis.**
3. The HCO_3 of 13 mEq/L is less than 24 mEq/L, so there is also a **metabolic acidosis.**

Q21-3: B

10 mEq/L.

Rationale: The normal anion gap is 12 mEq/L. The term *anion gap* refers to those ions (negatively charged molecules) in the bloodstream that we do not routinely measure, including phosphates, sulfates, organic acids, and negatively charged plasma proteins. One of the most abundant negatively charged ions in the blood is serum albumin. A normal serum albumin is 4.0 g/dL. For patients with hypoalbuminemia (low serum albumin), the normal or expected anion gap is smaller.

$$\text{Expected Anion Gap} = 12 - (2.5) * \left[4.0 \frac{g}{dL} - \text{Actual Serum Albumin} \right].$$

Therefore, for this patient,

$$\text{Expected Anion Gap} = 12 - [2.5 * (4 - 3.3)] = 12 - (2.5 * 0.7) = \sim 10 \text{ mEq/L}.$$

This is an important concept as patients with hypoalbuminemia may "hide" an anion gap acidosis if this correction is not performed.

Q21-4: C
Anion and non-anion gap acidosis.

Rationale:

1. Is there evidence for a chronic respiratory acid-base disorder that requires adjustment of the patient's "normal" HCO_3? No, the patient in this case has a diagnosis of chronic rejection of her lung transplant. This condition can be associated with either an obstructive or restrictive process and can be associated with chronic respiratory acidosis. However, in this case, there is no evidence that the patient has an underlying respiratory acidosis, either from the vignette or from the laboratory data provided. Therefore, we will assume a baseline $Paco_2$ of 40 mm Hg and an HCO_3 of 24 mEq/L.

2. Expected anion gap:

$$\text{Expected Anion Gap} = 12 - (2.5) * \left[4.0 \frac{g}{dL} - \text{Actual Serum Albumin} \right]$$

$$= 12 - (2.5 * [4.0 - 3.3])$$
$$= 12 - (2.5 * [0]) = \sim \mathbf{10 \text{ mEq/L}}.$$

3. Anion gap calculation:

$$\text{Serum Anion Gap} = [Na^+] - [HCO_3^-] - [Cl^-]$$
$$= 132 - (101 + 13) = 18 \text{ mEq/L, which is} > \mathbf{10 \text{ mEq/L}} \text{ (corrected)}$$
$$\rightarrow \textbf{anion gap acidosis is present.}$$

4. Delta-delta calculation:

$$\Delta\Delta = \frac{(\text{Actual Anion Gap} - \text{Expected Anion Gap})}{(\text{Baseline } HCO_3 - \text{Actual } HCO_3)}$$

$$= (18 - 10)/(24 - 13) = \mathbf{8/11, which is \sim 0.7.}$$

Delta-delta interpretation.	
Delta-Delta Value	Condition Present
< 0.4	Non-anion gap only
0.4–0.9	**Anion gap *and* non-anion gap acidosis**
1.0–2.0	Anion gap acidosis only
> 2.0	Anion gap acidosis and metabolic alkalosis

Q21-4: D
Lactic acidosis.

Rationale: The patient presents with likely pyelonephritis (with fever, flank pain, and associated history of such) and hypotension. The laboratory studies are most consistent with a lactic acidosis at the cause of the patient's anion gap acidosis. There is no evidence of acetaminophen toxicity, aspirin toxicity, or ketoacidosis. There is no serum osmolal gap (calculated in this case as 289 mOsm/L; the serum osmolal gap is therefore 1 mOsm/L).

$$\text{Calculated Serum Osmolality} = 2 * [Na^+] + \frac{[Glucose]}{18} + \frac{[BUN]}{2.8} + \frac{[EtOH]}{3.7}.$$

This is further supported by the elevated serum lactate and the lack of another reasonable cause.

Q21-5: C
27 mm Hg.

Rationale: Using the Winter formula, one can calculate what the expected arterial $Paco_2$ should be for a given serum HCO_3 if the patient's acidosis were completely compensated.

Respiratory Compensation for Acute Metabolic Acidosis (Winter Formula):

Expected $Paco_2$ = 1.5 * [Actual HCO_3] + 8 ± 2 (in mm Hg)
Expected $Paco_2$ = (1.5 * 13) + 8 = 19.5 + 8 = 27.5 ± 2 = ~(25 to 29) mm Hg.

Therefore, if the patient was appropriately compensating for the metabolic acidosis, we would expect the patient's $Paco_2$ to be between 25 and 29 mm Hg.

Q21-6: C
7.30.

Rationale: We would expect the patient's pH to be approximately 7.30 in this setting. For this case, we would apply the Henderson-Hasselbach equation (assuming a k_H of CO_2 is 0.0307 mmol/mm Hg), as follows:

Henderson-Hasselbalch Equation:

$$pH = 6.10 + \log\left(\frac{[HCO_3]}{0.03 * Pco_2}\right);$$

or,

$$pH = 7.61 + \log_{10}\left(\frac{[HCO_3]}{Paco_2}\right).$$

Therefore, the calculation is,

$$pH = 7.61 + \log_{10}(13/27) = 7.61 + (-0.32) = \mathbf{7.30}.$$

Recall that even with appropriate or "complete" compensation, the pH will not return to normal. This patient's respiratory acidosis is likely due to chronic rejection of the lung transplant allograft, leading to reduced respiratory reserve.

Q21-7: C
GI losses of bicarbonate secondary to ileal conduit.

Rationale: Recall that we can use either the urine anion gap (UAG) or urine osmolar gap (UOG) to qualitatively estimate urinary ammonium excretion. This is a case where the UAG alone is inconclusive. The patient's UAG is calculated as follows:

Urine Anion Gap:

$$UAG = [U_{Na}] + [U_K] - [U_{Cl}].$$

Therefore, for this patient,

$$UAG = U_{Na} + U_K - U_{Cl} = (10 + 12) - 53 = (-21).$$

Interpretation:

- A UAG that is greater than ~20 → reduced renal acid excretion (RTA).
- A UAG that is −20 → GI loss of HCO_3 (eg, diarrhea), although type 2 RTA is possible.
- A UAG between −20 and +10 is generally considered inconclusive.

The UAG can be inappropriately elevated in anion gap acidosis, a situation in which multiple unmeasured anions may be present in the urine (beta-hydroxybutyrate/acetoacetate [ketoacidosis], hippurate [toluene], HCO_3 [proximal RTA], D-lactate [D-lactic acidosis], L-lactate, 5-oxoproline [acetaminophen toxicity]). Therefore, in patients with a significant anion gap, the UOG is typically more useful. Here the UOG is calculated as follows:

Urine Osmolar Gap:

$$\text{Calculated Urine Osmolality} = 2*([Na^+]+[K^+])+\frac{[Urea]}{2.8}+\frac{[Glucose]}{18}$$

$$UOG = \text{Measured Urine Osmolality} - \text{Measured Urine Osmolality}$$

$$\text{Calculated Urine Osmolarity} = 2*([U_{Na}] + [U_K]) + (U_{Urea}(mg/dL)/2.8 + [U_{glucose}(mg/dL)/18]$$

$$\text{Calculated Urine Osmolarity} = 2*[10 + 12] + [122/2.8] + [0/18] = 87 \text{ mOsm/L}$$

$$UOG = 450 - 97 \text{ Osm/L} = 33 \text{ mOsm.}$$

Similar to the UAG, the UOG is used as a surrogate for the urine ammonium concentration. Therefore, a larger gap indicates increased urinary NH_4 excretion. In normal acid-base conditions, the UOG is between 10 and 100 mOsm/L. During a significant metabolic acidosis, patients with impaired renal tubular acidification (type 1 and type 4 RTA) are unable to excrete additional acid (NH_4), and therefore the osmolar gap does not change. Patients with an intact renal response to acidemia (ie, GI losses) should have a significant UOG (~ >300 to 400 mOsm/L) as a result of increased NH_4 excretion. The patient's non-anion gap acidosis therefore appears to be due to GI losses of HCO_3, likely from the existing ileal conduit, leading to chronic non-anion gap acidosis. This generally will occur when there has been prolonged contact time between the urine and the ileal conduit, usually occurring when the conduit becomes obstructed.

References

Cruz DN1, Huot SJ. Metabolic complications of urinary diversions: an overview. Am J Med. 1997;102:477.

Krajewski W, Piszczek R, Krajewska M, et al. Urinary diversion metabolic complications—underestimated problem. Adv Clin Exp Med. 2014;23:633.

Tanrikut C1, McDougal WS. Acid-base and electrolyte disorders after urinary diversion. World J Urol. 2004;22:168.

CASE 22

A 24-year-old man is being evaluated in the emergency department (ED) for confusion, weakness, and palpitations. He was brought in by EMS, who found the patient lying in the street outside a convenience store. He is unable to provide significant history regarding medical conditions, medications, or drug/alcohol use. On initial examination, he does not appear to have experienced any significant trauma. His BP is 110/80 and HR is 120, with frequent PVCs and short runs of nonsustained ventricular tachycardia on the monitor. He is tachypneic with RR of 28 and Sao_2 of 99% on 2 L NC. He is afebrile. A head CT scan and CXR are negative. His laboratory results are shown in the following table. At his previous ED visit last year, he had a Cr of 1.5, up from 1.0 3 years earlier.

Laboratory data.			
ABGs		Basic Metabolic Panel	
pH	7.28	Na	134 mEq/L
$Paco_2$	32 mm Hg	K	2.6 mEq/L
Pao_2	91 mm Hg	Cl	103 mEq/L
HCO_3	15 mEq/L	CO_2	15 mEq/L
		BUN	31 mg/dL
		Cr	2.0 mg/dL
		Glucose	77 mg/dL
		Albumin	4.0 g/dL
		EtOH	0 mg/dL

QUESTIONS

Q22-1: Define the patient's baseline acid-base status: Does this patient have an underlying chronic acid-base disorder that we need to account for in order to appropriately interpret the acute acid-base disorders?

A. There is no evidence for an underlying chronic respiratory or metabolic acid-base disorder in this patient, so we would assume a baseline $Paco_2$ of 40 mm Hg and an HCO_3 of 24 mEq/L.

B. While the patient has a condition predisposing him to a chronic acid-base disorder, there is insufficient information to estimate the patient's baseline $Paco_2$ and HCO_3 values; therefore, we will assume a baseline $Paco_2$ of 40 mm Hg and a baseline HCO_3 of 24 mEq/L.

C. The patient has an underlying acid-base condition, and we have sufficient information to estimate the patient's baseline $Paco_2$ and HCO_3 values.

Q22-2: What is/are the primary acid-base disturbance(s) occurring in this case?

A. Metabolic acidosis only
B. Respiratory acidosis only
C. Metabolic alkalosis only
D. Respiratory alkalosis only
E. Metabolic acidosis and a respiratory acidosis
F. Metabolic alkalosis and a respiratory alkalosis

Q22-3: How would the metabolic acidosis component be classified in this case?

A. Anion gap acidosis
B. Non-anion gap acidosis
C. Anion and non-anion gap acidosis
D. Anion gap acidosis and a metabolic alkalosis

Q22-4: The patient's additional laboratory studies demonstrate phosphorus of 4.4 mEq/L, lactate of 1.4 mmol/L, and negative serum beta-hydroxybutyrate (BHB). The patient's drug screen shows no ethyl alcohol ingestion, no acetaminophen, and no salicylates, and the urine drug screen is also negative. He is receiving potassium supplementation. What would be the most appropriate next step in the patient's evaluation?

A. Serum osmolal gap
B. Urine osmolar gap
C. Urine anion gap
D. Urine chloride
E. Stool studies

Q22-5: Laboratory testing returns the following values:

Serum EtOH	< 3 mg/dL
Serum acetaminophen level	< 5 mg/dL (ULN for therapeutic use 20 mg/dL)
Serum salicylates level	< 5 mg/dL (ULN for therapeutic use 30 mg/dL)
Serum osmolality	290 mOsm/kg
Serum L-lactate	1.4 mmol/L (ULN 2.0 mmol/L venous)
Beta-hydroxybutyrate (acetone)	< 0.18 mmol/L (ULN 0.18 mmol/L)
Serum glucose	77 mg/dL

What is the serum osmolal gap?

A. 0 mEq/L
B. 7 mEq/L
C. 14 mEq/L
D. 21 mEq/L

Q22-6: You decide to investigate the patient's non-anion gap acidosis. The patient's urine studies are as follows:

Urine Na	20 mEq/L
Urine K	10 mEq/L
Urine Cl	25 mEq/L
Urine urea	100 mg/dL
Urine glucose	30 mg/dL
Urine osmolality	130 mOsm/L
Urine pH	6.0
Urine RBCs	Many present
Urine WBCs	None
Urine protein	Moderate
Urine microscopic	Microscopic stones present

What is the cause of the patient's non-anion gap acidosis?

A. Type 1 (distal) RTA
B. Type 2 (proximal) RTA
C. GI losses of bicarbonate
D. Type 4 RTA

Q22-7: The patient's mother is contacted and lists a number of items she found in the patient's bedroom: Marijuana, alprazolam, citalopram, cigarettes, several cans of paint thinner, and multiple vials of model glue. She informs you that her son told her he was putting together models as a hobby. What is the likely etiology of the patient's current condition?

A. Methanol toxicity

B. Benzodiazepine overdose

C. Carbon monoxide poisoning

D. Toluene toxicity

E. Ethyl alcohol poisoning

Q22-8: Does the patient in this case demonstrate appropriate respiratory or metabolic compensation?

A. Yes, the respiratory compensation is appropriate.

B. No, a concomitant respiratory alkalosis is present.

C. No, a concomitant respiratory acidosis is present.

D. Yes, the metabolic compensation is appropriate.

E. No, a concomitant metabolic acidosis is present.

F. No, a concomitant metabolic alkalosis is present.

ANSWERS

Q22-1: A

There is no evidence for an underlying chronic respiratory or metabolic acid-base disorder in this patient, so we would assume a baseline $Paco_2$ of 40 mm Hg and an HCO_3 of 24 mEq/L.

Rationale: Ignoring these underlying chronic acid-base disorders can significantly alter the interpretation of a patient's acute acid-base status. This was demonstrated in the first case of the series. However, often, we do not have the necessary information (eg, prior ABG or VBG, or prior serum chemistry with an HCO_3) and are forced to assume the ongoing processes are all acute in nature. We are primarily concerned about chronic respiratory acid-base disorders, as these can significantly alter the patient's baseline or expected values for the serum HCO_3 and $Paco_2$, and we have reliable equations to predict the expected baseline values. The respiratory compensation for both chronic metabolic acidosis and alkalosis is generally poor, so there are no equations or rules to predict what the $Paco_2$ should be in these cases. While the baseline serum HCO_3 may be significantly off from our standard value of 24 mEq/L in these patients, we would assume a baseline $Paco_2$ of 40 mm Hg in patients with chronic metabolic processes. Once we identify the patient's baseline $Paco_2$ and HCO_3 values, we will need to use these values in the appropriate equations to identify the ongoing acute processes.

Q22-2: A

Metabolic acidosis only.

Rationale:

1. The pH is 7.28; therefore, the primary disorder is an **acidosis.**
2. The $Paco_2$ of 32 mm Hg is less than 40 mm Hg, so this is not the cause of acidosis.
3. The HCO_3 of 15 mEq/L is less than 24 mEq/L, so there is a **metabolic acidosis.**

Q22-3: C

Anion and non-anion gap acidosis.

Rationale:

1. Is there evidence for a chronic respiratory acid-base disorder that requires adjustment of the patient's "normal" HCO_3? No, there is no evidence for a chronic respiratory acid-base disorder, so we would assume a baseline $Paco_2$ of 40 mm Hg and an HCO_3 of 24 mEq/L.
2. Expected anion gap:

$$\text{Expected Anion Gap} = 12 - (2.5) * \left[4.0 \frac{g}{dL} - \text{Actual Serum Albumin} \right]$$

$$= 12 - (2.5 * [4.0 - 4.0])$$
$$= 12 - (2.5 * [0]) = \textbf{12 mEq/L.}$$

3. Anion gap calculation:

$$\text{Serum Anion Gap} = [Na^+] - [HCO_3^-] - [Cl^-]$$
$$134 - (103 + 15) = 16 \text{ mEq/L, which is} > 12 \text{ mEq/L}$$
$$\rightarrow \textbf{anion gap acidosis is present.}$$

4. Delta-delta calculation:

$$\Delta\Delta = \frac{(\text{Actual Anion Gap} - \text{Expected Anion Gap})}{(\text{Baseline HCO}_3 - \text{Actual HCO}_3)}$$

$$= (16 - 12)/(24 - 15) = \textbf{4/9, which is ~0.44.}$$

Delta-delta interpretation.	
Delta-Delta Value	**Condition Present**
< 0.4	Non-anion gap only
0.4–0.9	**Anion gap *and* non-anion gap acidosis**
1.0–2.0	Anion gap acidosis only
> 2.0	Anion gap acidosis and metabolic alkalosis

Therefore, there is both a high anion gap acidosis as well as a non-anion gap acidosis present.

Q22-4: A
Serum osmolal gap.

Rationale: In a patient with a high anion gap acidosis, the primary differential diagnoses include lactic acidosis, D-lactic acidosis (rare), diabetic/alcoholic/starvation ketoacidosis, acetaminophen toxicity, salicylate toxicity, renal failure, and organic acid ingestion (methanol/ethylene glycol). The patient's laboratory findings have ruled out the bulk of these conditions and organic acid ingestion. Organic acid ingestion is potentially life-threatening with significant morbidity when treatment is delayed. Therefore, the most appropriate step in this patient would be to rule out an organic acid ingestion.

Q22-5: B
7 mEq/L.

Rationale: The serum osmolal gap is the difference between the laboratory-measured ("true") serum osmolality and a "calculated" osmolality based on commonly measured compounds that are known to contribute to the serum osmolality. Therefore, similar to the serum anion gap, the serum osmolal gap represents the "unmeasured" compounds also contributing to the serum osmolality. The serum osmolal gap can be helpful in determining if an organic alcohol ingestion has occurred recently. The following are potential causes of an elevated serum osmolality.

Conditions associated with elevated serum osmolality.
With an Elevated Serum Anion Gap
1. Ethanol ingestion with alcohol ketoacidosis (acetone is an unmeasured osmole, in addition to ethanol)—the osmolality is usually elevated more so by the increased ethanol concentration, so the osmolal "gap" depends on whether the term for ethanol is included in the osmolality calculation*
2. Organic alcohol ingestions (methanol, ethylene glycol, diethylene glycol, propylene glycol)
3. Diabetic ketoacidosis—similar to ethanol ingestion, earlier, glucose and acetone contribute to the osmolality, since the glucose term is always included in the calculation
4. Salicylate toxicity
5. Renal failure—the BUN is nearly always included in the osmolality
Without an Elevated Serum Anion Gap
1. Hyperosmolar therapy (mannitol, glycerol)
2. Other organic solvent ingestion (eg, acetone)
3. Isopropyl alcohol ingestion (produces only acetone rather than an organic acid, so no anion gap is seen)
4. Hypertriglyceridemia
5. Hyperproteinemia
*A mildly elevated osmolal gap has been reported in the literature in patients with lactic acidosis in critical illness, particularly severe distributive shock. The pathology is not quite clear, although it likely is related to multiorgan failure—particularly involving the liver and kidneys—and the release of cellular components known to contribute to the osmolal gap. This is typically around 10 mOsm/L, although it may be as high as 20 to 25 mOsm/L.

Similar to the serum anion gap, the serum osmolal gap is determined by the difference between the "calculated" serum osmolality and the true measured serum osmolality. The equation for the serum osmolal gap typically includes factors for sodium, glucose, BUN, and ethanol, as these are readily measurable in most laboratories. Therefore, the serum osmolal gap will represent the osmolality of those "unmeasured" osmoles, including organic alcohols and acetone. The most common form is shown as follows:

$$\text{Calculated Serum Osmolality} = 2*[\text{Na}^+] + \frac{[\text{Glucose}]}{18} + \frac{[\text{BUN}]}{2.8} + \frac{[\text{EtOH}]}{3.7};$$

In which the units of measure are as follows: Na, mEq/L; glucose, mg/dL; BUN, mg/dL; and EtOH, mg/dL. The conversion factors are shown in the preceding equation as well. A normal serum osmolal gap is around −10 to +10 mOsm/L (or mOsm/kg).

Therefore, for this patient,

$$\begin{aligned}
\text{Calculated Serum Osmolality} &= [2*\text{Na}] + [\text{Glucose}/18] + [\text{BUN}/2.8] + [\text{EtOH}/3.7] \\
&= (2*134) + (77/18) + (31/2.8) + (0/3.7) \\
&= 283 \text{ mOsm/L.}
\end{aligned}$$

$$\begin{aligned}
\text{Serum Osmolal Gap} &= \text{Measured Serum Osmolality} - \text{Calculated Osmolality} \\
&= (290 - 283) = 7 \text{ mOsm/L, which is} < 10 \text{ mOsm/L} \\
&\rightarrow \textbf{normal serum osmolal gap.}
\end{aligned}$$

Therefore, the patient does not appear to have a serum osmolal gap, indicating that a recent ingestion of organic alcohol is not likely. However, note that in organic alcohol ingestions, the serum osmolal gap manifesting shortly after ingestion will slowly close, leading to a worsening serum anion gap as the alcohol is converted to organic acid. The only way to formally rule out an ingestion is through direct testing for metabolites of the suspected organic alcohol.

Q22-6: A
Type 1 (distal) RTA.

Rationale: Recall that we can use either the urine anion gap (UAG) or urine osmolar gap (UOG) to qualitatively estimate urinary ammonium excretion. This is a case where the UAG alone is inconclusive. The patient's UAG is calculated as follows:

$$UAG = [U_{Na}] + [U_K] - [UCl]$$

Therefore, for this patient,

$$UAG = U_{Na} + U_K - U_{Cl} = (20 + 10) - 25 = (+5) \text{ mEq/L}.$$

Interpretation:

- A UAG that is greater than ~10 → renal loss of HCO_3 (RTA).
- A UAG that is less than −20 → GI loss of HCO_3 (eg, diarrhea).
- A UAG between −20 and +10 is generally considered inconclusive.

The UAG can be inappropriately elevated in anion gap acidosis, a situation in which multiple unmeasured anions may be present in the urine (BHB/acetoacetate [ketoacidosis], hippurate [toluene], HCO_3 [proximal RTA], D-lactate [D-lactic acidosis], L-lactate, 5-oxoproline [acetaminophen toxicity]). Therefore, in patients with a significant anion gap, the UOG is typically more useful.

Here the UOG is:

$$\text{Calculated Urine Osmolality} = 2 * ([Na^+] + [K^+]) + \frac{[Urea]}{2.8} + \frac{[Glucose]}{18}$$

$$UOG = \text{Measured Urine Osmolality} - \text{Measured Urine Osmolality}$$

$$\text{Calculated Urine Osmolarity} = 2 * ([U_{Na}] + [U_K])$$
$$+ (U_{Urea} \text{ (mg/dL)}/2.8] + [U_{glucose} \text{ (mg/dL)}/18]$$

$$\text{Calculated Urine Osmolarity} = 2 * [20 + 10] + [100/2.8] + [30/18] = 97 \text{ mOsm/L}$$
$$UOG = 130 - 97 \text{ Osm/L} = 33 \text{ mOsm}.$$

Similar to the UAG, the UOG is used as a surrogate for the urine ammonium concentration. Therefore, a larger gap indicates increased urinary NH_4 excretion. In normal acid-base conditions, the UOG is between 10 and 100 mOsm/L. During a significant metabolic acidosis, patients with impaired renal tubular acidification (type 1 and type 4 RTA) are unable to excrete additional acid (NH_4), and therefore the osmolar gap does not change. Patients with an intact renal response to acidemia (ie, GI losses) should have a significant UOG ($\sim$ >300 to 400 mOsm/L) as a result of increased NH_4 excretion.

To determine the type of RTA, one can look at the urine pH, serum potassium, for evidence of kidney stones.

Diagnosis of RTA.			
	Type 1 RTA	**Type 2 RTA**	**Type 4 RTA**
Severity of metabolic acidosis, (HCO_3)	Severe (< 10–12 mEq/L typically)	Intermediate (12–20 mEq/L)	Mild (15–20 mEq/L)
Associated urine abnormalities	Urinary phosphate, calcium are increased; bone disease often present	Urine glucose, amino acids, phosphate, calcium may be elevated	
Urine pH	HIGH (> 5.5)	Low (acidic), until serum HCO_3 level exceeds the resorptive ability of the proximal tubule, then becomes alkalotic once reabsorptive threshold is crossed	Low (acidic)
Serum K^+	Low to normal; should correct with oral HCO_3 therapy	Classically low, although may be normal or even high with rare genetic defects; worsens with oral HCO_3 therapy	HIGH
Renal stones	Often	No	No
Renal tubular defect	Reduced NH_4 secretion in distal tubule	Reduced HCO_3 resorption in proximal tubule	Reduced H^+/K^+ exchange in distal and collecting tubule due to decreased aldosterone or aldosterone resistance
Urine anion gap	> 10	Negative	> 10
Urine osmolal gap	Reduced during acute acidosis		Reduced during acute acidosis

The patient's urine pH is 6.0 despite the acidosis and the serum potassium is low. This is consistent with a type 1 RTA (distal), which affects the ability of the kidney to acidify the urine. These patients also often have kidney stones as a complication. Hypokalemia is a common complication of distal RTAs, and in cases can lead to arrhythmias, cramping, and weakness, as seen here.

Q22-7: D
Toluene toxicity.

Rationale: The patient presented with an anion gap acidosis and a concomitant non-anion gap acidosis in the setting of having multiple industrial products containing toluene. Toluene is an aromatic hydrocarbon that produces the characteristic smell of paint thinners. It may be abused through recreational inhalation. Subacute use will usually produce a non-anion gap metabolic acidosis with a high urine osmolar gap and hypokalemia. Toluene is converted to benzyl alcohol, then to benzaldehyde, benzoic acid, then to hippuric acid, then to hippurate. In patients with intact renal function, the hippuric anion can be readily excreted as conjugates of sodium and potassium, leading to hypovolemia and hypokalemia, while preserving the serum anion gap. The volume depletion can eventually lead to renal failure, causing the accumulation of hippurate anions as renal acidification function declines, leading to the eventual development of a high anion gap acidosis. Additionally, chronic use of toluene also appears to contribute to the development of a type 1 distal RTA as well as chronic renal insufficiency.

In toluene toxicity, the urine anion gap underestimates the excretion of urinary ammonium as chloride is excreted with the hippurate anions in addition to ammonia. In this setting, the urine osmolar gap is more useful.

Causes of RTA.
Causes of Type 1 (Distal) RTA
Primary • Idiopathic or familial (may be recessive or dominant)
Secondary • Medications: Lithium, amphotericin, ifosfamide, NSAIDs • Rheumatologic disorders: Sjögren syndrome, SLE, RA • Hypercalciuria (idiopathic) or associated with vitamin D deficiency or hyperparathyroidism • Sarcoidosis • Obstructive uropathy • Wilson disease • Rejection of renal transplant allograft • *Toluene toxicity*
Causes of Type 2 (Proximal) RTA
Primary • Idiopathic • Familial (primarily recessive disorders) • Genetic: Fanconi syndrome, cystinosis, glycogen storage disease (type 1), Wilson disease, galactosemia
Secondary • Medications: Acetazolamide, topiramate, aminoglycoside antibiotics, ifosfamide, reverse transcriptase inhibitors (tenofovir) • Heavy metal poisoning: Lead, mercury, copper • Multiple myeloma or amyloidosis (secondary to light chain toxicity) • Sjögren syndrome • Vitamin D deficiency • Rejection of renal transplant allograft

(Continued)

Causes of RTA. (*continued*)
Causes of Type 4 RTA (Hypoaldosteronism or Aldosterone Resistance)
Primary
• Primary adrenal insufficiency • Inherited disorders associated with hypoaldosteronism • Pseudohypoaldosteronism (types 1 and 2)
Secondary
• Causes of hyporeninemic hypoaldosteronism such as renal disease (diabetic nephropathy), NSAID use, calcineurin inhibitors, volume expansion/volume overload • Causes of distal tubule voltage defects such as sickle cell disease, obstructive uropathy, SLE • Severe illness/septic shock • Angiotensin II–associated medications: ACE inhibitors, ARBs, direct renin inhibitors • Potassium-sparing diuretics: Spironolactone, amiloride, triamterene • Antibiotics: Trimethoprim, pentamidine

Q22-8: A

Yes, the respiratory compensation is appropriate.

Rationale: Using the Winter formula, one can calculate what the expected arterial $Paco_2$ should be for a given serum HCO_3 if the patient were completely compensated.

Respiratory Compensation for Acute Metabolic Acidosis (Winter Formula):

$$\text{Expected } Paco_2 = 1.5 * [\text{Actual } HCO_3] + 8 \pm 2 \text{ (in mm Hg)}$$
$$\text{Expected } Paco_2 = 1.5 * (\text{Actual } HCO_3) + 8 \, (\pm 2)$$
$$= (1.5 * 15) + 8 = 22.5 + 8 = 30.5 \pm 2 = (29 \text{ to } 33) \text{ mm Hg.}$$

This patient has an appropriate compensatory response to the metabolic acidosis.

References

Batlle D, Grupp M, Gaviria M, Kurtzman NA. Distal renal tubular acidosis with intact capacity to lower urinary pH. Am J Med. 1982;72:751.

Batlle D, Haque SK. Genetic causes and mechanisms of distal renal tubular acidosis. Nephrol Dial Transplant. 2012;27:3691.

Batlle DC, Hizon M, Cohen E, et al. The use of the urinary anion gap in the diagnosis of hyperchloremic metabolic acidosis. N Engl J Med. 1988;318:594.

Batlle DC, von Riotte A, Schlueter W. Urinary sodium in the evaluation of hyperchloremic metabolic acidosis. N Engl J Med. 1987;316:140.

Batlle DC, Sabatini S, Kurtzman NA. On the mechanism of toluene-induced renal tubular acidosis. Nephron. 1988;49:210.

Buckalew VM Jr, McCurdy DK, Ludwig GD, et al. Incomplete renal tubular acidosis. Physiologic studies in three patients with a defect in lowering urine pH. Am J Med. 1968;45:32.

Carlisle EJ, Donnelly SM, Vasuvattakul S, et al. Glue-sniffing and distal renal tubular acidosis: sticking to the facts. J Am Soc Nephrol. 1991;1:1019.

Dyck RF, Asthana S, Kalra J, et al. A modification of the urine osmolal gap: an improved method for estimating urine ammonium. Am J Nephrol. 1990;10:359.

Karet FE. Mechanisms in hyperkalemic renal tubular acidosis. J Am Soc Nephrol. 2009;20:251.

Kim GH, Han JS, Kim YS, et al. Evaluation of urine acidification by urine anion gap and urine osmolal gap in chronic metabolic acidosis. Am J Kidney Dis. 1996;27:42.

Lee Hamm L, Hering-Smith KS, Nakhoul NL. Acid-base and potassium homeostasis. Semin Nephrol. 2013;33:257.

Meregalli P, Lüthy C, Oetliker OH, Bianchetti MG. Modified urine osmolal gap: an accurate method for estimating the urinary ammonium concentration? Nephron. 1995;69:98.

Oh M, Carroll HJ. Value and determinants of urine anion gap. Nephron. 2002;90:252.

Rodríguez Soriano J. Renal tubular acidosis: the clinical entity. J Am Soc Nephrol. 2002;13:2160.

Taher SM, Anderson RJ, McCartney R, et al. Renal tubular acidosis associated with toluene "sniffing". N Engl J Med. 1974;290:765.

Tuchscherer J, Rehman H. Metabolic acidosis in toluene sniffing. CJEM. 2013;15:249.

CASE 23

A 53-year-old man with poorly controlled type 2 diabetes mellitus (insulin-dependent) presents to the emergency department after a motor vehicle accident. He has a large facial laceration as well as a fracture of the left femur. His urine toxicology screen is negative and his serum alcohol level is undetectable. He is quite tachypneic and in considerable pain. His vital signs are T 35.9°C, RR is 40, HR 140, and BP 75/50. His Hbg is 8.5 g/dL on presentation, which is 5 g/dL lower than his level 6 months earlier in clinic. His laboratory values are shown in the following table. He takes insulin, HCTZ, lisinopril, and pravastatin.

Laboratory data.			
ABGs		**Basic Metabolic Panel**	
pH	7.50	Na	136 mEq/L
$Paco_2$	22 mm Hg	K	5.8 mEq/L
Pao_2	91 mm Hg	Cl	104 mEq/L
HCO_3	17 mEq/L	CO_2	17 mEq/L
		BUN	44 mg/dL
		Cr	0.9 mg/dL
		Glucose	124 mg/dL
		Albumin	4 g/dL
		EtOH	0 mg/dL

QUESTIONS

Q23-1: Define the patient's baseline acid-base status: Does this patient have an underlying chronic acid-base disorder that we need to account for in order to appropriately interpret the acute acid-base disorders?

A. There is no evidence for an underlying chronic respiratory or metabolic acid-base disorder in this patient, so we would assume a baseline $Paco_2$ of 40 mm Hg and an HCO_3 of 24 mEq/L.

B. While the patient has a condition predisposing him to a chronic acid-base disorder, there is insufficient information to estimate the patient's baseline $Paco_2$ and HCO_3 values; therefore, we will assume a baseline $Paco_2$ of 40 mm Hg and a baseline HCO_3 of 24 mEq/L.

C. The patient has an underlying acid-base condition, and we have sufficient information to estimate the patient's baseline $Paco_2$ and HCO_3 values.

Q23-2: What is/are the primary acid-base disturbance(s) occurring in this case?

A. Metabolic acidosis only
B. Respiratory acidosis only
C. Respiratory alkalosis only
D. Metabolic alkalosis only
E. Metabolic acidosis and a respiratory acidosis
F. Metabolic alkalosis and a respiratory alkalosis

Q23-3: How would the metabolic acidosis component be classified in this case?

A. Anion gap acidosis
B. Non-anion gap acidosis
C. Anion and non-anion gap acidosis
D. Anion gap acidosis and a metabolic alkalosis

Q23-4: Laboratory testing returns the following results:

Serum EtOH	< 3 mg/dL
Serum acetaminophen level	< 5 mg/dL (ULN for therapeutic use 20 mg/dL)
Serum salicylates level	< 5 mg/dL (ULN for therapeutic use 30 mg/dL)
Serum osmolality	300 mOsm/kg
Serum L-lactate	4.5 mmol/L (ULN 2.0 mmol/L venous)
Beta-hydroxybutyrate (acetone)	< 0.18 mmol/L (ULN 0.18 mmol/L)
Serum glucose	124 mg/dL

What is the serum osmolal gap?

A. 0 mOsm/L
B. 4 mOsm/L
C. 22 mOsm/L
D. 59 mOsm/L

Q23-5: What is the likely source of the patient's metabolic acidosis?

A. Diabetic ketoacidosis
B. Lactic acidosis
C. Methanol ingestion
D. Acetaminophen ingestion
E. Aspirin ingestion

Q23-6: Which of the following is not a common cause of respiratory alkalosis?

A. Aspirin overdose
B. Liver failure
C. Pain/discomfort
D. Anxiety
E. Neuromuscular disorder (eg, ALS)

Q23-7: You decide to investigate the patient's non-anion gap acidosis. The patient's urine studies are as follows:

Urine Na	12 mEq/L
Urine K	32 mEq/L
Urine Cl	20 mEq/L
Urine pH	5.5

What is the cause of the patient's non-anion gap acidosis?

A. Type 1 (distal) RTA
B. Type 2 (proximal) RTA
C. GI losses of bicarbonate
D. Type 4 RTA

ANSWERS

Q23-1: A

There is no evidence for an underlying chronic respiratory or metabolic acid-base disorder in this patient, so we would assume a baseline $Paco_2$ of 40 mm Hg and an HCO_3 of 24 mEq/L.

Rationale: Ignoring these underlying chronic acid-base disorders can significantly alter the interpretation of a patient's acute acid-base status. This was demonstrated in the first case of the series. However, often, we do not have the necessary information (eg, prior ABG or VBG, or prior serum chemistry with an HCO_3) and are forced to assume the ongoing processes are all acute in nature. We are primarily concerned about chronic respiratory acid-base disorders, as this can significantly alter the patient's baseline or expected values for the serum HCO_3 and $Paco_2$, and we have reliable equations to predict the expected baseline values. The respiratory compensation for both chronic metabolic acidosis and alkalosis is generally poor, so there are no equations or rules to predict what the $Paco_2$ should be in these cases. While the baseline serum HCO_3 may be significantly off from our standard value of 24 mEq/L in these patients, we would assume a baseline $Paco_2$ of 40 mm Hg in patients with chronic metabolic processes. Once we identify the patient's baseline $Paco_2$ and HCO_3 values, we will need to use these values in the appropriate equations to identify the ongoing acute processes.

Q23-2: C

Respiratory alkalosis only.

Rationale:

1. The pH is 7.50; therefore, the primary disorder is an **alkalosis.**
2. The $Paco_2$ of 22 mm Hg is less than 40 mm Hg, so there is a **respiratory alkalosis.**
3. The HCO_3 of 14 mEq/L is less than 24 mEq/L, so there is no metabolic alkalosis.

Q23-3: C

Anion and non-anion gap acidosis.

Rationale:

1. Is there evidence for a chronic respiratory acid-base disorder that requires adjustment of the patient's "normal" HCO_3? No, there is no evidence for a chronic respiratory acid-base disorder in this patient, so we would assume a baseline $Paco_2$ of 40 mm Hg and an HCO_3 of 24 mEq/L.
2. Expected anion gap:

$$\text{Expected Anion Gap} = 12 - (2.5) * \left[4.0\, \frac{g}{dL} - \text{Actual Serum Albumin} \right]$$

$$= 12 - (2.5 * [4.0 - 4.0])$$

$$= 12 - (2.5 * [0]) = \textbf{12 mEq/L.}$$

3. Anion gap calculation:

$$\text{Serum Anion Gap} = [Na^+] - [HCO_3^-] - [Cl^-]$$
$$= 136 - (104 + 17) = 15 \text{ mEq/L, which is} > 12 \text{ mEq/L}$$
$$\rightarrow \textbf{anion gap acidosis is present.}$$

4. Delta-delta calculation:

$$\Delta\Delta = \frac{(\text{Actual Anion Gap} - \text{Expected Anion Gap})}{(\text{Baseline HCO}_3 - \text{Actual HCO}_3)}$$

$$= (15 - 12)/(24 - 17) = \textbf{3/7, which is} \sim\textbf{0.4.}$$

Delta-delta interpretation.	
Delta-Delta Value	Condition Present
< 0.4	Non-anion gap only
0.4–0.9	**Anion gap *and* non-anion gap acidosis**
1.0–2.0	Anion gap acidosis only
> 2.0	Anion gap acidosis and metabolic alkalosis

Q23-4: D
59 mOsm/L.

Rationale: Similar to the serum anion gap, the serum osmolal gap is determined by the difference between the "calculated" serum osmolality and the true measured serum osmolality. The equation for the serum osmolal gap typically includes factors for sodium, glucose, BUN, and ethanol, as these are readily measurable in most laboratories. Therefore, the serum osmolal gap will represent the osmolality of those "unmeasured" osmoles, including organic alcohols and acetone. The most common form is shown as follows:

$$\text{Calculated Serum Osmolality} = 2*[Na^+] + \frac{[\text{Glucose}]}{18} + \frac{[\text{BUN}]}{2.8} + \frac{[\text{EtOH}]}{3.7};$$

In which the units of measure are as follows: Na, mEq/L; glucose, mg/dL; BUN, mg/dL; and EtOH, mg/dL. The conversion factors are shown in the preceding equation as well. A normal serum osmolal gap is around −10 to +10 mOsm/L (or mOsm/kg).

Therefore, for this patient,

$$\text{Calculated Serum Osmolality} = [2*Na] + [\text{Glucose}/18] + [\text{BUN}/2.8] + [\text{EtOH}/3.7]$$
$$= (2*136) + (124/18) + (44/2.8) + (0/3.7)$$
$$= 295.$$

$$\text{Serum Osmolal Gap} = \text{Measured Serum Osmolality} - \text{Calculated Osmolality}$$
$$= (300 - 295) = 5, \text{ which is} < 10 \rightarrow \textit{no} \textbf{ serum osmolal gap.}$$

Q23-5: B
Lactic acidosis.

Rationale: The patient presents with hypotension following the loss of a significant blood volume related to the car accident, with a substantial drop in hemoglobin concentration. While lactic acidosis is most commonly associated with an infectious etiology, acute blood loss anemia can lead to distributive shock as well the development of a lactic acidosis. The patient's serum lactic level is significantly elevated, while the beta-hydroxybutyrate and the serum acetaminophen results are negative. There is no serum osmolal gap to suggest methanol ingestion. Given the presence of a metabolic acidosis and a concomitant respiratory alkalosis, aspirin toxicity would be high in the differential. However, since the patient has a negative serum salicylate level, this is not the cause.

Q23-6: E
Neuromuscular disease (eg, ALS).

Rationale: Neuromuscular disorders such as ALS are associated with respiratory acidosis, not alkalosis. Although patients may have tachypnea as they lack the muscle strength to take deep breaths. Patients with CNS insults such as stroke may have respiratory alkalosis due to issues with their respiratory center. Liver failure is associated with respiratory alkalosis due to an inability to clear toxins, which can stimulate the respiratory centers. Aspirin is also a stimulant of the respiratory center. Pulmonary embolism is another common cause of a respiratory alkalosis, and this patient's vignette is most consistent with an acute pulmonary embolism. The patient's vignette is most consistent with pain or discomfort as the cause of the respiratory alkalosis, as it is not merely a compensatory mechanism for the concomitant metabolic acidosis.

Q23-7: D
Type 4 RTA.

Rationale: Recall that we can use either the urine anion gap (UAG) or urine osmolar gap (UOG) to qualitatively estimate urinary ammonium excretion. This is a case where the UAG alone is inconclusive. The patient's UAG is calculated as follows:

$$UAG = [U_{Na}] + [U_K] + [U_{Cl}]$$
$$UAG = U_{Na} + U_K - U_{Cl} = (12 + 32) - 20 = (+24) \text{ mEq/L.}$$

Interpretation:

- A UAG that is greater than ~20 → reduced renal acid excretion (RTA).
- A UAG that is −20 → GI loss of HCO_3 (eg, diarrhea), although type 2 RTA is possible.
- A UAG between −20 and +10 is generally considered inconclusive.

This patient has an elevated UAG, which is concerning for a possible RTA as the cause of the patient's non-anion gap metabolic acidosis. However, this patient also has an anion gap acidosis. The UAG can be inappropriately elevated in anion gap acidosis, a situation in which multiple unmeasured anions may be present in the urine (beta-hydroxybutyrate/acetoacetate [ketoacidosis], hippurate [toluene], HCO_3 [proximal RTA], D-lactate [D-lactic acidosis], L-lactate, 5-oxoproline [acetaminophen toxicity]). Therefore, in patients with a significant anion gap, the UOG is typically more useful. However, we don't have the necessary information here to calculate the serum osmolal gap, so we will have to move forward with the information we have.

Diagnosis of RTA.			
	Type 1 RTA	Type 2 RTA	Type 4 RTA
Severity of metabolic acidosis, (HCO_3)	Severe (< 10–12 mEq/L typically)	Intermediate (12–20 mEq/L)	Mild (15–20 mEq/L)
Associated urine abnormalities	Urinary phosphate, calcium are increased; bone disease often present	Urine glucose, amino acids, phosphate, calcium may be elevated	
Urine pH	HIGH (> 5.5)	Low (acidic), until serum HCO_3 level exceeds the resorptive ability of the proximal tubule, then becomes alkalotic once reabsorptive threshold is crossed	Low (acidic)
Serum K^+	Low to normal; should correct with oral HCO_3 therapy	Classically low, although may be normal or even high with rare genetic defects; worsens with oral HCO_3 therapy	HIGH
Renal stones	Often	No	No
Renal tubular defect	Reduced NH_4 secretion in distal tubule	Reduced HCO_3 resorption in proximal tubule	Reduced H^+/K^+ exchange in distal and collecting tubule due to decreased aldosterone or aldosterone resistance
Urine anion gap	> 10	Negative	> 10
Urine osmolal gap	Reduced during acute acidosis		Reduced during acute acidosis

The patient's urine pH is 5.3 (acidic) and the UAG is positive (+24). Additionally, the patient has an elevated serum potassium level, most consistent with a type 4 RTA. Type 4 RTA is commonly seen in patients with hypoaldosteronism, including diabetes mellitus, renal insufficiency, NSAID use, ACE inhibitor use, calcineurin inhibitor use, severe illness, and primary adrenal insufficiency. This patient has a history of diabetes mellitus that is poorly controlled and is also taking an ACE inhibitor, both of which may be contributing.

Causes of renal tubular acidosis.
Causes of Type 1 (Distal) RTA
Primary   • Idiopathic or familial (may be recessive or dominant)
Secondary   • Medications: Lithium, amphotericin, ifosfamide, NSAIDs   • Rheumatologic disorders: Sjögren syndrome, SLE, RA   • Hypercalciuria (idiopathic) or associated with vitamin D deficiency or hyperparathyroidism   • Sarcoidosis   • Obstructive uropathy   • Wilson disease   • Rejection of renal transplant allograft   • Toluene toxicity
Causes of Type 2 (Proximal) RTA
Primary   • Idiopathic   • Familial (primarily recessive disorders)   • Genetic: Fanconi syndrome, cystinosis, glycogen storage disease (type 1), Wilson disease, galactosemia
Secondary   • Medications: Acetazolamide, topiramate, aminoglycoside antibiotics, ifosfamide, reverse transcriptase inhibitors (tenofovir)   • Heavy metal poisoning: Lead, mercury, copper   • Multiple myeloma or amyloidosis (secondary to light chain toxicity)   • Sjögren syndrome   • Vitamin D deficiency   • Rejection of renal transplant allograft
Causes of Type 4 RTA (Hypoaldosteronism or Aldosterone Resistance)
Primary   • Primary adrenal insufficiency   • Inherited disorders associated with hypoaldosteronism   • Pseudohypoaldosteronism (types 1 and 2)
Secondary   • Causes of hyporeninemic hypoaldosteronism such as renal disease (diabetic nephropathy), NSAID use, calcineurin inhibitors, volume expansion/volume overload   • Causes of distal tubule voltage defects such as sickle cell disease, obstructive uropathy, SLE   • Severe illness/septic shock   • Angiotensin II–associated medications: ACE inhibitors, ARBs, direct renin inhibitors   • Potassium-sparing diuretics: Spironolactone, amiloride, triamterene   • Antibiotics: Trimethoprim, pentamidine

References

Adeva-Andany M, López-Ojén M, Funcasta-Calderón R, et al. Comprehensive review on lactate metabolism in human health. Mitochondrion. 2014;17:76.

Arroliga AC, Shehab N, McCarthy K, Gonzales JP. Relationship of continuous infusion lorazepam to serum propylene glycol concentration in critically ill adults. Crit Care Med. 2004;32:1709.

Batlle D, Grupp M, Gaviria M, Kurtzman NA. Distal renal tubular acidosis with intact capacity to lower urinary pH. Am J Med. 1982;72:751.

Batlle D, Haque SK. Genetic causes and mechanisms of distal renal tubular acidosis. Nephrol Dial Transplant. 2012;27:3691.

Batlle DC, Hizon M, Cohen E, et al. The use of the urinary anion gap in the diagnosis of hyperchloremic metabolic acidosis. N Engl J Med. 1988;318:594.

Batlle DC, von Riotte A, Schlueter W. Urinary sodium in the evaluation of hyperchloremic metabolic acidosis. N Engl J Med. 1987;316:140.

Braden GL, Strayhorn CH, Germain MJ, et al. Increased osmolal gap in alcoholic acidosis. Arch Intern Med. 1993;153:2377.

Buckalew VM Jr, McCurdy DK, Ludwig GD, et al. Incomplete renal tubular acidosis. Physiologic studies in three patients with a defect in lowering urine pH. Am J Med. 1968;45:32.

Dyck RF, Asthana S, Kalra J, et al. A modification of the urine osmolal gap: an improved method for estimating urine ammonium. Am J Nephrol. 1990;10:359.

Gabow PA. Ethylene glycol intoxication. Am J Kidney Dis. 1988;11:277.

Gennari FJ. Current concepts. Serum osmolality. Uses and limitations. N Engl J Med. 1984;310:102.

Glasser L, Sternglanz PD, Combie J, Robinson A. Serum osmolality and its applicability to drug overdose. Am J Clin Pathol. 1973;60:695.

Karet FE. Mechanisms in hyperkalemic renal tubular acidosis. J Am Soc Nephrol. 2009;20:251.

Kim GH, Han JS, Kim YS, et al. Evaluation of urine acidification by urine anion gap and urine osmolal gap in chronic metabolic acidosis. Am J Kidney Dis. 1996;27:42.

Kraut JA, Kurtz I. Toxic alcohol ingestions: clinical features, diagnosis, and management. Clin J Am Soc Nephrol. 2008;3:208.

Kraut JA, Xing SX. Approach to the evaluation of a patient with an increased serum osmolal gap and high-anion-gap metabolic acidosis. Am J Kidney Dis. 2011;58:480.

Lee Hamm L, Hering-Smith KS, Nakhoul NL. Acid-base and potassium homeostasis. Semin Nephrol. 2013;33:257.

Levy B. Lactate and shock state: the metabolic view. Curr Opin Crit Care. 2006;12:315.

Lynd LD, Richardson KJ, Purssell RA, et al. An evaluation of the osmole gap as a screening test for toxic alcohol poisoning. BMC Emerg Med. 2008;8:5.

Madias NE. Lactic acidosis. Kidney Int. 1986;29:752.

Marraffa JM, Holland MG, Stork CM, et al. Diethylene glycol: widely used solvent presents serious poisoning potential. J Emerg Med. 2008;35:401.

Meregalli P, Lüthy C, Oetliker OH, Bianchetti MG. Modified urine osmolal gap: an accurate method for estimating the urinary ammonium concentration? Nephron. 1995;69:98.

Mikkelsen ME, Miltiades AN, Gaieski DF, et al. Serum lactate is associated with mortality in severe sepsis independent of organ failure and shock. Crit Care Med. 2009;37:1670.

Oh M, Carroll HJ. Value and determinants of urine anion gap. Nephron. 2002;90:252.

Purssell RA, Pudek M, Brubacher J, Abu-Laban RB. Derivation and validation of a formula to calculate the contribution of ethanol to the osmolal gap. Ann Emerg Med. 2001;38:653.

Robinson AG, Loeb JN. Ethanol ingestion—commonest cause of elevated plasma osmolality? N Engl J Med. 1971;284:1253.

Rodríguez Soriano J. Renal tubular acidosis: the clinical entity. J Am Soc Nephrol. 2002;13:2160.

Rose BD, Post TW. Clinical Physiology of Acid-Base and Electrolyte Disorders. 5e. New York, NY: McGraw Hill; 2001:583.

Schelling JR, Howard RL, Winter SD, Linas SL. Increased osmolal gap in alcoholic ketoacidosis and lactic acidosis. Ann Intern Med. 1990;113:580.

CASE 24

A 57-year-old white man who was previously diagnosed with ALS presents to the emergency department with a productive cough, fever, altered mental status, tachycardia, and hypotension. He is currently using noninvasive ventilation for 12 to 14 hours a day, but over the past few days has been having more issues with cough, congestion, and lethargy. His wife called EMS, and he was found to be febrile (38.7°C), tachycardic to the 120s, and hypotensive to 75/50. He was given 1 L NS en route to the hospital. He has taken no OTC or prescription medications. On examination, he has bronchial breath sounds and rhonchi in the right middle and lower lobe regions. His most recent clinic data, from 2 weeks prior, include an ABG with a baseline $Paco_2$ of 58 mm Hg and a serum HCO_3 of 30 mEq/L. His WBC count is 22,000 with a left shift. His baseline Cr is 0.6. His current laboratory results are shown in the following table:

Laboratory data.			
ABGs		Basic Metabolic Panel	
pH	7.14	Na	136 mEq/L
$Paco_2$	72 mm Hg	K	4.9 mEq/L
Pao_2	91 mm Hg	Cl	93 mEq/L
HCO_3	24 mEq/L	CO_2	24 mEq/L
		BUN	28 mg/dL
		Cr	1.2 mg/dL
		Glucose	124 mg/dL
		Albumin	3.1 g/dL
		EtOH	0 mg/dL

QUESTIONS

Q24-1: Define the patient's baseline acid-base status: Does this patient have an underlying chronic acid-base disorder that we need to account for in order to appropriately interpret the acute acid-base disorders?

A. There is no evidence for an underlying chronic respiratory or metabolic acid-base disorder in this patient, so we would assume a baseline $Paco_2$ of 40 mm Hg and an HCO_3 of 24 mEq/L.

B. While the patient has a condition predisposing him to a chronic acid-base disorder, there is insufficient information to estimate the patient's baseline $Paco_2$ and HCO_3 values; therefore, we will assume a baseline $Paco_2$ of 40 mm Hg and a baseline HCO_3 of 24 mEq/L.

C. The patient has an underlying acid-base condition, and we have sufficient information to estimate the patient's baseline $Paco_2$ and HCO_3 values.

Q24-2: What is/are the primary acid-base disturbance(s) occurring in this case?

A. Metabolic acidosis only
B. Respiratory acidosis only
C. Metabolic acidosis and a respiratory acidosis
D. Metabolic alkalosis and a respiratory alkalosis

Q24-3: For a perfectly healthy patient, a normal anion gap is assumed to be 12 mEq/L. What should be considered a normal anion gap in this patient?

A. 12 mEq/L
B. 10 mEq/L
C. 7 mEq/L
D. 4 mEq/L

Q24-4: How would the metabolic acidosis component be classified in this case?

A. Anion gap acidosis
B. Non-anion gap acidosis
C. Anion and non-anion gap acidosis
D. Anion gap acidosis and a metabolic alkalosis

Q24-5: Laboratory testing returns the following results:

Serum EtOH	< 3 mg/dL
Serum acetaminophen level	< 5 mg/dL (ULN for therapeutic use 20 mg/dL)
Serum salicylates level	< 5 mg/dL (ULN for therapeutic use 30 mg/dL)
Serum osmolality	291 mOsm/kg
Serum L-lactate	NA
Beta-hydroxybutyrate (acetone)	< 0.18 mmol/L (ULN 0.18 mmol/L)
Serum glucose	124 mg/dL

What is the serum osmolal gap?

A. 0 mOsm/L
B. 2 mOsm/L
C. 10 mOsm/L
D. 23 mOsm/L

Q24-6: Given the preceding information, what laboratory test should be performed next to determine the cause of the patient's anion gap acidosis?

A. Serum phosphate
B. Serum lactate
C. Serum acetaminophen level
D. Urine chloride
E. Urine anion gap

Q24-7: Based on previous laboratory findings, we know that this patient has a chronic respiratory acidosis with a baseline $Paco_2$ of 58 mm Hg. Additionally, the patient has an acute respiratory acidosis with the $Paco_2$ rising to 72 mm Hg. If the patient *did not have a concomitant metabolic acidosis*, what would one expect the serum HCO_3 to be if the patient was compensating fully for the acute and chronic portions of the respiratory acidosis?

A. 50 mEq/L
B. 25 mEq/L
C. 31 mEq/L
D. 28 mEq/L

ANSWERS

Q24-1: C

The patient has an underlying acid-base condition and we have sufficient information to estimate the patient's baseline $Paco_2$ and HCO_3 values. This patient has ALS, a neuromuscular disorder associated with hypercarbic respiratory failure as the disease progresses in nonventilated patients. He has a defined chronic respiratory acidosis per the vignette. Therefore, we need to adjust the baseline values for the patient's $Paco_2$ to 58 mm Hg, and the HCO_3 accordingly to 30 mEq/L.

Rationale: Ignoring these underlying chronic acid-base disorders can significantly alter the interpretation of a patient's acute acid-base status. This was demonstrated in the first case of the series. However, often, we do not have the necessary information (eg, prior ABG or VBG, or prior serum chemistry with an HCO_3) and are forced to assume the ongoing processes are all acute in nature. We are primarily concerned about chronic respiratory acid-base disorders, as these can significantly alter the patient's baseline or expected values for the serum HCO_3 and $Paco_2$, and we have reliable equations to predict the expected baseline values. The respiratory compensation for both chronic metabolic acidosis and alkalosis is generally poor, so there are no equations or rules to predict what the $Paco_2$ should be in these cases. While the baseline serum HCO_3 may be significantly off from our standard value of 24 mEq/L in these patients, we would assume a baseline $Paco_2$ of 40 mm Hg in patients with chronic metabolic processes. Once we identify the patient's baseline $Paco_2$ and HCO_3 values, we will need to use these values in the appropriate equations to identify the ongoing acute processes.

Q24-2: C

Metabolic acidosis and a respiratory acidosis.

Rationale:

1. The pH is 7.14; therefore, the primary disorder is an acidosis.
2. The $Paco_2$ of 72 mm Hg is greater than both the patient's baseline $Paco_2$ (58 mm Hg) as well as above the normal $Paco_2$ (40 mm Hg), indicating the presence of both **acute** and **chronic respiratory acidosis.**
3. The HCO_3 of 24 mEq/L, while typically normal, is significantly less than the patient's baseline HCO_3 of 30, so there is an **acute metabolic acidosis.**

Q24-3: B

10 mEq/L.

Rationale: The normal anion gap is 12 mEq/L. The term *anion gap* refers to those ions (negatively charged molecules) in the bloodstream that we do not routinely measure (or include in the calculation), including magnesium, potassium, phosphates, sulfates, organic acids, and negatively charged plasma proteins. One of the most abundant negatively charged ions in the blood is serum albumin. A normal serum albumin is 4.0 g/dL. For patients with hypoalbuminemia (low serum albumin), the normal or expected anion gap is smaller.

$$\text{Expected Anion Gap} = 12 - (2.5) * \left[4.0 \frac{g}{dL} - \text{Actual Serum Albumin} \right].$$

So for this patient,

$$\text{Expected Anion Gap} = 12 - [2.5 * (4 - 3.1)] = 12 - (2.5 * 0.9) = 9.75 \sim 10 \text{ mEq/L}.$$

This is an important concept as patients with hypoalbuminemia may "hide" an anion gap acidosis if this correction is not performed.

Q24-4: C
Anion and non-anion gap acidosis.

Rationale:

1. Is there evidence for a chronic respiratory acid-base disorder that requires adjustment of the patient's "normal" HCO_3? Yes, as we concluded earlier, this patient has a chronic respiratory acidosis and a baseline compensatory renal compensation. The baseline HCO_3 for this patient is therefore 30 mEq/L.
2. Expected anion gap:

$$\text{Expected Anion Gap} = 12 - (2.5) * \left[4.0 \frac{g}{dL} - \text{Actual Serum Albumin} \right]$$
$$= 12 - (2.5 * [4.0 - 3.1])$$
$$= 12 - (2.5 * [0.9]) = \textbf{10 mEq/L.}$$

3. Anion gap calculation:

$$\text{Serum Anion Gap} = [Na^+] - [HCO_3^-] - [Cl^-]$$
$$= 136 - (93 + 24) = 19, \text{ which is} > 10 \text{ mEq/L}$$
$$\rightarrow \textbf{anion gap acidosis is present.}$$

4. Delta-delta calculation:

$$\Delta\Delta = \frac{(\text{Actual Anion Gap} - \text{Expected Anion Gap})}{(\text{Baseline } HCO_3 - \text{Actual } HCO_3)}$$
$$= (19 - 10)/(30 - 24) = \textbf{9/6, which is} \sim \textbf{1.66.}$$

Delta-delta interpretation.	
Delta-Delta Value	**Condition Present**
< 0.4	Non-anion gap only
0.4–0.9	Anion gap *and* non-anion gap acidosis
1.0–2.0	**Anion gap acidosis only**
> 2.0	Anion gap acidosis and metabolic alkalosis

Q24-5: D
2 mOsm/L.

Rationale: Similar to the serum anion gap, the serum osmolal gap is determined by the difference between the "calculated" serum osmolality and the true measured serum osmolality. The equation for the serum osmolal gap typically includes factors for sodium, glucose, BUN, and ethanol, as these are readily measurable in most laboratories. Therefore, the serum osmolal gap will represent the osmolality of those "unmeasured" osmoles, including organic alcohols and acetone. The most common form is shown as follows:

$$\text{Calculated Serum Osmolality} = 2 * [Na^+] + \frac{[\text{Glucose}]}{18} + \frac{[BUN]}{2.8} + \frac{[EtOH]}{3.7};$$

In which the units of measure are as follows: Na, mEq/L; glucose, mg/dL; BUN, mg/dL; and EtOH, mg/dL. The conversion factors are shown in the preceding equation as well. A normal serum osmolal gap is around −10 to +10 mOsm/L (or mOsm/kg).

Therefore, for this patient,

$$\begin{aligned}
\text{Calculated Serum Osmolality} &= [2 * Na] + [\text{Glucose}/18] + [BUN/2.8] + [EtOH/3.7] \\
&= (2 * 136) + (124/18) + (28/2.8) + (0/3.7) \\
&= 288.9 \sim 289 \text{ mOsm/L}.
\end{aligned}$$

$$\begin{aligned}
\text{Serum Osmolal Gap} &= \text{Measured Serum Osmolality} - \text{Calculated Osmolality} \\
&= (291 - 289) = 2 \text{ mOsm/L, which is} < 10 \text{ mOsm/L} \\
&\rightarrow \textbf{no serum osmolal gap.}
\end{aligned}$$

Q24-6: B
Serum lactate.

Rationale: The patient has a high anion gap metabolic acidosis. He presented with hypotension in the setting of sepsis and the delta-delta ratio of 1.6 is a classic presentation of lactic acidosis. Although the patient has an acute kidney injury, this is not likely to be the cause of the high anion gap acidosis, as acute renal failure usually involves development of a non-anion gap metabolic acidosis initially, followed by the eventual development of an anion gap as the ability of the kidney to excrete anions worsens. Additionally, this patient's BUN is not significantly elevated. The patient does not take OTC medications, so an acetaminophen overdose is unlikely. The urine chloride is used to determine the etiology of a patient's metabolic alkalosis, while the urine anion gap (or urine osmolar gap) is used to determine the etiology of a non-anion gap metabolic acidosis.

Q24-7: C
31 mEq/L.

Rationale: Patients with neuromuscular disorders such as ALS will develop progressively worsening chronic respiratory acidosis as the disease progresses. While many patients may be temporized with noninvasive methods of mechanical ventilation prior to requiring invasive ventilation, patients with chronic respiratory failure have very little ventilatory reserve due to neuromuscular weakness and are often unable to compensate for any significant metabolic acidosis. Such is the case here, where this patient is unable to appropriately compensate for his metabolic acidosis for any significant period of time.

We know that the patient's baseline value for HCO_3 is 30 mEq/L and his baseline $Paco_2$ is 58 mm Hg. The baseline HCO_3 represents a compensatory metabolic alkalosis in response to the patient's chronic respiratory acidosis.

The appropriate HCO_3 for the *chronic* portion of respiratory acidosis is calculated as follows:

Expected $[HCO_3^-]$ = Normal $[HCO_3^-]$ + 0.35 * [Actual $Paco_2$ – Normal $Paco_2$]
Expected $[HCO_3^-]$ = 24 + 0.35 * [58 – 40 mm Hg] = 30 mEq/L.

To determine what the expected HCO_3 would be if the patient is fully compensating for the *acute* portion of the respiratory acidosis (ie, the increase from 58 mm Hg to 72 mm Hg), and assuming no concomitant metabolic acidosis or alkalosis, we would use the following calculation:

Expected $[HCO_3^-]$ = Baseline $[HCO_3^-]$ + 0.10 * [Actual $Paco_2$ – Baseline $Paco_2$]
Expected $[HCO_3^-]$ = 30 + 0.10 * [72 – 58 mm Hg] = 31.4 mEq/L.

References

Adrogué HJ, Madias NE. Secondary responses to altered acid-base status: the rules of engagement. J Am Soc Nephrol 2010; 21:920.

Berend K, de Vries AP, Gans RO. Physiological approach to assessment of acid-base disturbances. N Engl J Med. 2014 Oct 9;371(15):1434-45. doi: 10.1056/NEJMra1003327.

Feldman M, Soni N, Dickson B. Influence of hypoalbuminemia or hyperalbuminemia on the serum anion gap. J Lab Clin Med 2005; 146:317.

Gennari FJ. Current concepts. Serum osmolality. Uses and limitations. N Engl J Med 1984; 310:102.

Krapf R, Beeler I, Hertner D, Hulter HN. Chronic respiratory alkalosis. The effect of sustained hyperventilation on renal regulation of acid-base equilibrium. N Engl J Med 1991; 324:1394.

Kraut JA, Kurtz I. Toxic alcohol ingestions: clinical features, diagnosis, and management. Clin J Am Soc Nephrol 2008; 3:208.

Kraut JA, Nagami GT. The serum anion gap in the evaluation of acid-base disorders: what are its limitations and can its effectiveness be improved? Clin J Am Soc Nephrol 2013; 8:2018.

Martinu T, Menzies D, Dial S. Re-evaluation of acid-base prediction rules in patients with chronic respiratory acidosis. Can Respir J 2003; 10:311.

Purssell RA, Pudek M, Brubacher J, Abu-Laban RB. Derivation and validation of a formula to calculate the contribution of ethanol to the osmolal gap. Ann Emerg Med 2001;38 (6): 653–9. doi:10.1067/mem.2001.119455. PMID 11719745.

Weinberger SE, Schwartzstein RM, Weiss JW. Hypercapnia. N Engl J Med 1989; 321:1223.

West JB. Causes of carbon dioxide retention in lung disease. N Engl J Med 1971; 284:1232.

Williams MH Jr, Shim CS. Ventilatory failure. Etiology and clinical forms. Am J Med 1970; 48:477.

CASE 25

A 44-year-old black man presents with altered mental status, tachycardia, and moderate abdominal pain. His medical problems include IDDM, irritable bowel syndrome on SSRI therapy, hypertension on amlodipine and losartan, and hyperlipidemia on simvastatin. His wife reports that he stayed home from work 3 days ago due to a GI illness with frequent emesis. He was attempting to take fluids as tolerated but has not been able to tolerate much in the way of food intake. Over the past 24 hours, he has been complaining of diffuse achy or crampy abdominal pain, and his mentation has worsened slowly. His vital signs are as follows: T 36.6°C, RR 26, HR 130, and BP 95/60. He has a mild leukocytosis with WBCs of 14,000. His remaining laboratory values are listed as follows. On examination, he has a benign abdomen.

Laboratory data.			
ABGs		Basic Metabolic Panel	
pH	7.19	Na	131 mEq/L
$Paco_2$	24 mm Hg	K	5.7 mEq/L
Pao_2	91 mm Hg	Cl	77 mEq/L
HCO^3	9 mEq/L	CO_2	9 mEq/L
		BUN	44 mg/dL
		Cr	0.8 mg/dL
		Glucose	850 mg/dL
		Albumin	4.7 g/dL
		EtOH	0 g/dL

QUESTIONS

Q25-1: Define the patient's baseline acid-base status: Does this patient have an underlying chronic acid-base disorder that we need to account for in order to appropriately interpret the acute acid-base disorders?

A. There is no evidence for an underlying chronic respiratory or metabolic acid-base disorder in this patient, so we would assume a baseline $Paco_2$ of 40 mm Hg and an HCO_3 of 24 mEq/L.

B. While the patient has a condition predisposing him to a chronic acid-base disorder, there is insufficient information to estimate the patient's baseline $Paco_2$ and HCO_3 values; therefore, we will assume a baseline $Paco_2$ of 40 mm Hg and a baseline HCO_3 of 24 mEq/L.

C. The patient has an underlying acid-base condition, and we have sufficient information to estimate the patient's baseline $Paco_2$ and HCO_3 values.

Q25-2: What is/are the primary acid-base disturbance(s) occurring in this case?

A. Metabolic acidosis only
B. Respiratory acidosis only
C. Metabolic acidosis and a respiratory acidosis
D. Metabolic alkalosis and a respiratory alkalosis

Q25-3: What should be considered a normal anion gap in this patient?

A. 14 mEq/L
B. 12 mEq/L
C. 10 mEq/L
D. 4 mEq/L

Q25-4: How would the metabolic acidosis component be classified in this case?

A. Anion gap acidosis
B. Non-anion gap acidosis
C. Anion and non-anion gap acidosis
D. Anion gap acidosis and a metabolic alkalosis

Q25-5: The patient's measured serum osmolality is 332 mOsm/L. What is the expected serum osmolality?

A. 290 mOsm/L
B. 310 mOsm/L
C. 360 mOsm/L
D. 325 mOsm/L

Q25-6: The following studies are performed:

Serum EtOH	< 3 mg/dL
Serum acetaminophen level	< 5 mg/dL (ULN for therapeutic use 20 mg/dL)
Serum salicylates level	< 5 mg/dL (ULN for therapeutic use 30 mg/dL)
Serum osmolality	332 mOsm/kg
Serum L-lactate	2.1 mmol/L (ULN 2.0 mmol/L venous)
Beta-hydroxybutyrate (acetone)	2.31 mmol/L (ULN 0.18 mmol/L)
Serum glucose	850 mg/dL

What is the most likely cause of the patient's anion-gap metabolic acidosis?

A. Starvation ketoacidosis
B. Alcoholic ketoacidosis
C. Diabetic ketoacidosis
D. Lactic acidosis
E. Acute renal failure

Q25-7: Given the patient's elevated serum glucose, what is the patient's corrected serum sodium (Na)?

A. 120 mEq/L
B. 124 mEq/L
C. 135 mEq/L
D. 139 mEq/L
E. 143 mEq/L

Q25-8: Does the patient in this case demonstrate appropriate respiratory or metabolic compensation?

A. Yes, the respiratory compensation is appropriate.
B. No, a concomitant respiratory alkalosis is present.
C. No, a concomitant respiratory acidosis is present.
D. Yes, the metabolic compensation is appropriate.
E. No, a concomitant metabolic acidosis is present.
F. No, a concomitant metabolic alkalosis is present.

Q25-9: What is the most likely cause of the patient's concomitant metabolic alkalosis? The patient's urine studies are as follows:

Urine Na	10 mEq/L
Urine K	20 mEq/L
Urine Cl	6 mEq/L
Urine glucose	230 mg/dL
Urine pH	5.5

A. Emesis
B. Thiazide diuretic use
C. Milk-alkali ingestion
D. Therapeutic bicarbonate infusion

ANSWERS

Q25-1: A

There is no evidence for an underlying chronic respiratory or metabolic acid-base disorder in this patient, so we would assume a baseline $Paco_2$ of 40 mm Hg and an HCO_3 of 24 mEq/L.

Rationale: Ignoring these underlying chronic acid-base disorders can significantly alter the interpretation of a patient's acute acid-base status. This was demonstrated in the first case of the series. However, often, we do not have the necessary information (eg, prior ABG or VBG, or prior serum chemistry with an HCO_3) and are forced to assume the ongoing processes are all acute in nature. We are primarily concerned about chronic respiratory acid-base disorders, as these can significantly alter the patient's baseline or expected values for the serum HCO_3 and $Paco_2$, and we have reliable equations to predict the expected baseline values. The respiratory compensation for both chronic metabolic acidosis and alkalosis is generally poor, so there are no equations or rules to predict what the $Paco_2$ should be in these cases. While the baseline serum HCO_3 may be significantly off from our standard value of 24 mEq/L in these patients, we would assume a baseline $Paco_2$ of 40 mm Hg in patients with chronic metabolic processes. Once we identify the patient's baseline $Paco_2$ and HCO_3 values, we will need to use these values in the appropriate equations to identify the ongoing acute processes.

Q25-2: A

Metabolic acidosis only.

Rationale:

1. The pH is 7.19; therefore, the primary disorder is an **acidosis.**
2. The $Paco_2$ of 24 mm Hg is less than 40 mm Hg, so this is not the cause of the acidosis.
3. The HCO_3 of 9 mEq/L is less than 24 mEq/L, so there is a **metabolic acidosis.**

Q25-3: A

14 mEq/L.

Rationale: The normal anion gap is 12 mEq/L. The term *anion gap* refers to those ions (negatively charged molecules) in the bloodstream that we do not routinely measure, including phosphates, sulfates, organic acids, and negatively charged plasma proteins. One of the most abundant negatively charged ions in the blood is serum albumin. A normal serum albumin is 4.0 g/dL. For patients with hypoalbuminemia (low serum albumin), the normal or expected anion gap is smaller.

$$\text{Expected Anion Gap} = 12 - (2.5) * \left[4.0\,\frac{g}{dL} - \text{Actual Serum Albumin} \right].$$

So for this patient,

Expected Anion Gap = $12 - [2.5 * (4 - 4.7)] = 12 - (2.5 * -0.7) = 13.75 \sim 14$ mEq/L.

This is an unusual case in which the patient has an elevated serum albumin, likely secondary to hypovolemia and resultant hemoconcentration. Correcting for this patient's serum albumin returns an expected anion gap of 14 mEq/L rather than 12 mEq/L.

Q25-4: D
Anion gap acidosis and a metabolic alkalosis.

Rationale:

1. Is there evidence for a chronic respiratory acid-base disorder that requires adjustment of the patient's "normal" HCO_3? No, there is no evidence for a chronic respiratory acid-base disorder, so we would assume a baseline $Paco_2$ of 40 mm Hg and an HCO_3 of 24 mEq/L.

2. Expected anion gap:

$$\text{Expected Anion Gap} = 12 - (2.5) * \left[4.0 \, \frac{g}{dL} - \text{Actual Serum Albumin} \right]$$

$$= 12 - (2.5 * [4.0 - 4.7])$$
$$= 12 - (2.5 * [-0.7]) = \textbf{13.75} \sim \textbf{14 mEq/L.}$$

3. Anion gap calculation:

$$\text{Serum Anion Gap} = [Na^+] - [HCO_3^-] - [Cl^-]$$
$$= 131 - (77 + 9) = \textbf{45 mEq/L,} \text{ which is} > 14 \text{ mEq/L}$$
$$\rightarrow \textbf{anion gap acidosis is present.}$$

4. Delta-delta calculation:

$$\Delta\Delta = \frac{(\text{Actual Anion Gap} - \text{Expected Anion Gap})}{(\text{Baseline } HCO_3 - \text{Actual } HCO_3)}$$

$$= (45 - 14)/(24 - 9) = \textbf{31/15, which is} > \textbf{2.0.}$$

Delta-delta interpretation.	
Delta-Delta Value	Condition Present
< 0.4	Non-anion gap only
0.4–0.9	Anion gap *and* non-anion gap acidosis
1.0–2.0	Anion gap acidosis only
> 2.0	**Anion gap acidosis and metabolic alkalosis**

Q25-5: D
325 mOsm/L.

Rationale: To determine the patient's serum osmolal gap, we first need to determine the calculated serum osmolality. The serum osmolality may be calculated as follows:

$$\text{Calculated Serum Osmolality} = [2 * \text{Na}] + [\text{Glucose}/18] + [\text{BUN}/2.8] + [\text{EtOH}/3.7]$$
$$= (2 * 131) + (850/18) + (44/2.8) + (0/3.7)$$
$$= \textbf{325 mOsm/L.}$$

The serum osmolal gap is therefore,

$$\text{Serum Osmolal Gap} = \text{Measured Serum Osmolality} - \text{Calculated Osmolality}$$
$$= (332 - 325) = 8 \text{ mOsm/L, which is} > 10 \text{ mOsm/L}$$
$$\rightarrow \textbf{no serum osmolal gap.}$$

A normal serum osmolal gap is less than 10. There are four primary causes of an elevated osmolar gap:

1. Alcohol ingestion (ethanol, methanol, ethylene glycol, isopropyl alcohol)
2. Carbohydrate/sugars, namely mannitol
3. Hypertriglyceridemia
4. Hypergammaglobulinemia

This patient does not appear to have a serum osmolal gap.

Q25-6: C
Diabetic ketoacidosis.

Rationale: DKA is the most likely cause of this patient's anion-gap acidosis. The patient presented with an anion gap acidosis and a significantly elevated serum glucose level (850 mg/dL). Additional laboratory testing has demonstrated a negative serum acetaminophen level and a borderline normal serum lactate level. The patient has a normal serum osmolal gap as well. The positive serum beta-hydroxybutyrate and serum acetone levels confirm that a ketoacidosis is present. The patient has a negative EtOH, and there is no suggestion of prolonged starvation to suggest a starvation ketoacidosis.

Q25-7: E
143 mEq/L.

Rationale: Although we use the measured [Na] rather than the corrected [Na] for acid-base calculations, we can determine the predicted serum [Na] when corrected for hyperglycemia. Determining the corrected value can be helpful in identifying other potential causes for a patient's presentation. For example, a patient who recently presented in DKA had a normal serum sodium level, but when corrected, the serum sodium was significantly elevated.

$$\text{Corrected [Na]} = \text{Measured [Na]} + \left(1.6 * \frac{[\text{Serum Glucose} - 100]}{100} \right)$$

$$\text{Corrected [Na]} = 131 + \left(1.6 * \frac{850 - 100}{100} \right)$$

$$\text{Corrected [Na]} = 131 + 12 = 143 \text{ mEq/L.}$$

The correction for hypertriglyceridemia is as follows:

$$\text{Corrected [Na]} = \text{Measured [Na]} + 0.002 * [\text{Triglyceride (in mg/dL)}].$$

Q25-8: A
Yes, the respiratory compensation is appropriate.

Rationale: Using the Winter formula, one can calculate what the expected arterial $Paco_2$ should be for a given serum HCO_3 if the patient were completely compensated.

Respiratory Compensation for Acute Metabolic Acidosis (Winter Formula):

$$\text{Expected Paco}_2 = 1.5 * [\text{Actual HCO}_3^-] + 8 \pm 2 \text{ (in mm Hg)}$$
$$= (1.5 * 9) + 8 = 13.5 + 8 = 21.5 \pm 2 = (19.5 \text{ to } 23.5) \text{ mm Hg.}$$

This patient has an appropriate compensatory response to the metabolic acidosis.

Q25-9: A
Emesis.

Rationale: The vignette states that the patient has been experiencing significant emesis. The urine chloride is less than 10 mEq/L, which is most consistent with a chloride-responsive cause of metabolic alkalosis. This would include cystic fibrosis (CF), diuretic therapy, contraction alkalosis, hyperemesis, and post-hypercapnia response. The patient does not have a diagnosis of CF and is not currently on diuretics for his hypertension. Additionally, he has no recent known hypercapnic episodes. The cause is likely a combination of hyperemesis and contraction from the GI illness. The GI illness likely led to DKA, which further contributes to contraction via osmotic diuresis. Additionally, hyperglycemia can further worsen GI symptoms, including delayed gastric emptying.

Causes of metabolic alkalosis.
History: Rule Out the Following as Causes
• Alkali load ("milk-alkali" or calcium-alkali syndrome, oral sodium bicarbonate, IV sodium bicarbonate) • Genetic causes (CF) • Presence of hypercalcemia • IV β-lactam antibiotics • Laxative abuse (may also cause a metabolic acidosis depending on diarrheal HCO_3 losses)
If None of the Above, Then. . .
Urine Chloride < 20 mEq/L (Chloride-Responsive Causes)
• Loss of gastric acid (hyperemesis, NGT suctioning) • Prior diuretic use (in hours to days following discontinuation) • Post-hypercapnia • Villous adenoma • Congenital chloridorrhea • Chronic laxative abuse (may also cause a metabolic acidosis depending on diarrheal HCO_3 losses) • CF
OR
Urine Chloride > 20 mEq/L (Chloride-Resistant Causes)
Urine Chloride > 20 mEq/L, Lack of HTN, Urine Potassium < 30 mEq/L
• Hypokalemia or hypomagnesemia • Laxative abuse (if dominated by hypokalemia) • Bartter syndrome • Gitelman syndrome
Urine Chloride > 20 mEq/L, Lack of HTN, Urine Potassium > 30 mEq/L
• Current diuretic use
Urine Chloride > 20 mEq/L, Presence of HTN, Urine Potassium Variable but Usually > 30 mEq/L
Elevated plasma renin level: • Renal artery stenosis • Renin-secreting tumor • Renovascular disease
Low plasma renin, low plasma aldosterone: • Cushing syndrome • Exogenous mineralocorticoid use • Genetic disorder (11-hydoxylase or 17-hydrolyase deficiency, 11β-HSD deficiency) • Liddle syndrome • Licorice toxicity
Low plasma renin, high plasma aldosterone: • Primary hyperaldosteronism • Adrenal adenoma • Bilateral adrenal hyperplasia

References

Abreo K, Adlakha A, Kilpatrick S, et al. The milk-alkali syndrome. A reversible form of acute renal failure. Arch Intern Med. 1993;153:1005.

Barton CH, Vaziri ND, Ness RL, et al. Cimetidine in the management of metabolic alkalosis induced by nasogastric drainage. Arch Surg. 1979;114:70.

Bear R, Goldstein M, Phillipson E, et al. Effect of metabolic alkalosis on respiratory function in patients with chronic obstructive lung disease. Can Med Assoc J. 1977;117:900.

DeFronzo RA, Matzuda M, Barret E. Diabetic ketoacidosis: a combined metabolic-nephrologic approach to therapy. Diabetes Rev. 1994;2:209.

Fulop M, Murthy V, Michilli A, et al. Serum beta-hydroxybutyrate measurement in patients with uncontrolled diabetes mellitus. Arch Intern Med. 1999;159:381.

Galla JH, Gifford JD, Luke RG, Rome L. Adaptations to chloride-depletion alkalosis. Am J Physiol. 1991;261:R771.

Garella S, Chang BS, Kahn SI. Dilution acidosis and contraction alkalosis: review of a concept. Kidney Int. 1975;8:279.

Gennari FJ, Weise WJ. Acid-base disturbances in gastrointestinal disease. Clin J Am Soc Nephrol. 2008;3:1861.

Hamm LL, Nakhoul N, Hering-Smith KS. Acid-base homeostasis. Clin J Am Soc Nephrol. 2015;10:2232.

Hulter HN, Sebastian A, Toto RD, et al. Renal and systemic acid-base effects of the chronic administration of hypercalcemia-producing agents: calcitriol, PTH, and intravenous calcium. Kidney Int. 1982;21:445.

Khanna A, Kurtzman NA. Metabolic alkalosis. J Nephrol. 2006;19(suppl 9):S86.

Laski ME, Sabatini S. Metabolic alkalosis, bedside and bench. Semin Nephrol. 2006;26:404.

Luke RG, Galla JH. It is chloride depletion alkalosis, not contraction alkalosis. J Am Soc Nephrol. 2012;23:204.

Miller PD, Berns AS. Acute metabolic alkalosis perpetuating hypercarbia. A role for acetazolamide in chronic obstructive pulmonary disease. JAMA. 1977;238:2400.

Oster JR, Materson BJ, Rogers AI. Laxative abuse syndrome. Am J Gastroenterol. 1980;74:451.

Patel AM, Goldfarb S. Got calcium? Welcome to the calcium-alkali syndrome. J Am Soc Nephrol. 2010;21:1440.

Porter WH, Yao HH, Karounos DG. Laboratory and clinical evaluation of assays for beta-hydroxybutyrate. Am J Clin Pathol. 1997;107:353.

Rose BD, Post TW. Clinical Physiology of Acid-Base and Electrolyte Disorders. 5e. New York, NY: McGraw Hill; 2001:559; 809-815.

Schwartz WB, Van Ypersele de Strihou, Kassirer JP. Role of anions in metabolic alkalosis and potassium deficiency. N Engl J Med. 1968;279:630.

Shen T, Braude S. Changes in serum phosphate during treatment of diabetic ketoacidosis: predictive significance of severity of acidosis on presentation. Intern Med J. 2012;42:1347.

Sweetser LJ, Douglas JA, Riha RL, Bell SC. Clinical presentation of metabolic alkalosis in an adult patient with cystic fibrosis. Respirology. 2005;10:254.

Taki K, Mizuno K, Takahashi N, Wakusawa R. Disturbance of CO2 elimination in the lungs by carbonic anhydrase inhibition. Jpn J Physiol. 1986;36:523.

Turban S, Beutler KT, Morris RG, et al. Long-term regulation of proximal tubule acid-base transporter abundance by angiotensin II. Kidney Int. 2006;70:660.

Wachtel TJ, Tetu-Mouradjian LM, Goldman DL, et al. Hyperosmolarity and acidosis in diabetes mellitus: a three-year experience in Rhode Island. J Gen Intern Med. 1991;6:495.

CASE 26

A 42-year-old woman with a longstanding history of medical noncompliance, type 2 (insulin-dependent) diabetes, morbid obesity, osteoporosis, hypothyroidism, and prior cholecystectomy presents to the emergency department (ED) with diffuse abdominal pain, nausea, and encephalopathy. The patient is unable to provide any significant history, but her daughter reports she had been complaining of abdominal pain and poor appetite for the past 2 to 3 weeks that gradually worsened. The daughter also notes that her mother is very sedentary. At the ED, the patient undergoes a CT scan of the abdomen/pelvis that is concerning for ischemic bowel. She has no significant family or social history. Her vital signs on arrival are as follows: T 38.2°C, RR 28, HR 130, BP 80/50, and Sao_2 95%. The patient receives broad-spectrum antibiotics and is taken emergently to the operating room. Her laboratory findings are as follows:

Laboratory data.			
ABGs		Basic Metabolic Panel	
pH	7.32	Na	138 mEq/L
$Paco_2$	33 mm Hg	K	4.4 mEq/L
Pao_2	100 mm Hg	Cl	100 mEq/L
HCO_3	17 mEq/L	CO_2	17 mEq/L
		BUN	44 mg/dL
		Cr	1.1 mg/dL
		Glucose	100 mg/dL
		Albumin	3.0 g/dL
		EtOH	0 mg/dL

QUESTIONS

Q26-1: Define the patient's baseline acid-base status: Does this patient have an underlying chronic acid-base disorder that we need to account for in order to appropriately interpret the acute acid-base disorders?

A. There is no evidence for an underlying chronic respiratory or metabolic acid-base disorder in this patient, so we would assume a baseline $Paco_2$ of 40 mm Hg and an HCO_3 of 24 mEq/L.

B. While the patient has a condition predisposing her to a chronic acid-base disorder, there is insufficient information to estimate the patient's baseline $Paco_2$ and HCO_3 values; therefore, we will assume a baseline $Paco_2$ of 40 mm Hg and a baseline HCO_3 of 24 mEq/L.

C. The patient has an underlying acid-base condition, and we have sufficient information to estimate the patient's baseline $Paco_2$ and HCO_3 values.

Q26-2: What is/are the primary acid-base disturbance(s) occurring in this case?

A. Metabolic acidosis only
B. Respiratory acidosis only
C. Metabolic alkalosis only
D. Respiratory alkalosis only
E. Metabolic acidosis and a respiratory acidosis
F. Metabolic alkalosis and a respiratory alkalosis

Q26-3: For a perfectly healthy patient, a normal anion gap is assumed to be 12 mEq/L. What should be considered a normal anion gap in this patient?

A. 12 mEq/L
B. 9.5 mEq/L
C. 7 mEq/L
D. 4.5 mEq/L

Q26-4: How would the metabolic acidosis component be classified in this case?

A. Anion gap acidosis
B. Non-anion gap acidosis
C. Anion and non-anion gap acidosis
D. Anion gap acidosis and a metabolic alkalosis

Q26-5: Does the patient in this case demonstrate appropriate respiratory or metabolic compensation?

A. Yes, the respiratory compensation is appropriate.
B. No, a concomitant respiratory alkalosis is present.
C. No, a concomitant respiratory acidosis is present.
D. Yes, the metabolic compensation is appropriate.
E. No, a concomitant metabolic acidosis is present.
F. No, a concomitant metabolic alkalosis is present.

Q26-6: The patient returns from the operating room following resection of a small portion of ischemic bowel, washout of the abdominal cavity, and creation of an ostomy. She receives appropriate source control, antibiotic therapy, and fluid resuscitation, and her lactate, which was elevated on presentation returns to normal. Her renal function, which was mildly elevated on presentation also returns to normal; however, the patient's serum HCO_3 remains unexpectedly low. Additionally, the patient remains extremely weak on examination, despite improvement in her mental status. The output from her ostomy has been normal, and the patient is tolerating tube feedings currently at nutritional goal. The patient's basic metabolic panel is as follows:

Na	137 mEq/L
K	4.4 mEq/L
Cl	116 mEq/L
CO_2	17 mEq/L
BUN	12 mg/dL
Cr	0.4 mg/dL
Glucose	123 mg/dL
Albumin	2.2 g/dL
EtOH	0 mg/dL

The patient's ABG shows pH of 7.30 with $Paco_2$ of 35 mm Hg. How would the metabolic acidosis component be classified in this case?

A. Anion gap acidosis
B. Non-anion gap acidosis
C. Anion and non-anion gap acidosis
D. Anion gap acidosis and a metabolic alkalosis

Q26-7: You decide to investigate the patient's non-anion gap acidosis. The results of some additional studies are as follows:

Urine Na	32 mEq/L
Urine K	8 mEq/L
Urine Cl	28 mEq/L
Urine glucose	44 mg/dL
Urine pH	5.5
Urine RBCs	None
Urine WBCs	None
Urine protein	Moderate
Urine microscopic:	None
Other Pertinent Findings	
Serum K	3.3 mEq/L
Vitamin D (25-OH)	< 2 ng/mL (LLN 30 ng/mL)

What is the cause of the patient's non-anion gap acidosis?

A. Type 1 (distal) RTA
B. Type 2 (proximal) RTA
C. GI losses of bicarbonate
D. Type 4 RTA

ANSWERS

Q26-1: A

There is no evidence for an underlying chronic respiratory or metabolic acid-base disorder in this patient, so we would assume a baseline $Paco_2$ of 40 mm Hg and an HCO_3 of 24 mEq/L.

Rationale: Ignoring these underlying chronic acid-base disorders can significantly alter the interpretation of a patient's acute acid-base status. This was demonstrated in the first case of the series. However, often, we do not have the necessary information (eg, prior ABG or VBG, or prior serum chemistry with an HCO_3) and are forced to assume the ongoing processes are all acute in nature. We are primarily concerned about chronic respiratory acid-base disorders, as these can significantly alter the patient's baseline or expected values for the serum HCO_3 and $Paco_2$, and we have reliable equations to predict the expected baseline values. The respiratory compensation for both chronic metabolic acidosis and alkalosis is generally poor, so there are no equations or rules to predict what the $Paco_2$ should be in these cases. While the baseline serum HCO_3 may be significantly off from our standard value of 24 mEq/L in these patients, we would assume a baseline $Paco_2$ of 40 mm Hg in patients with chronic metabolic processes. Once we identify the patient's baseline $Paco_2$ and HCO_3 values, we will need to use these values in the appropriate equations to identify the ongoing acute processes.

Q26-2: A

Metabolic acidosis only.

Rationale:

1. The pH is 7.32; therefore, the primary disorder is an **acidosis.**
2. The $Paco_2$ of 33 mm Hg is less than 40 mm Hg, so this is not the cause of acidosis.
3. The HCO_3 of 17 mEq/L is less than 24 mEq/L, so there is a **metabolic acidosis.**

Q26-3: B

9.5 mEq/L.

Rationale: The normal anion gap is 12 mEq/L. The term *anion gap* refers to net charge of all ions in the bloodstream that we do not routinely measure (calcium, potassium, magnesium, phosphates, sulfates, organic acids, and negatively charged plasma proteins). One of the most abundant negatively charged ions in the blood is serum albumin. A normal serum albumin is 4.0 g/dL. For patients with hypoalbuminemia (low serum albumin), the normal or expected anion gap is smaller.

$$\text{Expected Anion Gap} = 12 - (2.5) * \left[4.0 \frac{\text{g}}{\text{dL}} - \text{Actual Serum Albumin} \right].$$

So for this patient,

$$\text{Expected Anion Gap} = 12 - [2.5 * (4 - 3)] = 12 - (2.5 * 1) = 9.5 \text{ mEq/L}.$$

This is an important concept as patients with hypoalbuminemia may "hide" an anion gap acidosis if this correction is not performed.

Q26-4: A
Anion gap acidosis.

Rationale:

1. Is there evidence for a chronic respiratory acid-base disorder that requires adjustment of the patient's "normal" HCO_3? No, there is no evidence for a chronic respiratory acid-base disorder, so we would assume a baseline $Paco_2$ of 40 mm Hg and an HCO_3 of 24 mEq/L.
2. Expected anion gap:

$$\text{Expected Anion Gap} = 12 - (2.5) * \left[4.0\,\frac{g}{dL} - \text{Actual Serum Albumin} \right]$$
$$= 12 - (2.5 * [4.0 - 3.0])$$
$$= 12 - (2.5 * [3.0]) = \mathbf{9.5\ mEq/L}.$$

3. Anion gap calculation:

$$\text{Serum Anion Gap} = [Na^+] - [HCO_3^-] - [Cl^-]$$
$$= 138 - (100 + 17) = 21 \text{ mEq/L, which is} > 9.5 \text{ mEq/L}$$
$$\rightarrow \textbf{anion gap acidosis is present.}$$

4. Delta-delta calculation:

$$\Delta\Delta = \frac{(\text{Actual Anion Gap} - \text{Expected Anion Gap})}{(\text{Baseline } HCO_3 - \text{Actual } HCO_3)}$$
$$= (21 - 9.5)/(24 - 17) = \mathbf{11.5/7,\ which\ is \sim 1.6.}$$

Delta-delta interpretation.	
Delta-Delta Value	Condition Present
< 0.4	Non-anion gap only
0.4–0.9	Anion gap *and* non-anion gap acidosis
1.0–2.0	**Anion gap acidosis only**
> 2.0	Anion gap acidosis and metabolic alkalosis

Therefore, this patient has an anion gap acidosis without evidence of a concomitant non-anion gap metabolic acidosis or a metabolic alkalosis. This a classic delta-delta value consistent with lactic acidosis, which is the likely cause of this patient's metabolic acidosis given the clinical history.

Q26-5: A
Yes, the respiratory compensation is appropriate.

Rationale: Using the Winter formula, one can calculate what the expected arterial $Paco_2$ should be for a given serum HCO_3 if the patient were completely compensated.

Respiratory Compensation for Acute Metabolic Acidosis (Winters Formula):

Expected $Paco_2$ = 1.5 * [Actual HCO_3] + 8 ± 2 (in mm Hg)
Expected $Paco_2$ = 1.5 * (Actual HCO_3) + 8 (± 2)
$= (1.5 * 17) + 8 = 25.5 + 8 = 33.5 ± 2 = (31$ to $35)$ mm Hg.

The patient's $Paco_2$ falls within this range (33 mm Hg). Therefore, this patient has an appropriate compensatory response to the metabolic acidosis.

Q26-6: B
Non-anion gap acidosis.

Rationale:

1. Expected anion gap:

Expected Anion Gap (AG) = 12 − (2.5 * [4.0 − Actual Albumin])
$= 12 − (2.5 * [4.0 − 2.2])$
$= 12 − (2.5 * [2.8]) = \textbf{7.5 mEq/L.}$

2. Anion gap calculation:

AG = Na − (Cl + HCO_3)
$137 − (116 + 17) = 4$ mEq/L, which is < 7.5 mEq/L → **no anion gap exists.**

Therefore, this patient has shifted from an anion gap acidosis to a non-anion gap acidosis.

Q26-7: B
Type 2 (proximal) RTA.

Rationale: Here, as no serum anion gap is present, it should be sufficient to evaluate the urine anion gap, which is more readily available at most facilities than the urine osmolar gap. The urine anion gap can help differentiate situations in which there is inadequate renal excretion of acids (type 1 [distal] and type 4 RTA) from situations in which there is appropriate urine acidification but other losses of HCO_3 (GI causes). However, it is not particularly useful for patients with a proximal RTA. Here the urine anion gap is calculated as follows:

Urine Anion Gap = $[U_{Na}] + [U_K] − [U_{Cl}]$.

Therefore, for this patient,

Urine Anion Gap = $U_{Na} + U_K − U_{Cl} = (32 + 8) − 28 = (+12)$ mEq/L.

Although the urine anion gap falls into an equivocal range, it is not as negative as would be expected in a patient with GI loss of HCO_3 as the predominant cause.

To determine the type of RTA, one can look at the urine pH and serum potassium for evidence of kidney stones.

Interpretation:

- A urine anion gap that is greater than ~20 mEq/L → reduced renal acid excretion (RTA).
- A urine anion gap that is less than −20 mEq/L → GI loss of HCO_3 (eg, diarrhea), although type 2 RTA is possible.
- A urine anion gap between −20 and +10 mEq/L is generally considered inconclusive.

Diagnosis of RTA.			
	Type 1 RTA	Type 2 RTA	Type 4 RTA
Severity of metabolic acidosis, (HCO_3)	Severe (< 10–12 mEq/L typically)	Intermediate (12–20 mEq/L)	Mild (15–20 mEq/L)
Associated urine abnormalities	Urinary phosphate, calcium are increased; bone disease often present	Urine glucose, amino acids, phosphate, calcium may be elevated	
Urine pH	HIGH (> 5.5)	Low (acidic), until serum HCO_3 level exceeds the resorptive ability of the proximal tubule; then becomes alkalotic once reabsorptive threshold is crossed	Low (acidic)
Serum K+	Low to normal; should correct with oral HCO_3 therapy	Classically low, although may be normal or even high with rare genetic defects; worsens with oral HCO_3 therapy	HIGH
Renal stones	Often	No	No
Renal tubular defect	Reduced NH_4 secretion in distal tubule	Reduced HCO_3 resorption in proximal tubule	Reduced H^+/K^+ exchange in distal and collecting tubule due to decreased aldosterone or aldosterone resistance
Urine anion gap	> 10	Negative	> 10
Urine osmolal gap	Reduced during acute acidosis		Reduced during acute acidosis

The patient's urine pH is acidic (pH 5.5) with hypokalemia and no renal stones. The pH makes a distal RTA (type 1) unlikely, and the low serum potassium makes a type 4 RTA unlikely as well. Importantly, the patient has an undetectable vitamin D level. Severe vitamin D deficiency (rickets) can impact proximal tubular function, leading to hypophosphatemia and hypocalcemia, with phosphaturia, glycosuria (as seen here), aminoaciduria, and tubular proteinuria. Additionally, it can also be associated with severe weakness and balance issues, among other complications. The treatment is generally supplementation with HCO_3, phosphate, and vitamin D. Although this can result from inherited genetic mutations, sporadic cases do occur. The mechanisms underlying how vitamin D level impacts HCO_3 resorption are not completely clear. The other primary cause of type 2 RTA is carbonic anhydrase inhibitor use.

Causes of renal tubular acidosis.
Causes of Type 1 (Distal) RTA
Primary
• Idiopathic or familial (may be recessive or dominant)
Secondary
• Medications: Lithium, amphotericin, ifosfamide, NSAIDs
• Rheumatologic disorders: Sjögren syndrome, SLE, RA
• Hypercalciuria (idiopathic) or associated with vitamin D deficiency or hyperparathyroidism
• Sarcoidosis
• Obstructive uropathy
• Wilson disease
• Rejection of renal transplant allograft
• Toluene toxicity
Causes of Type 2 (Proximal) RTA
Primary
• Idiopathic
• Familial (primarily recessive disorders)
• Genetic: Fanconi syndrome, cystinosis, glycogen storage disease (type 1), Wilson disease, galactosemia
Secondary
• Medications: Acetazolamide, topiramate, aminoglycoside antibiotics, ifosfamide, reverse transcriptase inhibitors (tenofovir)
• Heavy metal poisoning: Lead, mercury, copper
• Multiple myeloma or amyloidosis (secondary to light chain toxicity)
• Sjögren syndrome
• Vitamin D deficiency
• Rejection of renal transplant allograft
Causes of Type 4 RTA (Hypoaldosteronism or Aldosterone Resistance)
Primary
• Primary adrenal insufficiency
• Inherited disorders associated with hypoaldosteronism
• Pseudohypoaldosteronism (types 1 and 2)
Secondary
• Causes of hyporeninemic hypoaldosteronism such as renal disease (diabetic nephropathy), NSAID use, calcineurin inhibitors, volume expansion/volume overload
• Causes of distal tubule voltage defects such as sickle cell disease, obstructive uropathy, SLE
• Severe illness/septic shock
• Angiotensin II–associated medications: ACE inhibitors, ARBs, direct renin inhibitors
• Potassium-sparing diuretics: Spironolactone, amiloride, triamterene
• Antibiotics: Trimethoprim, pentamidine

References

Adrogué HJ, Madias NE. Secondary responses to altered acid-base status: the rules of engagement. J Am Soc Nephrol 2010; 21:920.

Batlle D, Chin-Theodorou J, Tucker BM. Metabolic Acidosis or Respiratory Alkalosis? Evaluation of a Low Plasma Bicarbonate Using the Urine Anion Gap. Am J Kidney Dis. 2017 Sep;70(3):440-444. doi: 10.1053/j.ajkd.2017.04.017. Epub 2017 Jun 7.

Batlle D, Grupp M, Gaviria M, Kurtzman NA. Distal renal tubular acidosis with intact capacity to lower urinary pH. Am J Med 1982; 72:751.

Batlle D, Haque SK. Genetic causes and mechanisms of distal renal tubular acidosis. Nephrol Dial Transplant 2012, 27:3691.

Batlle DC, Hizon M, Cohen E, Gutterman C, Gupta R. The use of the urinary anion gap in the diagnosis of hyperchloremic metabolic acidosis. N Engl J Med. 1988 Mar 10;318(10):594-9.

Batlle DC, von Riotte A, Schlueter W. Urinary sodium in the evaluation of hyperchloremic metabolic acidosis. N Engl J Med 1987; 316:140.

Berend K, de Vries AP, Gans RO. Physiological approach to assessment of acid-base disturbances. N Engl J Med. 2014 Oct 9;371(15):1434-45. doi: 10.1056/NEJMra1003327.

Buckalew VM Jr, McCurdy DK, Ludwig GD, et al. Incomplete renal tubular acidosis. Physiologic studies in three patients with a defect in lowering urine pH. Am J Med 1968; 45:32.

Dyck RF, Asthana S, Kalra J, et al. A modification of the urine osmolal gap: an improved method for estimating urine ammonium. Am J Nephrol 1990; 10:359.

Feldman M, Soni N, Dickson B. Influence of hypoalbuminemia or hyperalbuminemia on the serum anion gap. J Lab Clin Med 2005; 146:317.

Karet FE. Mechanisms in hyperkalemic renal tubular acidosis. J Am Soc Nephrol 2009; 20:251.

Kim GH, Han JS, Kim YS, et al. Evaluation of urine acidification by urine anion gap and urine osmolal gap in chronic metabolic acidosis. Am J Kidney Dis 1996; 27:42.

Kraut JA, Madias NE. Differential diagnosis of nongap metabolic acidosis: value of a systematic approach. Clin J Am Soc Nephrol. 2012 Apr;7(4):671-9. doi: 10.2215/CJN.09450911. Epub 2012 Mar 8.

Kraut JA, Nagami GT. The serum anion gap in the evaluation of acid-base disorders: what are its limitations and can its effectiveness be improved? Clin J Am Soc Nephrol 2013; 8:2018.

Lee Hamm L, Hering-Smith KS, Nakhoul NL. Acid-base and potassium homeostasis. Semin Nephrol 2013; 33:257.

Meregalli P, Lüthy C, Oetliker OH, Bianchetti MG. Modified urine osmolal gap: an accurate method for estimating the urinary ammonium concentration? Nephron 1995; 69:98.

Oh M, Carroll HJ. Value and determinants of urine anion gap. Nephron 2002; 90:252.

Rastegar M, Nagami GT. Non-Anion Gap Metabolic Acidosis: A Clinical Approach to Evaluation. Am J Kidney Dis. 2017 Feb;69(2):296-301. doi: 10.1053/j.ajkd.2016.09.013. Epub 2016 Oct 28.

Rodríguez Soriano J. Renal tubular acidosis: the clinical entity. J Am Soc Nephrol 2002; 13:2160.

CASE 27

A 66-year-old man with insulin-dependent diabetes mellitus (IDDM), tobacco use, and COPD (FEV$_1$ 1.95 L, 60% predicted) presents to the emergency department with a 1-day history of diarrhea, fatigue, and lightheadedness. He recently returned from a cruise and both he and his wife are ill. He reports minimal PO intake over the past 2 to 3 days. His serum glucose is 160 and his UA shows no ketones present. He has a baseline Cr of 1.0. He is hypotensive on presentation with HR 110 and BP 80/50. He has no history of chronic respiratory failure.

Laboratory data.			
ABGs		Basic Metabolic Panel	
pH	7.22	Na	135 mEq/L
Paco$_2$	52 mm Hg	K	3.0 mEq/L
Pao$_2$	80 mm Hg	Cl	102 mEq/L
HCO$_3$	13 mEq/L	CO$_2$	12 mEq/L
		BUN	44 mg/dL
		Cr	1.3 mg/dL
		Glucose	94 mg/dL
		Albumin	4.0 g/dL
		EtOH	0 mg/dL

QUESTIONS

Q27-1: Define the patient's baseline acid-base status: Does this patient have an underlying chronic acid-base disorder that we need to account for in order to appropriately interpret the acute acid-base disorders?

A. There is no evidence for an underlying chronic respiratory or metabolic acid-base disorder in this patient, so we would assume a baseline $Paco_2$ of 40 mm Hg and an HCO_3 of 24 mEq/L.

B. While the patient has a condition predisposing him to a chronic acid-base disorder, there is insufficient information to estimate the patient's baseline $Paco_2$ and HCO_3 values; therefore, we will assume a baseline $Paco_2$ of 40 mm Hg and a baseline HCO_3 of 24 mEq/L.

C. The patient has an underlying acid-base condition, and we have sufficient information to estimate the patient's baseline $Paco_2$ and HCO_3 values.

Q27-2: What is/are the primary acid-base disturbance(s) occurring in this case?

A. Metabolic acidosis only
B. Respiratory acidosis only
C. Metabolic acidosis and a respiratory acidosis
D. Metabolic alkalosis and a respiratory acidosis

Q27-3: How would the metabolic acidosis component be classified in this case?

A. Anion gap acidosis
B. Non-anion gap acidosis
C. Anion and non-anion gap acidosis
D. Anion gap acidosis and a metabolic alkalosis

Q27-4: The urine osmolal gap is 425 mOsm/L. The urine anion gap is −1 mEq/L. What is the most likely cause of the patient's non-anion gap metabolic acidosis?

A. Diarrhea
B. Type 1 RTA (distal renal tubular acidosis)
C. Type 4 RTA

Q27-5: The patient's laboratory data results are as follows:

Serum EtOH	< 3 mg/dL
Serum acetaminophen level	< 5 mg/dL (ULN for therapeutic use 20 mg/dL)
Serum salicylate level	< 5 mg/dL (ULN for therapeutic use 30 mg/dL)
Serum osmolality	298 mOsm/kg
Beta-hydroxybutyrate (acetone)	< 0.18 mmol/L (ULN 0.18 mmol/L)
Serum glucose	94 mg/dL
Serum phosphorus	2.9 mg/dL

What is the most likely cause of the patient's anion gap metabolic acidosis?

A. Methanol ingestion
B. Ethylene glycol ingestion
C. Lactic acidosis
D. Aspirin toxicity
E. Acetaminophen toxicity
F. Carbon monoxide poisoning

Q27-6: This patient also has a respiratory acidosis, which is most likely due to his underlying COPD, which limits his ability to compensate for a metabolic acidosis. What would be the expected $Paco_2$ for a patient with the same acute metabolic acidosis if he/she were compensating appropriately (ie, pH 7.40)?

A. 18 mm Hg
B. 20 mm Hg
C. 26 mm Hg
D. 34 mm Hg

ANSWERS

Q27-1: B

While the patient has a condition (COPD) predisposing him to a chronic acid-base disorder, there is insufficient information to estimate the patient's baseline $Paco_2$ and HCO_3 values; therefore, we will assume a baseline $Paco_2$ of 40 mm Hg and a baseline HCO_3 of 24 mEq/L.

Rationale: Ignoring these underlying chronic acid-base disorders can significantly alter the interpretation of a patient's acute acid-base status. This was demonstrated in the first case of the series. However, often we do not have the necessary information (eg, prior ABG or VBG, or prior serum chemistry with an HCO_3) and are forced to assume the ongoing processes are all acute in nature. We are primarily concerned about chronic respiratory acid-base disorders, as these can significantly alter the patient's baseline or expected values for the serum HCO_3 and $Paco_2$, and we have reliable equations to predict the expected baseline values. The respiratory compensation for both chronic metabolic acidosis and alkalosis is generally poor, so there are no equations or rules to predict what the $Paco_2$ should be in these cases. While the baseline serum HCO_3 may be significantly off from our standard value of 24 mEq/L in these patients, we would assume a baseline $Paco_2$ of 40 mm Hg in patients with chronic metabolic processes. Once we identify the patient's baseline $Paco_2$ and HCO_3 values, we will need to use these values in the appropriate equations to identify the ongoing acute processes.

Q27-2: C

Metabolic acidosis and respiratory acidosis.

Rationale:

1. The pH is 7.22; therefore, the primary disorder is an **acidosis**.
2. The $Paco_2$ of 52 mm Hg is greater than 40 mm Hg, so there is a **respiratory acidosis**.
3. The HCO_3 of 12 mEq/L is less than 24 mEq/L, so there is also a **metabolic acidosis**.

Q27-3: C

Anion and non-anion gap acidosis.

Rationale:

1. Is there evidence for a chronic acid-base disorder that requires adjustment of the patient's "normal" HCO_3? No, there is no evidence for a chronic acid-base disorder, so we would assume a baseline $Paco_2$ of 40 mm Hg and an HCO_3 of 24 mEq/L.
2. Expected anion gap:

$$\text{Expected Anion Gap} = 12 - (2.5) * \left[4.0 \frac{g}{dL} - \text{Actual Serum Albumin} \right]$$

$$= 12 - (2.5 * [4.0 - 4.0])$$
$$= 12 - (2.5 * [0]) = \textbf{12 mEq/L.}$$

3. Anion gap calculation:

$$Serum\ Anion\ Gap = [Na^+] - [HCO_3^-] - [Cl^-]$$
$$= 135 - (102 + 12) = 19\ mEq/L,\ which\ is > 12\ mEq/L$$
$$\rightarrow \textbf{anion gap acidosis is present.}$$

4. Delta-delta calculation: The delta-delta calculation helps determine if there is more than one type of metabolic acidosis occurring in a patient.

$$\Delta\Delta = \frac{(Actual\ Anion\ Gap - Expected\ Anion\ Gap)}{(Baseline\ HCO_3 - Actual\ HCO_3)}$$

$$= (19 - 12)/(24 - 12) = \textbf{7/12, which is < 1.}$$

Delta-delta interpretation.	
Delta-Delta Value	Condition Present
< 0.4	Non-anion gap only
0.4–1.0	**Anion gap *and* non-anion gap acidosis**
1.0–2.0	Anion gap acidosis only
> 2.0	Anion gap acidosis and metabolic alkalosis

This indicates that the decrease in the serum HCO_3 is out of proportion to degree of change in the anion gap. The ratio of 7/12 is ~0.6. So an anion gap acidosis and a non-anion gap acidosis are present.

Q27-4: A
Diarrhea.

Rationale: The loss of HCO_3 in diarrhea is the likely cause of the patient's non-anion gap acidosis. The urine anion gap is inconclusive, likely due to the patient's concomitant anion gap metabolic acidosis. The urine anion gap can be inappropriately elevated in anion gap acidosis, a situation in which multiple unmeasured anions may be present in the urine (beta-hydroxybutryate/acetoacetate [ketoacidosis], hippurate [toluene], HCO_3 [proximal RTA], D-lactate [D-lactic acidosis], L-lactate, 5-oxoproline [acetaminophen toxicity]). Therefore, in patients with a significant anion gap, the urine osmolar gap is typically more useful.

An alternative approach is to consider the urine osmolar gap. Here the urine osmolar gap is:

$$Calculated\ Urine\ Osmolality = 2*([Na^+]+[K^+]) + \frac{[Urea]}{2.8} + \frac{[Glucose]}{18}$$

$$Urine\ Osmolal\ Gap\ (UOG) = Measured\ Urine\ Osmolality - Calculated\ Urine\ Osmolality$$

Similar to the urine anion gap, the urine osmolar gap is used as a surrogate for the urine ammonium concentration. Therefore, a larger gap indicates increased urinary NH_4 excretion. In normal acid-base conditions, the urine osmolar gap is between 10 and 100 mOsm/L. During a significant metabolic acidosis, patients with impaired renal tubular acidification (type 1 and type 4 RTA) are unable to excrete additional acid (NH_4), and therefore the osmolar gap does not change. Patients with an intact renal response to acidemia (ie, GI losses) should have a significant urine osmolar gap ($\sim$ >300 to 400 mOsm/L) as a result of increased NH_4 excretion.

Therefore, the elevated urine osmolal gap supports a diagnosis of diarrhea as the cause. This is further supported by the low serum potassium.

Q27-5: C
Lactic acidosis.

Rationale: The patient's presentation with diarrhea, renal failure, hypotension, and tachycardia suggests an issue with tissue perfusion/oxygenation, so a lactic acidosis is the most likely cause. The other studies demonstrate no evidence of a ketoacidosis and no evidence of salicylate or acetaminophen toxicity. The serum osmolal gap is normal:

$$\text{Calculated Serum Osmolality} = 2*[Na^+] + \frac{[Glucose]}{18} + \frac{[BUN]}{2.8} + \frac{[EtOH]}{3.7}$$
$$= 2*[135] + [44/2.8] + [94/18] = 291 \text{ mOsm/L.}$$

$$\text{Serum Osmolal Gap (SOG)} = \text{Measured Serum Osmolality}$$
$$- \text{Calculated Serum Osmolality}$$
$$\text{SOG} = 298 \text{ mOsm/L} - 291 \text{ mOsm/L} = (+7) \text{ mOsm/L.}$$

This is less than 10, so the serum osmolal gap is normal. The patient's serum creatinine may be mildly elevated at 1.3; however, the BUN and phosphorus are not as elevated as one would expect if acute renal failure were the cause of the anion gap acidosis.

Carbon monoxide poisoning can be associated with a lactic acidosis due to systemic hypoxemia. Patients will typically have an elevated $Paco_2$ on ABG. This is diagnosed with a co-oximetry ABG study or pulse oximetry. The patient will typically have a history of relevant exposure such as smoke inhalation, use of an outdoor heating element in a closed space, exposure to car/motor exhaust in closed space, etc. However, this can occur from a malfunctioning gas stove or furnace as well and patients may become incapacitated prior to presentation, making diagnosis more difficult. A high index of suspicion is necessary to make the diagnosis if co-oximetry blood gases are not normally ordered or used in the clinical setting at the time of presentation.

Q27-6: C
26 mm Hg.

Rationale: Using the Winter formula, one can calculate what the expected arterial $Paco_2$ should be for a given serum HCO_3 if the patient were completely compensated.

Respiratory Compensation for Acute Metabolic Acidosis (Winter Formula):

$$\text{Expected Paco}_2 = 1.5*[\text{Actual HCO}_3^-] + 8 \pm 2 \text{ (in mm Hg)}$$
$$= (1.5*12) + 8 = 18 + 8 = 26 +/- 2 = \textbf{(24 to 28) mm Hg.}$$

References

Adeva-Andany M, López-Ojén M, Funcasta-Calderón R, et al. Comprehensive review on lactate metabolism in human health. Mitochondrion 2014; 17:76.

Adrogué HJ, Madias NE. Secondary responses to altered acid-base status: the rules of engagement. J Am Soc Nephrol 2010; 21:920.

Arroliga AC, Shehab N, McCarthy K, Gonzales JP. Relationship of continuous infusion lorazepam to serum propylene glycol concentration in critically ill adults. Crit Care Med 2004; 32:1709.

Berend K, de Vries AP, Gans RO. Physiological approach to assessment of acid-base disturbances. N Engl J Med. 2014 Oct 9;371(15):1434-45. doi: 10.1056/NEJMra1003327.

Braden GL, Strayhorn CH, Germain MJ, et al. Increased osmolal gap in alcoholic acidosis. Arch Intern Med 1993; 153:2377.

Feldman M, Soni N, Dickson B. Influence of hypoalbuminemia or hyperalbuminemia on the serum anion gap. J Lab Clin Med 2005; 146:317.

Gabow PA. Ethylene glycol intoxication. Am J Kidney Dis 1988; 11:277.

Gennari FJ. Current concepts. Serum osmolality. Uses and limitations. N Engl J Med 1984; 310:102.

Glasser L, et. al. Serum Osmolality and its applicability to drug overdose. Am. J. Clin. Path. 1973; 60:695.

Kraut JA, Kurtz I. Toxic alcohol ingestions: clinical features, diagnosis, and management. Clin J Am Soc Nephrol 2008; 3:208.

Kraut JA, Nagami GT. The serum anion gap in the evaluation of acid-base disorders: what are its limitations and can its effectiveness be improved? Clin J Am Soc Nephrol 2013; 8:2018.

Kraut JA, Xing SX. Approach to the evaluation of a patient with an increased serum osmolal gap and high-anion-gap metabolic acidosis. Am J Kidney Dis 2011; 58:480.

Levy B. Lactate and shock state: the metabolic view. Curr Opin Crit Care 2006; 12:315.

Lynd LD, Richardson KJ, Purssell RA, et al. An evaluation of the osmole gap as a screening test for toxic alcohol poisoning. BMC Emerg Med 2008; 8:5.

Madias NE. Lactic acidosis. Kidney Int 1986; 29:752.

Marraffa JM, Holland MG, Stork CM, et al. Diethylene glycol: widely used solvent presents serious poisoning potential. J Emerg Med 2008; 35:401.

Mikkelsen ME, Miltiades AN, Gaieski DF, et al. Serum lactate is associated with mortality in severe sepsis independent of organ failure and shock. Crit Care Med 2009; 37:1670.

Purssell RA, Pudek M, Brubacher J, Abu-Laban RB. Derivation and validation of a formula to calculate the contribution of ethanol to the osmolal gap. Ann Emerg Med 2001;38 (6): 653–9. doi:10.1067/mem.2001.119455. PMID 11719745.

Robinson AG, Loeb JN. Ethanol ingestion—commonest cause of elevated plasma osmolality? N Engl J Med 1971; 284:1253.

Schelling JR, Howard RL, Winter SD, Linas SL. Increased osmolal gap in alcoholic ketoacidosis and lactic acidosis. Ann Intern Med 1990; 113:580.

CASE 28

A 24-year-old woman with chronic migraines presents to the emergency department with altered mental status and what her husband describes as breathing that "looks uncomfortable." She has been having more issues with headaches over the past 2 days, but her husband notes no other problems. She takes no prescribed medications, has no history of illicit drug use, and drinks alcohol only socially. She does not smoke tobacco. She has a negative qualitative pregnancy test. Her neurologic examination demonstrates no focal motor or sensory deficits, although the patient is unable to cooperate with a complete examination. Her cardiopulmonary and abdominal examinations are normal. Her vital signs are T 37.0°C, RR 24, HR 85, BP 104/66, and Sao_2 96% on RA.

Laboratory data.			
ABGs		Basic Metabolic Panel	
pH	7.29	Na	144 mEq/L
$Paco_2$	15 mm Hg	K	3.8 mEq/L
Pao_2	100 mm Hg	Cl	108 mEq/L
HCO_3	16 mEq/L	CO_2	17 mEq/L
		BUN	12 mg/dL
		Cr	1.2 mg/dL
		Glucose	123 mg/dL
		Albumin	4.0 g/dL
		EtOH	0 mg/dL

QUESTIONS

Q28-1: Define the patient's baseline acid-base status: Does this patient have an underlying chronic acid-base disorder that we need to account for in order to appropriately interpret the acute acid-base disorders?

A. There is no evidence for an underlying chronic respiratory or metabolic acid-base disorder in this patient, so we would assume a baseline $Paco_2$ of 40 mm Hg and an HCO_3 of 24 mEq/L.

B. While the patient has a condition predisposing her to a chronic acid-base disorder, there is insufficient information to estimate the patient's baseline $Paco_2$ and HCO_3 values; therefore, we will assume a baseline $Paco_2$ of 40 mm Hg and a baseline HCO_3 of 24 mEq/L.

C. The patient has an underlying acid-base condition, and we have sufficient information to estimate the patient's baseline $Paco_2$ and HCO_3 values.

Q28-2: What is/are the primary acid-base disturbance(s) occurring in this case?

A. Metabolic acidosis only
B. Respiratory acidosis only
C. Metabolic acidosis and a respiratory acidosis
D. Metabolic alkalosis and a respiratory alkalosis

Q28-3: How would the metabolic acidosis component be classified in this case?

A. Anion gap acidosis
B. Non-anion gap acidosis
C. Anion and non-anion gap acidosis
D. Anion gap acidosis and a metabolic alkalosis

Q28-4: Does the patient in this case demonstrate appropriate respiratory compensation?

A. Yes, the respiratory compensation is appropriate.
B. No, a concomitant respiratory alkalosis is present.
C. No, a concomitant respiratory acidosis is present.
D. Yes, the metabolic compensation is appropriate.
E. No, a concomitant metabolic acidosis is present.
F. No, a concomitant metabolic alkalosis is present.

Q28-5: In patients with an anion gap metabolic acidosis *and* a concomitant respiratory alkalosis, what is the most appropriate test to order next?

A. Serum drug screen (EtOH, ASA, salicylates)
B. Serum lactate
C. Serum beta-hydroxybutyrate
D. Serum osmolality
E. Urine osmolality

ANSWERS

Q28-1: A

There is no evidence for an underlying chronic respiratory or metabolic acid-base disorder in this patient, so we would assume a baseline $Paco_2$ of 40 mm Hg and an HCO_3 of 24 mEq/L.

Rationale: Ignoring these underlying chronic acid-base disorders can significantly alter the interpretation of a patient's acute acid-base status. This was demonstrated in the first case of the series. However, often we do not have the necessary information (eg, prior ABG or VBG, or prior serum chemistry with an HCO_3) and are forced to assume the ongoing processes are all acute in nature. We are primarily concerned about chronic respiratory acid-base disorders, as these can significantly alter the patient's baseline or expected values for the serum HCO_3 and $Paco_2$, and we have reliable equations to predict the expected baseline values. The respiratory compensation for both chronic metabolic acidosis and alkalosis is generally poor, so there are no equations or rules to predict what the $Paco_2$ should be in these cases. While the baseline serum HCO_3 may be significantly off from our standard value 24 mEq/L in these patients, we would assume a baseline $Paco_2$ of 40 mm Hg in patients with chronic metabolic processes. Once we identify the patient's baseline $Paco_2$ and HCO_3 values, we will need to use these values in the appropriate equations to identify the ongoing acute processes.

Q28-2: A

Metabolic acidosis only.

Rationale:

1. The pH is 7.29; therefore, the primary disorder is an **acidosis.**
2. The $Paco_2$ of 15 mm Hg is less than 40 mm Hg, so this is **not the cause of acidosis.**
3. The HCO_3 of 14 mEq/L is less than 24 mEq/L, so there is a **metabolic acidosis.**

Q28-3: C

Anion gap metabolic acidosis.

Rationale:

1. Is there evidence for a chronic acid-base disorder that requires adjustment of the patient's "normal" HCO_3? No, there is no evidence for a chronic acid-base disorder, so we would assume a baseline $Paco_2$ of 40 mm Hg and an HCO_3 of 24 mEq/L.
2. Expected anion gap:

$$\text{Expected Anion Gap} = 12 - (2.5) * \left[4.0 \frac{g}{dL} - \text{Actual Serum Albumin} \right]$$

$$= 12 - (2.5 * [4.0 - 4.0])$$
$$= 12 - (2.5 * [0]) = \textbf{12 mEq/L.}$$

3. Anion gap calculation:

$$\text{Serum Anion Gap} = [Na^+] - [HCO_3^-] - [Cl^-]$$
$$= 144 - (108 + 17) = 19 \text{ mEq/L, which is} > 12 \text{ mEq/L}$$
$$\rightarrow \textbf{anion gap acidosis is present.}$$

4. Delta-delta calculation: The delta-delta calculation helps determine if there is more than one type of metabolic acidosis occurring in a patient.

$$\Delta\Delta = \frac{(\text{Actual Anion Gap} - \text{Expected Anion Gap})}{(\text{Baseline HCO}_3 - \text{Actual HCO}_3)}$$

$$= (19 - 12)/(24 - 17) = 7/7, \textbf{ which is} = \textbf{1.}$$

Delta-delta interpretation.	
Delta-Delta Value	Condition Present
< 0.4	Non-anion gap only
0.4–1.0	Anion gap *and* non-anion gap acidosis
1.0–2.0	**Anion gap acidosis only**
> 2.0	Anion gap acidosis and metabolic alkalosis

This indicates that the change in serum HCO_3 for this patient is what we would expect from the change in the anion gap. **This patient therefore has a pure anion gap metabolic acidosis.**

Q28-4: B
No, a concomitant respiratory alkalosis is present.

Rationale: Using the Winter formula, one can calculate what the expected arterial $Paco_2$ should be for a given serum HCO_3 if the patient were completely compensated.

Respiratory Compensation for Acute Metabolic Acidosis (Winter Formula):

$$\text{Expected Paco}_2 = 1.5 * [\text{Actual HCO}_3] + 8 \pm 2 \text{ (in mm Hg)}$$
$$= (1.5 * 17) + 8 = 25.5 + 8 = 33.5 +/- 2 = (31 \text{ to } 35) \text{ mm Hg.}$$

Since the patient's $Paco_2$ on presentation was lower than the expected range of 31 to 35 mm Hg, **this patient also has a concomitant respiratory alkalosis.**

Q28-5: A
Serum drug screen for ASA.

Rationale: All of the listed tests are appropriate for a patient with an anion gap metabolic acidosis. However, the concomitant respiratory alkalosis is a classic presentation of salicylate toxicity, when in adults salicylates directly stimulate the respiratory center. The presentation is more commonly seen with an overall alkalemia (pH > 7.45), but not in all cases. The patient has a normal blood pressure so a lactic acidosis is less useful at this point. Given the patient has a no history of diabetes or alcohol use and normal serum albumin, a ketoacidosis is unlikely. The urine osmolality is helpful in differentiating non-anion gap metabolic acidosis. The serum osmolality is a good thought; however, the respiratory alkalosis makes aspirin toxicity more likely.

References

Demeter SL, Cordasco EM. Hyperventilation syndrome and asthma. Am J Med. 1986;81:989.

Eichenholz A, Mulhausen RO, Redleaf PS. Nature of acid-base disturbance in salicylate intoxication. Metabolism. 1963;12:164.

Gabow PA, Anderson RJ, Potts DE, Schrier RW. Acid-base disturbances in the salicylate-intoxicated adult. Arch Intern Med. 1978;138:1481.

Gardner WN. The pathophysiology of hyperventilation disorders. Chest. 1996;109:516.

Hill JB. Salicylate intoxication. N Engl J Med. 1973;288:1110.

Nardi AE, Freire RC, Zin WA. Panic disorder and control of breathing. Respir Physiol Neurobiol. 2009;167:133.

Saisch SG, Wessely S, Gardner WN. Patients with acute hyperventilation presenting to an inner-city emergency department. Chest. 1996;110:952.

Temple AR. Acute and chronic effects of aspirin toxicity and their treatment. Arch Intern Med. 1981;141:364.

Thisted B, Krantz T, Strøom J, Sørensen MB. Acute salicylate self-poisoning in 177 consecutive patients treated in ICU. Acta Anaesthesiol Scand. 1987;31:312.

CASE 29

A 70-year-old man with severe COPD presents to the emergency department (ED) obtunded, with rapid shallow breathing. He is intubated in the ED. His wife reports that he has been experiencing worsening shortness of breath at home over the past 24 hours, with increased sputum production and some low-grade fevers. He is normotensive on admission to the ICU. His vital signs are T 37.6°C, RR 34, HR 121, BP 131/66, and Sao_2 92% on RA. A CTA pulmonary embolism (PE) protocol is negative for PE. His examination is notable for poor air movement throughout with near-absent breath sounds at the apices bilaterally. His CXR is notable for hyperinflation with diaphragm flattening. A review of his prior laboratory findings reveals a serum HCO_3 of 32 mEq/L at baseline 2 months earlier, when the patient was otherwise feeling well. The patient takes no illicit drugs and drinks no alcohol.

Laboratory data.			
ABGs		Basic Metabolic Panel	
pH	7.13	Na	124 mEq/L
$Paco_2$	112 mm Hg	K	3.1 mEq/L
Pao_2	70 mm Hg	Cl	79 mEq/L
HCO_3	37 mEq/L	CO_2	37 mEq/L
		BUN	21 mg/dL
		Cr	1.1 mg/dL
		Glucose	103 mg/dL
		Albumin	3.6 g/dL
		EtOH	0 mg/dL

QUESTIONS

Q29-1: Define the patient's baseline acid-base status: Does this patient have an underlying chronic acid-base disorder that we need to account for in order to appropriately interpret the acute acid-base disorders?

A. There is no evidence for an underlying chronic respiratory or metabolic acid-base disorder in this patient, so we would assume a baseline $Paco_2$ of 40 mm Hg and an HCO_3 of 24 mEq/L.

B. While the patient has a condition that predisposes him to a chronic acid-base disorder, there is insufficient information to estimate the patient's baseline $Paco_2$ and HCO_3 values; therefore, we will assume a baseline $Paco_2$ of 40 mm Hg and a baseline HCO_3 of 24 mEq/L.

C. The patient has an underlying acid-base condition, and we have sufficient information to estimate the patient's baseline $Paco_2$ and HCO_3 values.

Q29-2: What is the patient's baseline $Paco_2$ if we assume the baseline serum HCO_3 is 32 mEq/L, and that this represents appropriate renal compensation for a chronic respiratory acidosis at baseline?

A. 50 mm Hg
B. 55 mm Hg
C. 60 mm Hg
D. 70 mm Hg
E. 25 mmHg

Q29-3: What is/are the primary acute acid-base disturbance(s) occurring in this case?

A. Metabolic acidosis only
B. Respiratory acidosis only
C. Metabolic acidosis and a respiratory acidosis
D. Metabolic alkalosis and a respiratory acidosis

Q29-4: This patient has an acute respiratory acidosis on top of his chronic respiratory acidosis. Does the patient also have any metabolic acid-base disorders present?

A. No, the elevation in the patient's HCO_3 can be accounted for by appropriate compensation for his acute-on-chronic respiratory failure.

B. Yes, the patient also has a concomitant metabolic acidosis.

C. Yes, the patient also has a concomitant metabolic alkalosis.

Q29-5: Now, assume that the entire process is acute rather than acute-on-chronic. What would you expect the patient's pH and serum HCO_3 to be if the entire respiratory process was acute and there was appropriate compensation?

A. pH 7.20, HCO_3 50 mEq/L
B. pH 7.31, HCO_3 43 mEq/L
C. pH 7.06, HCO_3 31 mEq/L
D. pH 6.92, HCO_3 22 mEq/L

Q29-6: Which of the variable below should be used to guide the patient's ventilator settings?

A. Returning the $Paco_2$ to 40 mm Hg
B. Returning the pH to 7.40
C. Returning the HCO_3 to 24

ANSWERS

Q29-1: C

The patient has an underlying acid-base condition, and we have sufficient information to estimate the patient's baseline $Paco_2$ and HCO_3 values. The patient has chronic respiratory failure with a baseline HCO_3 of 32 mEq/L. We will use this information in the coming questions to define the patient's baseline prior to this acute presentation.

Rationale: Ignoring these underlying chronic acid-base disorders can significantly alter the interpretation of a patient's acute acid-base status. This was demonstrated in the first case of the series. However, often we do not have the necessary information (eg, prior ABG or VBG, or prior serum chemistry with an HCO_3) and are forced to assume the ongoing processes are all acute in nature. We are primarily concerned about chronic respiratory acid-base disorders, as these can significantly alter the patient's baseline or expected values for the serum HCO_3 and $Paco_2$, and we have reliable equations to predict the expected baseline values. The respiratory compensation for both chronic metabolic acidosis and alkalosis is generally poor, so there are no equations or rules to predict what the $Paco_2$ should be in these cases. While the baseline serum HCO_3 may be significantly off from our standard value of 24 mEq/L in these patients, we would assume a baseline $Paco_2$ of 40 mm Hg in patients with chronic metabolic processes. Once we identify the patient's baseline $Paco_2$ and HCO_3 values, we will need to use these values in the appropriate equations to identify the ongoing acute processes.

Q29-2: C

60 mm Hg.

Rationale: For this question, we will need to use the equation for metabolic compensation in chronic respiratory failure.

Metabolic Compensation for Chronic Respiratory Alkalosis:

$$\text{Expected } HCO_3 = \text{Baseline } HCO_3 + (0.40) [\text{Actual } Paco_2 - Paco_2]$$

Here, because we are examining the chronic component, the baseline values in the preceding equation will be the normal values ($Paco_2$ 40 mm Hg, HCO_3 24 mEq/L), and the expected/actual values are those seen at the patient's new baseline with his chronic respiratory insufficiency:

$$32 \text{ mEq/L} = 24 \text{ mEq/L} + (0.40) * [\text{Actual } Paco_2 - 40 \text{ mm Hg}]$$
$$32 - 24 = (0.40) * [\text{Actual } Paco_2 - 40 \text{ mm Hg})$$
$$\text{Actual } Paco_2 = 60 \text{ mm Hg}.$$

Therefore, we have defined the patient's **new** baseline, which is a $Paco_2$ of 60 mm Hg and a serum HCO_3 of 32 mEq/L.

Q29-3: B
Respiratory acidosis only.

Rationale:

1. The pH is 7.07; therefore, the primary disorder is an **acidosis**.
2. The $Paco_2$ of 107 mm Hg is greater than 60 mm Hg (patient's new baseline), so there is an **acute respiratory acidosis**.
3. The HCO_3 of 44 is greater than the baseline value of 32 mEq/L, so there is no metabolic acidosis.

Q29-4: A
No, the elevation in the patient's HCO_3 can be accounted for by appropriate compensation for his acute-on-chronic respiratory failure.

Rationale: To determine this, we will need to calculate what we expect the patient's $Paco_2$ with the acute process included.

Metabolic Compensation for Acute Respiratory Acidosis:

$$\text{Expected } HCO_3 = \text{Baseline } HCO_3 + (0.10) \, [\text{Actual } Paco_2 - \text{Baseline } Paco_2]$$

Here, we will use the patient's new baseline values ($Paco_2$ of 60 mm Hg and HCO_3 of 32 mEq/L), and the actual $Paco_2$ of 112 mm Hg.

$$\text{Expected } HCO_3 = 32 \text{ mEq/L} + (0.10) * [112 - 60] = 32 + (0.10) * [52] = 37 \text{ mEq/L}.$$

Since the patient's HCO_3 is 37 mEq/L, there is no associated metabolic acid-base disorder.

Q29-5: C
pH 7.06, HCO_3 31 mEq/L.

Rationale: For this question, we first need to determine what the patient's serum HCO_3 would be, then we will determine the pH. For this question, since there is no chronic respiratory acidosis, we would assume that the patient has a baseline $Paco_2$ of 40 mm Hg and a baseline HCO_3 of 24 mEq/L.

Metabolic Compensation for Acute Respiratory Acidosis:

$$\text{Expected } HCO_3 = \text{Baseline } HCO_3 + (0.10) \, [\text{Actual } Paco_2 - \text{Baseline } Paco_2]$$
$$= 24 \text{ mEq/L} + (0.10) * [112 - 40] = 24 + 14.4 = 31 \text{ mEq/L}.$$

Now, with the two values provided above ($Paco_2$ of 112 mm Hg and HCO_3 of 31 mEq/L), we can calculate the expected pH:

Henderson-Hasselbalch Equation

$$pH = 6.10 + \log\left(\frac{[HCO_3]}{0.03 * PaCO_2}\right),$$

or

$$pH = 7.61 + \log_{10}\left(\frac{[HCO_3]}{PaCO_2}\right).$$

So, here, the pH would be 7.06.

Also note that this patient would have a concomitant metabolic alkalosis, as his serum HCO_3 is more than that expected for simple compensation. Alternatively, if we assumed the entire respiratory process was chronic, we would expect the patient's serum HCO_3 to be 53 mEq/L (with a pH of 7.29), and this patient would then also have a metabolic acidosis (which would be a non-anion gap acidosis). This demonstrate, again, the importance of defining the patient's chronic acid-base disorders at the outset of the case in order to appropriately identify the acute processes.

Remember that the kidney requires time, usually 24 hours, to effectively compensate for an acute respiratory acidosis; this is unlike the lung, which can compensate almost instantaneously for a metabolic acidosis by increasing ventilation.

Q29-6: B
Returning the pH to 7.40.

Rationale: The pH is always the primary target for mechanical ventilation settings in respiratory acidosis. The target is to normalize the pH. The patient has a baseline $PaCO_2$ and HCO_3 (compensatory) that are abnormal due to his underlying lung disease. If you try to normalize the $PaCO_2$ to 40 mm Hg, the patient will become alkalotic until the kidneys can compensate and lose additional HCO_3 in the urine and normalize the HCO_3. In this case, when the patient is removed from mechanical ventilation, his baseline lung disease will lead to an acute increase in $PaCO_2$ and, as his HCO_3 has normalized, he will not be compensated and will likely require emergent reintubation. The pH and the $PaCO_2$ are typically the primary targets when fine-tuning mechanical ventilation settings.

References

Brackett NC Jr, Wingo CF, Muren O, Solano JT. Acid-base response to chronic hypercapnia in man. N Engl J Med. 1969;280:124.

Kelly AM, Kyle E, McAlpine R. Venous pCO(2) and pH can be used to screen for significant hypercarbia in emergency patients with acute respiratory disease. J Emerg Med. 2002;22:15.

Polak A, Haynie GD, Hays RM, Schwartz WB. Effects of chronic hypercapnia on electrolyte and acid-base equilibrium. I. Adaptation. J Clin Invest. 1961;40:1223.

Van Yperselle de Striho, Brasseur L, De Coninck JD. The "carbon dioxide response curve" for chronic hypercapnia in man. N Engl J Med. 1966;275:117.

Weinberger SE, Schwartzstein RM, Weiss JW. Hypercapnia. N Engl J Med. 1989;321:1223.

West JB. Causes of carbon dioxide retention in lung disease. N Engl J Med. 1971;284:1232.

Williams MH Jr, Shim CS. Ventilatory failure. Etiology and clinical forms. Am J Med. 1970;48:477.

CASE 30

A 65-year-old successful businessman with hypertension is brought to the emergency department from home with hypotension and shortness of breath. He recently traveled back from Asia following a business trip. Since returning home last evening, he has noted some lightheadedness and dyspnea with exertion, which has significantly progressed over the past 12 hours. His vitals signs are T 37.2°C, RR 28, HR 120, BP 90/50. He takes his amlodipine and HCTZ for his hypertension and maintains a 2-g salt diet. His baseline Cr is 0.8. His examination is notable for tachypnea, clear breath sounds throughout, sinus tachycardia, and no murmurs or rubs.

Laboratory data.			
ABGs		Basic Metabolic Panel	
pH	7.50	Na	144 mEq/L
$Paco_2$	22 mm Hg	K	4.0 mEq/L
Pao_2	114 mm Hg (85% Fio_2)	Cl	98 mEq/L
HCO_3	18 mEq/L	CO_2	17 mEq/L
		BUN	44 mg/dL
		Cr	1.9 mg/dL
		Glucose	89 mg/dL
		Albumin	4.0 g/dL
		EtOH	0 mg/dL

QUESTIONS

Q30-1: Define the patient's baseline acid-base status: Does this patient have an underlying chronic acid-base disorder that we need to account for in order to appropriately interpret the acute acid-base disorders?

A. There is no evidence for an underlying chronic respiratory or metabolic acid-base disorder in this patient, so we would assume a baseline $Paco_2$ of 40 mm Hg and an HCO_3 of 24 mEq/L.

B. While the patient has a condition predisposing him to a chronic acid-base disorder, there is insufficient information to estimate the patient's baseline $Paco_2$ and HCO_3 values; therefore, we will assume a baseline $Paco_2$ of 40 mm Hg and a baseline HCO_3 of 24 mEq/L.

C. The patient has an underlying acid-base condition, and we have sufficient information to estimate the patient's baseline $Paco_2$ and HCO_3 values.

Q30-2: What is/are the primary acid-base disturbance(s) occurring in this case?

A. Metabolic acidosis only
B. Respiratory acidosis only
C. Metabolic alkalosis only
D. Respiratory alkalosis only
E. Metabolic acidosis and a respiratory acidosis
F. Metabolic alkalosis and a respiratory alkalosis

Q30-3: Which of the following is not a common cause of respiratory alkalosis?

A. Aspirin overdose
B. Liver failure
C. Pulmonary embolism
D. Neuromuscular disorder (eg, ALS)
E. Pulmonary edema
F. Poorly controlled pain

Q30-4: How would the reduction in the patient's serum HCO_3 be classified in this case?

A. Anion gap acidosis.
B. Non-anion gap acidosis.
C. Anion and non-anion gap acidosis.
D. Anion gap acidosis and a metabolic alkalosis.
E. The reduction in the patient's HCO_3 represents an appropriate metabolic compensation to the respiratory alkalosis.

Q30-5: What laboratory testing would you order next in this patient to determine the source of the anion gap metabolic acidosis?

A. Serum osmolality
B. Serum lactate
C. Serum beta-hydroxybutyrate
D. Serum drug screen
E. Urine osmolality
F. Urine anion gap
G. Urine chloride

Q30-6: The urine chloride is elevated at 45 mEq/L. What is the most likely cause of the patient's concomitant metabolic alkalosis?

A. Hyperemesis due to gastroparesis from a low forward-flow state
B. Ongoing thiazide diuretic use
C. Prior thiazide diuretic use (several days prior)
D. Diarrhea
E. Angiotensin inhibitor use

ANSWERS

Q30-1: B

While the patient has a condition (chronic diuretic use) that could predispose him to a chronic acid-base disorder, there is insufficient information to estimate the patient's baseline $Paco_2$ and HCO_3 values; therefore, we will assume a baseline $Paco_2$ of 40 mm Hg and a baseline HCO_3 of 24 mEq/L.

Rationale: Ignoring these underlying chronic acid-base disorders can significantly alter the interpretation of a patient's acute acid-base status. This was demonstrated in the first case of the series. However, often, we do not have the necessary information (eg, prior ABG or VBG, or prior serum chemistry with an HCO_3) and are forced to assume the ongoing processes are all acute in nature. We are primarily concerned about chronic respiratory acid-base disorders, as these can significantly alter the patient's baseline or expected values for the serum HCO_3 and $Paco_2$, and we have reliable equations to predict the expected baseline values. The respiratory compensation for both chronic metabolic acidosis and alkalosis is generally poor, so there are no equations or rules to predict what the $Paco_2$ should be in these cases. While the baseline serum HCO_3 may be significantly off from our standard value of 24 mEq/L in these patients, we would assume a baseline $Paco_2$ of 40 mm Hg in patients with chronic metabolic processes. Once we identify the patient's baseline $Paco_2$ and HCO_3 values, we will need to use these values in the appropriate equations to identify the ongoing acute processes.

Q30-2: B

Respiratory alkalosis.

Rationale:

1. The pH is 7.50; therefore, the primary disorder is an **alkalosis**.
2. The $Paco_2$ of 22 mm Hg is less than 40 mm Hg, so **a respiratory alkalosis is present**.
3. The HCO_3 of 18 mEq/L is less than 24 mEq/L, so there is **no apparent metabolic alkalosis**.

Q30-3: D

ALS and other neuromuscular disease.

Rationale: Neuromuscular disorders such as ALS are associated with respiratory acidosis, not alkalosis. Although patients may have tachypnea, they lack the muscle strength to take deep breaths. Patients with CNS insults such as stroke may have respiratory alkalosis due to issues with their respiratory center. Liver failure is associated with respiratory alkalosis due to an inability to clear toxins, which can stimulate the respiratory centers. Aspirin is also a stimulant of the respiratory center. Pulmonary embolism (PE) is another common cause of a respiratory alkalosis, and this patient's vignette is most consistent with an acute PE.

Q30-4: D
Anion gap acidosis and a metabolic alkalosis.

Rationale:

1. Is there evidence for a chronic acid-base disorder that requires adjustment of the patient's "normal" HCO_3? No, there is no evidence for a chronic acid-base disorder, so we would assume a baseline $Paco_2$ of 40 mm Hg and an HCO_3 of 24 mEq/L.
2. Next, we need to determine if the reduction in the HCO_3 is simply an appropriate metabolic compensation, or if there is a concomitant metabolic acid-base disorder.

Metabolic Compensation for Acute Respiratory Alkalosis:

Expected HCO_3 = Baseline HCO_3 − (0.20) [Actual $Paco_2$ − Baseline $Paco_2$]
Expected HCO_3 = 24 mEq/L − (0.20) * [40 mm Hg − 22 mm Hg] = 20.5 mEq/L.

Since the serum HCO_3 is less than 20 mEq/L, a concomitant metabolic acidosis is present.

3. Expected anion gap:

$$\text{Expected Anion Gap} = 12 - (2.5) * \left[4.0 \frac{g}{dL} - \text{Actual Serum Albumin} \right]$$

$$= 12 - (2.5 * [4.0 - 4.0])$$
$$= 12 - (2.5 * [0]) = \textbf{12 mEq/L.}$$

4. Anion gap calculation:

$$\text{Serum Anion Gap} = [Na^+] - [HCO_3^-] - [Cl^-]$$
$$= 144 - (98 + 17) = 29 \text{ mEq/L which is} > 12 \text{ mEq/L}$$
$$\rightarrow \textbf{anion gap acidosis is present.}$$

5. Delta-delta calculation:

$$\Delta\Delta = \frac{(\text{Actual Anion Gap} - \text{Expected Anion Gap})}{(\text{Baseline HCO}_3 - \text{Actual HCO}_3)}$$

$$= (29 - 12)/(24 - 17) = \textbf{17/7, which is} > \textbf{2.}$$

Delta-delta interpretation.	
Delta-Delta Value	Condition Present
< 0.4	Non-anion gap only
0.4 – 0.9	Anion gap *and* non-anion gap acidosis
1.0 – 2.0	Anion gap acidosis only
> 2.0	**Anion gap acidosis and metabolic alkalosis**

This patient therefore has an **anion gap acidosis as well as a metabolic alkalosis**.

Q30-5: B
Serum lactate.

Rationale: This patient has an anion gap acidosis in the setting of hypotension from a likely PE. This is a low cardiac output state and is most consistent with a lactic acidosis secondary to cardiogenic shock. The serum osmolality, beta-hydroxybutyrate, and serum drug screen would be useful in the evaluation of an anion gap acidosis as well. The urine osmolality and urine anion gap are useful in differentiating causes of a non-anion gap metabolic acidosis, while the urine chloride is helpful in metabolic alkalosis.

Q30-6: B
Ongoing Thiazide diuretic use.

Rationale: Diuretics such as thiazides interfere with the resorption of chloride and sodium in the distal tubule, leading to increased loss of chloride compared with HCO_3. This patient is likely volume depleted (Na 144 indicates possible dehydration, along with the prerenal kidney failure and BUN/Cr ratio of about 20), and perhaps due to his low-sodium diet he has low dietary chloride intake. The combination of thiazide use, low-/no-salt diet, and dehydration have led to the rare state of metabolic alkalosis from thiazide use. The urine chloride is elevated here because of the patient's ongoing use of diuretics, leading to chloride-resistant metabolic alkalosis. As the direct effect of the diuretic wears off, the metabolic alkalosis can shift from a chloride-resistant to a chloride-responsive metabolic alkalosis. Options A and C are associated with a chloride-responsive metabolic alkalosis, whereas options D and E are associated with a non-anion gap metabolic acidosis.

References

Batlle D, Grupp M, Gaviria M, Kurtzman NA. Distal renal tubular acidosis with intact capacity to lower urinary pH. Am J Med. 1982;72:751.

Batlle D, Haque SK. Genetic causes and mechanisms of distal renal tubular acidosis. Nephrol Dial Transplant. 2012;27:3691.

Batlle DC, Hizon M, Cohen E, et al. The use of the urinary anion gap in the diagnosis of hyperchloremic metabolic acidosis. N Engl J Med. 1988;318:594.

Batlle DC, vonRiotte A, Schlueter W. Urinary sodium in the evaluation of hyperchloremic metabolic acidosis. N Engl J Med. 1987;316:140.

Buckalew VM Jr, McCurdy DK, Ludwig GD, et al. Incomplete renal tubular acidosis. Physiologic studies in three patients with a defect in lowering urine pH. Am J Med. 1968;45:32.

Karet FE. Mechanisms in hyperkalemic renal tubular acidosis. J Am Soc Nephrol. 2009;20:251.

Mélot C, Naeije R. Pulmonary vascular diseases. Compr Physiol. 2011;1:593.

Rodríguez Soriano J. Renal tubular acidosis: the clinical entity. J Am Soc Nephrol. 2002;13:2160.

Santolicandro A, Prediletto R, Fornai E, et al. Mechanisms of hypoxemia and hypocapnia in pulmonary embolism. Am J Respir Crit Care Med. 1995;152:336.

CASE 31

A 23-year-old man with IDDM who is noncompliant with his diabetes regimen presents to the emergency department with lethargy, abdominal pain, nausea, and malaise. The patient has a history of multiple prior admissions for diabetes-related complications, including gastroparesis and elevated blood glucose. His blood glucose on arrival is 340 mg/dL. His vital signs are T 36.1°C, RR 29, HR 133, BP 98/77, and Sao$_2$ 100% on RA. He has some mild abdominal tenderness on examination, but no rebound or guarding. He admits to poor compliance with his insulin regimen at home. He has sinus tachycardia and tachypnea on examination, but otherwise the cardiopulmonary examination is normal. He has no history of alcohol or illicit drug use. On review his Cr was 1.4 approximately 3 months prior at an outpatient clinic visit with the endocrinology service.

Laboratory data.			
ABGs		Basic Metabolic Panel	
pH	6.82	Na	129 mEq/L
Paco$_2$	16 mm Hg	K	6.2 mEq/L
Pao$_2$	93 mm Hg	Cl	90 mEq/L
HCO$_3$	< 5 mEq/L	CO$_2$	5 mEq/L
		BUN	44 mg/dL
		Cr	1.6 mg/dL
		Albumin	4.0 g/dL

QUESTIONS

Q31-1: Define the patient's baseline acid-base status: Does this patient have an underlying chronic acid-base disorder that we need to account for in order to appropriately interpret the acute acid-base disorders?

A. There is no evidence for an underlying, chronic respiratory or metabolic acid-base disorder in this patient, so we would assume a baseline $Paco_2$ of 40 mm Hg and an HCO_3 of 24 mEq/L.

B. While the patient has a condition predisposing him to a chronic acid-base disorder, there is insufficient information to estimate the patient's baseline $Paco_2$ and HCO_3 values; therefore, we will assume a baseline $Paco_2$ of 40 mm Hg and a baseline HCO_3 of 24 mEq/L.

C. The patient has an underlying acid-base condition, and we have sufficient information to estimate the patient's baseline $Paco_2$ and HCO_3 values.

Q31-2: What is/are the primary acid-base disturbance(s) occurring in this case?

A. Metabolic acidosis only
B. Respiratory acidosis only
C. Metabolic alkalosis only
D. Respiratory alkalosis only
E. Metabolic acidosis and a respiratory acidosis
F. Metabolic alkalosis and a respiratory alkalosis

Q31-3: How would the metabolic acidosis component be classified in this case?

A. Anion gap acidosis
B. Non-anion gap acidosis
C. Anion and non-anion gap acidosis
D. Anion gap acidosis and a metabolic alkalosis

Q31-4: Which of the following laboratory tests is most likely to confirm this patient's diagnosis?

A. Serum lactate
B. Serum beta-hydroxybutyrate
C. Urine anion gap
D. Urine osmolal gap
E. Serum drug screen

Q31-5: Does the patient in this case demonstrate appropriate respiratory compensation?

A. Yes, the respiratory compensation is appropriate.
B. No, a concomitant respiratory alkalosis is present.
C. No, a concomitant respiratory acidosis is present.
D. Yes, the metabolic compensation is appropriate.
E. No, a concomitant metabolic acidosis is present.
F. No, a concomitant metabolic alkalosis is present.

Q31-6: The patient has two large-bore IVs placed and is started on an insulin drip and is given 8 L of normal saline over the next 8 hours. His repeat lab values are now:

Laboratory data.					
ABGs			Basic Metabolic Panel		
pH	7.29		Na	148 mEq/L	
Paco$_2$	29 mm Hg		K	6.2 mEq/L	
Pao$_2$	101 mm Hg		Cl	124 mEq/L	
HCO^3	12 mEq/L		CO$_2$	13 mEq/L	
			BUN	22 mg/dL	
			Cr	1.0 mg/dL	
			Albumin	4.0 g/dL	

The patient still has a metabolic acidosis. How would the metabolic acidosis component be classified now?

A. Anion gap acidosis
B. Non-anion gap acidosis
C. Anion and non-anion gap acidosis
D. Anion gap acidosis and a metabolic alkalosis

Q31-7: Given the current lab values, is the patient still demonstrating an appropriate respiratory compensation?

A. Yes, the respiratory compensation is still appropriate.
B. No, a concomitant respiratory alkalosis is present.
C. No, a concomitant respiratory acidosis is present.

ANSWERS

Q31-1: B

While the patient has a condition (chronic renal insufficiency) predisposing him to a chronic acid-base disorder, there is insufficient information to estimate the patient's baseline $Paco_2$ and HCO_3 values; therefore, we will assume a baseline $Paco_2$ of 40 mm Hg and a baseline HCO_3 of 24 mEq/L.

Rationale: Ignoring these underlying chronic acid-base disorders can significantly alter the interpretation of a patient's acute acid-base status. This was demonstrated in the first case of the series. However, often, we do not have the necessary information (eg, prior ABG or VBG, or prior serum chemistry with an HCO_3) and are forced to assume the ongoing processes are all acute in nature. We are primarily concerned about chronic respiratory acid-base disorders, as these can significantly alter the patient's baseline or expected values for the serum HCO_3 and $Paco_2$, and we have reliable equations to predict the expected baseline values. The respiratory compensation for both chronic metabolic acidosis and alkalosis is generally poor, so there are no equations or rules to predict what the $Paco_2$ should be in these cases. While the baseline serum HCO_3 may be significantly off from our standard value of 24 mEq/L in these patients, we would assume a baseline $Paco_2$ of 40 mm Hg in patients with chronic metabolic processes. Once we identify the patient's baseline $Paco_2$ and HCO_3 values, we will need to use these values in the appropriate equations to identify the ongoing acute processes.

Q31-2: A

Metabolic acidosis only.

Rationale:

1. The pH is 6.82; therefore, the primary disorder is an **acidosis.**
2. The $Paco_2$ of 16 mm Hg is less than 40 mm Hg, so this is **not the cause of acidosis;**
3. The HCO_3 of 5 mEq/L is less than 24 mEq/L, so there is a **primary metabolic acidosis.**

Therefore, this patient has a primary metabolic acidosis.

Q31-3: A

Anion gap acidosis only.

Rationale:

1. Is there evidence for a chronic acid-base disorder that requires adjustment of the patient's "normal" HCO_3? No, there is no evidence for a chronic acid-base disorder, so we would assume a baseline $Paco_2$ of 40 mm Hg and an HCO_3 of 24 mEq/L.
2. Expected anion gap:

$$\text{Expected Anion Gap} = 12 - (2.5) * \left[4.0 \frac{g}{dL} - \text{Actual Serum Albumin} \right]$$

$$= 12 - (2.5 * [4.0 - 4.0])$$
$$= 12 - (2.5 * [0]) = \textbf{12 mEq/L.}$$

3. Anion gap calculation:

$$\text{Serum Anion Gap} = [Na^+] - [HCO_3^-] - [Cl^-]$$
$$= 129 - (90 + 5) = 34 \text{ mEq/L which is} > 12 \text{ mEq/L}$$
$$\rightarrow \textbf{anion gap acidosis is present.}$$

4. Delta-delta calculation:

$$\Delta\Delta = \frac{(\text{Actual Anion Gap} - \text{Expected Anion Gap})}{(\text{Baseline HCO}_3 - \text{Actual HCO}_3)}$$
$$= (34 - 12)/(24 - 5)$$
$$= 22/19, \textbf{ which is} > 1 \textbf{ but} < 2.$$

Delta-delta interpretation.	
Delta-Delta Value	Condition Present
< 0.4	Non-anion gap only
0.4–1.0	Anion gap *and* non-anion gap acidosis
1.0–2.0	**Anion gap acidosis only**
> 2.0	Anion gap acidosis and metabolic alkalosis

This patient has a pure anion gap metabolic acidosis.

Q31-4: B
Serum beta-hydroxybutyrate.

Rationale: This is a serum ketone assay that is used in the diagnosis of DKA, which is almost certainly the underlying cause of the patient's metabolic acidosis. While it would certainly be appropriate to obtain a serum lactate, serum drug screen (which typically includes ethanol, salicylate, and acetaminophen levels), and a serum osmolality, these are less likely causes in this particular patient, and the serum beta-hydroxybutyrate would be the most appropriate test. The urine anion and osmolal gaps would aid in differentiating causes of a non-anion gap metabolic acidosis.

Q31-5: A
Yes, the respiratory compensation is appropriate.

Rationale: Using the Winter formula, one can calculate what the expected arterial $Paco_2$ should be for a given serum bicarbonate if the patient were completely compensated.

$$\text{Expected Paco}_2 = 1.5 * [\text{Actual HCO}_3] + 8 \pm 2 \text{ (in mm Hg)}$$
$$= (1.5 * 5) + 8 = 7.5 + 8 = 15.5 +/- 2 = (13 \text{ to } 17) \text{ mm Hg.}$$

This patient has an appropriate compensatory respiratory alkalosis, as his $Paco_2$ falls within this range.

Q31-6: B

Non-anion gap acidosis.

Rationale:

1. Anion gap calculation:

$$\text{Serum Anion Gap} = [Na^+] - [HCO_3^-] - [Cl^-]$$
$$= 148 - (124 + 13) = 11 \text{ mEq/L which is} < 12 \text{ mEq/L}$$
$$\rightarrow \textbf{non-anion gap acidosis.}$$

This patient's anion gap acidosis has been replaced by a non-anion gap acidosis from volume resuscitation and appropriate treatment of DKA with IV insulin. This is a common finding during the treatment of DKA (and most commonly how the anion gap is closed). One should not necessarily expect normalization of the serum HCO_3 at the same time the anion gap is closed.

Q31-7: A

Yes, the respiratory compensation is still appropriate.

Rationale: Using the Winter formula, one can calculate what the expected arterial $Paco_2$ should be for a given serum HCO_3 if the patient were completely compensated.

Respiratory Compensation for Acute Metabolic Acidosis (Winter Formula):

$$\text{Expected } Paco_2 = 1.5 * [\text{Actual } HCO_3] + 8 \pm 2 \text{ (in mm Hg)}$$
$$= (1.5 * 13) + 8 = 19.5 + 8 = 27.5 +/- 2 = (25 \text{ to } 29) \text{ mm Hg.}$$

Again, this patient continues to have an appropriate respiratory compensation for the non-anion gap acidosis. Note that despite the anion gap closing, volume resuscitation has resulted in a non-anion gap acidosis and still requires some respiratory compensation.

References

DeFronzo RA, Matzuda M, Barret E. Diabetic ketoacidosis: a combined metabolic-nephrologic approach to therapy. Diabetes Rev. 1994;2:209.

Fulop M, Murthy V, Michilli A, et al. Serum beta-hydroxybutyrate measurement in patients with uncontrolled diabetes mellitus. Arch Intern Med. 1999;159:381.

Porter WH, Yao HH, Karounos DG. Laboratory and clinical evaluation of assays for beta-hydroxybutyrate. Am J Clin Pathol. 1997;107:353.

Rose BD, Post TW. Clinical Physiology of Acid-Base and Electrolyte Disorders, 5e. New York, NY: McGraw Hill; 2001:809.

Shen T, Braude S. Changes in serum phosphate during treatment of diabetic ketoacidosis: predictive significance of severity of acidosis on presentation. Intern Med J. 2012;42:1347.

Wachtel TJ, Tetu-Mouradjian LM, Goldman DL, et al. Hyperosmolarity and acidosis in diabetes mellitus: a three-year experience in Rhode Island. J Gen Intern Med. 1991;6:495.

CASE 32

A 31-year-old woman with refractory severe persistent asthma presents to the emergency department with a severe asthma exacerbation. She is very anxious, and wheezing is audible from the hallway. The patient is tachypneic and a CXR shows no infiltrate, no pneumothorax, and no other pathology. The patient takes albuterol, budesonide, salmeterol, and montelukast, in addition to over-the-counter fexofenadine (Allegra). She denies any recent environmental exposures or recent illicit drug or alcohol use. She does not smoke tobacco. Her vital signs on admission are T37.4°C, RR 24, HR 145, BP 155/89, and Sao_2 92% on 35% Fio_2 via nebulizer (continuous). She is afebrile.

Laboratory data.			
ABGs		**Basic Metabolic Panel**	
pH	7.33	Na	140 mEq/L
$Paco_2$	26 mm Hg	K	4.0 mEq/L
Pao_2	101 mm Hg	Cl	105 mEq/L
HCO_3	20 mEq/L	CO_2	20 mEq/L
		BUN	13 mg/dL
		Cr	1.0 mg/dL
		Glucose	129 mg/dL
		Albumin	3.9 g/dL
		EtOH	0 mg/dL

QUESTIONS

Q32-1: Define the patient's baseline acid-base status: Does this patient have an underlying chronic acid-base disorder that we need to account for in order to appropriately interpret the acute acid-base disorders?

A. There is no evidence for an underlying chronic respiratory or metabolic acid-base disorder in this patient, so we would assume a baseline $Paco_2$ of 40 mm Hg and an HCO_3 of 24 mEq/L.

B. While the patient has a condition predisposing her to a chronic acid-base disorder, there is insufficient information to estimate the patient's baseline $Paco_2$ and HCO_3 values; therefore, we will assume a baseline $Paco_2$ of 40 mm Hg and a baseline HCO_3 of 24 mEq/L.

C. The patient has an underlying acid-base condition, and we have sufficient information to estimate the patient's baseline $Paco_2$ and HCO_3 values.

Q32-2: What is/are the primary acid-base disturbance(s) occurring in this case?

A. Metabolic acidosis only
B. Respiratory acidosis only
C. Metabolic alkalosis only
D. Respiratory alkalosis only
E. Metabolic acidosis and a respiratory acidosis
F. Metabolic alkalosis and a respiratory alkalosis

Q32-3: How would the metabolic acidosis component be classified in this case?

A. Anion gap acidosis
B. Non-anion gap acidosis
C. Anion and non-anion gap acidosis
D. Anion gap acidosis and a metabolic alkalosis

Q32-4: What is the most likely cause of the patient's anion gap acidosis?

A. Organic alcohol ingestion
B. Salicylate toxicity
C. Acetaminophen toxicity
D. Lactic acidosis
E. DKA

Q32-5: The patient receives initial treatment, but she does not appear improved on repeat examination, and her wheezing is still quite prominent on examination. Her repeat laboratory values are as follows:

Laboratory data.			
ABGs		Basic Metabolic Panel	
pH	7.45	Na	140 mEq/L
Paco$_2$	35 mm Hg	K	4.0 mEq/L
Pao$_2$	101 mm Hg	Cl	105 mEq/L
HCO$_3$	24 mEq/L	CO$_2$	24 mEq/L
		BUN	13 mg/dL
		Cr	1.0 mg/dL

What is the primary acid-base disturbance now?

A. Metabolic acidosis only
B. Respiratory acidosis only
C. Metabolic alkalosis only
D. Respiratory alkalosis only
E. Metabolic acidosis and a respiratory acidosis
F. Metabolic alkalosis and a respiratory alkalosis

Q32-6: You go to check on the patient 2 hours later. She is difficult to arouse and her wheezing is still audible throughout on examination. You repeat her blood gas analysis:

Laboratory data.	
ABG	
pH	7.28
Paco$_2$	58 mm Hg
Pao$_2$	75 mm Hg
HCO$_3$	24 mEq/L

What is the primary acid-base disturbance now?

A. Metabolic acidosis only
B. Respiratory acidosis only
C. Metabolic alkalosis only
D. Respiratory alkalosis only
E. Metabolic acidosis and a respiratory acidosis
F. Metabolic alkalosis and a respiratory alkalosis

Q32-7: What likely accounts for the patient's new respiratory acidosis?

A. Neuromuscular disorder
B. Pulmonary edema
C. ARDS
D. Respiratory muscle fatigue due to asthma

ANSWERS

Q32-1: A

There is no evidence for an underlying chronic respiratory or metabolic acid-base disorder in this patient, so we would assume a baseline $Paco_2$ of 40 mm Hg and an HCO_3 of 24 mEq/L. Asthma, unlike COPD, is not commonly associated with chronic hypercarbic respiratory failure. However, this can develop over time if there is enough irreversible damage to the airways and lung parenchyma.

Rationale: Ignoring these underlying chronic acid-base disorders can significantly alter the interpretation of a patient's acute acid-base status. This was demonstrated in the first case of the series. However, often, we do not have the necessary information (eg, prior ABG or VBG, or prior serum chemistry with an HCO_3) and are forced to assume the ongoing processes are all acute in nature. We are primarily concerned about chronic respiratory acid-base disorders, as these can significantly alter the patient's baseline or expected values for the serum HCO_3 and $Paco_2$, and we have reliable equations to predict the expected baseline values. The respiratory compensation for both chronic metabolic acidosis and alkalosis is generally poor, so there are no equations or rules to predict what the $Paco_2$ should be in these cases. While the baseline serum HCO_3 may be significantly off from our standard value of 24 mEq/L in these patients, we would assume a baseline $Paco_2$ of 40 mm Hg in patients with chronic metabolic processes. Once we identify the patient's baseline $Paco_2$ and HCO_3 values, we will need to use these values in the appropriate equations to identify the ongoing acute processes.

Q32-2: A

Metabolic acidosis only.

Rationale:

1. The pH is 7.35; therefore, the primary disorder is an **acidosis.**
2. The $Paco_2$ of 25 mm Hg is less than 40 mm Hg, so this is **not the primary disorder.**
3. The HCO_3 of 20 mEq/L is less than 24 mEq/L, so there is a **primary metabolic acidosis.**

Q32-3: A

Anion gap acidosis.

Rationale:

1. Is there evidence for a chronic acid-base disorder that requires adjustment of the patient's "normal" HCO_3? No, there is no evidence for a chronic acid-base disorder, so we would assume a baseline $Paco_2$ of 40 mm Hg and an HCO_3 of 24 mEq/L.

2. Expected anion gap:

$$\text{Expected Anion Gap} = 12 - (2.5) * \left[4.0 \frac{g}{dL} - \text{Actual Serum Albumin} \right]$$

$$= 12 - (2.5 * [4.0 - 4.0])$$
$$= 12 - (2.5 * [0]) = \textbf{12 mEq/L.}$$

3. Anion gap calculation:

$$\text{Serum Anion Gap} = [Na^+] - [HCO_3^-] - [Cl^-]$$
$$= 140 - (105 + 20) = 15 \text{ mEq/L which is} > 12 \text{ mEq/L}$$
$$\rightarrow \textbf{anion gap acidosis is present.}$$

4. Delta-delta calculation:

$$\Delta\Delta = \frac{(\text{Actual Anion Gap} - \text{Expected Anion Gap})}{(\text{Baseline HCO}_3 - \text{Actual HCO}_3)}$$

$$= (16 - 12)/(24 - 20) = \textbf{5/5 which is} = \textbf{1.}$$

Delta-delta interpretation.	
Delta-Delta Value	Condition Present
< 0.4	Non-anion gap only
0.4–1.0	Anion gap and non-anion gap acidosis
1.0–2.0	**Anion gap acidosis only**
> 2.0	Anion gap acidosis and metabolic alkalosis

This patient therefore has an **anion gap acidosis.**

Q32-4: D
Lactic acidosis.

Rationale: The patient presents with findings concerning for a severe, acute asthma exacerbation, with considerable tachypnea and accessory muscle usage. This is often associated with a transient lactic acidosis due to the increased work of breathing.

Q32-5: B
Respiratory alkalosis only.

Rationale:

1. The pH is 7.45; therefore, the primary disorder is now an **alkalosis.**
2. The $Paco_2$ of 30 mm Hg is less than 40 mm Hg, so there is a **respiratory alkalosis.**
3. The HCO_3 of 24 mEq/L is equal to 24 mEq/L, so there is **no apparent metabolic alkalosis.**

Q32-6: B
Respiratory acidosis only.

Rationale:

1. The pH is 7.25; therefore, the primary disorder is now an **acidosis.**
2. The $Paco_2$ of 58 mm Hg is more than 40 mm Hg, so there is a **respiratory acidosis.**
3. The HCO_3 of 24 mEq/L is as expected (24), so there is **no apparent metabolic acidosis.**

Q32-7: D
Respiratory muscle fatigue.

Rationale: This is a classic presentation of a severe asthma attack or status asthmaticus. The patient initially presented with a metabolic acidosis, which was transient and the result of a mild lactic acidosis from increased work of breathing (similar to exercise). These transient lactic acidosis issues are often seen at the end of extreme exercise in athletes, during seizures, and during asthma exacerbations. As the bronchospasm from asthma does not resolve, the patient respiratory muscles become more and more fatigued and the patient eventually cannot keep up the work of breathing. The gradually rising $Paco_2$ is a warning sign of respiratory failure in an asthmatic patient who does not appear to be clinically improving (persistent audible wheezing). Although the patient may appear more comfortable, she is actually retaining CO_2, and becoming more obtunded. Additionally, as the pH decreases with worsening CO_2 retention, patients are more prone to hemodynamic demise, which lead back to distributive shock and a metabolic acidosis.

References

Schivo M, Phan C, Louie S, Harper RW. Critical asthma syndrome in the ICU. Clin Rev Allergy Immunol. 2015;48:31.

Weinberger SE, Schwartzstein RM, Weiss JW. Hypercapnia. N Engl J Med. 1989;321:1223.

West JB. Causes of carbon dioxide retention in lung disease. N Engl J Med. 1971;284:1232.

Williams MH Jr, Shim CS. Ventilatory failure. Etiology and clinical forms. Am J Med. 1970;48:477.

CASE 33

A 50-year-old man with cirrhosis secondary to chronic alcoholism presents to the emergency department for encephalopathy. He has not been taking his prescribed lactulose at home. His vital signs are T 36.0°C, RR 20, HR 108, BP 98/59 (about the patient's baseline), and Sao_2 99% on room air. He is mildly confused on examination, but in no distress. He takes lithium for bipolar disorder as well as albuterol PRN. He has diffuse abdominal distention without rebound or guarding. There is mild abdominal tenderness, which the patient states is baseline.

Laboratory data.			
ABGs		Basic Metabolic Panel	
pH	7.33	Na	131 mEq/L
$Paco_2$	25 mm Hg	K	3.1 mEq/L
Pao_2	100 mm Hg	Cl	113 mEq/L
HCO_3	15 mEq/L	CO_2	15 mEq/L
		BUN	5 mg/dL
		Cr	1.1 mg/dL
		Glucose	88 mg/dL
		Albumin	1.5 g/dL
		EtOH	0 mg/dL

QUESTIONS

Q33-1: Define the patient's baseline acid-base status: Does this patient have an underlying chronic acid-base disorder that we need to account for in order to appropriately interpret the acute acid-base disorders?

A. There is no evidence for an underlying chronic respiratory or metabolic acid-base disorder in this patient, so we would assume a baseline $Paco_2$ of 40 mm Hg and an HCO_3 of 24 mEq/L.

B. While the patient has a condition predisposing him to a chronic acid-base disorder, there is insufficient information to estimate the patient's baseline $Paco_2$ and HCO_3 values; therefore, we will assume a baseline $Paco_2$ of 40 mm Hg and a baseline HCO_3 of 24 mEq/L.

C. The patient has an underlying acid-base condition, and we have sufficient information to estimate the patient's baseline $Paco_2$ and HCO_3 values.

Q33-2: What is/are the primary acid-base disturbance(s) occurring in this case?

A. Metabolic acidosis only
B. Respiratory acidosis only
C. Metabolic alkalosis only
D. Respiratory alkalosis only
E. Metabolic acidosis and a respiratory acidosis
F. Metabolic alkalosis and a respiratory alkalosis

Q33-3: For a perfectly healthy patient a normal anion gap is assumed to be 12 mEq/L. What should be considered a normal anion gap in this patient?

A. 12 mEq/L
B. 10 mEq/L
C. 8 mEq/L
D. 5 mEq/L

Q33-4: How would the metabolic acidosis component be classified in this case?

A. Anion gap acidosis
B. Non-anion gap acidosis
C. Anion and non-anion gap acidosis
D. Anion gap acidosis and a metabolic alkalosis

Q33-5: You decide to investigate the patient's non-anion gap acidosis. The patient's urine studies are as follows:

Urine Na	15 mEq/L
Urine K	33 mEq/L
Urine Cl	12 mEq/L
Urine pH	8.1
Urine RBCs	None
Urine WBCs	None
Urine protein	None
Urine microscopic	Microscopic stones present

What is the cause of the patient's non-anion gap acidosis?

A. Type 1 (distal) RTA
B. Type 2 (proximal) RTA
C. GI losses of bicarbonate
D. Type 4 RTA

Q33-6: Which of the following studies would you order to determine the underlying cause of the patients distal (type 1) RTA?

A. Urine chloride
B. Transtubular potassium gradient
C. Kidney stone composition study
D. Serum uric acid
E. Serum lithium level

Q33-7: Does the patient in this case demonstrate appropriate respiratory compensation?

A. Yes, the respiratory compensation is appropriate.
B. No, a concomitant respiratory alkalosis is present.
C. No, a concomitant respiratory acidosis is present.

ANSWERS

Q33-1: B

While the patient has a condition predisposing him to a chronic acid-base disorder, there is insufficient information to estimate the patient's baseline $Paco_2$ and HCO_3 values; therefore, we will assume a baseline $Paco_2$ of 40 mm Hg and a baseline HCO_3 of 24 mEq/L. The patient has chronic alcoholism, which can be associated with cirrhosis and chronic acid-base disorders; however, we do not have sufficient information to make any conclusions regarding this possibility.

Rationale: Ignoring these underlying chronic acid-base disorders can significantly alter the interpretation of a patient's acute acid-base status. This was demonstrated in the first case of the series. However, often, we do not have the necessary information (eg, prior ABG or VBG, or prior serum chemistry with an HCO_3) and are forced to assume the ongoing processes are all acute in nature. We are primarily concerned about chronic respiratory acid-base disorders, as these can significantly alter the patient's baseline or expected values for the serum HCO_3 and $Paco_2$, and we have reliable equations to predict the expected baseline values. The respiratory compensation for both chronic metabolic acidosis and alkalosis is generally poor, so there are no equations or rules to predict what the $Paco_2$ should be in these cases. While the baseline serum HCO_3 may be significantly off from our standard value of 24 mEq/L in these patients, we would assume a baseline $Paco_2$ of 40 mm Hg in patients with chronic metabolic processes. Once we identify the patient's baseline $Paco_2$ and HCO_3 values, we will need to use these values in the appropriate equations to identify the ongoing acute processes.

Q33-2: A

Metabolic acidosis only.

Rationale:

1. The pH is 7.33; therefore, the primary disorder is an **acidosis.**
2. The $Paco_2$ of 25 mm Hg is less than 40 mm Hg, so this is **not the cause of acidosis.**
3. The HCO_3 of 15 mEq/L is less than 24 mEq/L, so there is a **primary metabolic acidosis.**

Q33-3: D

6.

Rationale: The normal anion gap is 12. The term *anion gap* refers to those ions (negatively charged molecules) in the bloodstream that we do not routinely measure, including phosphates, sulfates, organic acids, and negatively charged plasma proteins. One of the most abundant negatively charged ions in the blood is serum albumin. While we do measure serum albumin, it is not included in the standard calculation of an anion gap and is considered an "unmeasured anion." A normal serum albumin is 4.0 g/dL. For patients with hypoalbuminemia (low serum albumin), the normal or expected anion gap is smaller:

$$\text{Expected Anion Gap} = 12 - (2.5) * \left[4.0 \, \frac{g}{dL} - \text{Actual Serum Albumin} \right].$$

So for this patient:

Expected Anion Gap = 12 − [2.5 * (4 − 1.5)] = 12 − (2.5 * 2.5) = 5.75 ~6 mEq/L.

This is an important concept as patients with hypoalbuminemia may "hide" an anion gap acidosis if this correction is not performed.

Q33-4: B
Non-anion gap acidosis.

Rationale:

1. Is there evidence for a chronic acid-base disorder that requires adjustment of the patient's "normal" HCO_3? No, there is no evidence for a chronic acid-base disorder, so we would assume a baseline $Paco_2$ of 40 mm Hg and an HCO_3 of 24 mEq/L.
2. Expected anion gap:

$$\text{Expected Anion Gap} = 12 - (2.5) * \left[4.0\,\frac{g}{dL} - \text{Actual Serum Albumin} \right]$$
$$= 12 - (2.5 * [4.0 - 1.5])$$
$$= 12 - (2.5 * [2.5]) = \textbf{6 mEq/L.}$$

3. Anion gap calculation:

$$\text{Serum Anion Gap} = [Na^+] - [HCO_3^-] - [Cl^-]$$
$$= 131 - (113 + 15) = 3 \text{ mEq/L which is} > 6 \text{ mEq/L}$$
$$\rightarrow \textbf{non-anion gap acidosis only.}$$

As the patient has no anion gap the patient has an isolated anion gap acidosis. There is no need for the delta-delta calculation in this case.

Q33-5: A
Type 1 (distal) RTA.

Rationale: This patient has no anion gap acidosis, so we can use the urine anion gap in this case. The urine anion gap will help differentiate between GI loss of HCO_3 or renal loss of HCO_3.

$$\text{Urine Anion Gap (UAG)} = [U_{Na}] + [U_K] - [U_{Cl}]$$
$$= U_{Na} + U_K - U_{Cl} = (10 + 33) - 12 = (+31) \text{ mEq/L.}$$

A urine anion gap that is greater than +10 to 20 mEq/L is associated with reduced renal acid excretion (a type 1 or 4 RTA), while a urine anion gap that is less than −20 mEq/L is most commonly associated with GI loss of bicarbonate (eg, diarrhea), although type 2 RTA is possible. A urine anion gap between −20 and +10 mEq/L is generally considered inconclusive.

To determine the type of RTA, one can look at the urine pH, serum potassium, for evidence of kidney stones.

Evaluation of RTA.			
	Type 1 RTA	Type 2 RTA	Type 4 RTA
Severity of metabolic acidosis, (HCO$_3$)	Severe (<10–12 mEq/L typically)	Intermediate (12–20 mEq/L)	Mild (15–20 mEq/L)
Associated urine abnormalities	Urinary phosphate, calcium are increased; bone disease often present	Urine glucose, amino acids, phosphate, calcium may be elevated	
Urine pH	HIGH (> 5.5)	Low (acidic), until serum HCO$_3$ level exceeds the resorptive ability of the proximal tubule; then becomes alkalotic once reabsorptive threshold is crossed	Low (acidic)
Serum K$^+$	Low to normal; should correct with oral HCO$_3$ therapy	Classically low, although may be normal or even high with rare genetic defects; worsens with oral HCO$_3$ therapy	HIGH
Renal stones	Often	No	No
Renal tubular defect	Reduced NH$_4$ secretion in distal tubule	Reduced HCO$_3$ resorption in proximal tubule	Reduced H$^+$/K$^+$ exchange in distal and collecting tubule due to decreased aldosterone or aldosterone resistance
Urine anion gap	> 10	Negative initially; then positive when receiving serum HCO$_3$; then negative after therapy	> 10
Urine osmolal gap	Reduced (<150 mOsm/L) during acute acidosis	At baseline is < 100 mEq/L; unreliable during acidosis	Reduced (<150 mOm/L) during acute acidosis

The patient's urine pH is 8.0 (basic) despite the acidosis and the serum potassium is low. This is consistent with a type 1 RTA (distal), which affects the ability of the kidney to acidify the urine. These patients also often have kidney stones as a complication.

Q33-6: E
Serum lithium level.

Rationale: Lithium is a known potential cause of type 1 RTA. The patient has developed encephalopathy, which may be due to either the hepatic encephalopathy or lithium toxicity.

Causes of renal tubular acidosis.
Causes of Type 1 (Distal) RTA
Primary • Idiopathic or familial (may be recessive or dominant)
Secondary • Medications: Lithium, amphotericin, ifosfamide, NSAIDs • Rheumatologic disorders: Sjögren syndrome, SLE, RA • Hypercalciuria (idiopathic) or associated with vitamin D deficiency or hyperparathyroidism • Sarcoidosis • Obstructive uropathy • Wilson disease • Rejection of renal transplant allograft
Causes of Type 2 (Proximal) RTA
Primary • Idiopathic • Familial (primarily recessive disorders) • Genetic: Fanconi syndrome, cystinosis, glycogen storage disease (type 1), Wilson disease, galactosemia
Secondary • Medications: Acetazolamide, topiramate, aminoglycoside antibiotics, ifosfamide, reverse transcriptase inhibitors (tenofovir) • Heavy metal poisoning: Lead, mercury, copper • Multiple myeloma or amyloidosis (secondary to light chain toxicity) • Sjögren syndrome • Vitamin D deficiency • Rejection of renal transplant allograft
Causes of Type 4 RTA (Hypoaldosteronism or Aldosterone Resistance)
Primary • Primary adrenal insufficiency • Inherited disorders associated with hypoaldosteronism • Pseudohypoaldosteronism (types 1 and 2)
Secondary • Causes of hyporeninemic hypoaldosteronism such as renal disease (diabetic nephropathy), NSAID use, calcineurin inhibitors, volume expansion/volume overload • Causes of distal tubule voltage defects such as sickle cell disease, obstructive uropathy, SLE • Severe illness/septic shock • Angiotensin II-associated medications: ACE inhibitors, ARBs, direct renin inhibitors • Potassium-sparing diuretics: Spironolactone, amiloride, triamterene • Antibiotics: Trimethoprim, pentamidine

Q33-7: B
No, a concomitant respiratory alkalosis is present.

Rationale: Using the Winter formula, one can calculate what the expected arterial $Paco_2$ should be for a given serum HCO_3 if the patient were appropriately compensated for an acute metabolic acidosis.

Respiratory Compensation for Acute Metabolic Acidosis (Winter Formula):

$$\text{Expected } Paco_2 = 1.5 * [\text{Actual } HCO_3] + 8 \pm 2 \text{ (in mm Hg)}$$
$$= (1.5 * 15) + 8 = 22.5 + 8 = 30.5 +/- 2 = (29 \text{ to } 33) \text{ mm Hg.}$$

Since the patient's $Paco_2$ on presentation (25 mm Hg) was lower than the expected 29 to 33 mm Hg, the patient also has a relative respiratory alkalosis. This is likely due to his underlying cirrhosis in which toxins not cleared by the liver cause increased stimulation of the respiratory centers. It is very possible that this patient has a chronic respiratory alkalosis as well, but again this is unclear from the prompt.

References

Adrogué HJ, Madias NE. Secondary responses to altered acid-base status: the rules of engagement. J Am Soc Nephrol 2010; 21:920.

Batlle D, Chin-Theodorou J, Tucker BM. Metabolic Acidosis or Respiratory Alkalosis? Evaluation of a Low Plasma Bicarbonate Using the Urine Anion Gap. Am J Kidney Dis. 2017 Sep;70(3):440-444. doi: 10.1053/j.ajkd.2017.04.017. Epub 2017 Jun 7.

Batlle D, Grupp M, Gaviria M, Kurtzman NA. Distal renal tubular acidosis with intact capacity to lower urinary pH. Am J Med 1982; 72:751.

Batlle D, Haque SK. Genetic causes and mechanisms of distal renal tubular acidosis. Nephrol Dial Transplant 2012; 27:3691.

Batlle DC, Hizon M, Cohen E, Gutterman C, Gupta R. The use of the urinary anion gap in the diagnosis of hyperchloremic metabolic acidosis. N Engl J Med. 1988 Mar 10;318(10):594-9.

Batlle DC, von Riotte A, Schlueter W. Urinary sodium in the evaluation of hyperchloremic metabolic acidosis. N Engl J Med 1987; 316:140.

Berend K, de Vries AP, Gans RO. Physiological approach to assessment of acid-base disturbances. N Engl J Med. 2014 Oct 9;371(15):1434-45. doi: 10.1056/NEJMra1003327.

Buckalew VM Jr, McCurdy DK, Ludwig GD, et al. Incomplete renal tubular acidosis. Physiologic studies in three patients with a defect in lowering urine pH. Am J Med 1968; 45:32.

Feldman M, Soni N, Dickson B. Influence of hypoalbuminemia or hyperalbuminemia on the serum anion gap. J Lab Clin Med 2005; 146:317.

Karet FE. Mechanisms in hyperkalemic renal tubular acidosis. J Am Soc Nephrol 2009; 20:251.

Kraut JA, Madias NE. Differential diagnosis of nongap metabolic acidosis: value of a systematic approach. Clin J Am Soc Nephrol. 2012 Apr;7(4):671-9. doi: 10.2215/CJN.09450911. Epub 2012 Mar 8.

Kraut JA, Nagami GT. The serum anion gap in the evaluation of acid-base disorders: what are its limitations and can its effectiveness be improved? Clin J Am Soc Nephrol 2013; 8:2018.

Rastegar M, Nagami GT. Non-Anion Gap Metabolic Acidosis: A Clinical Approach to Evaluation. Am J Kidney Dis. 2017 Feb;69(2):296-301. doi: 10.1053/j.ajkd.2016.09.013. Epub 2016 Oct 28.

Rodríguez Soriano J. Renal tubular acidosis: the clinical entity. J Am Soc Nephrol 2002; 13:2160.

CASE 34

A 66-year-old man with IDDM, COPD, coronary artery disease, hypertension, and gout, who is a resident of a nursing home, presents with hypotension, rigors, and malaise. He is febrile (T 38.5°C). His other vital signs are RR 27, HR 121, BP 74/50, and Sao_2 90% on RA. He is started on antibiotics and a pan culture is obtained. His examination demonstrates mild flank tenderness bilaterally, as well as an irregularly irregular rhythm, moderate expiratory wheezing, and encephalopathy. He has no lower extremity edema and no JVD.

Laboratory data.			
ABGs		Basic Metabolic Panel	
pH	7.10	Na	139 mEq/L
$Paco_2$	50 mm Hg	K	6.6 mEq/L
Pao_2	60 mm Hg	Cl	108 mEq/L
HCO_3	14 mEq/L	CO_2	14 mEq/L
		BUN	5 mg/dL
		Cr	0.8 mg/dL
		Glucose	141 mg/dL
		Albumin	2.8 g/dL
		EtOH	0 mg/dL

QUESTIONS

Q34-1: Define the patient's baseline acid-base status: Does this patient have an underlying chronic acid-base disorder that we need to account for in order to appropriately interpret the acute acid-base disorders?

A. There is no evidence for an underlying chronic respiratory or metabolic acid-base disorder in this patient, so we would assume a baseline $Paco_2$ of 40 mm Hg and an HCO_3 of 24 mEq/L.

B. While the patient has a condition predisposing him to a chronic acid-base disorder, there is insufficient information to estimate the patient's baseline $Paco_2$ and HCO_3 values; therefore, we will assume a baseline $Paco_2$ of 40 mm Hg and a baseline HCO_3 of 24 mEq/L.

C. The patient has an underlying acid-base condition, and we have sufficient information to estimate the patient's baseline $Paco_2$ and HCO_3 values.

Q34-2: What is/are the primary acid-base disturbance(s) occurring in this case?

A. Metabolic acidosis only
B. Respiratory acidosis only
C. Metabolic alkalosis only
D. Respiratory alkalosis only
E. Metabolic acidosis and a respiratory acidosis
F. Metabolic alkalosis and a respiratory alkalosis

Q34-3: For a perfectly healthy patient a normal anion gap is assumed to be 12. What should be considered a normal anion gap in this patient?

A. 12 mEq/L
B. 9 mEq/L
C. 7 mEq/L
D. 4 mEq/L

Q34-4: How would the metabolic acidosis component be classified in this case?

A. Anion gap acidosis
B. Non-anion gap acidosis
C. Anion and non-anion gap acidosis
D. Anion gap acidosis and a metabolic alkalosis

Q34-5: The following laboratory values are noted:

Serum EtOH	< 3 mg/dL
Serum acetaminophen level	< 5 mg/dL (ULN for therapeutic use 20 mg/dL)
Serum salicylates level	< 5 mg/dL (ULN for therapeutic use 30 mg/dL)
Beta-hydroxybutyrate (acetone)	< 0.18 mmol/L (ULN 0.18 mmol/L)
Serum lactate	8.7 mmol/L (ULN 2.0 mmol/L venous)

Which of the following laboratory findings is most likely to reveal the source of the patient's anion gap acidosis?

A. Serum brain natriuretic peptide (BNP)
B. Serum creatinine kinase
C. Serum osmolality
D. Blood and urine cultures
E. Serum uric acid

Q34-6: You decide to investigate the patient's non-anion gap acidosis. The patient's urine studies are as follows:

Urine Na	20 mEq/L
Urine K	33 mEq/L
Urine Cl	31 mEq/L
Urine urea	313 mg/dL
Urine glucose	0 mg/dL
Urine osmolality	301 mOsm/L
Urine pH	5.3
Urine RBCs	Many
Urine WBCs	Many
Urine protein	Trace
Urine microscopic	None

What is the cause of the patient's non-anion gap acidosis?

A. Type 1 (distal) RTA
B. Type 2 (proximal) RTA
C. GI losses of bicarbonate
D. Type 4 RTA

ANSWERS

Q34-1: B

While the patient has a condition (COPD) predisposing him to a chronic acid-base disorder, there is insufficient information to estimate the patient's baseline $Paco_2$ and HCO_3 values; therefore, we will assume a baseline $Paco_2$ of 40 mm Hg and a baseline HCO_3 of 24 mEq/L.

Rationale: Ignoring these underlying chronic acid-base disorders can significantly alter the interpretation of a patient's acute acid-base status. This was demonstrated in the first case of the series. However, often, we do not have the necessary information (eg, prior ABG or VBG, or prior serum chemistry with an HCO_3) and are forced to assume the ongoing processes are all acute in nature. We are primarily concerned about chronic respiratory acid-base disorders, as these can significantly alter the patient's baseline or expected values for the serum HCO_3 and $Paco_2$, and we have reliable equations to predict the expected baseline values. The respiratory compensation for both chronic metabolic acidosis and alkalosis is generally poor, so there are no equations or rules to predict what the $Paco_2$ should be in these cases. While the baseline serum HCO_3 may be significantly off from our standard value of 24 mEq/L in these patients, we would assume a baseline $Paco_2$ of 40 mm Hg in patients with chronic metabolic processes. Once we identify the patient's baseline $Paco_2$ and HCO_3 values, we will need to use these values in the appropriate equations to identify the ongoing acute processes.

Q34-2: E

Metabolic acidosis and a respiratory acidosis.

Rationale:

1. The pH is 7.10; therefore, the primary disorder is an **acidosis.**
2. The $Paco_2$ of 50 mm Hg is greater than 40 mm Hg, so there is a **respiratory acidosis.**
3. The HCO_3 of 14 is less than 24, so there is also a **metabolic acidosis.**

This is a mixed primary metabolic acidosis and respiratory acidosis. The patient's respiratory acidosis is most likely related to his underlying COPD. We will further investigate the patient's metabolic acidosis in this case.

Q34-3: B

9 mEq/L.

Rationale: The normal anion gap is 12 mEq/L. The term *anion gap* refers to those ions (negatively charged molecules) in the bloodstream that we do not routinely measure, including phosphates, sulfates, organic acids, and negatively charged plasma proteins. One of the most abundant negatively charged ions in the blood is serum albumin. A normal serum albumin is 4.0 g/dL. For patients with hypoalbuminemia (low serum albumin), the normal or expected anion gap is smaller:

$$\text{Expected Anion Gap} = 12 - (2.5) * \left[4.0 \frac{g}{dL} - \text{Actual Serum Albumin} \right].$$

Therefore, for this patient:

$$\text{Expected Anion Gap} = 12 - [2.5 * (4 - 2.8)] = 12 - (2.5 * 1.2) = 9 \text{ mEq/L}.$$

This is an important concept as patients with hypoalbuminemia may "hide" an anion gap acidosis if this correction is not performed.

Q34-4: C
Anion and non-anion gap acidosis.

Rationale:

1. Is there evidence for a chronic acid-base disorder that requires adjustment of the patient's "normal" HCO_3? No, there is no evidence for a chronic acid-base disorder, so we would assume a baseline $Paco_2$ of 40 mm Hg and an HCO_3 of 24 mEq/L.
2. Expected anion gap:

$$\text{Expected Anion Gap} = 12 - (2.5) * \left[4.0 \frac{g}{dL} - \text{Actual Serum Albumin} \right]$$
$$= 12 - (2.5 * [4.0 - 2.8])$$
$$= 12 - (2.5 * [1.2]) = \mathbf{9 \text{ mEq/L.}}$$

3. Anion gap calculation:

$$\text{Serum Anion Gap} = [Na^+] - [HCO_3^-] - [Cl^-]$$
$$= 139 - (108 + 14) = 17 \text{ mEq/L, which is} > 12 \text{ mEq/L}$$
$$\rightarrow \textbf{anion gap acidosis is present.}$$

4. Delta-delta calculation:

$$\Delta\Delta = \frac{(\text{Actual Anion Gap} - \text{Expected Anion Gap})}{(\text{Baseline } HCO_3 - \text{Actual } HCO_3)}$$
$$= (17 - 9)/(24 - 14) = \mathbf{8/10, \text{ which is } 0.8 \text{ and} < 1.}$$

Delta-delta interpretation.	
Delta-Delta Value	Condition Present
< 0.4	Non-anion gap only
0.4–1.0	**Anion gap *and* non-anion gap acidosis**
1.0–2.0	Anion gap acidosis only
> 2.0	Anion gap acidosis and metabolic alkalosis

This patient therefore has both an anion gap acidosis and a non-anion gap acidosis.

Q34-5: D
Blood and urine cultures.

Rationale: The patient has an anion gap acidosis and presented with fever, rigors, hypotension, and flank tenderness. His presentation is most concerning for sepsis secondary to a urinary tract infection and/or pyelonephritis. The patient also has IDDM, so DKA would also be a concern. Given the fever and encephalopathy, there is also the potential for acetaminophen or aspirin toxicity if the patient is self-administering. The additional laboratory data provided in this question rule out these possibilities, and the serum lactate is quite elevated, supporting this as well. Additionally, there is no acute renal failure present at this time to suggest that as the potential cause. In terms of the other listed options, a serum BNP might be useful if we were concerned about lactic acidosis secondary to cardiogenic shock. A serum creatine kinase would be useful if we were concerned about rhabdomyolysis, neuroleptic malignant syndrome, or serotonin syndrome. A serum osmolality would be useful to determine if methanol or ethylene glycol ingestion were the source; however, this seems unlikely in this case. A serum uric acid would aid in a diagnosis of tumor lysis syndrome or perhaps an acute gout flare; however, the latter is not generally associated with a lactic acidosis.

Q34-6: C
Type 4 (distal) RTA.

Rationale: The urine anion gap is (+22) mEq/L. However, the urine anion gap can be inappropriately elevated in anion gap acidosis, a situation in which multiple unmeasured anions may be present in the urine (beta-hydroxybutyrate/acetoacetate [ketoacidosis], hippurate [toluene], bicarbonate [proximal RTA], D-lactate [D-lactic acidosis], L-lactate, 5-oxoproline [acetaminophen toxicity]). Therefore, in patients with a significant anion gap, the urine osmolar gap is typically more useful. Since the patient has an anion gap acidosis, we should use the serum osmolal gap first to determine if the patient has a type 1 or 4 RTA.

$$\text{Calculated Urine Osmolality} = 2 * ([Na^+] + [K^+]) + \frac{[Urea]}{2.8} + \frac{[Glucose]}{18}$$

$$= 218 \text{ mOsm/L}$$

$$\text{Urine Osmolal Gap (UOG)} = \text{Measured Urine Osmolality} - \text{Measured Urine Osmolality}$$

$$\text{UOG} = 301 - 218 = (+83) \text{ mOsm/L.}$$

Similar to the urine anion gap, the urine osmolar gap is used as a surrogate for the urine ammonium concentration. Therefore, a larger gap indicates increased urinary NH_4 excretion. In normal acid-base conditions, the urine osmolar gap is between 10 and 100 mOsm/L. During a significant metabolic acidosis, patients with impaired renal tubular acidification (type 1 and type 4 RTA) are unable to excrete additional acid (NH_4), and therefore the osmolar gap does not change. Patients with an intact renal response to acidemia (ie, GI losses) should have a significant urine osmolar gap ($\sim$ >300 to 400 mOsm/L) as a result of increased NH_4 excretion. This patient has an inappropriately low serum osmolal gap; therefore, the patient likely has either a type 1 or type 4 RTA.

NAGMA.

Cause of NAGMA

Evaluation Strategy

1. History (acute or chronic issues, medications, altered GI anatomy, genetic diseases, etc). Also, is the patient receiving an acid load, such as TPN?

2. Does the patient have chronic renal insufficiency? If so, this alone may be responsible for the non-anion gap acidosis.

3. Calculate urine anion gap and urine osmolal gap. The urine anion gap may be of limited value in patients with severe serum anion gap acidosis, as it may be falsely elevated. Similarly, the urine osmolal gap may be inappropriately elevated in patients with a significant serum osmolal gap (particularly due to mannitol).

4. Note the serum potassium as well as the urine pH.

5. If proximal RTA is suspected, look for evidence of other inappropriate compounds in the urine (amino acids, elevated phosphate, glucosuria) and calculate the fractional resorption of sodium bicarbonate (should be > 15%). Also check serum for evidence of dysfunctional of the PTH-vitamin D-calcium axis.

Cause of NAGMA

Low Serum Potassium
GI: Diarrhea, pancreaticoduodenal fistula, urinary intestinal diversion
Renal: Type 1 RTA (distal), type 2 RTA (proximal)
Medications/Exposures: Carbonic anhydrase inhibitors, toluene
Other: D-lactic Acidosis

High (or Normal) Serum Potassium
GI: Elevated ileostomy output
Renal: Type 4 RTA or chronic kidney disease
Medications: NSAIDs, antibiotics (trimethoprim, pentamidine), heparin, ACE inhibitors/ARBs/aldosterone antagonists (spironolactone), acid administration (TPN)

Evaluation of RTA.

	Type 1 RTA	Type 2 RTA	Type 4 RTA
Severity of metabolic acidosis, (HCO_3)	Severe (< 10–12 mEq/L typically)	Intermediate (12–20 mEq/L)	Mild (15–20 mEq/L)
Associated urine abnormalities	Urinary phosphate, calcium increased; bone disease often present	Urine glucose, amino acids, phosphate, calcium may be elevated	
Urine pH	HIGH (> 5.5)	Low (acidic), until serum HCO_3 level exceeds resorptive ability of proximal tubule; then becomes alkalotic once reabsorptive threshold is crossed	Low (acidic)
Serum K+	Low to normal; should correct with oral HCO_3 therapy	Classically low, although may be normal or even high with rare genetic defects; worsens with oral bicarbonate therapy	HIGH
Renal stones	Often	No	No

(Continued)

Evaluation of RTA. (*continued*)			
	Type 1 RTA	Type 2 RTA	Type 4 RTA
Renal tubular defect	Reduced NH_4 secretion in distal tubule	Reduced HCO_3 resorption in proximal tubule	Reduced H^+/K^+ exchange in distal and collecting tubules due to decreased aldosterone or aldosterone resistance
Urine anion gap	> 10	Negative initially; then positive when receiving serum HCO_3; then negative after therapy	> 10
Urine osmolal gap	Reduced (< 150 mOsm/L) during acute acidosis	At baseline < 100 mEq/L; unreliable during acidosis	Reduced (< 150 mOsm/L) during acute acidosis

The patient's urine pH is 5.0 (acidic) and the serum potassium is elevated at 6.6. This is consistent with a type 4 RTA (distal), in which the H^+/K^+ transporter is ineffective. This is a common complication of diabetic nephropathy and sickle cell disease, as well as a potential complication of several medications (eg, ACE inhibitors, trimethoprim, etc).

Causes of renal tubular acidosis.
Causes of Type 1 (Distal) RTA
Primary • Idiopathic or familial (may be recessive or dominant)
Secondary • Medications: Lithium, amphotericin, ifosfamide, NSAIDs • Rheumatologic disorders: Sjögren syndrome, SLE, RA • Hypercalciuria (idiopathic) or associated with vitamin D deficiency or hyperparathyroidism • Sarcoidosis • Obstructive uropathy • Wilson disease • Rejection of renal transplant allograft • Toluene toxicity
Causes of Type 2 (Proximal) RTA
Primary • Idiopathic • Familial (primarily recessive disorders) • Genetic: Fanconi syndrome, cystinosis, glycogen storage disease (type 1), Wilson disease, galactosemia
Secondary • Medications: Acetazolamide, topiramate, aminoglycoside antibiotics, ifosfamide, reverse transcriptase inhibitors (tenofovir) • Heavy metal poisoning: Lead, mercury, copper • Multiple myeloma or amyloidosis (secondary to light chain toxicity) • Sjögren syndrome • Vitamin D deficiency • Rejection of renal transplant allograft

(Continued)

Causes of renal tubular acidosis. (*continued*)
Causes of Type 4 RTA (Hypoaldosteronism or Aldosterone Resistance)
Primary • Primary adrenal insufficiency • Inherited disorders associated with hypoaldosteronism • Pseudohypoaldosteronism (types 1 and 2)
Secondary • Causes of hyporeninemic hypoaldosteronism such as renal disease (diabetic nephropathy), NSAID use, calcineurin inhibitors, volume expansion/volume overload • Causes of distal tubule voltage defects such as sickle cell disease, obstructive uropathy, SLE • Severe illness/septic shock • Angiotensin II–associated medications: ACE inhibitors, ARBs, direct renin inhibitors • Potassium-sparing diuretics: Spironolactone, amiloride, triamterene • Antibiotics: Trimethoprim, pentamidine

References

Adeva-Andany M, López-Ojén M, Funcasta-Calderón R, et al. Comprehensive review on lactate metabolism in human health. Mitochondrion. 2014;17:76.

Batlle D, Chin-Theodorou J, Tucker BM. Metabolic acidosis or respiratory alkalosis? Evaluation of a low plasma bicarbonate using the urine anion gap. Am J Kidney Dis. 2017;70:440.

Batlle D, Grupp M, Gaviria M, Kurtzman NA. Distal renal tubular acidosis with intact capacity to lower urinary pH. Am J Med. 1982;72:751.

Batlle D, Haque SK. Genetic causes and mechanisms of distal renal tubular acidosis. Nephrol Dial Transplant. 2012;27:3691.

Batlle DC, Hizon M, Cohen E, et al. The use of the urinary anion gap in the diagnosis of hyper-chloremic metabolic acidosis. N Engl J Med. 1988;318:594.

Batlle DC, von Riotte A, Schlueter W. Urinary sodium in the evaluation of hyperchloremic metabolic acidosis. N Engl J Med. 1987;316:140.

Bern M. Clinically significant pseudohyponatremia. Am J Hematol. 2006;81:558.

Buckalew VM Jr, McCurdy DK, Ludwig GD, et al. Incomplete renal tubular acidosis. Physiologic studies in three patients with a defect in lowering urine pH. Am J Med. 1968;45:32.

Corey HE. Stewart and beyond: new models of acid-base balance. Kidney Int. 2003;64:777.

Dyck RF, Asthana S, Kalra J, et al. A modification of the urine osmolal gap: an improved method for estimating urine ammonium. Am J Nephrol. 1990;10:359.

Faradji-Hazan V, Oster JR, Fedeman DG, et al. Effect of pyridostigmine bromide on serum bromide concentration and the anion gap. J Am Soc Nephrol. 1991;1:1123.

Feldman M, Soni N, Dickson B. Influence of hypoalbuminemia or hyperalbuminemia on the serum anion gap. J Lab Clin Med. 2005;146:317.

Fenves AZ, Kirkpatrick HM 3rd, Patel VV, et al. Increased anion gap metabolic acidosis as a result of 5-oxoproline (pyroglutamic acid): a role for acetaminophen. Clin J Am Soc Nephrol. 2006;1:441.

Fernandez PC, Cohen RM, Feldman GM. The concept of bicarbonate distribution space: the crucial role of body buffers. Kidney Int. 1989;36:747.

Forni LG, McKinnon W, Lord GA, et al. Circulating anions usually associated with the Krebs cycle in patients with metabolic acidosis. Crit Care. 2005;9:R591.

Karet FE. Mechanisms in hyperkalemic renal tubular acidosis. J Am Soc Nephrol. 2009;20:251.

Kim GH, Han JS, Kim YS, et al. Evaluation of urine acidification by urine anion gap and urine osmolal gap in chronic metabolic acidosis. Am J Kidney Dis. 1996;27:42.

Komaru Y, Inokuchi R, Ueda Y, et al. Use of the anion gap and intermittent hemodialysis following continuous hemodiafiltration in extremely high dose acute-on-chronic lithium poisoning: A case report. Hemodial Int. 2018;22:E15.

Kraut JA, Kurtz I. Toxic alcohol ingestions: clinical features, diagnosis, and management. Clin J Am Soc Nephrol. 2008;3:208.

Kraut JA, Madias NE. Differential diagnosis of nongap metabolic acidosis: value of a systematic approach. Clin J Am Soc Nephrol. 2012;7:671.

Kraut JA, Nagami GT. The serum anion gap in the evaluation of acid-base disorders: what are its limitations and can its effectiveness be improved? Clin J Am Soc Nephrol. 2013;8:2018.

Kraut JA, Xing SX. Approach to the evaluation of a patient with an increased serum osmolal gap and high-anion-gap metabolic acidosis. Am J Kidney Dis. 2011;58:480.

Lee Hamm L, Hering-Smith KS, Nakhoul NL. Acid-base and potassium homeostasis. Semin Nephrol. 2013;33:257.

Levy B. Lactate and shock state: the metabolic view. Curr Opin Crit Care. 2006;12:315.

Lu J, Zello GA, Randell E, et al. Closing the anion gap: contribution of D-lactate to diabetic ketoacidosis. Clin Chim Acta. 2011;412:286.

Madias NE. Lactic acidosis. Kidney Int. 1986;29:752.

Madias NE, Ayus JC, Adrogué HJ. Increased anion gap in metabolic alkalosis: the role of plasma-protein equivalency. N Engl J Med. 1979;300:1421.

Meregalli P, Lüthy C, Oetliker OH, Bianchetti MG. Modified urine osmolal gap: an accurate method for estimating the urinary ammonium concentration? Nephron. 1995;69:98.

Mikkelsen ME, Miltiades AN, Gaieski DF, et al. Serum lactate is associated with mortality in severe sepsis independent of organ failure and shock. Crit Care Med. 2009;37:1670.

Murray T, Long W, Narins RG. Multiple myeloma and the anion gap. N Engl J Med. 1975;292:574.

Oh M, Carroll HJ. Value and determinants of urine anion gap. Nephron. 2002;90:252.

Pierce NF, Fedson DS, Brigham KL, et al. The ventilatory response to acute base deficit in humans. Time course during development and correction of metabolic acidosis. Ann Intern Med. 1970;72:633.

Rastegar M, Nagami GT. Non-anion gap metabolic acidosis: a clinical approach to evaluation. Am J Kidney Dis. 2017;69:296.

Relman AS. What are acids and bases? Am J Med. 1954;17:435.

Rodríguez Soriano J. Renal tubular acidosis: the clinical entity. J Am Soc Nephrol. 2002;13:2160.

Schwartz WB, Relman AS. A critique of the parameters used in the evaluation of acid-base disorders. "Whole-blood buffer base" and "standard bicarbonate" compared with blood pH and plasma bicarbonate concentration. N Engl J Med. 1963;268:1382.

Zimmer BW, Marcus RJ, Sawyer K, Harchelroad F. Salicylate intoxication as a cause of pseudohyperchloremia. Am J Kidney Dis. 2008;51:346.

CASE 35

A 55-year-old woman with a history of adrenal insufficiency, hypothyroidism, and hypertension presents with altered mental status in the setting of a pneumonia. She has been hypotensive and tachycardic. She is intubated in the emergency department. Her initial BP was 80/40, with HR 130 and T 39.0°C. Her WBC count is 18,000/μL with 10% band forms present. Her RR was 10 prior to intubation. Her TSH returns normal. She reportedly has not been taking her medications for the past 3 days. The cardiopulmonary edema demonstrates sinus tachycardia as well as rhonchorous breath sounds over the left lower and mid-lung fields. She takes no OTC medications, drinks no alcohol, and does not use illicit drugs.

Laboratory data.			
ABGs		Basic Metabolic Panel	
pH	7.10	Na	140 mEq/L
$Paco_2$	50 mm Hg	K	5.6 mEq/L
Pao_2	55 mm Hg	Cl	110 mEq/L
HCO_3	14 mEq/L	CO_2	14 mEq/L
		BUN	24 mg/dL
		Cr	2.0 mg/dL
		Glucose	68 mg/dL
		Albumin	4.0 g/dL
		EtOH	0 mg/dL

QUESTIONS

Q35-1: Define the patient's baseline acid-base status: Does this patient have an underlying chronic acid-base disorder that we need to account for in order to appropriately interpret the acute acid-base disorders?

A. There is no evidence for an underlying chronic respiratory or metabolic acid-base disorder in this patient, so we would assume a baseline $Paco_2$ of 40 mm Hg and an HCO_3 of 24 mEq/L.

B. While the patient has a condition predisposing her to a chronic acid-base disorder, there is insufficient information to estimate the patient's baseline $Paco_2$ and HCO_3 values; therefore, we will assume a baseline $Paco_2$ of 40 mm Hg and a baseline HCO_3 of 24 mEq/L.

C. The patient has an underlying acid-base condition, and we have sufficient information to estimate the patient's baseline $Paco_2$ and HCO_3 values.

Q35-2: What is/are the primary acid-base disturbance(s) occurring in this case?

A. Metabolic acidosis only
B. Respiratory acidosis only
C. Metabolic alkalosis only
D. Respiratory alkalosis only
E. Metabolic acidosis and a respiratory acidosis
F. Metabolic alkalosis and a respiratory alkalosis

Q35-3: How would the metabolic acidosis component be classified in this case?

A. Anion gap acidosis
B. Non-anion gap acidosis
C. Anion and non-anion gap acidosis
D. Anion gap acidosis and a metabolic alkalosis

Q35-4: What laboratory test would you order next to evaluate the cause of the patient's anion gap acidosis?

A. Serum drug screen
B. Serum osmolality
C. Serum beta-hydroxybutyrate (BHB) or acetone
D. Serum lactate
E. Urine osmolality
F. Urine chloride
G. Serum cortisol

Q35-5: The patient's urine studies are as follows:

Urine Na	32 mEq/L
Urine K	49 mEq/L
Urine Cl	61 mEq/L
Urine urea	332 mg/dL
Urine glucose	0 mg/dL
Urine osmolality	410 mOsm/L
Urine pH	5.5
Urine RBCs	None
Urine WBCs	None
Urine protein	None
Urine microscopic	None
Fractional excretion of HCO_3	4%

What is the likely cause of the patient's non-anion gap acidosis?

A. Diarrhea
B. Autoimmune disease
C. Aminoglycoside use
D. Primary adrenal insufficiency

Q35-6: This patient also has a respiratory acidosis, which is likely due to respiratory muscle fatigue (which may, in part, be due to ongoing adrenal insufficiency as well). If the patient had an appropriate compensatory respiratory response, what would you expect the patient's $Paco_2$ to be?

A. 18 mm Hg
B. 20 mm Hg
C. 28 mm Hg
D. 34 mm Hg

ANSWERS

Q35-1: B

While the patient has a condition predisposing her to a chronic acid-base disorder, there is insufficient information to estimate the patient's baseline $Paco_2$ and HCO_3 values; therefore, we will assume a baseline $Paco_2$ of 40 mm Hg and a baseline HCO_3 of 24 mEq/L. This patient does have chronic adrenal insufficiency; however, she is on appropriate maintenance medication which should prevent a baseline acid-base disorder.

Rationale: Ignoring these underlying chronic acid-base disorders can significantly alter the interpretation of a patient's acute acid-base status. This was demonstrated in the first case of the series. However, often, we do not have the necessary information (eg, prior ABG or VBG, or prior serum chemistry with an HCO_3) and are forced to assume the ongoing processes are all acute in nature. We are primarily concerned about chronic respiratory acid-base disorders, as these can significantly alter the patient's baseline or expected values for the serum HCO_3 and $Paco_2$, and we have reliable equations to predict the expected baseline values. The respiratory compensation for both chronic metabolic acidosis and alkalosis is generally poor, so there are no equations or rules to predict what the $Paco_2$ should be in these cases. While the baseline serum HCO_3 may be significantly off from our standard value of 24 mEq/L in these patients, we would assume a baseline $Paco_2$ of 40 mm Hg in patients with chronic metabolic processes. Once we identify the patient's baseline $Paco_2$ and HCO_3 values, we will need to use these values in the appropriate equations to identify the ongoing acute processes.

Q35-2: E

Metabolic acidosis and a respiratory acidosis.

Rationale:

1. The pH is 7.10; therefore, the primary disorder is an **acidosis.**
2. The $Paco_2$ of 50 mm Hg is greater than 40 mm Hg, so there is a **respiratory acidosis**.
3. The HCO_3 of 13 mEq/L is less than 24 mEq/L, so there is also a **metabolic acidosis**.

Therefore, this patient has both a primary metabolic acidosis and a respiratory acidosis.

Q35-3: C

Anion and non-anion gap acidosis.

Rationale:

1. Is there evidence for a chronic acid-base disorder that requires adjustment of the patient's "normal" HCO_3? No, there is no evidence for a chronic acid-base disorder, so we would assume a baseline $Paco_2$ of 40 mm Hg and an HCO_3 of 24 mEq/L.

2. Expected anion gap:

$$\text{Expected Anion Gap} = 12 - (2.5) * \left[4.0\,\frac{g}{dL} - \text{Actual Serum Albumin} \right]$$

$$= 12 - (2.5 * [4.0 - 4.0])$$
$$= 12 - (2.5 * [0]) = \textbf{12 mEq/L.}$$

3. Anion gap calculation:

$$\text{Serum Anion Gap} = [Na^+] - [HCO_3^-] - [Cl^-]$$
$$= 140 - (110 + 14) = 16\ \text{mEq/L, which is} > 12\ \text{mEq/L}$$
$$\rightarrow \textbf{anion gap acidosis is present.}$$

4. Delta-delta calculation:

$$\Delta\Delta = \frac{(\text{Actual Anion Gap} - \text{Expected Anion Gap})}{(\text{Baseline HCO}_3 - \text{Actual HCO}_3)}$$

$$= (16 - 12)/(24 - 13) = \textbf{4/9, which is} > \textbf{0.4 but} < \textbf{1.}$$

Delta-delta interpretation.	
Delta-Delta Value	Condition Present
< 0.4	Non-anion gap only
0.4–1.0	**Anion gap *and* non-anion gap acidosis**
1.0–2.0	Anion gap acidosis only
> 2.0	Anion gap acidosis and metabolic alkalosis

Therefore, this patient has both an anion gap acidosis as well as a non-anion gap metabolic acidosis.

Q35-4: D
Serum lactate.

Rationale: The patient's presentation with fever, elevated WBC count, tachycardia, and hypotension in the setting of sepsis is most consistent with lactic acidosis, so a serum lactate is the most appropriate next study. Acute adrenal insufficiency in the setting of sepsis could also be contributing to the distributive shock present.

Q35-5: D
Primary adrenal insufficiency. Adrenal insufficiency is consistent with the development of a type 4 RTA.

Rationale:

NAGMA
Cause of NAGMA
Evaluation Strategy   1. History (acute or chronic issues, medications, altered GI anatomy, genetic diseases, etc). Also, is the patient receiving an acid load, such as TPN?   2. Does the patient have chronic renal insufficiency? If so, this alone may be responsible for the non-anion gap acidosis.   3. Calculate urine anion gap and urine osmolal gap. The urine anion gap may be of limited value in patients with severe serum anion gap acidosis, as it may be falsely elevated. Similarly, the urine osmolal gap may be inappropriately elevated in patients with a significant serum osmolal gap (particularly due to mannitol).   4. Note the serum potassium as well as the urine pH.   5. If proximal RTA is suspected, look for evidence of other inappropriate compounds in the urine (amino acids, elevated phosphate, glucosuria), and calculate the fractional resorption of sodium HCO_3 (should be > 15%). Also check serum for evidence of dysfunction of the PTH–vitamin D–calcium axis.
Cause of NAGMA
Low Serum Potassium   GI: Diarrhea, pancreaticoduodenal fistula, urinary intestinal diversion   Renal: Type 1 RTA (distal), type 2 RTA (proximal)   Medications/exposures: Carbonic anhydrase inhibitors, toluene   Other: D-Lactic acidosis   ***High (or Normal) Serum Potassium***   GI: Elevated ileostomy output   Renal: Type 4 RTA or CKD   Medications: NSAIDs; antibiotics (trimethoprim, pentamidine); heparin; ACE inhibitors, ARBs, aldosterone antagonists (spironolactone); acid administration (TPN)

The urine anion gap is (+20) mEq/L. However, the urine anion gap can be inappropriately elevated in anion gap acidosis, a situation in which multiple unmeasured anions may be present in the urine (BHB/acetoacetate [ketoacidosis], hippurate [toluene], HCO_3 [proximal RTA], D-lactate [D-lactic acidosis], L-lactate, 5-oxoproline [acetaminophen toxicity]). Therefore, in patients with a significant anion gap, the urine osmolar gap is typically more useful. Since the patient has an anion gap acidosis, we should use the serum osmolal gap first to determine if the patient has a type 1 or 4 RTA.

$$\text{Calculated Urine Osmolality} = 2 * ([Na^+] + [K^+]) + \frac{[Urea]}{2.8} + \frac{[Glucose]}{18}$$

$$= 328 \text{ mOsm/L}$$

$$\text{Urine Osmolal Gap (UOG)} = \text{Measured Urine Osmolality} - \text{Measured Urine Osmolality}$$

$$\text{UOG} = 410 - 328 = (+82) \text{ mOsm/L.}$$

Similar to the urine anion gap, the urine osmolar gap is used as a surrogate for the urine ammonium concentration. Therefore, a larger gap indicates increased urinary NH_4 excretion. In normal acid-base conditions, the urine osmolar gap is between 10 and 100 mOsm/L. During a significant metabolic acidosis, patients with impaired renal tubular acidification (type 1 and type 4 RTA) are unable to excrete additional acid (NH_4), and therefore the osmolar gap does not change. Patients with an intact renal response to acidemia (ie, GI losses) should have a significant urine osmolar gap (~ >300 to 400 mOsm/L) as a result of increased NH_4 excretion. This patient has an inappropriately low serum osmolal gap; therefore, the patient likely has either a type 1 or type 4 RTA. Now we can use the collateral information to make a diagnosis.

Evaluation of RTA.			
	Type 1 RTA	Type 2 RTA	Type 4 RTA
Severity of metabolic acidosis, (HCO_3)	Severe (< 10–12 mEq/L typically)	Intermediate (12–20 mEq/L)	Mild (15–20 mEq/L)
Associated urine abnormalities	Urinary phosphate, calcium increased; bone disease often present	Urine glucose, amino acids, phosphate, calcium may be elevated	
Urine pH	HIGH (> 5.5)	Low (acidic), until serum HCO_3 level exceeds resorptive ability of proximal tubule; then becomes alkalotic once reabsorptive threshold is crossed	Low (acidic)
Serum K^+	Low to normal; should correct with oral HCO_3 therapy	Classically low, although may be normal or even high with rare genetic defects; worsens with oral HCO_3 therapy	HIGH
Renal stones	Often	No	No
Renal tubular defect	Reduced NH_4 secretion in distal tubule	Reduced HCO_3 resorption in proximal tubule	Reduced H^+/K^+ exchange in distal and collecting tubules due to decreased aldosterone or aldosterone resistance
Urine anion gap	> 10	Negative initially; then positive when receiving serum HCO_3; then negative after therapy	> 10
Urine osmolal gap	Reduced (< 150 mOsm/L) during acute acidosis	At baseline < 100 mEq/L; unreliable during acidosis	Reduced (< 150 mOsm/L) during acute acidosis

The patient's urine pH is 5.5 (acidic) and the serum potassium is elevated at 5.6. This is consistent with a type 4 RTA (distal), in which the H^+/K^+ transporter is ineffective. The patient has adrenal insufficiency, and while the patient may be taking the maintenance medication at home, the patient also has septic shock and is not able to respond appropriately to this increased level of systemic stress. Patients require stress-dose steroids in such circumstances to prevent these complications.

Of the choices provided, only adrenal insufficiency is associated with a type 4 RTA.

Causes of renal tubular acidosis.
Causes of Type 1 (Distal) RTA
Primary • Idiopathic or familial (may be recessive or dominant)
Secondary • Medications: Lithium, amphotericin, ifosfamide, NSAIDs • Rheumatologic disorders: Sjögren syndrome, SLE, RA • Hypercalciuria (idiopathic) or associated with vitamin D deficiency or hyperparathyroidism • Sarcoidosis • Obstructive uropathy • Wilson disease • Rejection of renal transplant allograft • Toluene toxicity
Causes of Type 2 (Proximal) RTA
Primary • Idiopathic • Familial (Recessive disorders primarily) • Genetic: Fanconi syndrome, cystinosis, glycogen storage disease (type 1), Wilson disease, galactosemia
Secondary • Medications: Acetazolamide, topiramate, aminoglycoside antibiotics, ifosfamide, reverse transcriptase inhibitors (tenofovir) • Heavy metal poisoning: Lead, mercury, copper • Multiple myeloma or amyloidosis (secondary to light chain toxicity) • Sjögren syndrome • Vitamin D deficiency • Rejection of renal transplant allograft
Causes of Type 4 RTA (Hypoaldosteronism or Aldosterone Resistance)
Primary • Primary adrenal insufficiency • Inherited disorders associated with hypoaldosteronism • Pseudohypoaldosteronism (types 1 and 2)
Secondary • Causes of hyporeninemic hypoaldosteronism such as renal disease (diabetic nephropathy), NSAID use, calcineurin inhibitors, volume expansion/volume overload • Causes of distal tubule voltage defects such as sickle cell disease, obstructive uropathy, SLE • Severe illness/septic shock • Angiotensin II–associated medications: ACE inhibitors, ARBs, direct renin inhibitors • Potassium-sparing diuretics: Spironolactone, amiloride, triamterene • Antibiotics: Trimethoprim, pentamidine

Q35-6: C
28 mm Hg.

Rationale: Using the Winter formula, one can calculate what the expected arterial $Paco_2$ should be for a given serum HCO_3 if the patient were completely compensated.

Respiratory Compensation for Acute Metabolic Acidosis (Winter Formula):

$$\text{Expected } Paco_2 = 1.5 * [\text{Actual } HCO_3] + 8 \pm 2 \text{ (in mm Hg)}$$
$$= (1.5 * 13) + 8 = 19.5 + 8 = 27.5 \pm 2 = (26 \text{ to } 30) \text{ mm Hg.}$$

We would expect a patient with appropriate compensatory respiratory alkalosis to have a $Paco_2$ of 28 mm Hg.

References

Adeva-Andany M, López-Ojén M, Funcasta-Calderón R, et al. Comprehensive review on lactate metabolism in human health. Mitochondrion. 2014;17:76.

Arlt W. The approach to the adult with newly diagnosed adrenal insufficiency. J Clin Endocrinol Metab. 2009;94:1059.

Arlt W, Society for Endocrinology Clinical Committee. Society for Endocrinology Endocrine Emergency Guidance: emergency management of acute adrenal insufficiency (adrenal crisis) in adult patients. Endocr Connect. 2016;5:G1.

Batlle D, Chin-Theodorou J, Tucker BM. Metabolic acidosis or respiratory alkalosis? Evaluation of a low plasma bicarbonate using the urine anion gap. Am J Kidney Dis. 2017;70:440.

Batlle D, Grupp M, Gaviria M, Kurtzman NA. Distal renal tubular acidosis with intact capacity to lower urinary pH. Am J Med. 1982;72:751.

Batlle D, Haque SK. Genetic causes and mechanisms of distal renal tubular acidosis. Nephrol Dial Transplant. 2012;27:3691.

Batlle DC, Hizon M, Cohen E, et al. The use of the urinary anion gap in the diagnosis of hyperchloremic metabolic acidosis. N Engl J Med. 1988;318:594.

Batlle DC, von Riotte A, Schlueter W. Urinary sodium in the evaluation of hyperchloremic metabolic acidosis. N Engl J Med. 1987;316:140.

Buckalew VM Jr, McCurdy DK, Ludwig GD, et al. Incomplete renal tubular acidosis. Physiologic studies in three patients with a defect in lowering urine pH. Am J Med. 1968;45:32.

Dyck RF, Asthana S, Kalra J, et al. A modification of the urine osmolal gap: an improved method for estimating urine ammonium. Am J Nephrol. 1990;10:359.

Hahner S, Allolio B. Therapeutic management of adrenal insufficiency. Best Pract Res Clin Endocrinol Metab. 2009;23:167.

Iwasaku M, Shinzawa M, Tanaka S, et al. Clinical characteristics of adrenal crisis in adult population with and without predisposing chronic adrenal insufficiency: a retrospective cohort study. BMC Endocr Disord. 2017;17:58.

Karet FE. Mechanisms in hyperkalemic renal tubular acidosis. J Am Soc Nephrol. 2009;20:251.

Kim GH, Han JS, Kim YS, et al. Evaluation of urine acidification by urine anion gap and urine osmolal gap in chronic metabolic acidosis. Am J Kidney Dis. 1996;27:42.

Kraut JA, Madias NE. Differential diagnosis of nongap metabolic acidosis: value of a systematic approach. Clin J Am Soc Nephrol. 2012;7:671.

Lee Hamm L, Hering-Smith KS, Nakhoul NL. Acid-base and potassium homeostasis. Semin Nephrol. 2013;33:257.

Levy B. Lactate and shock state: the metabolic view. Curr Opin Crit Care. 2006;12:315.

Loriaux DL, Fleseriu M. Relative adrenal insufficiency. Curr Opin Endocrinol Diabetes Obes. 2009;16:392.

Madias NE. Lactic acidosis. Kidney Int. 1986;29:752.

Meregalli P, Lüthy C, Oetliker OH, Bianchetti MG. Modified urine osmolal gap: an accurate method for estimating the urinary ammonium concentration? Nephron. 1995;69:98.

Mikkelsen ME, Miltiades AN, Gaieski DF, et al. Serum lactate is associated with mortality in severe sepsis independent of organ failure and shock. Crit Care Med. 2009;37:1670.

Oh M, Carroll HJ. Value and determinants of urine anion gap. Nephron 2002; 90:252.

Ono Y, Ono S, Yasunaga H, et al. Clinical features and practice patterns of treatment for adrenal crisis: a nationwide cross-sectional study in Japan. Eur J Endocrinol. 2017;176:329.

Rastegar M, Nagami GT. Non-anion gap metabolic acidosis: a clinical approach to evaluation. Am J Kidney Dis. 2017;69:296.

Rodríguez Soriano J. Renal tubular acidosis: the clinical entity. J Am Soc Nephrol 2002;13:2160.

Weant KA, Sasaki-Adams D, Dziedzic K, et al. Acute relative adrenal insufficiency after aneurysmal subarachnoid hemorrhage. Neurosurgery. 2008;63:645; discussion 649.

CASE 36

A 34-year-old 34-week gravid woman presents with 1 to 2 days of nausea and emesis after eating food at a cookout with family. Two other family members also are sick with a stomach illness. She is afebrile and mildly tachycardic, with HR to the 110s, RR 24, and BP 125/66. Her urine dipstick is positive for ketones. Her abdominal examination is benign. She has no significant medical history, takes no medications, and does not drink alcohol. She denies any illicit drug use.

Laboratory data.			
ABGs		Basic Metabolic Panel	
pH	7.30	Na	144 mEq/L
$Paco_2$	25 mm Hg	K	4.0 mEq/L
Pao_2	101 mm Hg	Cl	98 mEq/L
HCO_3	17 mEq/L	CO_2	17 mEq/L
		BUN	20 mg/dL
		Cr	1.0 mg/dL
		Glucose	121 mg/dL
		Albumin	4.0 g/dL
		EtOH	0 mg/dL

QUESTIONS

Q36-1: Define the patient's baseline acid-base status: Does this patient have an underlying chronic acid-base disorder that we need to account for in order to appropriately interpret the acute acid-base disorders?

A. There is no evidence for an underlying chronic respiratory or metabolic acid-base disorder in this patient, so we would assume a baseline $Paco_2$ of 40 mm Hg and an HCO_3 of 24 mEq/L.

B. While the patient has a condition predisposing her to a chronic acid-base disorder, there is insufficient information to estimate the patient's baseline $Paco_2$ and HCO_3 values; therefore, we will assume a baseline $Paco_2$ of 40 mm Hg and a baseline HCO_3 of 24 mEq/L.

C. The patient has an underlying acid-base condition, and we have sufficient information to estimate the patient's baseline $Paco_2$ and HCO_3 values.

Q36-2: What is/are the primary acid-base disturbance(s) occurring in this case?

A. Metabolic acidosis only
B. Respiratory acidosis only
C. Metabolic alkalosis only
D. Respiratory alkalosis only
E. Metabolic acidosis and a respiratory acidosis
F. Metabolic alkalosis and a respiratory alkalosis

Q36-3: How would the metabolic acidosis component be classified in this case?

A. Anion gap acidosis
B. Non-anion gap acidosis
C. Anion and non-anion gap acidosis
D. Anion gap acidosis and a metabolic alkalosis

Q36-4: Does the patient in this case demonstrate appropriate respiratory compensation?

A. Yes, the respiratory compensation is appropriate.
B. No, a concomitant respiratory alkalosis is present.
C. No, a concomitant respiratory acidosis is present.
D. Yes, the metabolic compensation is appropriate.
E. No, a concomitant metabolic acidosis is present.
F. No, a concomitant metabolic alkalosis is present.

Q36-5: Match the following acid-base disorders in this patient to the most likely etiology (use each acid-base disorder only once):

A. Anion gap acidosis
B. Metabolic alkalosis
C. Respiratory alkalosis
— Maternal ketosis
— Hyperemesis
— Lactic acidosis
— Aspirin overdose
— Pregnancy
— Renal tubular acidosis

Q36-6: Which of the following would be considered a normal ABG for a pregnant patient in the third trimester?

A. pH 7.48, $Paco_2$ 30, HCO_3 28
B. pH 7.42, $Paco_2$ 30, HCO_3 21
C. pH 7.36, $Paco_2$ 42, HCO_3 21
D. pH 7.33, $Paco_2$ 44, HCO_3 26

ANSWERS

Q36-1: B

While the patient has a condition (pregnancy) that predisposes her to a chronic acid-base disorder, there is insufficient information to estimate the patient's baseline $Paco_2$ and HCO_3 values; therefore, we will assume a baseline $Paco_2$ of 40 mm Hg and a baseline HCO_3 of 24 mEq/L.

Rationale: Ignoring these underlying chronic acid-base disorders can significantly alter the interpretation of a patient's acute acid-base status. This was demonstrated in the first case of the series. However, often, we do not have the necessary information (eg, prior ABG or VBG, or prior serum chemistry with an HCO_3) and are forced to assume the ongoing processes are all acute in nature. We are primarily concerned about chronic respiratory acid-base disorders, as these can significantly alter the patient's baseline or expected values for the serum HCO_3 and $Paco_2$, and we have reliable equations to predict the expected baseline values. The respiratory compensation for both chronic metabolic acidosis and alkalosis is generally poor, so there are no equations or rules to predict what the $Paco_2$ should be in these cases. While the baseline serum HCO_3 may be significantly off from our standard value of 24 mEq/L in these patients, we would assume a baseline $Paco_2$ of 40 mm Hg in patients with chronic metabolic processes. Once we identify the patient's baseline $Paco_2$ and HCO_3 values, we will need to use these values in the appropriate equations to identify the ongoing acute processes.

Q36-2: A

Metabolic acidosis only.

Rationale:

1. The pH is 7.30; therefore, the primary disorder is a **primary acidosis.**
2. The $Paco_2$ of 25 mm Hg is less than 40 mm Hg, so there is **no respiratory acidosis.**
3. The HCO_3 of 17 mEq/L is less than 24 mEq/L, so there is a **metabolic acidosis.**

Therefore, this patient has a primary metabolic acidosis only.

Q36-3: D

Anion gap acidosis and a metabolic alkalosis.

Rationale:

1. Is there evidence for a chronic acid-base disorder that requires adjustment of the patient's "normal" HCO_3? No, there is no evidence for a chronic acid-base disorder, so we would assume a baseline $Paco_2$ of 40 mm Hg and an HCO_3 of 24 mEq/L.

2. Expected anion gap:

$$\text{Expected Anion Gap} = 12 - (2.5) * \left[4.0 \frac{g}{dL} - \text{Actual Serum Albumin} \right]$$
$$= 12 - (2.5 * [4.0 - 4.0])$$
$$= 12 - (2.5 * [0]) = \textbf{12 mEq/L.}$$

3. Anion gap calculation:

$$\text{Serum Anion Gap} = [Na^+] - [HCO_3^-] - [Cl^-]$$
$$= 144 - (98 + 17) = \textbf{29 mEq/L,} \text{ which is > than 12 mEq/L}$$
$$\rightarrow \textbf{anion gap acidosis is present.}$$

4. Delta-delta calculation:

$$\Delta\Delta = \frac{(\text{Actual Anion Gap} - \text{Expected Anion Gap})}{(\text{Baseline HCO}_3 - \text{Actual HCO}_3)}$$
$$= (29 - 12)/(24 - 17) = \textbf{17/7, which is > 2.}$$

Delta-delta interpretation.	
Delta-Delta Value	Condition Present
< 0.4	Non-anion gap only
0.4–1.0	Anion gap *and* non-anion gap acidosis
1.0–2.0	Anion gap acidosis only
> 2.0	**Anion gap acidosis and metabolic alkalosis**

This indicates that the patient has an anion gap acidosis as well as a metabolic alkalosis.

Q36-4: B
No, a concomitant respiratory alkalosis is present.

Rationale: Using the Winter formula, one can calculate what the expected arterial $Paco_2$ should be for a given serum HCO_3 if the patient were completely compensated.

Respiratory Compensation for Acute Metabolic Acidosis (Winter Formula):

$$\text{Expected Paco}_2 = 1.5 * [\text{Actual HCO}_3] + 8 \pm 2 \text{ (in mm Hg)}$$
$$= (1.5 * 17) + 8 = 25.5 + 8 = 33.5 \pm 2 = (31 \text{ to } 35) \text{ mm Hg.}$$

Since the patient's $Paco_2$ of **25 mm Hg** on presentation was lower than the expected range of 31 to 35 mm Hg, this patient also has a **concomitant respiratory alkalosis.**

Q36-5:
A. Maternal ketosis
B. Hyperemesis
— Lactic acidosis
— Aspirin overdose
C. Pregnancy
— Renal tubular acidosis

Rationale: This patient has a triple disorder. The patient's acute anion gap acidosis is most likely to due to maternal ketosis. In pregnancy, fasting ketosis can develop over a much shorter time (12 to 16 hours) period than in nongravid patients (> 24 hours). This patient has not been eating or drinking due to nausea and emesis. The metabolic alkalosis is due to hyperemesis and loss of gastric acid. In terms of respiratory disorders, this patient has a $Paco_2$ that is lower than expected, so this is not merely a compensatory respiratory alkalosis. This patient also has an overlying respiratory alkalosis that is likely due to pregnancy.

Q36-6: B
pH 7.42, $Paco_2$ 30, HCO_3 21.

Rationale: During the third trimester, increased progesterone and altered lung volumes due to extrathoracic restriction lead to a mild chronic respiratory alkalosis, which is appropriately compensated for by a metabolic acidosis.

References

Chesnutt AN. Physiology of normal pregnancy. Crit Care Clin. 2004;20:609.

Elkus R, Popovich J Jr. Respiratory physiology in pregnancy. Clin Chest Med. 1992;13:555.

Hegewald MJ, Crapo RO. Respiratory physiology in pregnancy. Clin Chest Med. 2011;32:1.

Lindinger MI, Heigenhauser GJ. Effects of gas exchange on acid-base balance. Compr Physiol. 2012;2:2203.

Prowse CM, Gaensler EA. Respiratory and acid-base changes during pregnancy. Anesthesiology. 1965;26:381.

CASE 37

A 70-year-old man with congestive heart failure is transferred to the ICU with worsening shortness of breath. His examination demonstrates inspiratory crackles throughout the bilateral lung fields, and he is hypoxemic, requiring a partial rebreather mask. The patient's vitals signs are T 35.9C, RR 29, HR 86, BP 80/30, Sao_2 95% on 4L/min supplemental O_2. The patients extremities are edematous bilaterally and cold to the touch. You review his chart and his last echocardiogram shows an ejection fraction of 15%. He has been treated for the past 24 hours with loop diuretics in an effort to improve his dyspnea. He does not use tobacco and does not drink alcohol. Home medications include metoprolol, spironolactone, and lisinopril.

Laboratory data.			
ABGs		Basic Metabolic Panel	
pH	7.24	Na	129 mEq/L
$Paco_2$	19 mm Hg	K	5.6 mEq/L
Pao_2	66 mm Hg	Cl	80 mEq/L
HCO_3	13 mEq/L	CO_2	10 mEq/L
		BUN	44 mg/dL
		Cr	1.9 mg/dL
		Glucose	103 mg/dL
		Albumin	2.0 g/dL
		EtOH	0 mg/dL

QUESTIONS

Q37-1: Define the patient's baseline acid-base status: Does this patient have an underlying chronic acid-base disorder that we need to account for in order to appropriately interpret the acute acid-base disorders?

A. There is no evidence for an underlying chronic respiratory or metabolic acid-base disorder in this patient, so we would assume a baseline $Paco_2$ of 40 mm Hg and an HCO_3 of 24 mEq/L.

B. While the patient has a condition predisposing him to a chronic acid-base disorder, there is insufficient information to estimate the patient's baseline $Paco_2$ and HCO_3 values; therefore, we will assume a baseline $Paco_2$ of 40 mm Hg and a baseline HCO_3 of 24 mEq/L.

C. The patient has an underlying acid-base condition, and we have sufficient information to estimate the patient's baseline $Paco_2$ and HCO_3 values.

Q37-2: What is/are the primary acid-base disturbance(s) occurring in this case?

A. Metabolic acidosis only
B. Respiratory acidosis only
C. Metabolic acidosis and a respiratory acidosis
D. Metabolic alkalosis and a respiratory alkalosis

Q37-3: How would the metabolic acidosis component be classified in this case?

A. Anion gap acidosis
B. Non-anion gap acidosis
C. Anion and non-anion gap acidosis
D. Anion gap acidosis and a metabolic alkalosis

Q37-4: Why do we use the serum HCO_3 from the basic metabolic panel (BMP) rather than the serum HCO_3 from the ABG?

A. The BMP provides information about the anion gap, so we use this HCO_3 to be more accurate when calculating the anion gap.

B. The HCO_3 in the BMP is a direct measurement, whereas the HCO_3 in the ABG is not a direct measurement but rather a calculated value.

C. The HCO_3 in the BMP is independent of the $Paco_2$ and therefore more accurate.

Q37-5: Does the patient in this case demonstrate appropriate respiratory compensation?

A. Yes, the respiratory compensation is appropriate.
B. No, a concomitant respiratory alkalosis is present.
C. No, a concomitant respiratory acidosis is present.

Q37-6: Match the following acid-base disorders in this patient to the most likely etiology (use each acid-base disorder only once):

A. Anion gap acidosis
B. Metabolic alkalosis
C. Respiratory alkalosis
— Heart failure-related pulmonary edema
— COPD
— Lactic acidosis
— Aspirin overdose
— Diuresis
— Renal tubular acidosis

ANSWERS

Q37-1: B

While the patient has a condition that potentially predisposes him to a chronic acid-base disorder (congestive heart failure), there is insufficient information to estimate the patient's baseline $Paco_2$ and HCO_3 values; therefore, we will assume a baseline $Paco_2$ of 40 mm Hg and a baseline HCO_3 of 24 mEq/L.

Rationale: Ignoring these underlying chronic acid-base disorders can significantly alter the interpretation of a patient's acute acid-base status. This was demonstrated in the first case of the series. However, often, we do not have the necessary information (eg, prior ABG or VBG, or prior serum chemistry with an HCO_3) and are forced to assume the ongoing processes are all acute in nature. We are primarily concerned about chronic respiratory acid-base disorders, as these can significantly alter the patient's baseline or expected values for the serum HCO_3 and $Paco_2$, and we have reliable equations to predict the expected baseline values. The respiratory compensation for both chronic metabolic acidosis and alkalosis is generally poor, so there are no equations or rules to predict what the $Paco_2$ should be in these cases. While the baseline serum HCO_3 may be significantly off from our standard value of 24 mEq/L in these patients, we would assume a baseline $Paco_2$ of 40 mm Hg in patients with chronic metabolic processes. Once we identify the patient's baseline $Paco_2$ and HCO_3 values, we will need to use these values in the appropriate equations to identify the ongoing acute processes.

Q37-2: A

Metabolic acidosis only.

Rationale:

1. The pH is 7.24; therefore, the primary disorder is an **acidosis.**
2. The $Paco_2$ of 29 mm Hg is less than 40 mm Hg, so there is **no respiratory acidosis.**
3. The HCO_3 of 13 is less than 24, so there is a **metabolic acidosis.**

Q37-3: D

Anion gap acidosis and a metabolic alkalosis.

Rationale:

1. Is there evidence for a chronic acid-base disorder that requires adjustment of the patient's "normal" HCO_3? No, there is no evidence for a chronic acid-base disorder, so we would assume a baseline $Paco_2$ of 40 mm Hg and an HCO_3 of 24 mEq/L.
2. Expected anion gap:

$$\text{Expected Anion Gap} = 12 - (2.5) * \left[4.0\, \frac{g}{dL} - \text{Actual Serum Albumin} \right]$$
$$= 12 - (2.5 * [4.0 - 2.0])$$
$$= 12 - (2.5 * [2]) = \textbf{7 mEq/L.}$$

3. Anion Gap Calculation:

$$\text{Serum Anion Gap} = [Na^+] - [HCO_3^-] - [Cl^-]$$
$$= 129 - (80 + 12) = \mathbf{37}, \text{ which is > than 7}$$
$$\rightarrow \textbf{anion gap acidosis is present.}$$

4. Delta-delta calculation:

$$\Delta\Delta = \frac{(\text{Actual Anion Gap} - \text{Expected Anion Gap})}{(\text{Baseline HCO}_3 - \text{Actual HCO}_3)}$$

$$= (37 - 7)/(24 - 10) = \mathbf{30/14}, \text{ which is > 2.}$$

Delta-delta interpretation.	
Delta-Delta Value	Condition Present
< 0.4	Non-anion gap only
0.4–1.0	Anion gap *and* non-anion gap acidosis
1.0–2.0	Anion gap acidosis only
> 2.0	**Anion gap acidosis and metabolic alkalosis**

This indicates that the patient has an **anion gap acidosis as well as a metabolic alkalosis.**

Q37-4: B

The HCO₃ in the BMP is a direct measurement, whereas the HCO₃ in the ABG is not a direct measurement but rather a calculated value.

Rationale: The HCO_3 on the ABG is a calculated value based on the pH and $Paco_2$, so it is not as accurate as the HCO_3 directly measured from the metabolic panel. It may be used as a surrogate for quick calculations when a BMP is not available, but again this calculation is dependent on several assumptions being correct.

Q37-5: B

No, a concomitant respiratory alkalosis is present.

Rationale: Using the Winter formula, one can calculate what the expected arterial $Paco_2$ should be for a given serum HCO_3 if the patient were completely compensated.

Respiratory Compensation for Acute Metabolic Acidosis (Winter Formula):

$$\text{Expected Paco}_2 = 1.5 * [\text{Actual HCO}_3] + 8 \pm 2 \text{ (in mm Hg)}$$
$$= (1.5 * 10) + 8 = 15 + 8 = 23 \pm 2 = (21 \text{ to } 25) \text{ mm Hg.}$$

Since the patient's $Paco_2$ on presentation to the ICU (**19 mm Hg**) is lower than the expected range of 21 to 25 mm Hg, this patient also has an **overlying respiratory alkalosis.**

Q37-6:
C. Heart failure-related pulmonary edema
— COPD
A. Lactic acidosis
— Aspirin overdose
B. Diuresis
— Renal tubular acidosis

Rationale: This patient has a triple disorder. The patient's anion gap acidosis is likely due to lactic acidosis from congestive heart failure. The cold, edematous extremities and low BP with a history of congestive heart failure with low ejection fraction are suggestive of this etiology. The patient's metabolic alkalosis is likely a result of overdiuresis. Given the patient's low albumin and his total body volume overload, he likely does not shift fluid quickly from the extravascular to intravascular space for diuresis and is intravascularly dry. The high BUN to Cr ratio would support this. Note that if one did not correct the expected anion gap for the patient's low albumin, this would have been missed. The respiratory alkalosis is likely due to the patient's pulmonary edema, apparent on examination.

References

Byrd JB, Turcu AF, Auchus RJ. Primary aldosteronism. Circulation. 2018;138:823.

Chhokar VS, Sun Y, Bhattacharya SK, et al. Hyperparathyroidism and the calcium paradox of aldosteronism. Circulation. 2005;111:871.

Corry DB, Tuck ML. Secondary aldosteronism. Endocrinol Metab Clin North Am. 1995;24:511.

Frangiosa A, De Santo LS, Anastasio P, De Santo NG. Acid-base balance in heart failure. J Nephrol. 2006;19(suppl 9):S115.

Khanna A, Kurtzman NA. Metabolic alkalosis. J Nephrol. 2006;19(suppl 9):S86.

Oster JR, Preston RA, Materson BJ. Fluid and electrolyte disorders in congestive heart failure. Semin Nephrol. 1994;14:485.

Radó JP, Marosi J, Takó J. High doses of spironolactone (Aldactone, SC-14266, Verospirone) alone and in combination with triamterene and-or diuretics in the treatment of refractory edema associated with secondary hyperaldosteronism. Endokrinologie. 1970;57:46.

Romani JD. The secondary hyperaldosteronism of cardiac insufficiency. Pathogenic study and physiopathological implications. Presse Med. 1960;68:441.

Seller RH, Ramirez O, Brest AN. Secondary aldosteronism in refractory edema. GP. 1967;35:104.

Soifer JT, Kim HT. Approach to metabolic alkalosis. Emerg Med Clin North Am. 2014;32:453.

Urso C, Brucculeri S, Caimi G. Acid-base and electrolyte abnormalities in heart failure: pathophysiology and implications. Heart Fail Rev. 2015;20:493.

Weber KT, Villarreal D. Aldosterone and antialdosterone therapy in congestive heart failure. Am J Cardiol. 1993;71:3A.

CASE 38

A 66-year-old man from Western Virginia with a history of alcoholism, tobacco abuse, COPD, hypertension, and hyperlipidemia presents to the emergency department with complaints of blurry vision. His family noted the patient was not "acting himself" for the past few hours and was experiencing falls and issues with vision at home. The patient reports blurry vision and states that he sees flashing lights. He is somewhat delirious and not able to complete a history. His medical record shows a primary care visit approximately 6 years ago, at which time the patient was noncompliant with all medications. His wife is unavailable to provide collateral history at this point. His vital signs are T 37.6°C, RR 23, HR 98, BP 129/78, and Sao_2 94% on RA. His prior laboratory values show no evidence of chronic respiratory failure.

Laboratory data.			
ABGs		Basic Metabolic Panel	
pH	7.18	Na	140 mEq/L
$Paco_2$	48 mm Hg	K	4.1 mEq/L
Pao_2	110 mm Hg	Cl	104 mEq/L
HCO_3	12 mEq/L	CO_2	12 mEq/L
		BUN	20 mg/dL
		Cr	1.6 mg/dL
		Glucose	119 mg/dL
		Albumin	4.0 g/dL
		EtOH	0 mg/dL

QUESTIONS

Q38-1: Define the patient's baseline acid-base status: Does this patient have an underlying chronic acid-base disorder that we need to account for in order to appropriately interpret the acute acid-base disorders?

A. There is no evidence for an underlying chronic respiratory or metabolic acid-base disorder in this patient, so we would assume a baseline $Paco_2$ of 40 mm Hg and an HCO_3 of 24 mEq/L.

B. While the patient has a condition that potentially predisposes him to a chronic acid-base disorder, there is insufficient information to estimate the patient's baseline $Paco_2$ and HCO_3 values; therefore, we will assume a baseline $Paco_2$ of 40 mm Hg and a baseline HCO_3 of 24 mEq/L.

C. The patient has an underlying acid-base condition, and we have sufficient information to estimate the patient's baseline $Paco_2$ and HCO_3 values.

Q38-2: What is/are the primary acid-base disturbance(s) occurring in this case?

A. Metabolic acidosis only
B. Respiratory acidosis only
C. Metabolic alkalosis only
D. Respiratory alkalosis only
E. Metabolic acidosis and a respiratory acidosis
F. Metabolic alkalosis and a respiratory alkalosis

Q38-3: How would the metabolic acidosis component be classified in this case?

A. Anion gap acidosis
B. Non-anion gap acidosis
C. Anion and non-anion gap acidosis
D. Anion gap acidosis and a metabolic alkalosis

Q38-4: Does the patient in this case demonstrate appropriate respiratory compensation?

A. Yes, the respiratory compensation is appropriate.
B. No, a concomitant respiratory alkalosis is present.
C. No, a concomitant respiratory acidosis is present.

Q38-5: What laboratory test would you order next to further evaluate the cause of the patient's anion gap acidosis?

A. Serum lactate
B. Serum osmolality
C. Serum drug screen for ASA level
D. Serum beta-hydroxybutyrate (BHA) and acetone

Q38-6: The patient's EtOH level is 0. The glucose level is 119 mg/dL. The measured serum osmolality is 326. What is the osmolar gap?

A. 10 mOsm/L
B. 22 mOsm/L
C. 31 mOsm/L
D. 6 mOsm/L

Q38-7: Match the following acid-base disorders in this patient to the most likely etiology (use each acid-base disorder only once):

A. Anion gap acidosis
B. Respiratory acidosis
— Methanol ingestion
— Lactic acidosis
— Aspirin overdose
— Diuretic overdose
— Renal tubular acidosis
— COPD

Q38-8: You order a serum methanol test, but results will not be available for 24 hours. What is the next best step?

A. Have family search for source of possible methanol or ethylene glycol ingestion at home and report back.
B. Contact the state health department.
C. Obtain an ophthalmology consultation and brain MRI.
D. Initiate fomepizole/ethanol infusion and dialysis.

ANSWERS

Q38-1: B

While the patient has a condition that potentially predisposes him to a chronic acid-base disorder, there is insufficient information to estimate the patient's baseline $Paco_2$ and HCO_3 values; therefore, we will assume a baseline $Paco_2$ of 40 mm Hg and a baseline HCO_3 of 24 mEq/L.

Rationale: Ignoring these underlying chronic acid-base disorders can significantly alter the interpretation of a patient's acute acid-base status. This was demonstrated in the first case of the series. However, often, we do not have the necessary information (eg, prior ABG or VBG, or prior serum chemistry with an HCO_3) and are forced to assume the ongoing processes are all acute in nature. We are primarily concerned about chronic respiratory acid-base disorders, as these can significantly alter the patient's baseline or expected values for the serum HCO_3 and $Paco_2$, and we have reliable equations to predict the expected baseline values. The respiratory compensation for both chronic metabolic acidosis and alkalosis is generally poor, so there are no equations or rules to predict what the $Paco_2$ should be in these cases. While the baseline serum HCO_3 may be significantly off from our standard value of 24 mEq/L in these patients, we would assume a baseline $Paco_2$ of 40 mm Hg in patients with chronic metabolic processes. Once we identify the patient's baseline $Paco_2$ and HCO_3 values, we will need to use these values in the appropriate equations to identify the ongoing acute processes.

Q38-2: E

Metabolic acidosis and a respiratory Acidosis.

Rationale:

1. The pH is 7.18, therefore the primary disorder is an **acidosis.**
2. The $Paco_2$ of 48 mm Hg is greater than 40 mm Hg, so there is a **respiratory acidosis.**
3. The HCO_3 of 12 mEq/L is less than 24 mEq/L, so there is a **metabolic acidosis.**

Therefore, this patient has both a primary respiratory and metabolic acidosis.

Q38-3: A

Anion gap acidosis.

Rationale:

1. Is there evidence for a chronic acid-base disorder that requires adjustment of the patient's "normal" HCO_3? No, there is no evidence for a chronic acid-base disorder, so we would assume a baseline $Paco_2$ of 40 mm Hg and an HCO_3 of 24 mEq/L.
2. Expected anion gap:

$$\text{Expected Anion Gap} = 12 - (2.5) * \left[4.0 \, \frac{\text{g}}{\text{dL}} - \text{Actual Serum Albumin} \right]$$

$$= 12 - (2.5 * [4.0 - 4.0])$$
$$= 12 - (2.5 * [0]) = \textbf{12 mEq/L.}$$

3. Anion gap calculation:

$$\text{Serum Anion Gap} = [Na^+] - [HCO_3^-] - [Cl^-]$$
$$= 140 - (104 + 12) = \textbf{24 mEq/L,} \text{ which is} > \text{than 12 mEq/L}$$
$$\rightarrow \textbf{anion gap acidosis is present.}$$

4. Delta-delta calculation:

$$\Delta\Delta = \frac{(\text{Actual Anion Gap} - \text{Expected Anion Gap})}{(\text{Baseline HCO}_3 - \text{Actual HCO}_3)}$$

$$= (24 - 12)/(24 - 12) = \textbf{12/12, which is} \sim\textbf{1, pure anion gap acidosis.}$$

Delta-delta interpretation.	
Delta-Delta Value	**Condition Present**
< 0.4	Non-anion gap only
0.4–0.9	Anion gap *and* non-anion gap acidosis
1.0–2.0	**Anion gap acidosis only**
> 2.0	Anion gap acidosis and metabolic alkalosis

Therefore, this patient has a pure anion gap acidosis as the cause of the metabolic acidosis component.

Q38-4: C
No, a concomitant respiratory acidosis is present.

Rationale: Using the Winter formula, one can calculate what the expected arterial $Paco_2$ should be for a given serum HCO_3 if the patient were completely compensated.

Respiratory Compensation for Acute Metabolic Acidosis (Winter Formula):

$$\text{Expected Paco}_2 = 1.5 * [\text{Actual HCO}_3] + 8 \pm 2 \text{ (in mm Hg)}$$
$$= (1.5 * 12) + 8 = 18 + 8 = 26 \pm 2 = (24 \text{ to } 28) \text{ mm Hg.}$$

Since the patient's $Paco_2$ of **48 mm Hg** on presentation was higher than the expected range of 24 to 28 mm Hg, this patient also has an **overlying respiratory acidosis.**

Q38-5: B
Serum osmolality.

Rationale: The patient's symptoms of blurry vision are concerning for a high serum osmolality condition. His blood glucose level of 119 mg/dL would not lead to blurry vision even if the patient developed DKA. Therefore, the best test to order next would be a serum osmolality.

Q38-6: C
31 mOsm/L.

Rationale: Similar to the serum anion gap, the serum osmolal gap is determined by the difference between the "calculated" serum osmolality and the true, measured serum osmolality. The equation for the serum osmolal gap (SOG) typically includes factors for sodium, glucose, BUN, and ethanol, as these are readily measurable in most laboratories. Therefore, the SOG will represent the osmolality of those "unmeasured" osmoles, including organic alcohols and acetone. The most common form is given as follows:

$$\text{Calculated Serum Osmolality} = 2*[Na^+] + \frac{[Glucose]}{18} + \frac{[BUN]}{2.8} + \frac{[EtOH]}{3.7}$$
$$= 2*[140] + [119/18] + 20/2.8] + [0/3.7] = 295 \text{ mOsm/L.}$$

$$\text{Serum Osmolal Gap (SOG)} = \text{Measured Serum Osmolality}$$
$$- \text{Calculated Serum Osmolality}$$
$$\text{SOG} = 326 \text{ mOsm/L} - 295 = 31 \text{ mOsm/L.}$$

The following table summarizes potential causes of an elevated serum osmolality.

With an Elevated Serum Anion Gap
1. Ethanol ingestion with alcohol ketoacidosis (acetone is an unmeasured osmole, in addition to ethanol)—the osmolality is usually elevated more so by the increased ethanol concentration, so the osmolal "gap" depends on whether the term for ethanol is included in the osmolality calculation.*
2. Organic alcohol ingestions (methanol, ethylene glycol, diethylene glycol, propylene glycol)
3. DKA similar to ethanol ingestion, glucose and acetone contribute to the osmolality, since the glucose term is always included in the calculation
4. Salicylate toxicity
5. Renal failure—the BUN is nearly always included in the osmolality
Without an Elevated Serum Anion Gap
1. Hyperosmolar therapy (mannitol, glycerol)
2. Other organic solvent ingestion (eg, acetone)
3. Isopropyl alcohol ingestion (produces only acetone rather than an organic acid, so no anion gap is seen)
4. Hypertriglyceridemia
5. Hyperproteinemia

*A mildly elevated osmolal gap has been reported in the literature in patients with lactic acidosis in critical illness, particularly severe distributive shock. The pathology is not quite clear, although it likely is related to multiorgan failure—particularly involving the liver and kidneys—and the release of cellular components known to contribute to the osmolal gap. This is typically around 10 mOsm, although it may be as high as 20–25 mOsm/L.

In this patient, we would be primarily worried about methanol ingestion given the neurologic and vision symptoms.

Q38-7:

A. Methanol ingestion
— Lactic acidosis
— Aspirin overdose
— Diuretic overdose
— Renal tubular acidosis
B. COPD

Rationale: This patient has a primary anion gap acidosis secondary to methanol ingestion, causing blindness. The patient has underlying COPD, which has limited his ability to compensate for this metabolic acidosis, and he is more likely to tire out and develop a respiratory acidosis, which is present in this case.

Q38-8: D
Initiate fomepizole/ethanol infusion and dialysis.

Rationale: Treatment should never be delayed in a case of suspected methanol or ethylene glycol ingestion while awaiting confirmation. The elevated osmolar gap along with suspicion of ingestion based on the blurred vision is sufficient evidence in this case. The severe morbidity associated with untreated methanol (blindness) or ethylene glycol (renal failure) necessitates immediate action, so fomepizole (preferred if available) or ethanol infusion and intermittent dialysis are essential now.

References

Church AS, Witting MD. Laboratory testing in ethanol, methanol, ethylene glycol, and isopropanol toxicities. J Emerg Med. 1997;15:687.

Eder AF, Dowdy YG, Gardiner JA, et al. Serum lactate and lactate dehydrogenase in high concentrations interfere in enzymatic assay of ethylene glycol. Clin Chem. 1996;42:1489.

Hoffman RS, Smilkstein MJ, Howland MA, Goldfrank LR. Osmol gaps revisited: normal values and limitations. J Toxicol Clin Toxicol. 1993;31:81.

Höjer J. Severe metabolic acidosis in the alcoholic: differential diagnosis and management. Hum Exp Toxicol. 1996;15:482.

Liesivuori J, Savolainen II. Methanol and formic acid toxicity: biochemical mechanisms. Pharmacol Toxicol. 1991;69:157.

Lynd LD, Richardson KJ, Purssell RA, et al. An evaluation of the osmole gap as a screening test for toxic alcohol poisoning. BMC Emerg Med. 2008;8:5.

Malandain H, Cano Y. Interferences of glycerol, propylene glycol, and other diols in the enzymatic assay of ethylene glycol. Eur J Clin Chem Clin Biochem. 1996;34:651.

Purssell RA, Pudek M, Brubacher J, Abu-Laban RB. Derivation and validation of a formula to calculate the contribution of ethanol to the osmolal gap. Ann Emerg Med. 2001;38:653.

Shirey T, Sivilotti M. Reaction of lactate electrodes to glycolate. Crit Care Med. 1999;27:2305.

Sivilotti ML. Methanol intoxication. Ann Emerg Med. 2000;35:313.

CASE 39

A 33-year-old obese woman with IDDM, hyperlipidemia, and hypertension presents to the emergency department with abdominal distention and diffuse abdominal pain of 24 hours duration. She is febrile to 39.2°C, with RR 28, HR 110, BP 140/70, and Sao$_2$ 95% on RA. On physical examination, diffuse tenderness without rebound or guarding is present. Hbg is 16 g/dL, WBC count 8000/mL, and blood glucose 450 mg/dL on admission. Lipase is 34,000 U/L (normal range 23 to 85 U/L).

Laboratory data.			
ABGs		**Basic Metabolic Panel**	
pH	7.10	Na	131 mEq/L
Paco$_2$	22 mm Hg	K	5.6 mEq/L
Pao$_2$	100 mm Hg	Cl	95 mEq/L
HCO$_3$	5 mEq/L	CO$_2$	5 mEq/L
		BUN	25 mg/dL
		Cr	0.7 mg/dL
		Glucose	450 mg/dL
		Albumin	4.0 g/dL
		EtOH	0 mg/dL

QUESTIONS

Q39-1: Define the patient's baseline acid-base status: Does this patient have an underlying chronic acid-base disorder that we need to account for in order to appropriately interpret the acute acid-base disorders?

A. There is no evidence for an underlying chronic respiratory or metabolic acid-base disorder in this patient, so we would assume a baseline $Paco_2$ of 40 mm Hg and an HCO_3 of 24 mEq/L.

B. While the patient has a condition that potentially predisposes her to a chronic acid-base disorder, there is insufficient information to estimate the patient's baseline $Paco_2$ and HCO_3 values; therefore, we will assume a baseline $Paco_2$ of 40 mm Hg and a baseline HCO_3 of 24 mEq/L.

C. The patient has an underlying acid-base condition, and we have sufficient information to estimate the patient's baseline $Paco_2$ and HCO_3 values.

Q39-2: What is/are the primary acid-base disturbance(s) occurring in this case?

A. Metabolic acidosis only
B. Respiratory acidosis only
C. Metabolic alkalosis only
D. Respiratory alkalosis only
E. Metabolic acidosis and a respiratory acidosis
F. Metabolic alkalosis and a respiratory alkalosis

Q39-3: How would the metabolic acidosis component be classified in this case?

A. Anion gap acidosis
B. Non-anion gap acidosis
C. Anion and non-anion gap acidosis
D. Anion gap acidosis and a metabolic alkalosis

Q39-4: Does the patient in this case demonstrate appropriate respiratory compensation?

A. Yes, the respiratory compensation is appropriate.
B. No, a concomitant respiratory alkalosis is present.
C. No, a concomitant respiratory acidosis is present.

Q39-5: The patient is placed on IV insulin, IV fluids, and electrolyte protocol. He has been appropriately treated for his DKA and his blood glucose is now 101 mg/dL. However, his serum Na remains low at 129 and serum HCO_3 remains 5 with a high anion gap acidosis. Additional laboratory findings are as follows:

Serum EtOH	< 3 mg/dL
Serum acetaminophen level	< 5 mg/dL (ULN for therapeutic use 20 mg/dL)
Serum salicylates level	< 5 mg/dL (ULN for therapeutic use 30 mg/dL)
Serum osmolality	423 mOsm/kg
Serum L-lactate	1.8 mmol/L (ULN 2.0 mmol/L venous)
Beta-hydroxybutyrate (acetone)	< 0.18 mmol/L (ULN 0.18 mmol/L)
Serum glucose	101 mg/dL

You check an ABG and the pH is 7.40 with an estimated HCO_3 of 22. What is the most likely source of this patient's acid-base disorder now?

A. Methanol toxicity
B. Ethylene glycol toxicity
C. Hyperlipidemia
D. Hyperproteinemia

ANSWERS

Q39-1: B

While the patient has a condition (diabetes mellitus) that potentially predisposes her to a chronic acid-base disorder, there is insufficient information to estimate the patient's baseline $Paco_2$ and HCO_3 values; therefore, we will assume a baseline $Paco_2$ of 40 mm Hg and a baseline HCO_3 of 24 mEq/L.

Rationale: Ignoring these underlying chronic acid-base disorders can significantly alter the interpretation of a patient's acute acid-base status. This was demonstrated in the first case of the series. However, often, we do not have the necessary information (eg, prior ABG or VBG, or prior serum chemistry with an HCO_3) and are forced to assume the ongoing processes are all acute in nature. We are primarily concerned about chronic respiratory acid-base disorders, as these can significantly alter the patient's baseline or expected values for the serum HCO_3 and $Paco_2$, and we have reliable equations to predict the expected baseline values. The respiratory compensation for both chronic metabolic acidosis and alkalosis is generally poor, so there are no equations or rules to predict what the $Paco_2$ should be in these cases. While the baseline serum HCO_3 may be significantly off from our standard value of 24 mEq/L in these patients, we would assume a baseline $Paco_2$ of 40 mm Hg in patients with chronic metabolic processes. Once we identify the patient's baseline $Paco_2$ and HCO_3 values, we will need to use these values in the appropriate equations to identify the ongoing acute processes.

Q39-2: A

Metabolic acidosis only.

Rationale:

1. The pH is 7.10; therefore, the primary disorder is an **acidosis**.
2. The $Paco_2$ of 22 mm Hg is less than 40 mm Hg, so there is **no respiratory acidosis**.
3. The HCO_3 of 5 is less than 24, so there is a **metabolic acidosis**.

Therefore, this patient has a primary metabolic acidosis.

Q39-3: A

Anion gap acidosis.

Rationale:

1. Is there evidence for a chronic acid-base disorder that requires adjustment of the patient's "normal" HCO_3? No, there is no evidence for a chronic acid-base disorder, so we would assume a baseline $Paco_2$ of 40 mm Hg and an HCO_3 of 24 mEq/L.
2. Expected anion gap:

$$\text{Expected Anion Gap} = 12 - (2.5) * \left[4.0\,\frac{g}{dL} - \text{Actual Serum Albumin} \right]$$

$$= 12 - (2.5 * [4.0 - 4.0])$$
$$= 12 - (2.5 * [0]) = \textbf{12 mEq/L}.$$

3. Anion gap calculation:

$$\text{Serum Anion Gap} = [Na^+] - [HCO_3^-] - [Cl^-]$$
$$= 131 - (95 + 5) = \textbf{31 mEq/L,} \text{ which is} > 12 \text{ mEq/L}$$
$$\rightarrow \textbf{anion gap acidosis is present.}$$

4. Delta-delta calculation:

$$\Delta\Delta = \frac{(\text{Actual Anion Gap} - \text{Expected Anion Gap})}{(\text{Baseline HCO}_3 - \text{Actual HCO}_3)}$$

$(31 - 12)/(24 - 5) = $ **19/19, which is ~1, pure anion gap acidosis.**

Delta-delta interpretation.	
Delta-Delta Value	Condition Present
< 0.4	Non-anion gap only
0.4–0.9	Anion gap *and* non-anion gap acidosis
1.0–2.0	**Anion gap acidosis only**
> 2.0	Anion gap acidosis and metabolic alkalosis

Therefore, this patient's primary metabolic acidosis is a due to a pure anion gap acidosis.

Q39-4: C
No, a concomitant respiratory acidosis is present.

Rationale: Using the Winter formula, one can calculate what the expected arterial $Paco_2$ should be for a given serum HCO_3 if the patient were appropriately compensated.

Respiratory Compensation for Acute Metabolic Acidosis (Winter Formula):

$$\text{Expected Paco}_2 = 1.5 * [\text{Actual HCO}_3] + 8 \pm 2 \text{ (in mm Hg)}$$
$$= (1.5 * 5) + 8 = 7.5 + 8 = 15 \pm 2 = (13 \text{ to } 17) \text{ mm Hg.}$$

Since the patient's $Paco_2$ on presentation of **22 mm Hg** was higher than the expected range of 13 to 17 mm Hg, this patient also has a **concomitant respiratory acidosis.**

Q39-5: C
Hyperlipidemia.

Rationale: In rare cases, patients with severe hypertriglyceridemia (> 2000 mg/dL) may present with acute pancreatitis, and this can cause a false anion gap acidosis due to interference with normal assays. This patient presented with acute pancreatitis leading to DKA on presentation (true acidosis on presentation given the pH), but following the treatment of DKA the patient's serum HCO_3 was spuriously low due to interference of the lipids with the assay for serum HCO_3. The ABG demonstrated a pH of 7.40 with a normal estimated HCO_3, which was correct. This is supported by the pseudo-hyponatremia as well, which is a common side effect of hypertriglyceridemia. If the patient's serum were to be ultracentrifuged to remove the lipids, the serum HCO_3 would be correct. Hyperlipidemia to this degree is usually visible when blood is drawn. This patient would likely receive plasmapheresis acutely.

References

DeFronzo RA, Matzuda M, Barret E. Diabetic ketoacidosis: a combined metabolic-nephrologic approach to therapy. Diabetes Rev. 1994;2:209.

Elisaf M, Merkouropoulos M, Tsianos EV, Siamopoulos KC. Acid-base and electrolyte abnormalities in alcoholic patients. Miner Electrolyte Metab. 1994;20:274.

Fulop M, Murthy V, Michilli A, et al. Serum beta-hydroxybutyrate measurement in patients with uncontrolled diabetes mellitus. Arch Intern Med. 1999;159:381.

Goldwasser P, Manjappa NG, Luhrs CA, Barth RH. Pseudohypobicarbonatemia caused by an endogenous assay interferent: a new entity. Am J Kidney Dis. 2011;58:617.

Igbinedion SO, Pandit S, Mavuram MS, Boktor M. Pseudohyponatraemia secondary to hyperlipidaemia in obstructive jaundice. BMJ Case Rep. 2017;2017. pii: bcr-2017-221984.

Porter WH, Yao HH, Karounos DG. Laboratory and clinical evaluation of assays for beta-hydroxybutyrate. Am J Clin Pathol. 1997;107:353.

Rifkin SI, Shaub B. Factitious hypobicarbonatemia associated with profound hyperlipidemia. Ren Fail. 2014;36:1155.

Rose BD, Post TW. Clinical Physiology of Acid-Base and Electrolyte Disorders, 5e. New York, NY: McGraw Hill; 2001:809.

Shen T, Braude S. Changes in serum phosphate during treatment of diabetic ketoacidosis: predictive significance of severity of acidosis on presentation. Intern Med J. 2012;42:1347.

Stein H. Spuriously low serum bicarbonate levels in patients with hyperlipidemia: a report of 4 cases. Am J Kidney Dis. 2019;73:131.

Turchin A, Seifter JL, Seely EW. Clinical problem-solving. Mind the gap. N Engl J Med. 2003;349:1465.

Wachtel TJ, Tetu-Mouradjian LM, Goldman DL, et al. Hyperosmolarity and acidosis in diabetes mellitus: a three-year experience in Rhode Island. J Gen Intern Med. 1991;6:495.

CASE 40

A 55-year-old man with a history of alcoholism presents to the emergency department with respiratory failure. He was found unconscious at home, with emesis on his clothes and covering his face. He was hypoxemic and was intubated on arrival. His vital signs are T 38.6°C, RR 25, HR 122, BP 104/66, and Sao_2 99% on 40% Fio_2. His WBC count is 26,400/mL and his CXR shows a large infiltrate in the right lower and middle lobes. No one is available to provide collateral information.

Laboratory data.			
ABGs		Basic Metabolic Panel	
pH	6.97	Na	121 mEq/L
$Paco_2$	55 mm Hg	K	2.9 mEq/L
Pao_2	133 mm Hg	Cl	70 mEq/L
HCO_3	11 mEq/L	CO_2	11 mEq/L
		BUN	33 mg/dL
		Cr	0.2 mg/dL
		Glucose	167 mg/dL
		Albumin	2.1 g/dL
		EtOH	0 mg/dL

QUESTIONS

Q40-1: Define the patient's baseline acid-base status: Does this patient have an underlying chronic acid-base disorder that we need to account for in order to appropriately interpret the acute acid-base disorders?

A. There is no evidence for an underlying chronic respiratory or metabolic acid-base disorder in this patient, so we would assume a baseline $Paco_2$ of 40 mm Hg and an HCO_3 of 24 mEq/L.

B. While the patient has a condition that potentially predisposes him to a chronic acid-base disorder, there is insufficient information to estimate the patient's baseline $Paco_2$ and HCO_3 values; therefore, we will assume a baseline $Paco_2$ of 40 mm Hg and a baseline HCO_3 of 24 mEq/L.

C. The patient has an underlying acid-base condition, and we have sufficient information to estimate the patient's baseline $Paco_2$ and HCO_3 values.

Q40-2: What is/are the primary acid-base disturbance(s) occurring in this case?

A. Metabolic acidosis only
B. Respiratory acidosis only
C. Metabolic acidosis and a respiratory acidosis
D. Metabolic alkalosis and a respiratory alkalosis

Q40-3: For a perfectly healthy patient, a normal anion gap is assumed to be 12 mEq/L. What should be considered a normal anion gap in this patient?

A. 12 mEq/L
B. 10 mEq/L
C. 7 mEq/L
D. 4 mEq/L

Q40-4: How would the metabolic acidosis component be classified in this case?

A. Anion gap acidosis
B. Non-anion gap acidosis
C. Anion and non-anion gap acidosis
D. Anion gap acidosis and a metabolic alkalosis

Q40-5: The following laboratory results are returned for this patient:

Serum EtOH	< 3 mg/dL
Serum acetaminophen level	< 5 mg/dL (ULN for therapeutic use 20 mg/dL)
Serum salicylates level	< 5 mg/dL (ULN for therapeutic use 30 mg/dL)
Serum osmolality	271 mOsm/kg
Serum L-lactate	1.1 mmol/L (ULN 2.0 mmol/L venous)
Beta-hydroxybutyrate (acetone)	5.66 mmol/L (ULN 0.18 mmol/L)
Serum glucose	167 mg/dL

What is the most likely cause of the patient's anion gap acidosis?

A. DKA
B. Sepsis from pneumonia
C. Salicylate toxicity
D. Alcoholic ketoacidosis

Q40-6: What test may help differentiate the cause of the patient's metabolic alkalosis?

A. Urine osmolar gap
B. Urine chloride
C. Urine anion gap
D. Urine sodium
E. Serum chloride
F. Fractional excretion of bicarbonate
G. Fractional excretion of urea

ANSWERS

Q40-1: B

While the patient has a condition that potentially predisposes him to a chronic acid-base disorder, there is insufficient information to estimate the patient's baseline $Paco_2$ and HCO_3 values; therefore, we will assume a baseline $Paco_2$ of 40 mm Hg and a baseline HCO_3 of 24 mEq/L.

Rationale: Ignoring these underlying chronic acid-base disorders can significantly alter the interpretation of a patient's acute acid-base status. This was demonstrated in the first case of the series. However, often, we do not have the necessary information (eg, prior ABG or VBG, or prior serum chemistry with an HCO_3) and are forced to assume the ongoing processes are all acute in nature. We are primarily concerned about chronic respiratory acid-base disorders, as these can significantly alter the patient's baseline or expected values for the serum HCO_3 and $Paco_2$, and we have reliable equations to predict the expected baseline values. The respiratory compensation for both chronic metabolic acidosis and alkalosis is generally poor, so there are no equations or rules to predict what the $Paco_2$ should be in these cases. While the baseline serum HCO_3 may be significantly off from our standard value of 24 mEq/L in these patients, we would assume a baseline $Paco_2$ of 40 mm Hg in patients with chronic metabolic processes. Once we identify the patient's baseline $Paco_2$ and HCO_3 values, we will need to use these values in the appropriate equations to identify the ongoing acute processes.

Q40-2: C

Metabolic acidosis and respiratory acidosis.

Rationale:

1. The pH is 6.97; therefore, the primary disorder is an **acidosis.**
2. The $Paco_2$ of 55 mm Hg is greater than 40 mm Hg, so there is a **respiratory acidosis.**
3. The HCO_3 of 5 mEq/L is less than 24 mEq/L, so there is a **metabolic acidosis.**

Q40-3: C

7 mEq/L.

Rationale: The normal anion gap is 12 mEq/L. The term "anion gap" refers to those ions (negatively charged molecules) in the bloodstream that we do not routinely measure, including phosphates, sulfates, organic acids, and negatively charged plasma proteins. One of the most abundant negatively charged ions in the blood is serum albumin. A normal serum albumin is 4.0 g/dL. For patients with hypoalbuminemia (low serum albumin), the normal or expected anion gap is smaller:

$$\text{Expected Anion Gap} = 12 - (2.5) * \left[4.0 \, \frac{\text{g}}{\text{dL}} - \text{Actual Serum Albumin} \right].$$

Therefore, for this patient:

$$\text{Expected Anion Gap} = 12 - [2.5 * (4 - 2.1)] = 12 - (2.5 * 1.9) = 7 \text{ mEq/L}.$$

This is an important concept as patients with hypoalbuminemia may "hide" an anion gap acidosis if this correction is not performed.

Q40-4: D

Anion gap acidosis and a metabolic alkalosis.

Rationale:

1. Is there evidence for a chronic acid-base disorder that requires adjustment of the patient's "normal" HCO_3? No, there is no evidence for a chronic acid-base disorder, so we would assume a baseline $Paco_2$ of 40 mm Hg and an HCO_3 of 24 mEq/L.
2. Expected anion gap:

$$\text{Expected Anion Gap} = 12 - (2.5) * \left[4.0 \frac{g}{dL} - \text{Actual Serum Albumin} \right]$$
$$= 12 - (2.5 * [4.0 - 2.1])$$
$$= 12 - (2.5 * [1.9]) = \textbf{7 mEq/L.}$$

3. Anion gap calculation:

$$\text{Serum Anion Gap} = [Na^+] - [HCO_3^-] - [Cl^-]$$
$$= 121 - (70 + 11) = \textbf{40 mEq/L}, \text{ which is} > 7 \text{ mEq/L}$$
$$\rightarrow \textbf{anion gap acidosis is present.}$$

4. Delta-delta calculation:

$$\Delta\Delta = \frac{(\text{Actual Anion Gap} - \text{Expected Anion Gap})}{(\text{Baseline } HCO_3 - \text{Actual } HCO_3)}$$
$$= (40 - 7)/(24 - 10) = \textbf{33/14, which is} > \textbf{2.0.}$$

Delta-delta interpretation.	
Delta-Delta Value	**Condition Present**
< 0.4	Non-anion gap only
0.4–0.9	Anion gap *and* non-anion gap acidosis
1.0–2.0	Anion gap acidosis only
> 2.0	**Anion gap acidosis and metabolic alkalosis**

Therefore, **an anion gap acidosis and a metabolic alkalosis exist.**

Q40-5: D
Alcoholic ketoacidosis.

Rationale: This patient has an anion gap acidosis with normal lactate, negative ASA and acetaminophen, and low glucose levels. His positive serum acetone and beta-hydroxybutyrate are the likely result of alcoholic ketoacidosis. The presentation is often difficult to differentiate from DKA, although patients with DKA typically have a prior diagnosis of diabetes (however, note that DKA can be the presenting symptom of diabetes, as well). The history of alcoholism should push one toward a diagnosis of alcoholic ketoacidosis.

The serum osmolal gap is calculated as follows:

$$\text{Calculated Serum Osmolality} = 2*[Na^+] + \frac{[\text{Glucose}]}{18} + \frac{[\text{BUN}]}{2.8} + \frac{[\text{EtOH}]}{3.7}$$
$$= 2*[121] + [167/18] + [33/2.8] = 263 \text{ mOsm/L}$$

$$\text{Serum Osmolal Gap (SOG)} = \text{Measured Serum Osmolality}$$
$$- \text{Calculated Serum Osmolality}$$

$$\text{SOG} = 271 \text{ mOsm/L} - 263 = (+8) \text{ mOsm/L.}$$

Q40-6: B
Urine chloride.

Rationale: The urine chloride can help differentiate causes of metabolic alkalosis. A urine chloride less than 10 mEq/L is associated with diuretic use, hyperemesis, villous adenoma, and in patients compensating for chronic hypercapnia. A urine chloride greater than 20 mEq/L is associated with a number of congenital conditions (Bartter syndrome, Gittleman syndrome, Liddle syndrome), primary hyperaldosteronism, renal artery stenosis, and renin-secreting tumors.

This patient most likely has a metabolic alkalosis due to hyperemesis given the presentation.

Causes of metabolic alkalosis.
History
Rule Out the Following as Causes • Alkali load ("milk-alkali" or calcium-alkali syndrome, oral sodium bicarbonate, intravenous sodium bicarbonate) • Genetic causes (CF) • Presence of hypercalcemia • Intravenous β-lactam antibiotics • Laxative abuse (may also cause a metabolic acidosis depending on diarrheal HCO_3 losses)

(Continued)

Causes of metabolic alkalosis. (*continued*)
If None of the Above, Then. . .
Urine Chloride < 20 mEq/L (*chloride-responsive causes*): • Loss of gastric acid (hyperemesis, NGT suctioning) • Prior diuretic use (in hours to days following discontinuation) • Post-hypercapnia • Villous adenoma • Congenital chloridorrhea • Chronic laxative abuse (may also cause a metabolic acidosis depending on diarrheal HCO_3 losses) • CF
OR: Urine Chloride > 20 mEq/L (*chloride-resistant causes*):
Urine Chloride > 20 mEq/L, Lack of HTN, Urine Potassium < 30 mEq/L
• Hypokalemia or hypomagnesemia • Laxative abuse (if dominated by hypokalemia) • Bartter syndrome • Gitelman syndrome
Urine Chloride > 20 mEq/L, Lack of HTN, Urine Potassium > 30 mEq/L
• Current diuretic use
Urine Chloride > 20 mEq/L, Presence of HTN, Urine Potassium Variable but Usually > 30 mEq/L
Elevated plasma renin level: • Renal artery stenosis • Renin-secreting tumor • Renovascular disease
Low plasma renin, low plasma aldosterone: • Cushing syndrome • Exogenous mineralocorticoid use • Genetic disorder (11-hydoxylase or 17-hydrolyase deficiency, 11β-HSD deficiency) • Liddle syndrome • Licorice toxicity
Low plasma renin, high plasma aldosterone: • Primary hyperaldosteronism • Adrenal adenoma • Bilateral adrenal hyperplasia

References

Abreo K, Adlakha A, Kilpatrick S, et al. The milk-alkali syndrome. A reversible form of acute renal failure. Arch Intern Med. 1993;153:1005.

Arroliga AC, Shehab N, McCarthy K, Gonzales JP. Relationship of continuous infusion lorazepam to serum propylene glycol concentration in critically ill adults. Crit Care Med. 2004;32:1709.

Barton CH, Vaziri ND, Ness RL, et al. Cimetidine in the management of metabolic alkalosis induced by nasogastric drainage. Arch Surg. 1979;114:70.

Bear R, Goldstein M, Phillipson E, et al. Effect of metabolic alkalosis on respiratory function in patients with chronic obstructive lung disease. Can Med Assoc J. 1977;117:900.

Braden GL, Strayhorn CH, Germain MJ, et al. Increased osmolal gap in alcoholic acidosis. Arch Intern Med. 1993;153:2377.

Gabow PA. Ethylene glycol intoxication. Am J Kidney Dis. 1988;11:277.

Galla JH, Gifford JD, Luke RG, Rome L. Adaptations to chloride-depletion alkalosis. Am J Physiol. 1991;261:R771.

Garella S, Chang BS, Kahn SI. Dilution acidosis and contraction alkalosis: review of a concept. Kidney Int. 1975;8:279.

Gennari FJ. Current concepts. Serum osmolality. Uses and limitations. N Engl J Med. 1984;310:102.

Gennari FJ, Weise WJ. Acid-base disturbances in gastrointestinal disease. Clin J Am Soc Nephrol. 2008;3:1861.

Glasser L, Sternglanz PD, Combie J, Robinson A. Serum osmolality and its applicability to drug overdose. Am J Clin Pathol. 1973;60:695.

Hamm LL, Nakhoul N, Hering-Smith KS. Acid-base homeostasis. Clin J Am Soc Nephrol. 2015;10:2232.

Hulter HN, Sebastian A, Toto RD, et al. Renal and systemic acid-base effects of the chronic administration of hypercalcemia-producing agents: calcitriol, PTH, and intravenous calcium. Kidney Int. 1982;21:445.

Jenkins DW, Eckle RE, Craig JW. Alcoholic ketoacidosis. JAMA. 1971;217:177.

Khanna A, Kurtzman NA. Metabolic alkalosis. J Nephrol. 2006;19(suppl 9):S86.

Kraut JA, Xing SX. Approach to the evaluation of a patient with an increased serum osmolal gap and high-anion-gap metabolic acidosis. Am J Kidney Dis. 2011;58:480.

Kraut JA, Kurtz I. Toxic alcohol ingestions: clinical features, diagnosis, and management. Clin J Am Soc Nephrol. 2008;3:208.

Laski ME, Sabatini S. Metabolic alkalosis, bedside and bench. Semin Nephrol. 2006;26:404.

Levy LJ, Duga J, Girgis M, Gordon EE. Ketoacidosis associated with alcoholism in nondiabetic subjects. Ann Intern Med. 1973;78:213.

Luke RG, Galla JH. It is chloride depletion alkalosis, not contraction alkalosis. J Am Soc Nephrol. 2012;23:204.

Lynd LD, Richardson KJ, Purssell RA, et al. An evaluation of the osmole gap as a screening test for toxic alcohol poisoning. BMC Emerg Med. 2008;8:5.

Marraffa JM, Holland MG, Stork CM, et al. Diethylene glycol: widely used solvent presents serious poisoning potential. J Emerg Med. 2008;35:401.

Miller PD, Berns AS. Acute metabolic alkalosis perpetuating hypercarbia. A role for acetazolamide in chronic obstructive pulmonary disease. JAMA. 1977;238:2400.

Oster JR, Materson BJ, Rogers AI. Laxative abuse syndrome. Am J Gastroenterol.1980;74:451.

Palmer BF, Clegg DJ. Electrolyte disturbances in patients with chronic alcohol-use disorder. N Engl J Med. 2017;377:1368.

Patel AM, Goldfarb S. Got calcium? Welcome to the calcium-alkali syndrome. J Am Soc Nephrol. 2010;21:1440.

Purssell RA, Pudek M, Brubacher J, Abu-Laban RB. Derivation and validation of a formula to calculate the contribution of ethanol to the osmolal gap. Ann Emerg Med. 2001;38:653.

Reichard GA Jr, Owen OE, Haff AC, et al. Ketone-body production and oxidation in fasting obese humans. J Clin Invest. 1974;53:508.

Robinson AG, Loeb JN. Ethanol ingestion—commonest cause of elevated plasma osmolality? N Engl J Med. 1971;284:1253.

Rose BD, Post TW. Clinical Physiology of Acid-Base and Electrolyte Disorders. 5e. New York, NY: McGraw Hill; 2001:559.

Schelling JR, Howard RL, Winter SD, Linas SL. Increased osmolal gap in alcoholic ketoacidosis and lactic acidosis. Ann Intern Med. 1990;113:580.

Schwartz WB, Van Ypersele de Strihou C, Kassirer JP. Role of anions in metabolic alkalosis and potassium deficiency. N Engl J Med. 1968;279:630.

Sweetser LJ, Douglas JA, Riha RL, Bell SC. Clinical presentation of metabolic alkalosis in an adult patient with cystic fibrosis. Respirology. 2005;10:254.

Taki K, Mizuno K, Takahashi N, Wakusawa R. Disturbance of CO_2 elimination in the lungs by carbonic anhydrase inhibition. Jpn J Physiol. 1986;36:523.

Toth HL, Greenbaum LA. Severe acidosis caused by starvation and stress. Am J Kidney Dis. 2003;42:E16.

Turban S, Beutler KT, Morris RG, et al. Long-term regulation of proximal tubule acid-base transporter abundance by angiotensin II. Kidney Int. 2006;70:660.

CASE 41

A 44-year-old man with a history of alcohol withdrawal complicated by seizures and drug use presents to the emergency department (ED). He is combative and is intubated in the ED for his own safety. Following intubation, his vital signs are normal. He has a nonfocal examination and all imaging is negative for acute pathology, including a CXR and a head CT scan. You are called in the ICU by the provider in the ED, who provides the details of the patient's care to this point. Transfer to the ICU is then arranged and you assume care of the patient. The patient has peripheral IVs placed and is started on normal saline. The patient's laboratory findings are as follows:

Laboratory data.			
ABGs		Basic Metabolic Panel	
pH	7.47	Na	156 mEq/L
$Paco_2$	33 mm Hg	K	1.4 mEq/L
Pao_2	288 mm Hg	Cl	137 mEq/L
HCO_3	26 mEq/L	CO_2	10 mEq/L
Na	138 mEq/L	BUN	< 5 mg/dL
K	4.8 mEq/L	Cr	0.1 mg/dL
Lactate	1.8 mmol/L	Glucose	23 mg/dL
		Albumin	1.8 g/dL
		EtOH	134 mg/dL

QUESTIONS

Q41-1: What is the most likely cause of the discrepancy between the patient's ABG findings (with Na, K, lactate, Hbg) and the values on his basic metabolic panel (BMP)?

A. Wrong patient's ABG matched with current patient's BMP (or vice versa)
B. Hyperproteinemia
C. Ethylene glycol toxicity
D. Dilution with normal saline
E. Alcoholic ketoacidosis

Q41-2: Define the patient's baseline acid-base status: Does this patient have an underlying chronic acid-base disorder that we need to account for in order to appropriately interpret the acute acid-base disorders?

A. There is no evidence for an underlying chronic respiratory or metabolic acid-base disorder in this patient, so we would assume a baseline $Paco_2$ of 40 mm Hg and an HCO_3 of 24 mEq/L.
B. While the patient has a condition that potentially predisposes him to a chronic acid-base disorder, there is insufficient information to estimate the patient's baseline $Paco_2$ and HCO_3 values; therefore, we will assume a baseline $Paco_2$ of 40 mm Hg and a baseline HCO_3 of 24 mEq/L.
C. The patient has an underlying acid-base condition, and we have sufficient information to estimate the patient's baseline $Paco_2$ and HCO_3 values.

Q41-3: The patient is transferred to the ICU for further management of his alcohol-related issues. He is started on thiamine and folate, but remains combative and does not follow commands. On hospitalization day 1 (HD1), he develops symptoms consistent with alcohol withdrawal and is started on a lorazepam infusion at 10 mg/h due to continued delirium tremens. However, on HD3, he is noted to be very tachypneic on the ventilator, with mild hypotension. Laboratory results from the morning bloodwork are as follows:

Laboratory data.			
ABGs		Basic Metabolic Panel	
pH	7.05	Na	141 mEq/L
$Paco_2$	19 mm Hg	K	6.0 mEq/L
Pao_2	101 mm Hg	Cl	100 mEq/L
HCO_3	5 mEq/L	CO_2	6 mEq/L
		BUN	10 mg/dL
		Cr	0.7 mg/dL
		Albumin	4.0 g/dL

What is/are the primary acid-base disorder(s)?

A. Metabolic acidosis only
B. Respiratory acidosis only
C. Metabolic acidosis and a respiratory acidosis
D. Metabolic alkalosis and a respiratory alkalosis

Q41-4: How would the metabolic acidosis component be classified in this case?

A. Anion gap acidosis
B. Non-anion gap acidosis
C. Anion and non-anion gap acidosis
D. Anion gap acidosis and a metabolic alkalosis

Q41-5: Does the patient in this case demonstrate appropriate respiratory compensation?

A. Yes, the respiratory compensation is appropriate.
B. No, a concomitant respiratory alkalosis is present.
C. No, a concomitant respiratory acidosis is present.

Q41-6: The following laboratory findings are reported:

Serum EtOH	< 3 mg/dL
Serum acetaminophen level	< 5 mg/dL (ULN for therapeutic use 20 mg/dL)
Serum salicylates level	< 5 mg/dL (ULN for therapeutic use 30 mg/dL)
Serum osmolality	337 mOsm/kg
Serum L-lactate	6.7 mmol/L (ULN 2.0 mmol/L venous)
Beta-hydroxybutyrate (acetone)	< 0.18 mmol/L (ULN 0.18 mmol/L)
Serum glucose	141 mg/dL

What would you do next?

A. Broaden antibiotics.
B. Start antiepileptic drugs (AEDs) for possible seizure.
C. Stop the lorazepam infusion.
D. Change the ventilator settings.

Q41-7: What other test may be helpful in this patient with propylene glycol toxicity?

A. Serum brain natriuretic peptide (BNP)
B. Serum D-lactate
C. Serum C-reactive protein
D. Urine drug screen
E. Urine metanephrines

Q41-8: The patient's lorazepam infusion is stopped and he is transitioned to phenobarbital for management of alcohol withdrawal. His acid-base issues resolve, and the patient is maintained on fentanyl and a high-dose propofol infusion for continued agitation. There is concern for permanent encephalopathy as the patient is unable to follow commands. A brain MRI shows damage to the bilateral mammary bodies, and the patient is scheduled for tracheostomy. On HD11, the patient develops tachypnea once again, with associated hypotension and hyperkalemia. His laboratory findings are as follows:

Laboratory data.			
ABGs		Basic Metabolic Panel	
pH	7.11	Na	140 mEq/L
Paco$_2$	22 mm Hg	K	6.7 mEq/L
Pao$_2$	101 mm Hg	Cl	100 mEq/L
HCO$_3$	5 mEq/L	CO$_2$	10 mEq/L
		BUN	44 mg/dL
		Cr	2.3 mg/dL
		Glucose	125 mg/dL
		Albumin	4.0 g/dL
		EtOH	0 mg/dL
		CK	22,000 IU/L
		Triglycerides	4500 mg/dL
		WBC	5000/mL

What acid-base disturbance(s) is/are present now?

A. Metabolic acidosis, both anion gap and non-anion gap, with respiratory alkalosis
B. Metabolic acidosis, anion gap only, with respiratory acidosis
C. Metabolic acidosis, non-anion gap only, with appropriate compensation
D. Metabolic acidosis, anion gap only, with appropriate compensation

Q41-9: What would you do next?

A. Start antibiotics.
B. Restart lorazepam infusion.
C. Stop propofol infusion.
D. Start fomepizole infusion.
E. Start AED infusion.

ANSWERS

Q41-1: D
Dilution with normal saline.

Rationale: When there are such large discrepancies between a patient's venous blood studies and his/her ABG, there are two likely possibilities: (1) systematic error (eg, wrong patient); or (2) assay interference from a substance in the blood (eg, triglycerides). Substances such as triglycerides or elevated protein levels from malignancies can interfere with measurement of electrolytes and serum HCO_3 concentrations, and can cause both pseudohyponatremia and "pseudo-anion gap acidosis." However, in this case, the anion gap is normal and the sodium is elevated. A patient with ethylene glycol toxicity or alcoholic ketoacidosis would be expected to have an abnormal ABG to correlate with the BMP. In this case, the patient's venous blood was likely drawn from a vein proximal to the site of normal saline infusion, which can lead to the dilution of blood with normal saline and the patient's very abnormal ABG. This is further supported by the drastic differences in Hbg and K, as well.

Q41-2: B
While the patient has a condition that potentially predisposes him to a chronic acid-base disorder, there is insufficient information to estimate the patient's baseline $Paco_2$ and HCO_3 values; therefore, we will assume a baseline $Paco_2$ of 40 mm Hg and a baseline HCO_3 of 24 mEq/L.

Rationale: Ignoring these underlying chronic acid-base disorders can significantly alter the interpretation of a patient's acute acid-base status. This was demonstrated in the first case of the series. However, often, we do not have the necessary information (eg, prior ABG or VBG, or prior serum chemistry with an HCO_3) and are forced to assume the ongoing processes are all acute in nature. We are primarily concerned about chronic respiratory acid-base disorders, as these can significantly alter the patient's baseline or expected values for the serum HCO_3 and $Paco_2$, and we have reliable equations to predict the expected baseline values. The respiratory compensation for both chronic metabolic acidosis and alkalosis is generally poor, so there are no equations or rules to predict what the $Paco_2$ should be in these cases. While the baseline serum HCO_3 may be significantly off from our standard value 24 of mEq/L in these patients, we would assume a baseline $Paco_2$ of 40 mm Hg in patients with chronic metabolic processes. Once we identify the patient's baseline $Paco_2$ and HCO_3 values, we will need to use these values in the appropriate equations to identify the ongoing acute processes.

Q41-3: A
Metabolic acidosis only.

Rationale:

1. The pH is 7.05; therefore, the primary disorder is an **acidosis.**
2. The $Paco_2$ of 19 mm Hg is less than 40 mm Hg, so there is a **no respiratory acidosis.**
3. The HCO_3 of 6 mEq/L is less than 24 mEq/L, so there is a **metabolic acidosis.**

Therefore, this patient has a primary metabolic acidosis.

Q41-4: A

Anion gap acidosis.

Rationale:

1. Is there evidence for a chronic acid-base disorder that requires adjustment of the patient's "normal" HCO_3? No, there is no evidence for a chronic acid-base disorder, so we would assume a baseline $Paco_2$ of 40 mm Hg and an HCO_3 of 24 mEq/L.
2. Expected anion gap:

$$\text{Expected Anion Gap} = 12 - (2.5) * \left[4.0 \frac{g}{dL} - \text{Actual Serum Albumin} \right]$$
$$= 12 - (2.5 * [4.0 - 4.0])$$
$$= 12 - (2.5 * [0]) = \textbf{12 mEq/L.}$$

3. Anion gap calculation:

$$\text{Serum Anion Gap} = [Na^+] - [HCO_3^-] - [Cl^-]$$
$$= 141 - (100 + 5) = \textbf{36 mEq/L,} \text{ which is } > 12 \text{ mEq/L}$$
$$\rightarrow \textbf{anion gap acidosis is present.}$$

4. Delta-delta calculation:

$$\Delta\Delta = \frac{(\text{Actual Anion Gap} - \text{Expected Anion Gap})}{(\text{Baseline } HCO_3 - \text{Actual } HCO_3)}$$
$$= (36 - 12)/(24 - 5) = \textbf{24/18, which is } \sim \textbf{1.33.}$$

Delta-delta interpretation.	
Delta-Delta Value	Condition Present
< 0.4	Non-anion gap only
0.4–0.9	Anion gap *and* non-anion gap acidosis
1.0–2.0	**Anion gap acidosis only**
> 2.0	Anion gap acidosis and metabolic alkalosis

Therefore, this patient's primary metabolic acidosis is caused by a pure anion gap acidosis.

Q41-5: A

Yes, the respiratory compensation is appropriate.

Rationale: Using the Winter formula, one can calculate what the expected arterial $Paco_2$ should be for a given serum HCO_3 if the patient were appropriately compensated.

Respiratory Compensation for Acute Metabolic Acidosis (Winter Formula):

$$\text{Expected Paco}_2 = 1.5 * [\text{Actual } HCO_3] + 8 \pm 2 \text{ (in mm Hg)}$$
$$= (1.5 * 6) + 8 = 9 + 8 = 17 \pm 2 = (15 \text{ to } 19) \text{ mm Hg.}$$

Since the patient's $Paco_2$ on presentation of **19 mm Hg** was within the expected range of 15 to 19 mm Hg, this patient is appropriately compensating for the **metabolic acidosis**.

Q41-6: C
Stop the lorazepam infusion.

Rationale: In this case, the patient has a severe anion gap acidosis with appropriate respiratory compensation. Option D, changing the ventilator settings, will not likely help much in this case as the patient's $Paco_2$ is close to minimal. Seizure activity can certainly cause a transient lactic acidosis but does not account for the patient's serum osmolal gap. An infection is always a significant risk in the ICU and antibiotics are a good thought, but again an infection does not account for the patient's serum osmolal gap.

The osmolal gap is calculated as follows:

$$\text{Calculated Serum Osmolality} = 2 * [Na^+] + \frac{[\text{Glucose}]}{18} + \frac{[\text{BUN}]}{2.8} + \frac{[\text{EtOH}]}{3.7}$$

$$= 293 \text{ mOsm/L}$$

$$\text{Serum Osmolal Gap (SOG)} = \text{Measured Serum Osmolality}$$

$$- \text{Calculated Serum Osmolality}$$

$$\text{SOG} = 337 \text{ mOsm/L} - 293 \text{ mOsm/L} = (+44) \text{ mOsm/L}.$$

The following table summarizes potential causes of an elevated serum osmolality.

With an Elevated Serum Anion Gap
1. Ethanol ingestion with alcohol ketoacidosis (acetone is an unmeasured osmole, in addition to ethanol)— the osmolality is usually elevated more so by the increased ethanol concentration, so the osmolal "gap" depends on whether the term for ethanol is included in the osmolality calculation*
2. Organic alcohol ingestions (methanol, ethylene glycol, diethylene glycol, propylene glycol)
3. DKA—similar to ethanol ingestion, glucose and acetone contribute to the osmolality, since the glucose term is always included in the calculation
4. Salicylate toxicity
5. Renal failure—the BUN is nearly always included in the osmolality
Without an Elevated Serum Anion Gap
1. Hyperosmolar therapy (mannitol, glycerol)
2. Other organic solvent ingestion (eg, acetone)
3. Isopropyl alcohol ingestion (produces only acetone rather than an organic acid, so no anion gap is seen)
4. Hypertriglyceridemia
5. Hyperproteinemia
*A mildly elevated osmolal gap has been reported in the literature in patients with lactic acidosis in critical illness, particularly severe distributive shock. The pathology is not quite clear, although it likely is related to multiorgan failure—particularly involving the liver and kidneys—and the release of cellular components known to contribute to the osmolal gap. This is typically around 10 mOsm, although it may be as high as 20–25 mOsm/L.

The elevated osmolar gap is most likely caused by either a sugar source (mannitol, sorbitol) or an organic alcohol (ethylene glycol, methanol). The patient has been intubated for several days and does not have access to ethylene glycol, isopropyl alcohol, or methanol. A review of the medications shows he is on lorazepam infusion, which uses propylene glycol as a carrier. At high rates, this can lead to an anion gap acidosis. As propylene glycol is metabolized by the body, it is converted into lactate, giving rise to an elevated lactate level as seen here. While most cases of propylene glycol toxicity can be treated conservatively with fluids, severe cases may require initiation of fomepizole and intermittent dialysis.

Q41-7: B
Serum D-lactate.

Rationale: D-Lactate is produced from the metabolism of propylene glycol.

Q41-8: D
Metabolic acidosis, anion gap only, with appropriate compensation.

Rationale: Using the steps from previous questions:

1. There is an acidosis, with no respiratory component, but a metabolic component. So there is a **metabolic acidosis**.
2. There is an **anion gap acidosis** (anion gap is now 30).
3. The delta-delta is 18/14, ~ 1.3, so this a **pure anion gap acidosis.**
4. The expected compensatory $Paco_2$ is 21 to 25 mm Hg, so there is **appropriate respiratory compensation**.

Q41-9: C
Stop propofol infusion.

Rationale: This patient has propofol infusion syndrome, a rare and complex syndrome associated with long-term infusion of propofol (usually > 48 to 72 hours) at high doses (> 70 mcg/kg/min). The mortality associated with this condition is extremely high. The syndrome is associated with a high anion gap lactic acidosis that is otherwise unexplained, cardiac dysfunction, hypertriglyceridemia, shock liver, acute renal failure, rhabdomyolysis, and hyperkalemia. This patient's propofol infusion should be discontinued immediately. Treatment is primarily with discontinuation of propofol, vigorous fluids and electrolyte repletion, and renal replacement therapy. The role of sodium HCO_3 infusion is questionable.

References

Cannon ML, Glazier SS, Bauman LA. Metabolic acidosis, rhabdomyolysis, and cardiovascular collapse after prolonged propofol infusion. J Neurosurg. 2001;95:1053.

Jahn A, Bodreau C, Farthing K, Elbarbry F. Assessing propylene glycol toxicity in alcohol withdrawal patients receiving intravenous benzodiazepines: a one-compartment pharmacokinetic model. Eur J Drug Metab Pharmacokinet. 2018;43:423.

Kraut JA, Kurtz I. Toxic alcohol ingestions: clinical features, diagnosis, and management. Clin J Am Soc Nephrol. 2008;3:208.

Kraut JA, Xing SX. Approach to the evaluation of a patient with an increased serum osmolal gap and high-anion-gap metabolic acidosis. Am J Kidney Dis. 2011;58:480.

Mirrakhimov AE, Voore P, Halytskyy O, et al. Propofol infusion syndrome in adults: a clinical update. Crit Care Res Pract. 2015;2015:260385.

Parker MG, Fraser GL, Watson DM, Riker RR. Removal of propylene glycol and correction of increased osmolar gap by hemodialysis in a patient on high dose lorazepam infusion therapy. Intensive Care Med. 2002;28:81.

Sabsovich I, Rehman Z, Yunen J, Coritsidis G. Propofol infusion syndrome: a case of increasing morbidity with traumatic brain injury. Am J Crit Care. 2007;16:82.

Wilson KC, Reardon C, Theodore AC, Farber HW. Propylene glycol toxicity: a severe iatrogenic illness in ICU patients receiving IV benzodiazepines: a case series and prospective, observational pilot study. Chest. 2005;128:1674.

Wong JM. Propofol infusion syndrome. Am J Ther. 2010;17:487.

Zar T, Graeber C, Perazella MA. Recognition, treatment, and prevention of propylene glycol toxicity. Semin Dial. 2007;20:217.

Zar T, Yusufzai I, Sullivan A, Graeber C. Acute kidney injury, hyperosmolality and metabolic acidosis associated with lorazepam. Nat Clin Pract Nephrol. 2007;3:515.

CASE 42

A 33-year-old man with no known health problems is transferred to the ICU from the emergency department (ED). He presented to the ED encephalopathic with a fever to 40.6°C and hypoxemic respiratory failure. His flu swab was positive for influenza A. The patient was hypotensive on arrival and tachycardic, with RR 22, BP 70/30, HR 140, and Sao_2 87% on Room Air. He was intubated in the ED because of his altered mental status. His wife reports that he has been sick for the past few days and has not been eating or drinking much, with frequent diarrhea. An LP in the ED was negative for bacterial meningitis, with normal CSF OP. His CXR shows bilateral fluffy infiltrates throughout the lung fields.

Laboratory data.			
ABGs		Basic Metabolic Panel	
pH	7.31	Na	140 mEq/L
$Paco_2$	19 mm Hg	K	4.5 mEq/L
Pao_2	48 mm Hg	Cl	106 mEq/L
HCO_3	17 mEq/L	CO_2	17 mEq/L
		BUN	23 mg/dL
		Cr	2.3 mg/dL
		Glucose	101 mg/dL
		Albumin	4.0 g/dL
		EtOH	0 mg/dL

QUESTIONS

Q42-1: Define the patient's baseline acid-base status: Does this patient have an underlying chronic acid-base disorder that we need to account for in order to appropriately interpret the acute acid-base disorders?

A. There is no evidence for an underlying chronic respiratory or metabolic acid-base disorder in this patient, so we would assume a baseline $Paco_2$ of 40 mm Hg and an HCO_3 of 24 mEq/L.

B. While the patient has a condition that potentially predisposes him to a chronic acid-base disorder, there is insufficient information to estimate the patient's baseline $Paco_2$ and HCO_3 values; therefore, we will assume a baseline $Paco_2$ of 40 mm Hg and a baseline HCO_3 of 24 mEq/L.

C. The patient has an underlying acid-base condition, and we have sufficient information to estimate the patient's baseline $Paco_2$ and HCO_3 values.

Q42-2: What is/are the primary acid/base disturbance(s) occurring in this case?

A. Metabolic acidosis only
B. Respiratory acidosis only
C. Metabolic acidosis and a respiratory acidosis
D. Metabolic alkalosis and a respiratory alkalosis

Q42-3: How would the metabolic acidosis component be classified in this case?

A. Anion gap acidosis
B. Non-anion gap acidosis
C. Anion and non-anion gap acidosis
D. Anion gap acidosis and a metabolic alkalosis

Q42-4: Does the patient demonstrate appropriate respiratory compensation?

A. Yes, the respiratory compensation is appropriate.
B. No, a concomitant respiratory alkalosis is present.
C. No, a concomitant respiratory acidosis is present.

Q42-5: Laboratory testing returns the following serum and urine results:

Serum Values	
Serum EtOH	< 3 mg/dL
Serum acetaminophen level	< 5 mg/dL (ULN for therapeutic use 20 mg/dL)
Serum salicylates level	< 5 mg/dL (ULN for therapeutic use 30 mg/dL)
Serum osmolality	296 mOsm/kg
Serum L-lactate	4.0 mmol/L (ULN 2.0 mmol/L venous)
Beta-hydroxybutyrate (acetone)	< 0.18 mmol/L (ULN 0.18 mmol/L)
Serum glucose	101 mg/dL
Urine Values	
Urine Na	8 mEq/L
Urine K	10 mEq/L
Urine Cl	41 mEq/L
Urine urea	332 mg/dL
Urine glucose	0 mg/dL
Urine osmolality	784 mOsm/L
Urine pH	5.3
Urine RBCs	None
Urine WBCs	None
Urine protein	None
Urine microscopic	None

What are the causes of the patient's anion gap and non-anion gap acidosis?

A. Lactic acidosis, renal failure
B. Acetaminophen toxicity, diarrhea
C. DKA, renal tubular acidosis (RTA)
D. Lactic acidosis, diarrhea

Q42-6: The patient is admitted to the ICU where he is diagnosed with severe ARDS as a result of influenza. He is given paralytic drugs and placed on ARDS protocol ventilator settings. After several hours, two ABGs are stable; his other laboratory results are as follows:

Laboratory data.				
ABGs		Basic Metabolic Panel		
pH	7.27	Na	140 mEq/L
$Paco_2$	55 mm Hg	K	4.0 mEq/L
Pao_2	65 mm Hg	Cl	105 mEq/L
HCO_3	26 mEq/L	CO_2	26 mEq/L
		BUN	10 mg/dL
		Cr	1.0 mg/dL

What acid-base disturbances are present now?

A. Metabolic acidosis, both anion gap and non-anion gap, with respiratory alkalosis
B. Respiratory acidosis with anion gap acidosis only
C. Respiratory acidosis with appropriate renal compensation
D. Respiratory acidosis with an overlying metabolic alkalosis

Q42-7: After reviewing the patient's most recent ABG, you ask the respiratory therapist to change the ventilator settings to help the patient remove additional CO_2 to normalize the pH. The respiratory therapist informs you that the patient is on the maximum safe ventilator settings for his body size with tidal volumes and peak pressures at the upper limits for lung protective ventilation. What do you do next?

A. Start an HCO_3 infusion
B. Discuss the need for ECMO
C. Change the sedation settings
D. Initiate diuretic therapy
E. Continue current settings

ANSWERS

Q42-1: A

There is no evidence for an underlying chronic respiratory or metabolic acid-base disorder in this patient, so we would assume a baseline $Paco_2$ of 40 mm Hg and an HCO_3 of 24 mEq/L.

Rationale: Ignoring these underlying chronic acid-base disorders can significantly alter the interpretation of a patient's acute acid-base status. This was demonstrated in the first case of the series. However, often, we do not have the necessary information (eg, prior ABG or VBG, or prior serum chemistry with an HCO_3) and are forced to assume the ongoing processes are all acute in nature. We are primarily concerned about chronic respiratory acid-base disorders, as these can significantly alter the patient's baseline or expected values for the serum HCO_3 and $Paco_2$, and we have reliable equations to predict the expected baseline values. The respiratory compensation for both chronic metabolic acidosis and alkalosis is generally poor, so there are no equations or rules to predict what the $Paco_2$ should be in these cases. While the baseline serum HCO_3 may be significantly off from our standard value of 24 mEq/L in these patients, we would assume a baseline $Paco_2$ of 40 mm Hg in patients with chronic metabolic processes. Once we identify the patient's baseline $Paco_2$ and HCO_3 values, we will need to use these values in the appropriate equations to identify the ongoing acute processes.

Q42-2: A

Metabolic acidosis only.

Rationale:

1. The pH is 7.31; therefore, the primary disorder is an **acidosis.**
2. The $Paco_2$ of 19 mm Hg is less than 40 mm Hg, so there is **no respiratory acidosis.**
3. The HCO_3 of 17 mEq/L is less than 24 mEq/L, so there is a **metabolic acidosis.**

Q42-3: C

Anion gap acidosis and a non-anion gap acidosis.

Rationale:

1. Is there evidence for a chronic acid-base disorder that requires adjustment of the patient's "normal" HCO_3? No, there is no evidence for a chronic acid-base disorder, so we would assume a baseline $Paco_2$ of 40 mm Hg and an HCO_3 of 24 mEq/L.
2. Expected anion gap:

$$\text{Expected Anion Gap} = 12 - (2.5) * \left[4.0 \frac{g}{dL} - \text{Actual Serum Albumin} \right]$$
$$= 12 - (2.5 * [4.0 - 4.0])$$
$$= 12 - (2.5 * [0]) = \textbf{12 mEq/L.}$$

3. Anion gap calculation:

$$\text{Serum Anion Gap} = [Na^+] - [HCO_3^-] - [Cl^-]$$
$$= 140 - (106 + 17) = \textbf{17 mEq/L, which is} > 12 \text{ mEq/L}$$
$$\rightarrow \textbf{anion gap acidosis is present.}$$

4. Delta-delta calculation:

$$\Delta\Delta = \frac{(\text{Actual Anion Gap} - \text{Expected Anion Gap})}{(\text{Baseline } HCO_3 - \text{Actual } HCO_3)}$$
$$= (17 - 12)/(24 - 17) = \textbf{5/7, which is} \sim \textbf{0.7.}$$

Delta-delta interpretation.	
Delta-Delta Value	Condition Present
< 0.4	Non-anion gap only
0.4–1.0	**Anion gap *and* non-anion gap acidosis**
1.0–2.0	Anion gap acidosis only
> 2.0	Anion gap acidosis and metabolic alkalosis

Q42-4: B
No, a concomitant respiratory alkalosis is present.

Rationale: Using the Winter formula, one can calculate what the expected arterial $Paco_2$ should be for a given serum HCO_3 if the patient were completely compensated.

Respiratory Compensation for Acute Metabolic Acidosis (Winter Formula):

$$\text{Expected } Paco_2 = 1.5 * [\text{Actual } HCO_3] + 8 \pm 2 \text{ (in mm Hg)}$$
$$= (1.5 * 17) + 8 = 33.5 + 8 = 33.5 \pm 2 = (31 \text{ to } 35) \text{ mm Hg.}$$

Since the patient's $Paco_2$ on presentation of **19 mm Hg** was lower than the expected range of 31 to 35 mm Hg, **this patient has an overlying respiratory alkalosis.**

Q42-5: D
Lactic acidosis, diarrhea.

Rationale: The workup for the patient's anion gap acidosis showed only an elevated lactate level, and the presentation is consistent with this as the cause of his anion gap acidosis. The only outstanding calculation is to ensure there is no serum osmolal gap:

$$\text{Calculated Serum Osmolality} = 2 * [Na^+] + \frac{[\text{Glucose}]}{18} + \frac{[\text{BUN}]}{2.8} + \frac{[\text{EtOH}]}{3.7}$$
$$= 294 \text{ mOsm/L}$$
$$\text{Serum Osmolal Gap (SOG)} = \text{Measured Serum Osmolality} - \text{Calculated Serum Osmolality}$$
$$\text{SOG} = 296 - 294 \text{ mOsm/L} = (+2) \text{ mOsm/L.}$$

The urine osmolar gap (UOG) is negative (−23 mEq/L), indicating increased urinary excretion of NH_4 (ie, increased urinary acid excretion), which is consistent with a GI cause for the non-anion gap acidosis. The urine anion gap can be inappropriately elevated in anion gap acidosis, a situation in which multiple unmeasured anions may be present in the urine (beta-hydroxybutyrate/acetoacetate [ketoacidosis], hippurate [toluene], HCO_3 [proximal RTA], D-lactate [D-lactic acidosis], L-lactate, 5-oxoproline [acetaminophen toxicity]). Therefore, in patients with a significant anion gap, the UOG is typically more useful.

$$\text{Calculated Urine Osmolality} = 2 * [U_{Na} + U_K] + \frac{[U_{BUN}]}{2.8} + \frac{[U_{glucose}]}{18}$$

$$= 155 \text{ mOsm/L}$$

$$\text{SOG} = \text{Measured Serum Osmolality} - \text{Calculated Serum Osmolality}$$

$$\text{UOG} = 784 - 155 \text{ mOsm/L} = (+629) \text{ mOsm/L}.$$

Similar to the urine anion gap, the UOG is used as a surrogate for the urine ammonium concentration. Therefore, a larger gap indicates increased urinary NH_4 excretion. In normal acid-base conditions, the UOG is between 10 and 100 mOsm/L. During a significant metabolic acidosis, patients with impaired renal tubular acidification (type 1 and type 4 RTA) are unable to excrete additional acid (NH_4), and therefore the osmolar gap does not change. Patients with an intact renal response to acidemia (ie, GI losses) should have a significant UOG (~ >300 to 400 mOsm/L) as a result of increased NH_4 excretion. Therefore, for this patient, both the urine anion gap and the UOG are negative, so the likely cause for the NAGMA is diarrhea.

Q42-6: C

Respiratory acidosis with appropriate renal compensation.

Rationale: Using the steps from previous questions for this case:

1. There is an acidosis, with a respiratory component, but no metabolic acidosis. So there is a **respiratory acidosis** as the primary component.
2. There is no anion gap acidosis (the anion gap is 9).
3. The delta-delta calculation is not useful here.
4. The expected compensatory HCO_3 in the acute phase is as follows:

Metabolic Compensation for Acute Respiratory Acidosis:

$$\text{Expected } HCO_3 = \text{Baseline } HCO_3 + (0.10) [\text{Actual } Paco_2 - \text{Baseline } Paco_2]$$
$$= 24 + [0.10 * (55 - 40)] = 24 + 1.5 = 25.5 \text{ or } 26 \text{ mEq/L}.$$

Since this patient has a HCO_3 of 26 mEq/L, he is **compensating appropriately** and no additional non-anion gap metabolic acidosis or metabolic alkalosis is present.

Q42-7: E
Continue current settings.

Rationale: The patient is currently receiving appropriate mechanical ventilation settings per ARDS protocols. Under these protocols, it is safer to allow patients to have a respiratory acidosis and maintain lower ventilator settings (eg, tidal volumes of 4 to 6 mL/kg ideal body weight, peak pressure < 30 cm H_2O) than to use unsafe ventilator settings to normalize the pH, as these high settings are known to cause additional lung injury. This policy is called "permissive hypercapnia," and as long as patients tolerate the mild acidosis from a cardiovascular standpoint, they will be allowed to have a pH between 7.20 and 7.40 to enable the lower ventilator settings.

An HCO_3 infusion would potentially worsen the situation, as a large portion of the HCO_3 infused is converted directly to CO_2, and the patient's $Paco_2$ may actually worsen. This patient is being adequately ventilated and oxygenated on conventional mechanical ventilation currently, so ECMO is not yet indicated. There is no mention of issues with sedation as the patient is appropriately paralyzed. Diuresis is more likely to improve oxygenation than ventilation.

References

Adeva-Andany M, López-Ojén M, Funcasta-Calderón R, et al. Comprehensive review on lactate metabolism in human health. Mitochondrion. 2014;17:76.

Batlle D, Chin-Theodorou J, Tucker BM. Metabolic acidosis or respiratory alkalosis? Evaluation of a low plasma bicarbonate using the urine anion gap. Am J Kidney Dis. 2017;70:440.

Batlle D, Grupp M, Gaviria M, Kurtzman NA. Distal renal tubular acidosis with intact capacity to lower urinary pH. Am J Med. 1982;72:751.

Batlle D, Haque SK. Genetic causes and mechanisms of distal renal tubular acidosis. Nephrol Dial Transplant. 2012;27:3691.

Batlle DC, Hizon M, Cohen E, et al. The use of the urinary anion gap in the diagnosis of hyperchloremic metabolic acidosis. N Engl J Med. 1988;318:594.

Batlle DC, von Riotte A, Schlueter W. Urinary sodium in the evaluation of hyperchloremic metabolic acidosis. N Engl J Med. 1987;316:140.

Buckalew VM Jr, McCurdy DK, Ludwig GD, et al. Incomplete renal tubular acidosis. Physiologic studies in three patients with a defect in lowering urine pH. Am J Med. 1968;45:32.

Dyck RF, Asthana S, Kalra J, et al. A modification of the urine osmolal gap: an improved method for estimating urine ammonium. Am J Nephrol. 1990;10:359.

Karet FE. Mechanisms in hyperkalemic renal tubular acidosis. J Am Soc Nephrol. 2009;20:251.

Kim GH, Han JS, Kim YS, et al. Evaluation of urine acidification by urine anion gap and urine osmolal gap in chronic metabolic acidosis. Am J Kidney Dis. 1996;27:42.

Kraut JA, Madias NE. Differential diagnosis of nongap metabolic acidosis: value of a systematic approach. Clin J Am Soc Nephrol. 2012;7:671.

Lee Hamm L, Hering-Smith KS, Nakhoul NL. Acid-base and potassium homeostasis. Semin Nephrol 2013; 33:257.

Levy B. Lactate and shock state: the metabolic view. Curr Opin Crit Care. 2006;12:315.

Madias NE. Lactic acidosis. Kidney Int. 1986;29:752.

Meregalli P, Lüthy C, Oetliker OH, Bianchetti MG. Modified urine osmolal gap: an accurate method for estimating the urinary ammonium concentration? Nephron. 1995;69:98.

Mikkelsen ME, Miltiades AN, Gaieski DF, et al. Serum lactate is associated with mortality in severe sepsis independent of organ failure and shock. Crit Care Med. 2009;37:1670.

Oh M, Carroll HJ. Value and determinants of urine anion gap. Nephron. 2002;90:252.

Rastegar M, Nagami GT. Non-anion gap metabolic acidosis: a clinical approach to evaluation. Am J Kidney Dis. 2017;69:296.

Rodríguez Soriano J. Renal tubular acidosis: the clinical entity. J Am Soc Nephrol. 2002;13:2160.

CASE 43

A 45-year-old woman with systemic lupus erythematosus (SLE) and CKD presents to the emergency department from home with right lower quadrant abdominal pain, nausea, and fever. She is febrile to 38°C, with RR 28, BP 150/110, HR 110, and Sao_2 97% on Room Air. She takes hydroxychloroquine for SLE. Her baseline Cr is 2.3 and her BUN was 43 last week in clinic, with a serum HCO_3 of 24 mEq/L. She is writhing in pain.

Laboratory data.			
ABGs		Basic Metabolic Panel	
pH	7.48	Na	136 mEq/L
$Paco_2$	18 mm Hg	K	6.4 mEq/L
Pao_2	109 mm Hg	Cl	106 mEq/L
HCO_3	6 mEq/L	CO_2	6 mEq/L
		BUN	160 mg/dL
		Cr	8.8 mg/dL
		Glucose	124 mg/dL
		Albumin	2.8 g/dL
		EtOH	0 mg/dL

QUESTIONS

Q43-1: Define the patient's baseline acid-base status: Does this patient have an underlying chronic acid-base disorder that we need to account for in order to appropriately interpret the acute acid-base disorders?

A. There is no evidence for an underlying chronic respiratory or metabolic acid-base disorder in this patient, so we would assume a baseline $Paco_2$ of 40 mm Hg and an HCO_3 of 24 mEq/L.

B. While the patient has a condition that potentially predisposes her to a chronic acid-base disorder, there is insufficient information to estimate the patient's baseline $Paco_2$ and HCO_3 values; therefore, we will assume a baseline $Paco_2$ of 40 mm Hg and a baseline HCO_3 of 24 mEq/L.

C. The patient has an underlying acid-base condition, and we have sufficient information to estimate the patient's baseline $Paco_2$ and HCO_3 values.

Q43-2: What is/are the primary acid/base disturbance(s) occurring in this case?

A. Metabolic acidosis only
B. Respiratory acidosis only
C. Metabolic alkalosis only
D. Respiratory alkalosis only
E. Metabolic acidosis and a respiratory acidosis
F. Metabolic alkalosis and a respiratory alkalosis

Q43-3: The patient's serum salicylate level is undetectable. What is the likely cause of her respiratory alkalosis?

A. Pulmonary embolism
B. Uncontrolled pain or anxiety
C. COPD
D. Opioid overdose

Q43-4: How would the metabolic acidosis component be classified in this case?

A. Anion gap acidosis
B. Non-anion gap acidosis
C. Anion and non-anion gap acidosis
D. Anion gap acidosis and a metabolic alkalosis

Q43-5: The patient's laboratory tests return the following results:

Serum EtOH	< 3 mg/dL
Serum acetaminophen level	< 5 mg/dL (ULN for therapeutic use 20 mg/dL)
Serum salicylates level	< 5 mg/dL (ULN for therapeutic use 30 mg/dL)
Serum osmolality	341 mOsm/kg
Serum L-lactate	1.1 mmol/L (ULN 2.0 mmol/L venous)
Beta-hydroxybutyrate (acetone)	< 0.18 mmol/L (ULN 0.18 mmol/L)
Serum glucose	124 mg/dL
Urine osmolal gap	110 mOsm/L
Urine pH	5.5

What is the likely cause of the patient's anion and non-anion gap acidosis?
A. Lactic acidosis
B. Acetaminophen toxicity
C. Toluene toxicity
D. DKA
E. Acute renal failure (uremic acidosis)
F. RTA

Q43-6: What is this patient's HCO_3 deficit, assuming the following?

HCO_3 space (L)	0.4 L/kg (lean body weight)
Lean body weight (kg)	70 kg
Desired HCO_3 (mEq/L)	24
Current HCO_3 (mEq/L)	6

A. 672 mEq
B. 504 mEq
C. 448 mEq
D. 168 mEq

Q43-7: How many hours would it take to replete this patient's HCO_3 to a *target level of 12 mEq/L* (assuming a volume of distribution of 56 L) if you were administering a sodium bicarbonate infusion (150 mEq/L in D_5W) at 125 mL/h?
A. 12 hours
B. 18 hours
C. 24 hours
D. 27 hours
E. 36 hours

ANSWERS

Q43-1: A

There is no evidence for an underlying chronic respiratory or metabolic acid-base disorder in this patient, so we would assume a baseline $Paco_2$ of 40 mm Hg and an HCO_3 of 24 mEq/L. Despite having considerable CKD at baseline, the patient appeared to have a normal HCO_3 recently in clinic.

Rationale: Ignoring these underlying chronic acid-base disorders can significantly alter the interpretation of a patient's acute acid-base status. This was demonstrated in the first case of the series. However, often, we do not have the necessary information (eg, prior ABG or VBG, or prior serum chemistry with an HCO_3) and are forced to assume the ongoing processes are all acute in nature. We are primarily concerned about chronic respiratory acid-base disorders, as these can significantly alter the patient's baseline or expected values for the serum HCO_3 and $Paco_2$, and we have reliable equations to predict the expected baseline values. The respiratory compensation for both chronic metabolic acidosis and alkalosis is generally poor, so there are no equations or rules to predict what the $Paco_2$ should be in these cases. While the baseline serum HCO_3 may be significantly off from our standard value of 24 mEq/L in these patients, we would assume a baseline $Paco_2$ of 40 mm Hg in patients with chronic metabolic processes. Once we identify the patient's baseline $Paco_2$ and HCO_3 values, we will need to use these values in the appropriate equations to identify the ongoing acute processes.

Q43-2: D

Respiratory alkalosis only.

Rationale:

1. The pH is 7.48; therefore, the primary disorder is an **alkalosis.**
2. The $Paco_2$ of 18 mm Hg is less than 40 mm Hg, so there is a **respiratory alkalosis.**
3. The HCO_3 of 6 mEq/L is less than 24, so there is **no metabolic alkalosis.**

Q43-3: B

Uncontrolled pain or anxiety.

Rationale: This patient presented with symptoms consistent with acute appendicitis. The respiratory alkalosis is not solely a compensatory mechanism for the metabolic acidosis that is present as the pH is alkalotic. The respiratory alkalosis may be due to pain and hyperventilation.

Q43-4: C

Anion gap acidosis and a non-anion gap acidosis.

Rationale:

1. Is there evidence for a chronic acid-base disorder that requires adjustment of the patient's "normal" HCO_3? No, there is no evidence for a chronic acid-base disorder, so we would assume a baseline $Paco_2$ of 40 mm Hg and an HCO_3 of 24 mEq/L.

2. Expected anion gap:

$$\text{Expected Anion Gap} = 12 - (2.5) * \left[4.0 \frac{g}{dL} - \text{Actual Serum Albumin} \right]$$

$$= 12 - (2.5 * [4.0 - 2.8])$$
$$= 12 - (2.5 * [1.2]) = \textbf{9 mEq/L.}$$

3. Anion gap calculation:

$$\text{Serum Anion Gap} = [Na^+] - [HCO_3^-] - [Cl^-]$$
$$= 136 - (106 + 6) = \textbf{24 mEq/L,} \text{ which is} > 9 \text{ mEq/L}$$
$$\rightarrow \textbf{anion gap acidosis is present.}$$

4. Delta-delta calculation:

$$\Delta\Delta = \frac{(\text{Actual Anion Gap} - \text{Expected Anion Gap})}{(\text{Baseline HCO}_3 - \text{Actual HCO}_3)}$$

$$= (24 - 9)/(24 - 6) = \textbf{15/18, which is} \sim \textbf{0.833.}$$

Delta-delta interpretation.	
Delta-Delta Value	Condition Present
< 0.4	Non-anion gap only
0.4–1.0	**Anion gap *and* non-anion gap acidosis**
1.0–2.0	Anion gap acidosis only
> 2.0	Anion gap acidosis and metabolic alkalosis

The delta-delta is between 0.4 and 1, so an anion gap and a non-anion gap acidosis exist.

Q43-5: E
Acute renal failure (uremic acidosis).

Rationale: The patient's acute renal failure-on-CKD is the likely cause with the acute renal failure causing acute accumulation of acid anions (eg, phosphate, sulphate). This is supported by the hyperkalemia. There is no lactic acidosis, no organic acid ingestion, no ASA or acetaminophen toxicity, and no evidence of a ketoacidosis present. The serum osmolal gap, which takes into account the uremia, is normal.

$$\text{Calculated Serum Osmolality} = 2 * [Na^+] + \frac{[Glucose]}{18} + \frac{[BUN]}{2.8} + \frac{[EtOH]}{3.7}$$

$$= 336 \text{ mOsm/L}$$

$$\text{Serum Osmolal Gap (SOG)} = \text{Measured Serum Osmolality}$$
$$- \text{Calculated Serum Osmolality}$$

$$\text{SOG} = 341 - 336 \text{ mOsm/L} = (+5) \text{ mOsm/L.}$$

The patient's non-anion gap acidosis is likely a complex process including acute-on-chronic renal failure. This is also likely the cause of the patients non-anion gap acidosis, as the urine osmolal gap is abnormal (pointing toward a type 1 or type 4 RTA), with an acidic urine pH and elevated serum potassium. This is consistent with a type 4 RTA, which can be caused by either SLE or renal failure.

Causes of RTA.
Causes of Type 1 (Distal) RTA
Primary • Idiopathic or familial (may be recessive or dominant)
Secondary • Medications: Lithium, amphotericin, ifosfamide, NSAIDs • Rheumatologic disorders: Sjögren syndrome, SLE, RA • Hypercalciuria (idiopathic) or associated with vitamin D deficiency or hyperparathyroidism • Sarcoidosis • Obstructive uropathy • Wilson disease • Rejection of renal transplant allograft • Toluene toxicity
Causes of Type 2 (Proximal) RTA
Primary • Idiopathic • Familial (primarily recessive disorders) • Genetic: Fanconi syndrome, cystinosis, glycogen storage disease (type 1), Wilson disease, galactosemia **Secondary** • Medications: Acetazolamide, topiramate, aminoglycoside antibiotics, ifosfamide, reverse transcriptase inhibitors (tenofovir) • Heavy metal poisoning: Lead, mercury, copper • Multiple myeloma or amyloidosis (secondary to light chain toxicity) • Sjögren syndrome • Vitamin D deficiency • Rejection of renal transplant allograft
Causes of Type 4 RTA (Hypoaldosteronism or Aldosterone Resistance)
Primary • Primary adrenal insufficiency • Inherited disorders associated with hypoaldosteronism • Pseudohypoaldosteronism (types 1 and 2) **Secondary** • Causes of hyporeninemic hypoaldosteronism such as renal disease (diabetic nephropathy), NSAID use, calcineurin inhibitors, volume expansion/volume overload • Causes of distal tubule voltage defects such as sickle cell disease, obstructive uropathy, SLE • Severe illness/septic shock • Angiotensin II–associated medications: ACE inhibitors, ARBs, direct renin inhibitors • Potassium-sparing diuretics: Spironolactone, amiloride, triamterene • Antibiotics: Trimethoprim, pentamidine

Q43-6: B
504 mEq.

Rationale: Using the steps presented earlier, the HCO_3 deficit and space can be calculated as follows:

Bicarbonate Deficit and Space:

$$HCO_3^- \text{ Space} = [0.4] * LBW \text{ (in kg)} = 28$$
$$HCO_3^- \text{ Deficit} = HCO_3^- \text{ Space} * HCO_3^- \text{ Deficit/L}$$
$$= 28 * (24 - 6 \text{ mEq/L})$$
$$= (28 \text{ L}) * (18 \text{ mEq/L})$$
$$= 504 \text{ mEq.}$$

This patient has a deficiency of 504 mEq of HCO_3 overall. This was calculated using a static equation for the HCO_3 deficit. However, the HCO_3 space is actually dynamic and changes with the HCO_3 concentration. The dynamic equation for the volume of distribution is as follows:

$$HCO_3^- \text{ Space} = \left[0.4 + \left(\frac{2.4}{HCO_3^-}\right)\right] * LBW \text{ (in kg)};$$

Where the HCO_3 is the starting concentration. In this case, the HCO_3 space would be:

$$HCO_3^- \text{ Space} = \left[0.4 + \left(\frac{2.4}{[6]}\right)\right] * 70 = (0.4 + 0.4) * 70 = 56L;$$

Which effectively doubles the HCO_3 space and the HCO_3 deficit (now 1008 mEq/L).

Q43-7: B
18 hours.

Rationale: To get the goal of 12 mEq/L, the deficit is 336 mEq of HCO_3 when using the 56-L volume of distribution. Each 1-L bag of sodium bicarbonate solution has 150 mEq, so the patient needs 2.24 L of this fluid. If it is administered at 125 mL/h (0.125 L/h), this would take 18 hours to complete. Generally, if the serum HCO_3 is less than 10 to 12 mEq/L, the HCO_3 is replaced until a target of 12 mEq/L with sodium bicarbonate as rapidly as needed, and then the HCO_3 up to a level greater than 15 mEq/L over an 18- to 24-hour period.

References

Bailey JL. Metabolic acidosis: an unrecognized cause of morbidity in the patient with chronic kidney disease. Kidney Int. 2005;68(suppl 96):S15.

Halperin ML, Ethier JH, Kamel KS. Ammonium excretion in chronic metabolic acidosis: benefits and risks. Am J Kidney Dis. 1989;14:267.

Koda-Kimble M, Young LY, et al. Handbook of Applied Therapeutics. Philadelphia, PA: Lippincott Williams & Wilkins; 2006:P10.3(1104).

Kraut JA, Kurtz I. Metabolic acidosis of CKD: diagnosis, clinical characteristics, and treatment. Am J Kidney Dis. 2005;45:978.

Krieger NS, Frick KK, Bushinsky DA. Mechanism of acid-induced bone resorption. Curr Opin Nephrol Hypertens. 2004;13:423.

Warnock DG. Uremic acidosis. Kidney Int. 1988;34:278.

Widmer B, Gerhardt RE, Harrington JT, Cohen JJ. Serum electrolyte and acid base composition. The influence of graded degrees of chronic renal failure. Arch Intern Med. 1979;139:1099.

CASE 44

A 44-year-old woman is brought to the emergency department by her family. She has encephalopathy and ataxia, and is tachypneic on presentation, with T 37.9°C, RR 28, HR 112, BP 150/80, and Sao$_2$ 99% on Room Air. She has a history of HTN; morbid obesity with recent gastric bypass complicated by small intestine ischemia, requiring small bowel resection 3 months prior; and stage 2 CKD with baseline Cr of 1.6. She has been experiencing nausea and emesis since yesterday when she attended a bake sale.

Laboratory data.			
ABGs		Basic Metabolic Panel	
pH	7.17	Na	140 mEq/L
Paco$_2$	13 mm Hg	K	4.0 mEq/L
Pao$_2$	90 mm Hg	Cl	84 mEq/L
HCO$_3$	5 mEq/L	CO$_2$	5 mEq/L
		BUN	14 mg/dL
		Cr	1.6 mg/dL
		Glucose	137 mg/dL
		Albumin	4.0 g/dL
		EtOH	0 mg/dL

QUESTIONS

Q44-1: Define the patient's baseline acid-base status: Does this patient have an underlying chronic acid-base disorder that we need to account for in order to appropriately interpret the acute acid-base disorders?

A. There is no evidence for an underlying chronic respiratory or metabolic acid-base disorder in this patient, so we would assume a baseline $Paco_2$ of 40 mm Hg and an HCO_3 of 24 mEq/L.

B. While the patient has a condition predisposing her to a chronic acid-base disorder, there is insufficient information to estimate the patient's baseline $Paco_2$ and HCO_3 values; therefore, we will assume a baseline $Paco_2$ of 40 mm Hg and a baseline HCO_3 of 24 mEq/L.

C. The patient has an underlying acid-base condition, and we have sufficient information to estimate the patient's baseline $Paco_2$ and HCO_3 values.

Q44-2: What is/are the primary acid/base disturbance(s) occurring in this case?

A. Metabolic acidosis only
B. Respiratory acidosis only
C. Metabolic alkalosis only
D. Respiratory alkalosis only
E. Metabolic acidosis and a respiratory acidosis
F. Metabolic alkalosis and a respiratory alkalosis

Q44-3: How would the metabolic acidosis component be classified in this case?

A. Anion gap acidosis
B. Non-anion gap acidosis
C. Anion and non-anion gap acidosis
D. Anion gap acidosis and a metabolic alkalosis

Q44-4: Does the patient in this case demonstrate appropriate respiratory compensation?

A. Yes, the respiratory compensation is appropriate.
B. No, a concomitant respiratory alkalosis is present.
C. No, a concomitant respiratory acidosis is present.

Q44-5: Laboratory testing returns the following results:

Serum EtOH	< 3 mg/dL
Serum acetaminophen level	< 5 mg/dL (ULN for therapeutic use 20 mg/dL)
Serum salicylates level	< 5 mg/dL (ULN for therapeutic use 30 mg/dL)
Serum osmolality	300 mOsm/kg
Serum L-lactate	1.0 mmol/L (ULN 2.0 mmol/L venous)
Beta-hydroxybutyrate (acetone)	< 0.18 mmol/L (ULN 0.18 mmol/L)
Serum glucose	137 mg/dL
Serum phosphorus	3.3 mg/dL
Urine drug screen	Negative

What is the likely cause of the patient's anion gap acidosis?

A. L-Lactic acidosis
B. Acetaminophen toxicity
C. D-Lactic acidosis
D. DKA
E. Acute renal failure (uremic acidosis)
F. Ethylene glycol toxicity

Q44-6: The urine chloride is 8 mEq/L. What is the likely cause of the patient's metabolic alkalosis?

A. Hyperemesis
B. Milk-alkali syndrome
C. Congenital renal disorder (eg, Gittleman syndrome)

ANSWERS

Q44-1: B

While the patient has a condition predisposing her to a chronic acid-base disorder, there is insufficient information to estimate the patient's baseline $Paco_2$ and HCO_3 values; therefore, we will assume a baseline $Paco_2$ of 40 mm Hg and a baseline HCO_3 of 24 mEq/L.

Rationale: Ignoring these underlying chronic acid-base disorders can significantly alter the interpretation of a patient's acute acid-base status. This was demonstrated in the first case of the series. However, often, we do not have the necessary information (eg, prior ABG or VBG, or prior serum chemistry with an HCO_3) and are forced to assume the ongoing processes are all acute in nature. We are primarily concerned about chronic respiratory acid-base disorders, as these can significantly alter the patient's baseline or expected values for the serum HCO_3 and $Paco_2$, and we have reliable equations to predict the expected baseline values. The respiratory compensation for both chronic metabolic acidosis and alkalosis is generally poor, so there are no equations or rules to predict what the $Paco_2$ should be in these cases. While the baseline serum HCO_3 may be significantly off from our standard value of 24 mEq/L in these patients, we would assume a baseline $Paco_2$ of 40 mm Hg in patients with chronic metabolic processes. Once we identify the patient's baseline $Paco_2$ and HCO_3 values, we will need to use these values in the appropriate equations to identify the ongoing acute processes.

Q44-2: A

Metabolic acidosis only.

Rationale:

1. The pH is 7.22; therefore, the primary disorder is an **acidosis.**
2. The $Paco_2$ of 12 mm Hg is less than 40 mm Hg, so there is **no respiratory acidosis.**
3. The HCO_3 of 5 mEq/L is less than 24 mEq/L, so there is a **metabolic acidosis.**

Q44-3: D

Anion gap acidosis and a metabolic alkalosis.

Rationale:

1. Is there evidence for a chronic acid-base disorder that requires adjustment of the patient's "normal" HCO_3? No, there is no evidence for a chronic acid-base disorder, so we would assume a baseline $Paco_2$ of 40 mm Hg and an HCO_3 of 24 mEq/L.
2. Expected anion gap:

$$\text{Expected Anion Gap} = 12 - (2.5) * \left[4.0\,\frac{g}{dL} - \text{Actual Serum Albumin} \right]$$

$$= 12 - (2.5 * [4.0 - 4.0])$$

$$= 12 - (2.5 * [0]) = \textbf{12 mEq/L.}$$

3. Anion gap calculation:

$$\text{Serum Anion Gap} = [Na^+] - [HCO_3^-] - [Cl^-]$$
$$= 140 - (84 + 5) = \textbf{51 mEq/L,} \text{ which is} > 12 \text{ mEq/L}$$
$$\rightarrow \textbf{anion gap acidosis is present.}$$

4. Delta-delta calculation:

$$\Delta\Delta = \frac{(\text{Actual Anion Gap} - \text{Expected Anion Gap})}{(\text{Baseline HCO}_3 - \text{Actual HCO}_3)}$$
$$= (51 - 12)/(24 - 5) = 39/19 = \textbf{2.06, which is} > \textbf{2.}$$

Delta-delta interpretation.	
Delta-Delta Value	Condition Present
< 0.4	Non-anion gap only
0.4–1.0	Anion gap *and* non-anion gap acidosis
1.0–2.0	Anion gap acidosis only
> 2.0	**Anion gap acidosis and metabolic alkalosis**

The delta-delta is greater than 2, so there is an anion gap acidosis and a metabolic alkalosis.

Q44-4: A
Yes, the respiratory compensation is appropriate.

Rationale: Using the Winter formula, one can calculate what the expected arterial $Paco_2$ should be for a given serum HCO_3 if the patient were completely compensated.

Respiratory Compensation for Acute Metabolic Acidosis (Winter Formula):

$$\text{Expected Paco}_2 = 1.5 * [\text{Actual HCO}_3] + 8 \pm 2 \text{ (in mm Hg)}$$
$$= (1.5 * 5) + 8 = 7.5 + 8 = 15.5 \pm 2 = (13 \text{ to } 17) \text{ mm Hg.}$$

Since the patient's $Paco_2$ on presentation of **13 mm Hg** is within the expected range of 13 to 17 mm Hg, this patient has **appropriate compensation.**

Q44-5: C
D-Lactic acidosis.

Rationale: The patient has a high anion gap acidosis, with negative diagnostic testing for L-lactate, negative ketoacidosis, negative serum osmolal gap that would be consistent with ethylene glycol or methanol toxicity, negative drug screen ruling out ASA and acetaminophen, no uremia, and no significant renal failure. In patients with short gut syndrome, heavy carbohydrate loads can be converted quickly to L-lactate, overloading the ability of the body to clear D-lactate. Neurologic symptoms are common.

The serum osmolal gap is calculated as follows:

$$\text{Calculated Serum Osmolality} = 2*[Na^+] + \frac{[Glucose]}{18} + \frac{[BUN]}{2.8} + \frac{[EtOH]}{3.7}$$
$$= 293 \text{ mOsm/L}$$
$$\text{Serum Osmolal Gap} = 300 \text{ mOsm/L} - 293 \text{ mOsm/L} = (+7) \text{ mOsm/L}.$$

Depending on the clinical laboratory, the test for L-lactate may be stereospecific and will only detect L-lactate but not D-lactate (as in this case). A high index of suspicion is necessary in such cases to make the diagnosis. Patients with short bowel syndrome, patients with large infusions of propylene glycol, and those with DKA are at increased risk for D-lactic acidosis. In patients with short gut syndrome or small bowel resection, an increased load of carbohydrates is delivered to the large intestine. These compounds are usually broken down in the small bowel and absorbed. When delivered to the large bowel, these carbohydrates can be metabolized by bacteria in the large bowel, yielding D-lactate as a product. This is readily absorbed in the large bowel, but, unlike L-lactate, cannot be converted to pyruvate by lactate dehydrogenase. Therefore it must be secreted by the kidney. While this is usually accomplished in a rapid manner that prevents the accumulation of D-lactate, a large ingestion of carbohydrates can overwhelm the ability of kidneys to clear the D-lactate. The neurologic effects of D-lactic acidosis seem to be independent of D-lactate itself, indicating that other toxic metabolites may be produced through a similar mechanism.

Q44-6: A
Hyperemesis.

Rationale: The patient's urine chloride is very low, so this is considered a chloride-responsive alkalosis; the low urinary chloride indicates the body is tightly holding onto chloride rather than excreting it, so the patient is likely chloride-depleted. Conditions that lead to a chloride-depletion state include hyperemesis and diuretic use. Chloride-resistant states have a urine chloride greater than 20 to 30 mEq/L and include congenital renal conditions (Bartter syndrome) and milk-alkali syndrome.

Causes of metabolic alkalosis.
History: Rule Out the Following as Causes
• Alkali load ("milk-alkali" or calcium-alkali syndrome, oral sodium bicarbonate, IV sodium bicarbonate) • Genetic causes (CF) • Presence of hypercalcemia • IV β-lactam antibiotics • Laxative abuse (may also cause a metabolic acidosis depending on diarrheal HCO$_3$ losses)

(Continued)

Causes of metabolic alkalosis. (*continued*)
If None of the Above, Then. . .
Urine Chloride < 20 mEq/L (Chloride-Responsive Causes) • Loss of gastric acid (hyperemesis, NGT suctioning) • Prior diuretic use (in hours to days following discontinuation) • Post-hypercapnia • Villous adenoma • Congenital chloridorrhea • Chronic laxative abuse (may also cause a metabolic acidosis depending on diarrheal HCO_3 losses) • CF
OR
Urine Chloride > 20 mEq/L (Chloride-Resistant Causes)
Urine Chloride > 20 mEq/L, Lack of HTN, Urine Potassium < 30 mEq/L
• Hypokalemia or hypomagnesemia • Laxative abuse (if dominated by hypokalemia) • Bartter syndrome • Gitelman syndrome
Urine Chloride > 20 mEq/L, Lack of HTN, Urine Potassium > 30 mEq/L
• Current diuretic use
Urine Chloride > 20 mEq/L, Presence of HTN, Urine Potassium Variable but Usually > 30 mEq/L
***Elevated plasma renin level*:** • Renal artery stenosis • Renin-secreting tumor • Renovascular disease
***Low plasma renin, low plasma aldosterone*:** • Cushing syndrome • Exogenous mineralocorticoid use • Genetic disorder (11-hydoxylase or 17-hydrolyase deficiency, 11β-HSD deficiency) • Liddle syndrome • Licorice toxicity
***Low plasma renin, high plasma aldosterone*:** • Primary hyperaldosteronism • Adrenal adenoma • Bilateral adrenal hyperplasia

References

Abreo K, Adlakha A, Kilpatrick S, et al. The milk-alkali syndrome. A reversible form of acute renal failure. Arch Intern Med. 1993;153:1005.

Adeva-Andany M, López-Ojén M, Funcasta-Calderón R, et al. Comprehensive review on lactate metabolism in human health. Mitochondrion. 2014;17:76.

Barton CH, Vaziri ND, Ness RL, et al. Cimetidine in the management of metabolic alkalosis induced by nasogastric drainage. Arch Surg. 1979;114:70.

Bear R, Goldstein M, Phillipson E, et al. Effect of metabolic alkalosis on respiratory function in patients with chronic obstructive lung disease. Can Med Assoc J. 1977;117:900.

Coronado BE, Opal SM, Yoburn DC. Antibiotic-induced D-lactic acidosis. Ann Intern Med. 1995;122:839.

Galla JH, Gifford JD, Luke RG, Rome L. Adaptations to chloride-depletion alkalosis. Am J Physiol. 1991;261:R771.

Garella S, Chang BS, Kahn SI. Dilution acidosis and contraction alkalosis: review of a concept. Kidney Int. 1975;8:279.

Gennari FJ, Weise WJ. Acid-base disturbances in gastrointestinal disease. Clin J Am Soc Nephrol. 2008;3:1861.

Halperin ML, Kamel KS. D-lactic acidosis: turning sugar into acids in the gastrointestinal tract. Kidney Int. 1996;49:1.

Hamm LL, Nakhoul N, Hering-Smith KS. Acid-base homeostasis. Clin J Am Soc Nephrol. 2015;10:2232.

Hulter HN, Sebastian A, Toto RD, et al. Renal and systemic acid-base effects of the chronic administration of hypercalcemia-producing agents: calcitriol, PTH, and intravenous calcium. Kidney Int. 1982;21:445.

Jorens PG, Demey HE, Schepens PJ, et al. Unusual D-lactic acid acidosis from propylene glycol metabolism in overdose. J Toxicol Clin Toxicol. 2004;42:163.

Khanna A, Kurtzman NA. Metabolic alkalosis. J Nephrol. 2006;19(suppl 9):S86.

Laski ME, Sabatini S. Metabolic alkalosis, bedside and bench. Semin Nephrol. 2006;26:404.

Levy B. Lactate and shock state: the metabolic view. Curr Opin Crit Care. 2006;12:315.

Luke RG, Galla JH. It is chloride depletion alkalosis, not contraction alkalosis. J Am Soc Nephrol. 2012;23:204.

Madias NE. Lactic acidosis. Kidney Int. 1986;29:752.

Mikkelsen ME, Miltiades AN, Gaieski DF, et al. Serum lactate is associated with mortality in severe sepsis independent of organ failure and shock. Crit Care Med. 2009;37:1670.

Miller PD, Berns AS. Acute metabolic alkalosis perpetuating hypercarbia. A role for acetazolamide in chronic obstructive pulmonary disease. JAMA. 1977;238:2400.

Oster JR, Materson BJ, Rogers AI. Laxative abuse syndrome. Am J Gastroenterol. 1980;74:451.

Patel AM, Goldfarb S. Got calcium? Welcome to the calcium-alkali syndrome. J Am Soc Nephrol. 2010;21:1440.

Rose BD, Post TW. Clinical Physiology of Acid-Base and Electrolyte Disorders. 5e. New York, NY: McGraw Hill; 2001:559.

Schwartz WB, Van Ypersele de Strihou, Kassirer JP. Role of anions in metabolic alkalosis and potassium deficiency. N Engl J Med. 1968;279:630.

Stolberg L, Rolfe R, Gitlin N, et al. d-Lactic acidosis due to abnormal gut flora: diagnosis and treatment of two cases. N Engl J Med. 1982;306:1344.

Sweetser LJ, Douglas JA, Riha RL, Bell SC. Clinical presentation of metabolic alkalosis in an adult patient with cystic fibrosis. Respirology. 2005;10:254.

Taki K, Mizuno K, Takahashi N, Wakusawa R. Disturbance of CO2 elimination in the lungs by carbonic anhydrase inhibition. Jpn J Physiol. 1986;36:523.

Tsao YT, Tsai WC, Yang SP. A life-threatening double gap metabolic acidosis. Am J Emerg Med. 2008;26:385.e5.

Turban S, Beutler KT, Morris RG, et al. Long-term regulation of proximal tubule acid-base transporter abundance by angiotensin II. Kidney Int. 2006;70:660.

Uchida H, Yamamoto H, Kisaki Y, et al. D-lactic acidosis in short-bowel syndrome managed with antibiotics and probiotics. J Pediatr Surg. 2004;39:634.

Uribarri J, Oh MS, Carroll HJ. D-lactic acidosis. A review of clinical presentation, biochemical features, and pathophysiologic mechanisms. Medicine (Baltimore). 1998;77:73.

CASE 45

The following are general questions that review common causes and laboratory testing for various acid-base disorders.

QUESTIONS

Q45-1: What are the potential causes of an anion gap metabolic acidosis? (Place an "X" next to each possible cause.)

	Lactic acidosis		Methanol		Hyperkalemia
	Renal tubular acidosis		Ethylene glycol		DKA
	Alcoholic ketoacidosis		Diuretic use		Isoniazid use
	Diarrhea		Starvation ketosis		Bactrim use
	Renal failure		Bartter syndrome		Carbon monoxide
	Lithium		Uremia		Adrenal insufficiency
	Salicylate toxicity		Cystic fibrosis		Cyanide
	Ureteral diversion		Paraldehyde toxicity		Hyperemesis

Q45-2: What are potential causes of non-anion gap metabolic acidosis? (Place an "X" next to each possible cause.)

	TPN		Isoniazid
	Lactic acidosis		Acetazolamide use
	Renal tubular acidosis		COPD
	Hyperemesis		Methanol
	Progesterone		Diarrhea
	Hyperchloremic fluids		Ethylene glycol
	Opioid overdose		DKA
	Aminoglycoside use		Pancreatic diversion

Q45-3: What are the potential causes of respiratory acidosis (place an "X" next to each possible cause) and respiratory alkalosis (place an "O" next to each cause)?

	COPD		Salicylate overdose
	Respiratory muscle fatigue		Pulmonary edema
	Progesterone		Opioid overdose
	Asthma		Pain
	Anxiety		Poor gas exchange
	Neuromuscular disorder		Cirrhosis

Q45-4: What are the causes of a metabolic alkalosis? (Place an "X" next to each possible cause.)

	Lactic acidosis		Methanol		Milk-alkali syndrome
	Renal tubular acidosis		Ethylene glycol		DKA
	Volume contraction		Diuretic use		Hypercalcemia
	Diarrhea		Cushing syndrome		Sulfamethoxazole-trimethoprim use
	Renal failure		Bartter syndrome		Carbon monoxide
	Laxative abuse		Uremia		Licorice
	Salicylate toxicity		Refeeding syndrome		Cyanide
	Ureteral diversion		Gitelman syndrome		Hyperemesis

Q45-5: What are the causes of an elevated serum osmolal gap? (Place an "X" next to each possible cause.) Assume we account only for Na, BUN, and glucose in the calculation.

	Ethanol		Hyperlipidemia		Hypernatremia
	DKA		Opioid overdose		Hyperproteinemia
	Mannitol		Sorbitol		Hypercalcemia
	Starvation ketosis		Lithium overdose		Hyperkalemia
	Ethylene glycol		TCA overdose		Isopropyl alcohol
	RTA		Acetaminophen		Hyperphosphatemia
	Methanol		Diuretic use		Propylene glycol

Q45-6: Which of the causes of an elevated serum osmolal gap listed in Q45-5 are also causes of an *anion gap* acidosis?

Q45-7: Which test is most helpful in determining the cause of a non-anion gap acidosis?

A. Lactate
B. Serum osmolal gap
C. Urine anion gap
D. Urine chloride

Q45-8: Which test is most helpful in determining the cause of a metabolic alkalosis?

A. Lactate
B. Serum osmolal gap
C. Urine anion gap
D. Urine chloride

ANSWERS

Q45-1:

X	Lactic acidosis	X	Methanol		Hyperkalemia
	Renal tubular acidosis	X	Ethylene glycol	X	DKA
X	Alcoholic ketoacidosis		Diuretic use	X	Isoniazid use
	Diarrhea	X	Starvation ketosis		Bactrim use
X	Renal failure		Bartter syndrome	X	Carbon monoxide
	Lithium	X	Uremia		Adrenal insufficiency
X	Salicylate toxicity		Cystic fibrosis	X	Cyanide
	Ureteral diversion	X	Paraldehyde toxicity		Hyperemesis

Rationale:

Causes of anion gap acidosis.	
Common	Less Common
Lactic acidosis (including transient)	Cyanide poisoning
Renal failure ("uremia")	Carbon monoxide poisoning
Diabetic ketoacidosis	Aminoglycosides
Alcoholic ketoacidosis	Phenformin use
Starvation ketoacidosis	D-Lactic acidosis
Salicylate poisoning (ASA)	Paraldehyde
Acetaminophen poisoning (paracetamol)	Iron
Organic alcohol poisoning (ethylene glycol, methanol, propylene glycol)	Isoniazid
Toluene poisoning ("glue-sniffing")	Inborn errors of metabolism

Or, one may use a mnemonic such as **(CAT) MUDPILES:**

C – cyanide, carbon monoxide
A – alcoholic ketoacidosis
T – toluene toxicity
M – methanol
U – uremia/renal failure
D – DKA
P – paraldehyde, paracetamol (acetaminophen or 5-oxoproline)
I – isoniazid
L – lactic acidosis (L- and D-isoforms)
E – ethylene glycol
S – salicylates

Q45-2:

X	TPN		Isoniazid
	Lactic acidosis	X	Acetazolamide use
X	Renal tubular acidosis		COPD
	Hyperemesis		Methanol
	Progesterone	X	Diarrhea
X	Hyperchloremic fluids		Ethylene glycol
	Opioid overdose		DKA
X	Aminoglycoside use	X	Pancreatic diversion

Rationale:

Cause of NAGMA.

Low Serum Potassium

GI: Diarrhea, pancreaticoduodenal fistula, urinary intestinal diversion
Renal: Type 1 RTA (distal), type 2 RTA (proximal)
Medications/exposures: Carbonic anhydrase inhibitors, toluene
Other: D-Lactic acidosis

High (or Normal) Serum Potassium

GI: Elevated ileostomy output
Renal: Type 4 RTA or CKD
Medications: NSAIDs; antibiotics (trimethoprim, pentamidine); heparin; ACE inhibitors, ARBs, aldosterone antagonists (spironolactone); acid administration (TPN)

Causes of renal tubular acidosis.

Causes of Type 1 (Distal) RTA

Primary
· Idiopathic or familial (may be recessive or dominant)

Secondary
· Medications: Lithium, amphotericin, ifosfamide, NSAIDs
· Rheumatologic disorders: Sjögren syndrome, SLE, RA
· Hypercalciuria (idiopathic) or associated with vitamin D deficiency or hyperparathyroidism
· Sarcoidosis
· Obstructive uropathy
· Wilson disease
· Rejection of renal transplant allograft
· Toluene toxicity

Causes of Type 2 (Proximal) RTA

Primary
· Idiopathic
· Familial (primarily recessive disorders)
· Genetic: Fanconi syndrome, cystinosis, glycogen storage disease (type 1), Wilson disease, galactosemia

(Continued)

Causes of renal tubular acidosis. (*continued*)
Secondary
• Medications: Acetazolamide, topiramate, aminoglycoside antibiotics, ifosfamide, reverse transcriptase inhibitors (tenofovir)
• Heavy metal poisoning: Lead, mercury, copper
• Multiple myeloma or amyloidosis (secondary to light chain toxicity)
• Sjögren syndrome
• Vitamin D deficiency
• Rejection of renal transplant allograft
Causes of Type 4 RTA (Hypoaldosteronism or Aldosterone Resistance)
Primary
• Primary adrenal insufficiency
• Inherited disorders associated with hypoaldosteronism
• Pseudohypoaldosteronism (types 1 and 2)
Secondary
• Causes of hyporeninemic hypoaldosteronism such as renal disease (diabetic nephropathy), NSAID use, calcineurin inhibitors, volume expansion/volume overload
• Causes of distal tubule voltage defects such as sickle cell disease, obstructive uropathy, SLE
• Severe illness/septic shock
• Angiotensin II–associated medications: ACE inhibitors, ARBs, direct renin inhibitors
• Potassium-sparing diuretics: Spironolactone, amiloride, triamterene
• Antibiotics: Trimethoprim, pentamidine

Q45-3:

X	COPD	O	Salicylate overdose
X	Respiratory muscle fatigue	O	Pulmonary edema
O	Progesterone	X	Opioid overdose
X	Asthma	O	Pain
O	Anxiety	X	Poor gas exchange
X	Neuromuscular disorder	O	Cirrhosis

Q45-4:

	Lactic acidosis		Methanol	X	Milk-alkali syndrome
	Renal tubular acidosis		Ethylene glycol		DKA
X	Volume contraction	X	Diuretic use		Hypercalcemia
	Diarrhea	X	Cushing syndrome		Sulfamethoxazole-trimethoprim use
	Renal failure	X	Bartter syndrome		Carbon monoxide
X	Laxative abuse		Uremia	X	Licorice
	Salicylate toxicity	X	Refeeding syndrome		Cyanide
	Ureteral diversion	X	Gitelman syndrome	X	Hyperemesis

Rationale:

Causes of metabolic alkalosis.
History: Rule Out the Following as Causes
• Alkali load ("milk-alkali" or calcium-alkali syndrome, oral sodium bicarbonate, IV sodium bicarbonate)   • Genetic causes (cystic fibrosis [CF])   • Presence of hypercalcemia   • IV β-lactam antibiotics   • Laxative abuse (may also cause a metabolic acidosis depending on diarrheal HCO_3 losses)
If None of the Above, Then. . .
Urine Chloride < 20 mEq/L (Chloride-Responsive Causes)   • Loss of gastric acid (hyperemesis, NGT suctioning)   • Prior diuretic use (in hours to days following discontinuation)   • Post-hypercapnia   • Villous adenoma   • Congenital chloridorrhea   • Chronic laxative abuse (may also cause a metabolic acidosis depending on diarrheal HCO_3 losses)   • CF
OR
Urine Chloride > 20 mEq/L (Chloride-Resistant Causes)
Urine Chloride > 20 mEq/L, Lack of HTN, Urine Potassium < 30 mEq/L
• Hypokalemia or hypomagnesemia   • Laxative abuse (if dominated by hypokalemia)   • Bartter syndrome   • Gitelman syndrome
Urine Chloride > 20 mEq/L, Lack of HTN, Urine Potassium > 30 mEq/L
• Current diuretic use
Urine Chloride > 20 mEq/L, Presence of HTN, Urine Potassium Variable but Usually > 30 mEq/L
Elevated plasma renin level: • Renal artery stenosis   • Renin-secreting tumor   • Renovascular disease
Low plasma renin, low plasma aldosterone:• Cushing syndrome   • Exogenous mineralocorticoid use   • Genetic disorder (11-hydoxylase or 17-hydrolyase deficiency, 11β-HSD deficiency)   • Liddle syndrome   • Licorice toxicity
Low plasma renin, high plasma aldosterone: • Primary hyperaldosteronism   • Adrenal adenoma   • Bilateral adrenal hyperplasia

Q45-5: For rationale, please see the table following Q45-6.

X	Ethanol	X	Hyperlipidemia		Hypernatremia
	DKA		Opioid overdose	X	Hyperproteinemia
X	Mannitol	X	Sorbitol		Hypercalcemia
	Starvation ketosis		Lithium overdose		Hyperkalemia
X	Ethylene glycol		TCA overdose	X	Isopropyl alcohol
	RTA		Acetaminophen		Hyperphosphatemia
X	Methanol		Diuretic use	X	Propylene glycol

Q45-6: Ethylene glycol; Propylene glycol; Methanol

Important: Note that isopropyl alcohol does not cause an anion gap. Ethanol itself does not usually cause an anion gap acidosis, but rather ketoacidosis associated with alcoholism. If a patient with acute alcohol ingestion has a significant anion gap, another source/ingestion should be sought. Hyperlipidemia and hyperproteinemia may cause a false anion gap acidosis due to lab interference.

Rationale: The following are potential causes of an elevated serum osmolality:

Conditions associated with elevated serum osmolality.
With an Elevated Serum Anion Gap
1. Ethanol ingestion with alcoholic ketoacidosis (acetone is an unmeasured osmole, in addition to ethanol)—the osmolality is usually elevated more so by the increased ethanol concentration, so the osmolal "gap" depends on whether the term for ethanol is included in the osmolality calculation*
2. Organic alcohol ingestions (methanol, ethylene glycol, diethylene glycol, propylene glycol)
3. DKA—similar to ethanol ingestion, glucose and acetone contribute to the osmolality since the glucose terms is always included in the calculation
4. Salicylate toxicity.
5. Renal failure—the BUN is nearly always included in the osmolality
Without an Elevated Serum Anion Gap
1. Hyperosmolar therapy (mannitol, glycerol)
2. Other organic solvent ingestion (eg, acetone)
3. Isopropyl alcohol ingestion (produces only acetone rather than an organic acid, so no anion gap is seen)
4. Hypertriglyceridemia
5. Hyperproteinemia
*A mildly elevated osmolal gap has been reported in the literature in patients with lactic acidosis in critical illness, particularly severe distributive shock. The pathology is not quite clear, although it is likely related to multiorgan failure—particularly the liver and kidneys—and the release of cellular components known to contribute to the osmolal gap. The serum osmolal gap in this situation is typically around 10, although may be as high as 20 to 25 mOsm/L.

Q45-7: C
Urine anion gap.

Rationale: A negative urine anion gap is associated with a GI source of HCO_3 loss (diarrhea) or a renal loss of HCO_3 (type 2/proximal RTA, amyloidosis, multiple myeloma, acetazolamide use). The positive urine anion gap is associated with a poor renal acid excretion (type 1/distal or type 4 RTA, early renal failure).

Q45-8: D
Urine chloride.

Rationale: A urine chloride less than 20 mEq is consistent with a chloride-responsive cause (hyperemesis, diuretic Use), whereas a urine chloride greater than 20 mEq is consistent with a congenital renal disorder (Bartter, Gitelman) or hyperaldosteronism (see metabolic alkalosis figure above).

References

Abreo K, Adlakha A, Kilpatrick S, et al. The milk-alkali syndrome. A reversible form of acute renal failure. Arch Intern Med. 1993;153:1005.

Arroliga AC, Shehab N, McCarthy K, Gonzales JP. Relationship of continuous infusion lorazepam to serum propylene glycol concentration in critically ill adults. Crit Care Med. 2004;32:1709.

Barton CH, Vaziri ND, Ness RL, et al. Cimetidine in the management of metabolic alkalosis induced by nasogastric drainage. Arch Surg. 1979;114:70.

Batlle D, Chin-Theodorou J, Tucker BM. Metabolic acidosis or respiratory alkalosis? Evaluation of a low plasma bicarbonate using the urine anion gap. Am J Kidney Dis. 2017;70:440.

Batlle D, Grupp M, Gaviria M, Kurtzman NA. Distal renal tubular acidosis with intact capacity to lower urinary pH. Am J Med. 1982;72:751.

Batlle D, Haque SK. Genetic causes and mechanisms of distal renal tubular acidosis. Nephrol Dial Transplant. 2012;27:3691.

Batlle DC, Hizon M, Cohen E, et al. The use of the urinary anion gap in the diagnosis of hyperchloremic metabolic acidosis. N Engl J Med. 1988;318:594.

Batlle DC, von Riotte A, Schlueter W. Urinary sodium in the evaluation of hyperchloremic metabolic acidosis. N Engl J Med. 1987;316:140.

Bear R, Goldstein M, Phillipson E, et al. Effect of metabolic alkalosis on respiratory function in patients with chronic obstructive lung disease. Can Med Assoc J. 1977;117:900.

Bern M. Clinically significant pseudohyponatremia. Am J Hematol. 2006;81:558.

Braden GL, Strayhorn CH, Germain MJ, et al. Increased osmolal gap in alcoholic acidosis. Arch Intern Med. 1993;153:2377.

Buckalew VM Jr, McCurdy DK, Ludwig GD, et al. Incomplete renal tubular acidosis. Physiologic studies in three patients with a defect in lowering urine pH. Am J Med. 1968;45:32.

Corey HE. Stewart and beyond: new models of acid-base balance. Kidney Int. 2003;64:777.

Demeter SL, Cordasco EM. Hyperventilation syndrome and asthma. Am J Med. 1986;81:989.

Dyck RF, Asthana S, Kalra J, et al. A modification of the urine osmolal gap: an improved method for estimating urine ammonium. Am J Nephrol. 1990;10:359.

Faradji-Hazan V, Oster JR, Fedeman DG, et al. Effect of pyridostigmine bromide on serum bromide concentration and the anion gap. J Am Soc Nephrol. 1991;1:1123.

Feldman M, Soni N, Dickson B. Influence of hypoalbuminemia or hyperalbuminemia on the serum anion gap. J Lab Clin Med 2005;146:317.

Fenves AZ, Kirkpatrick HM 3rd, Patel VV, et al. Increased anion gap metabolic acidosis as a result of 5-oxoproline (pyroglutamic acid): a role for acetaminophen. Clin J Am Soc Nephrol. 2006;1:441.

Fernandez PC, Cohen RM, Feldman GM. The concept of bicarbonate distribution space: the crucial role of body buffers. Kidney Int. 1989;36:747.

Forni LG, McKinnon W, Lord GA, et al. Circulating anions usually associated with the Krebs cycle in patients with metabolic acidosis. Crit Care. 2005;9:R591.

Gabow PA. Ethylene glycol intoxication. Am J Kidney Dis. 1988;11:277.

Galla JH, Gifford JD, Luke RG, Rome L. Adaptations to chloride-depletion alkalosis. Am J Physiol. 1991;261:R771.

Gardner WN. The pathophysiology of hyperventilation disorders. Chest 1996;109:516.

Garella S, Chang BS, Kahn SI. Dilution acidosis and contraction alkalosis: review of a concept. Kidney Int. 1975;8:279.

Gennari FJ. Current concepts. Serum osmolality. Uses and limitations. N Engl J Med. 1984;310:102.

Gennari FJ, Weise WJ. Acid-base disturbances in gastrointestinal disease. Clin J Am Soc Nephrol. 2008;3:1861.

Glasser L, Sternglanz PD, Combie J, Robinson A. Serum osmolality and its applicability to drug overdose. Am J Clin Patholol. 1973;60:695.

Hamm LL, Nakhoul N, Hering-Smith KS. Acid-base homeostasis. Clin J Am Soc Nephrol. 2015;10:2232.

Hulter HN, Sebastian A, Toto RD, et al. Renal and systemic acid-base effects of the chronic administration of hypercalcemia-producing agents: calcitriol, PTH, and intravenous calcium. Kidney Int. 1982;21:445.

Karet FE. Mechanisms in hyperkalemic renal tubular acidosis. J Am Soc Nephrol. 2009;20:251.

Khanna A, Kurtzman NA. Metabolic alkalosis. J Nephrol. 2006;19(suppl 9):S86.

Kim GH, Han JS, Kim YS, et al. Evaluation of urine acidification by urine anion gap and urine osmolal gap in chronic metabolic acidosis. Am J Kidney Dis. 1996;27:42.

Komaru Y, Inokuchi R, Ueda Y, et al. Use of the anion gap and intermittent hemodialysis following continuous hemodiafiltration in extremely high dose acute-on-chronic lithium poisoning: A case report. Hemodial Int. 2018;22:E15.

Kraut JA, Kurtz I. Toxic alcohol ingestions: clinical features, diagnosis, and management. Clin J Am Soc Nephrol. 2008;3:208.

Kraut JA, Madias NE. Differential diagnosis of nongap metabolic acidosis: value of a systematic approach. Clin J Am Soc Nephrol. 2012;7:671.

Kraut JA, Nagami GT. The serum anion gap in the evaluation of acid-base disorders: what are its limitations and can its effectiveness be improved? Clin J Am Soc Nephrol. 2013;8:2018.

Kraut JA, Xing SX. Approach to the evaluation of a patient with an increased serum osmolal gap and high-anion-gap metabolic acidosis. Am J Kidney Dis. 2011;58:480.

Laski ME, Sabatini S. Metabolic alkalosis, bedside and bench. Semin Nephrol. 2006;26:404.

Lee Hamm L, Hering-Smith KS, Nakhoul NL. Acid-base and potassium homeostasis. Semin Nephrol. 2013;33:257.

Lu J, Zello GA, Randell E, et al. Closing the anion gap: contribution of D-lactate to diabetic ketoacidosis. Clin Chim Acta. 2011;412:286.

Luke RG, Galla JH. It is chloride depletion alkalosis, not contraction alkalosis. J Am Soc Nephrol. 2012;23:204.

Lynd LD, Richardson KJ, Purssell RA, et al. An evaluation of the osmole gap as a screening test for toxic alcohol poisoning. BMC Emerg Med. 2008;8:5.

Madias NE, Ayus JC, Adrogué HJ. Increased anion gap in metabolic alkalosis: the role of plasma-protein equivalency. N Engl J Med. 1979;300:1421.

Marraffa JM, Holland MG, Stork CM, et al. Diethylene glycol: widely used solvent presents serious poisoning potential. J Emerg Med. 2008;35:401.

Meregalli P, Lüthy C, Oetliker OH, Bianchetti MG. Modified urine osmolal gap: an accurate method for estimating the urinary ammonium concentration? Nephron. 1995;69:98.

Miller PD, Berns AS. Acute metabolic alkalosis perpetuating hypercarbia. A role for acetazolamide in chronic obstructive pulmonary disease. JAMA. 1977;238:2400.

Murray T, Long W, Narins RG. Multiple myeloma and the anion gap. N Engl J Med. 1975;292:574.

Nardi AE, Freire RC, Zin WA. Panic disorder and control of breathing. Respir Physiol Neurobiol. 2009;167:133.

Oh M, Carroll HJ. Value and determinants of urine anion gap. Nephron. 2002;90:252.

Oster JR, Materson BJ, Rogers AI. Laxative abuse syndrome. Am J Gastroenterol. 1980;74:451.

Patel AM, Goldfarb S. Got calcium? Welcome to the calcium-alkali syndrome. J Am Soc Nephrol. 2010;21:1440.

Pierce NF, Fedson DS, Brigham KL, et al. The ventilatory response to acute base deficit in humans. Time course during development and correction of metabolic acidosis. Ann Intern Med. 1970;72:633.

Purssell RA, Pudek M, Brubacher J, Abu-Laban RB. Derivation and validation of a formula to calculate the contribution of ethanol to the osmolal gap. Ann Emerg Med. 2001;38:653.

Rastegar M, Nagami GT. Non-anion gap metabolic acidosis: a clinical approach to evaluation. Am J Kidney Dis. 2017;69:296.

Relman AS. What are acids and bases? Am J Med. 1954;17:435.

Robinson AG, Loeb JN. Ethanol ingestion–commonest cause of elevated plasma osmolality? N Engl J Med. 1971;284:1253.

Rodríguez Soriano J. Renal tubular acidosis: the clinical entity. J Am Soc Nephrol. 2002;13:2160.

Rose BD, Post TW. Clinical Physiology of Acid-Base and Electrolyte Disorders. 5e. New York, NY: McGraw Hill; 2001:559

Saisch SG, Wessely S, Gardner WN. Patients with acute hyperventilation presenting to an inner-city emergency department. Chest. 1996;110:952.

Schelling JR, Howard RL, Winter SD, Linas SL. Increased osmolal gap in alcoholic ketoacidosis and lactic acidosis. Ann Intern Med. 1990;113:580.

Schwartz WB, Relman AS. A critique of the parameters used in the evaluation of acid-base disorders. "Whole-blood buffer base" and "standard bicarbonate" compared with blood pH and plasma bicarbonate concentration. N Engl J Med. 1963;268:1382.

Schwartz WB, Van Ypersele de Strihou, Kassirer JP. Role of anions in metabolic alkalosis and potassium deficiency. N Engl J Med. 1968;279:630.

Sweetser LJ, Douglas JA, Riha RL, Bell SC. Clinical presentation of metabolic alkalosis in an adult patient with cystic fibrosis. Respirology. 2005;10:254.

Taki K, Mizuno K, Takahashi N, Wakusawa R. Disturbance of CO2 elimination in the lungs by carbonic anhydrase inhibition. Jpn J Physiol. 1986;36:523.

Turban S, Beutler KT, Morris RG, et al. Long-term regulation of proximal tubule acid-base transporter abundance by angiotensin II. Kidney Int. 2006;70:660.

Weinberger SE, Schwartzstein RM, Weiss JW. Hypercapnia. N Engl J Med. 1989;321:1223.

West JB. Causes of carbon dioxide retention in lung disease. N Engl J Med. 1971;284:1232.

Williams MH Jr, Shim CS. Ventilatory failure. Etiology and clinical forms. Am J Med. 1970;48:477.

Zimmer BW, Marcus RJ, Sawyer K, Harchelroad F. Salicylate intoxication as a cause of pseudohy-perchloremia. Am J Kidney Dis. 2008;51:346.

CASE 46

A 78-year-old female nursing home resident with dementia presents with fevers, hypotension, and lethargy. Her vital signs are as follows: T 39.4°C, RR 10, HR 130, BP 60/40 and Sao₂ 96% on room air. Her urine is cloudy and foul-smelling. The patient also reportedly has been experiencing diarrhea. She takes only PRN medications, which include acetaminophen, furosemide, and polyethylene glycol 3350 (MiraLAX). She has not taken any PRN medications in the past 48 hours per nursing home records. She has a history of chronic venous insufficiency, GERD, and migraine headaches.

Laboratory data.			
ABGs		Basic Metabolic Panel	
pH	7.13	Na	140 mEq/L
$Paco_2$	37 mm Hg	K	4 mEq/L
Pao_2	100 mm Hg	Cl	107 mEq/L
HCO_3	12 mEq/L	CO_2	12 mEq/L
		BUN	44 mg/dL
		Cr	3.6 mg/dL
		Glucose	100 mg/dL
		Albumin	3.0 g/dL
		EtOH	0 mg/dL

QUESTIONS

Q46-1: **Define the patient's baseline acid-base status: Does this patient have an underlying chronic acid-base disorder that we need to account for in order to appropriately interpret the acute acid-base disorders?**

A. There is no evidence for an underlying chronic respiratory or metabolic acid-base disorder in this patient, so we would assume a baseline $Paco_2$ of 40 mm Hg and an HCO_3 of 24 mEq/L.

B. While the patient has a condition predisposing her to a chronic acid-base disorder, there is insufficient information to estimate the patient's baseline $Paco_2$ and HCO_3 values; therefore, we will assume a baseline $Paco_2$ of 40 mm Hg and a baseline HCO_3 of 24 mEq/L.

C. The patient has an underlying acid-base condition, and we have sufficient information to estimate the patient's baseline $Paco_2$ and HCO_3 values.

Q46-2: **What is/are the primary acid-base disturbance(s) occurring in this case?**

A. Metabolic acidosis only
B. Respiratory acidosis only
C. Metabolic acidosis and a respiratory acidosis
D. Metabolic alkalosis and a respiratory alkalosis
E. Metabolic alkalosis only
F. Respiratory alkalosis only

Q46-3: **How would the metabolic acidosis component be classified in this case?**

A. Anion gap acidosis
B. Non-anion gap acidosis
C. Anion and non-anion gap acidosis
D. Anion gap acidosis and a metabolic alkalosis

Q46-4: **Does the patient in this case demonstrate appropriate respiratory or metabolic compensation?**

A. Yes, the respiratory compensation is appropriate.
B. No, a concomitant respiratory alkalosis is present.
C. No, a concomitant respiratory acidosis is present.
D. Yes, the metabolic compensation is appropriate.
E. No, a concomitant metabolic acidosis is present.
F. No, a concomitant metabolic alkalosis is present.

Q46-5: What test would you order next to determine the cause of the patient's anion gap acidosis?

A. Serum lactate
B. Serum phosphorus
C. Urine drug screen
D. Serum beta-hydroxybutyrate (BHA) and acetone
E. Serum toluene level
F. Urine osmolarity
G. Urine anion gap

Q46-6: The patient's serum lactate is 12.7 mmol/L. The urine electrolytes are as follows:

Urine Na	10 mEq/L
Urine K	21 mEq/L
Urine Cl	35 mEq/L
Urine urea	145 mg/dL
Urine glucose	0 mg/dL
Urine osmolality	671 mOsm/L
Urine pH	5.5
Urine RBCs	Many
Urine WBCs	Many
Urine protein	Trace
Urine microscopic	No stones

What is the most likely cause of the patient's non-anion gap acidosis?

A. Diarrhea
B. Type 1 RTA (distal tubule)
C. Type 2I RTA (proximal tubule)
D. Type 4 RTA (distal tubule/collecting duct)

ANSWERS

Q46-1: A

There is no evidence for an underlying chronic respiratory or metabolic acid-base disorder in this patient, so we would assume a baseline $Paco_2$ of 40 mm Hg and an HCO_3 of 24 mEq/L.

Rationale: Ignoring these underlying chronic acid-base disorders can significantly alter the interpretation of a patient's acute acid-base status. This was demonstrated in the first case of the series. However, often, we do not have the necessary information (eg, prior ABG or VBG, or prior serum chemistry with an HCO_3) and are forced to assume the ongoing processes are all acute in nature. We are primarily concerned about chronic respiratory acid-base disorders, as these can significantly alter the patient's baseline or expected values for the serum HCO_3 and $Paco_2$, and we have reliable equations to predict the expected baseline values. The respiratory compensation for both chronic metabolic acidosis and alkalosis is generally poor, so there are no equations or rules to predict what the $Paco_2$ should be in these cases. While the baseline serum HCO_3 may be significantly off from our standard value of 24 mEq/L in these patients, we would assume a baseline $Paco_2$ of 40 mm Hg in patients with chronic metabolic processes. Once we identify the patient's baseline $Paco_2$ and HCO_3 values, we will need to use these values in the appropriate equations to identify the ongoing acute processes.

Q46-2: A

Metabolic acidosis only.

Rationale:

1. The pH is 7.13; therefore, the primary disorder is an **acidosis.**
2. The $Paco_2$ of 37 mm Hg is less than 40 mm Hg, so **no primary respiratory issue is present.**
3. The HCO_3 of 12 mEq/L is less than 24 mEq/L, so there is **a metabolic acidosis.**

Q46-3: C

Anion and non-anion gap acidosis.

Rationale:

1. Is there evidence for a chronic acid-base disorder that requires adjustment of the patient's "normal" HCO_3? No, there is no evidence for a chronic acid-base disorder, so we would assume a baseline $Paco_2$ of 40 mm Hg and an HCO_3 of 24 mEq/L.
2. Expected anion gap:

$$\text{Expected Anion Gap} = 12 - (2.5) * \left[4.0\,\frac{g}{dL} - \text{Actual Serum Albumin} \right]$$
$$= 12 - (2.5 * [4.0 - 3.0])$$
$$= 12 - (2.5 * [1]) = 9.5, \text{ which is} \sim 10 \text{ mEq/L.}$$

3. Anion gap calculation:

$$Serum\ Anion\ Gap = [Na^+] - [HCO_3^-] - [Cl^-]$$
$$140 - (107 + 12) = \textbf{21 mEq/L,}\ \text{which is} > 10\ mEq/L$$
$$\rightarrow \textbf{anion gap acidosis is present.}$$

4. Delta-delta calculation:

$$\Delta\Delta = \frac{(\text{Actual Anion Gap} - \text{Expected Anion Gap})}{(\text{Baseline HCO}_3 - \text{Actual HCO}_3)}$$
$$= (21 - 10)/(24 - 12) = \textbf{11/12, which is 0.9.}$$

Delta-delta interpretation.	
Delta-Delta Value	Condition Present
< 0.4	Non-anion gap only
0.4–0.9	**Anion gap *and* non-anion gap acidosis**
1.0–2.0	Anion gap acidosis only
> 2.0	Anion gap acidosis and metabolic alkalosis

Q46-4: C
No, a concomitant respiratory acidosis is present.

Rationale: Using the Winter formula, one can calculate what the expected arterial $Paco_2$ should be for a given serum HCO_3 if the patient were completely compensated.

$$\text{Expected Paco}_2 = 1.5 * [\text{Actual HCO}_3] + 8 \pm 2\ (\text{in mm Hg})$$
$$= (1.5 * 12) + 8 = 18 + 8 = 26 \pm 2 = \textbf{(24 to 28) mm Hg.}$$

This patient's $Paco_2$ of 37 mm Hg is **higher** than the expected range, and therefore a concomitant **respiratory acidosis** exists.

Q46-5: A
Serum lactate.

Rationale: The patient's presentation with hypotension is concerning for a low perfusion state and lactic acidosis should be suspected first. The normal glucose is highly uncommon for DKA and the patient has no known history of diabetes per the vignette. A serum osmolarity and drug study are good options if the lactate is normal. (Note that acetaminophen toxicity can cause a lactic acidosis as well.) The urine osmolarity and urine anion gap are more useful for non-anion gap acidosis.

Q46-6: A
Diarrhea.

Rationale: This is a case where the urine anion gap alone is inconclusive due to the severe anion gap acidosis:

$$\text{Urine Anion Gap (UAG)} = [U_{Na}] + [U_K] - [U_{Cl}].$$

Therefore, for this patient,

$$\text{UAG} - (10 + 21) \quad 35 = (-4) \text{ mEq/L}.$$

A UAG that is greater than 20 mEq/L is associated with reduced renal acid excretion (type 1 or 4 RTA), while a urine anion gap that is less than −20 mEq/L is most commonly associated with GI loss of HCO_3 (eg, diarrhea), although type 2 RTA is possible. A UAG between −20 and +10 mEq/L is generally considered inconclusive. The UAG can be inappropriately elevated in anion gap acidosis, a situation in which multiple unmeasured anions may be present in the urine (BHB/acetoacetate [ketoacidosis], hippurate [toluene], HCO_3 [proximal RTA], D-lactate [D-lactic acidosis], L-lactate [lactic acidosis], 5-oxoproline [acetaminophen toxicity]). Therefore, in patients with a significant anion gap, the urine osmolar gap is typically more useful.

Here the urine osmolar gap is as follows:

$$\text{Calculated Urine Osmolality} = 2 * ([Na^+] + [K^+]) + \frac{[\text{Urea}]}{2.8} + \frac{[\text{Glucose}]}{18}$$
$$= 2 * (10 + 21) + [145/2.8] + [0/18] = 113 \text{ mOsm/L}$$

$$\text{Osmolal Gap (UOG)} = \text{Measured Urine Osmolality}$$
$$- \text{Measured Urine Osmolality}$$

$$\text{UOG} = 671 \text{ mOsm/L} - 113 \text{ mOsm/L} = 557 \text{ mOsm/L}.$$

Similar to the UAG, the UOG is used as a surrogate for the urine ammonium concentration. Therefore, a larger gap indicates increased urinary NH_4 excretion. In normal acid-base conditions, the UOG is between 10 and 100 mOsm/L. During a significant metabolic acidosis, patients with impaired renal tubular acidification (type 1 and type 4 RTA) are unable to excrete additional acid (NH_4), and therefore the osmolar gap does not change. Patients with an intact renal response to acidemia (ie, GI losses) should have a significant UOG (~ > 300 to 400 mOsm/L) as a result of increased NH_4 excretion. Therefore, the likely cause of this patient's non-anion gap acidosis is diarrhea.

References

Adeva-Andany M, López-Ojén M, Funcasta-Calderón R, et al. Comprehensive review on lactate metabolism in human health. Mitochondrion. 2014;17:76.

Batlle D, Chin-Theodorou J, Tucker BM. Metabolic acidosis or respiratory alkalosis? Evaluation of a low plasma bicarbonate using the urine anion gap. Am J Kidney Dis. 2017;70:440.

Batlle D, Grupp M, Gaviria M, Kurtzman NA. Distal renal tubular acidosis with intact capacity to lower urinary pH. Am J Med. 1982;72:751.

Batlle D, Haque SK. Genetic causes and mechanisms of distal renal tubular acidosis. Nephrol Dial Transplant. 2012;27:3691.

Batlle DC, Hizon M, Cohen E, et al. The use of the urinary anion gap in the diagnosis of hyperchloremic metabolic acidosis. N Engl J Med. 1988;318:594.

Batlle DC, von Riotte A, Schlueter W. Urinary sodium in the evaluation of hyperchloremic metabolic acidosis. N Engl J Med. 1987;316:140.

Buckalew VM Jr, McCurdy DK, Ludwig GD, et al. Incomplete renal tubular acidosis. Physiologic studies in three patients with a defect in lowering urine pH. Am J Med. 1968;45:32.

Dyck RF, Asthana S, Kalra J, et al. A modification of the urine osmolal gap: an improved method for estimating urine ammonium. Am J Nephrol. 1990; 10:359.

Karet FE. Mechanisms in hyperkalemic renal tubular acidosis. J Am Soc Nephrol. 2009;20:251.

Kim GH, Han JS, Kim YS, et al. Evaluation of urine acidification by urine anion gap and urine osmolal gap in chronic metabolic acidosis. Am J Kidney Dis. 1996;27:42.

Kraut JA, Madias NE. Differential diagnosis of nongap metabolic acidosis: value of a systematic approach. Clin J Am Soc Nephrol. 2012;7:671.

Lee Hamm L, Hering-Smith KS, Nakhoul NL. Acid-base and potassium homeostasis. Semin Nephrol. 2013;33:257.

Levy B. Lactate and shock state: the metabolic view. Curr Opin Crit Care. 2006;12:315.

Madias NE. Lactic acidosis. Kidney Int. 1986;29:752.

Meregalli P, Lüthy C, Oetliker OH, Bianchetti MG. Modified urine osmolal gap: an accurate method for estimating the urinary ammonium concentration? Nephron. 1995;69:98.

Mikkelsen ME, Miltiades AN, Gaieski DF, et al. Serum lactate is associated with mortality in severe sepsis independent of organ failure and shock. Crit Care Med. 2009;37:1670.

Oh M, Carroll HJ. Value and determinants of urine anion gap. Nephron. 2002;90:252.

Rastegar M, Nagami GT. Non-anion gap metabolic acidosis: a clinical approach to evaluation. Am J Kidney Dis. 2017;69:296.

Rodríguez Soriano J. Renal tubular acidosis: the clinical entity. J Am Soc Nephrol. 2002;13:2160.

CASE 47

A 44-year-old male patient with coronary artery disease, tobacco abuse, HTN, and back pain presents to the emergency department from home with altered mental status. His wife reports that he fell recently while doing yardwork. He has a history of peptic ulcer disease and never uses NSAIDs. He has an allergy to acetaminophen. He is afebrile, with RR 30, HR 112, BP 110/70, and Sao_2 99% on RA.

Laboratory data.			
ABGs		Basic Metabolic Panel	
pH	7.51	Na	140 mEq/L
$Paco_2$	22 mm Hg	K	4 mEq/L
Pao_2	100 mm Hg	Cl	104 mEq/L
HCO_3	17 mEq/L	CO_2	17 mEq/L
		BUN	21 mg/dL
		Cr	1 mg/dL
		Glucose	100 mg/dL
		Albumin	4.0 g/dL
		EtOH	0 mg/dL

QUESTIONS

Q47-1: Define the patient's baseline acid-base status: Does this patient have an underlying chronic acid-base disorder that we need to account for in order to appropriately interpret the acute acid-base disorders?

A. There is no evidence for an underlying chronic respiratory or metabolic acid-base disorder in this patient, so we would assume a baseline $Paco_2$ of 40 mm Hg and an HCO_3 of 24 mEq/L.

B. While the patient has a condition predisposing him to a chronic acid-base disorder, there is insufficient information to estimate the patient's baseline $Paco_2$ and HCO_3 values; therefore, we will assume a baseline $Paco_2$ of 40 mm Hg and a baseline HCO_3 of 24 mEq/L.

C. The patient has an underlying acid-base condition, and we have sufficient information to estimate the patient's baseline $Paco_2$ and HCO_3 values.

Q47-2: What is/are the primary acid-base disturbance(s) occurring in this case?

A. Metabolic acidosis only
B. Respiratory acidosis only
C. Metabolic acidosis and a respiratory acidosis
D. Metabolic alkalosis and a respiratory alkalosis
E. Metabolic alkalosis only
F. Respiratory alkalosis only

Q47-3: The patient has an HCO_3 of 17 mEq/L. How would you classify the metabolic acidosis that is present?

A. Anion gap acidosis
B. Non-anion gap acidosis
C. Anion and non-anion gap acidosis
D. Anion gap acidosis and a metabolic alkalosis
E. There is appropriate metabolic compensation for the respiratory alkalosis

Q47-4: Laboratory testing returns the following results:

Serum EtOH	< 3 mg/dL
Serum acetaminophen level	< 5 mg/dL (ULN for therapeutic use 20 mg/dL)
Serum osmolality	298 mOsm/kg
Serum L-lactate	2.9 mmol/L (ULN 2.0 mmol/L venous)
Beta-hydroxybutyrate (acetone)	0.41 mmol/L (ULN 0.18 mmol/L)
Serum glucose	100 mg/dL

What is the most likely cause of the patient's acid-base disorder?

A. Acetaminophen overdose
B. Aspirin overdose
C. Opioid overdose
D. Benzodiazepine overdose
E. Toluene exposure
F. Aminoglycoside exposure

Q47-5: Now, assume the patient's respiratory alkalosis is chronic rather than the acute condition we considered earlier (remember, chronic aspirin toxicity also exists). What serum HCO_3 would you expect if the patient is appropriately compensating for a chronic respiratory alkalosis with $Paco_2$ of 22 mm Hg?

A. 6 mEq/L
B. 13 mEq/L
C. 17 mEq/L
D. 21 mEq/L
E. 28 mEq/L
F. 35 mEq/L

ANSWERS

Q47-1: A

There is no evidence for an underlying chronic respiratory or metabolic acid-base disorder in this patient, so we would assume a baseline $Paco_2$ of 40 mm Hg and an HCO_3 of 24 mEq/L.

Rationale: Ignoring these underlying chronic acid-base disorders can significantly alter the interpretation of a patient's acute acid-base status. This was demonstrated in the first case of the series. However, often, we do not have the necessary information (eg, prior ABG or VBG, or prior serum chemistry with an HCO_3) and are forced to assume the ongoing processes are all acute in nature. We are primarily concerned about chronic respiratory acid-base disorders, as these can significantly alter the patient's baseline or expected values for the serum HCO_3 and $Paco_2$, and we have reliable equations to predict the expected baseline values. The respiratory compensation for both chronic metabolic acidosis and alkalosis is generally poor, so there are no equations or rules to predict what the $Paco_2$ should be in these cases. While the baseline serum HCO_3 may be significantly off from our standard value of 24 mEq/L in these patients, we would assume a baseline $Paco_2$ of 40 mm Hg in patients with chronic metabolic processes. Once we identify the patient's baseline $Paco_2$ and HCO_3 values, we will need to use these values in the appropriate equations to identify the ongoing acute processes.

Q47-2: F

Respiratory alkalosis only.

Rationale:

1. The pH is 7.51; therefore, the primary disorder is an **alkalosis.**
2. The $Paco_2$ of 22 mm Hg is less than 40 mm Hg, so there is a **respiratory alkalosis.**
3. The HCO_3 of 17 is less than 24, so there is **no metabolic alkalosis present.**

Q47-3: A

Anion gap acidosis only.

Rationale:

1. Is there evidence for a chronic acid-base disorder that requires adjustment of the patient's "normal" HCO_3? No, there is no evidence for a chronic acid-base disorder, so we would assume a baseline $Paco_2$ of 40 mm Hg and an HCO_3 of 24 mEq/L.
2. Next, we need to determine if the reduction in the HCO_3 is simply an appropriate metabolic compensation, or if there is a concomitant metabolic acid-base disorder.

Metabolic Compensation for Acute Respiratory Alkalosis:

Expected HCO_3 = Baseline HCO_3 − (0.20) [Actual $Paco_2$ − Baseline $Paco_2$]
Expected HCO_3 = 24 mEq/L − (0.20) * [40 mm Hg − 22 mm Hg] = 20.5 mEq/L

Since the serum HCO_3 is less than 20 mEq/L, a concomitant metabolic acidosis is present.

3. Expected anion gap:

$$\text{Expected Anion Gap} = 12 - (2.5) * \left[4.0 \frac{g}{dL} - \text{Actual Serum Albumin} \right]$$

$$= 12 - (2.5 * [4.0 - 4.0])$$
$$= 12 - (2.5 * [0]) = \textbf{12 mEq/L.}$$

4. Anion gap calculation:

$$\text{Serum Anion Gap} = [Na^+] - [HCO_3^-] - [Cl^-]$$
$$= 140 - (104 + 17) = \textbf{19 mEq/L,} \text{ which is } > 12 \text{ mEq/L}$$
$$\rightarrow \textbf{anion gap acidosis is present.}$$

5. Delta-delta calculation:

$$\Delta\Delta = \frac{(\text{Actual Anion Gap} - \text{Expected Anion Gap})}{(\text{Baseline } HCO_3 - \text{Actual } HCO_3)}$$

$$= (19 - 12)/(24 - 17) = 7/7, \textbf{ which is 1.0.}$$

Delta-Delta interpretation.	
Delta-Delta Value	Condition Present
< 0.4	Non-anion gap only
0.4–0.9	Anion gap *and* non-anion gap acidosis
1.0–2.0	**Anion gap acidosis only**
> 2.0	Anion gap acidosis and metabolic alkalosis

Q47-4: B
Aspirin overdose.

Rationale: The patient's respiratory alkalosis and anion gap acidosis is a classic presentation of aspirin toxicity. The acetaminophen level is negative. The serum lactate and ketones can be elevated in salicylate toxicity as a result of aspirin interfering with normal metabolic pathways. The calculated serum osmolality is as follows:

$$\text{Calculated Serum Osmolality} = 2 * [Na^+] + \frac{[Glucose]}{18} + \frac{[BUN]}{2.8} + \frac{[EtOH]}{3.7}$$

$$= 2 * [140] + [100/18] + [21/2.8] = 293 \text{ mOsm/L}$$

$$\text{Serum Osmolal Gap (SOG)} = \text{Measured Serum Osmolality} - \text{Calculated Serum Osmolality}$$

$$\text{SOG} = 298 \text{ mOsm/L} - 293 = (+5) \text{ mOsm/L;}$$
$$\text{therefore, there is no serum osmolal gap.}$$

Opioid and benzodiazepine overdose as associated with respiratory acidosis, while toluene toxicity is associated with either an anion gap or non-anion gap metabolic acidosis. Aminoglycoside exposure is associated with a non-anion gap acidosis or a metabolic alkalosis. The only options listed for this question that can explain the abnormalities in this case is aspirin toxicity.

Q47-5: C
17 mEq/L.

Rationale: If the patient had a *chronic* respiratory alkalosis, the expected compensatory drop in the HCO_3 is calculated as follows:

$$\text{Expected } HCO_3 = \text{Baseline } HCO_3 + (0.4) [\text{Actual } Paco_2 - \text{Baseline } Paco_2]$$
$$= 24 - [(40 - 22) * 0.4] = 24 - (18 * 0.4) = 24 - 7 = \mathbf{17 \text{ mm Hg}.}$$

Chronic aspirin toxicity can present in a similar manner to acute toxicity, or the symptoms may be milder in nature. Patients with chronic salicylate toxicity may also have salicylate levels in the therapeutic range.

References

Eichenholz A, Mulhausen RO, Redleaf PS. Nature of acid-base disturbance in salicylate intoxication. Metabolism. 1963;12:164.

Fertel BS, Nelson LS, Goldfarb DS. The underutilization of hemodialysis in patients with salicylate poisoning. Kidney Int. 2009;75:1349.

Gabow PA, Anderson RJ, Potts DE, Schrier RW. Acid-base disturbances in the salicylate-intoxicated adult. Arch Intern Med. 1978;138:1481.

Hill JB. Salicylate intoxication. N Engl J Med. 1973;288:1110.

Karsh J. Adverse reactions and interactions with aspirin. Considerations in the treatment of the elderly patient. Drug Saf. 1990;5:317.

Temple AR. Acute and chronic effects of aspirin toxicity and their treatment. Arch Intern Med. 1981;141:364.

Thisted B, Krantz T, Strøom J, Sørensen MB. Acute salicylate self-poisoning in 177 consecutive patients treated in ICU. Acta Anaesthesiol Scand. 1987;31:312.

CASE 48

A 43-year-old man with HTN, obesity, IDDM, and possibly early diabetic nephropathy presents with nausea, emesis, and chest pain of 3 days' duration. He has a troponin level of 0.66 ng/mL and a CK-MB of 22 IU/L, with a normal serum CK (CK-MB% is 8%). The patient's vital signs are T 35.9°C, RR 28, HR 120, BP 108/66, Sao_2 97% on room air. He is warm and dry on examination. The CXR is clear. His point-of-care blood glucose is > 600 mg/dL. He is interactive but falls asleep easily when not stimulated. His abdominal examination reveals mild tenderness to palpation without rebound or guarding. He denies chest pain.

Laboratory data.			
ABGs		Basic Metabolic Panel	
pH	7.02	Na	131 mEq/L
$Paco_2$	20 mm Hg	K	5.6 mEq/L
Pao_2	100 mm Hg	Cl	70 mEq/L
HCO_3	6 mEq/L	CO_2	5 mEq/L
		BUN	22 mg/dL
		Cr	1 mg/dL
		Glucose	688 mg/dL
		Albumin	4.0 g/dL
		EtOH	0 mg/dL

QUESTIONS

Q48-1: Define the patient's baseline acid-base status: Does this patient have an underlying chronic acid-base disorder that we need to account for in order to appropriately interpret the acute acid-base disorders?

A. There is no evidence for an underlying chronic respiratory or metabolic acid-base disorder in this patient, so we would assume a baseline $Paco_2$ of 40 mm Hg and an HCO_3 of 24 mEq/L.

B. While the patient has a condition predisposing him to a chronic acid-base disorder, there is insufficient information to estimate the patient's baseline $Paco_2$ and HCO_3 values; therefore, we will assume a baseline $Paco_2$ of 40 mm Hg and a baseline HCO_3 of 24 mEq/L.

C. The patient has an underlying acid-base condition, and we have sufficient information to estimate the patient's baseline $Paco_2$ and HCO_3 values.

Q48-2: What is/are the primary acid-base disturbance(s) occurring in this case?

A. Metabolic acidosis only
B. Respiratory acidosis only
C. Metabolic acidosis and a respiratory acidosis
D. Metabolic alkalosis and a respiratory alkalosis
E. Metabolic alkalosis only
F. Respiratory alkalosis only

Q48-3: The patient has an HCO_3 of 5 mEq/L. How would you classify the metabolic acidosis that is present?

A. Anion gap acidosis
B. Non-anion gap acidosis
C. Anion and non-anion gap acidosis
D. Anion gap acidosis and a metabolic alkalosis

Q48-4: Does the patient in this case demonstrate appropriate respiratory or metabolic compensation?

A. Yes, the respiratory compensation is appropriate.
B. No, a concomitant respiratory alkalosis is present.
C. No, a concomitant respiratory acidosis is present.
D. Yes, the metabolic compensation is appropriate.
E. No, a concomitant metabolic acidosis is present.
F. No, a concomitant metabolic alkalosis is present.

Q48-5: The patient's serum osmolality is measured at 310 mOsm/L. What test would you order next to determine the cause of the patient's anion gap acidosis?

A. Serum lactate
B. Serum phosphorus
C. Urine drug screen
D. Serum beta-hydroxybutyrate (BHA) and acetone
E. Serum toluene level
F. Urine osmolarity
G. Urine anion gap

Q48-6: The urine electrolytes are as follows:

Urine Na	10 mEq/L
Urine K	21 mEq/L
Urine Cl	6 mEq/L
Urine pH	5.5

What is the most likely cause of the patient's metabolic alkalosis?

A. Hyperemesis
B. Bartter syndrome
C. Liddle syndrome
D. Hyperaldosteronism

ANSWERS

Q48-1: B

While the patient has a condition (diabetic nephropathy) predisposing him to a chronic acid-base disorder, there is insufficient information to estimate the patient's baseline $Paco_2$ and HCO_3 values; therefore, we will assume a baseline $Paco_2$ of 40 mm Hg and a baseline HCO_3 of 24 mEq/L.

Rationale: Ignoring these underlying chronic acid-base disorders can significantly alter the interpretation of a patient's acute acid-base status. This was demonstrated in the first case of the series. However, often, we do not have the necessary information (eg, prior ABG or VBG, or prior serum chemistry with a HCO_3) and are forced to assume the ongoing processes are all acute in nature. We are primarily concerned about chronic respiratory acid-base disorders, as these can significantly alter the patient's baseline or expected values for the serum HCO_3 and $Paco_2$, and we have reliable equations to predict the expected baseline values. The respiratory compensation for both chronic metabolic acidosis and alkalosis is generally poor, so there are no equations or rules to predict what the $Paco_2$ should be in these cases. While the baseline serum HCO_3 may be significantly off from our standard value of 24 mEq/L in these patients, we would assume a baseline $Paco_2$ of 40 mm Hg in patients with chronic metabolic processes. Once we identify the patient's baseline $Paco_2$ and HCO_3 values, we will need to use these values in the appropriate equations to identify the ongoing acute processes.

Q48-2: A

Metabolic acidosis only.

Rationale:

1. The pH is 7.02; therefore, the primary disorder is an **acidosis**.
2. The $Paco_2$ of 20 mm Hg is less than 40 mm Hg, so **respiratory acidosis is not the primary issue.**
3. The HCO_3 of 5 mEq/L is less than 24 mEq/L, so there is **a metabolic acidosis.**

Q48-3: D

Anion gap acidosis and a metabolic alkalosis.

Rationale:

1. Is there evidence for a chronic acid-base disorder that requires adjustment of the patient's "normal" HCO_3? No, there is no evidence for a chronic acid-base disorder, so we would assume a baseline $Paco_2$ of 40 mm Hg and an HCO_3 of 24 mEq/L.

2. Expected anion gap:

$$\text{Expected Anion Gap} = 12 - (2.5) * \left[4.0\,\frac{g}{dL} - \text{Actual Serum Albumin} \right]$$
$$= 12 - (2.5 * [4.0 - 4.0])$$
$$= 12 - (2.5 * [0]) = \textbf{12 mEq/L.}$$

3. Anion gap calculation:

$$\text{Serum Anion Gap} = [\text{Na}^+] - [\text{HCO}_3^-] - [\text{Cl}^-]$$
$$= 131 - (70 + 5) = \textbf{56 mEq/L,} \text{ which is} > 12 \text{ mEq/L}$$
$$\rightarrow \textbf{anion gap acidosis is present.}$$

4. Delta-delta calculation:

$$\Delta\Delta = \frac{(\text{Actual Anion Gap} - \text{Expected Anion Gap})}{(\text{Baseline HCO}_3 - \text{Actual HCO}_3)}$$
$$= (56 - 12)/(24 - 5) = \textbf{44/19, which is} \sim \textbf{2.3.}$$

Delta-delta interpretation.	
Delta-Delta Value	Condition Present
< 0.4	Non-anion gap only
0.4–0.9	Anion gap *and* non-anion gap acidosis
1.0–2.0	Anion gap acidosis only
> 2.0	**Anion gap acidosis and metabolic alkalosis**

Q48-4: C
No, a concomitant respiratory acidosis is present.

Rationale: Using the Winter formula, one can calculate what the expected arterial Paco_2 should be for a given serum HCO_3 if the patient were completely compensated.

Respiratory Compensation for Acute Metabolic Acidosis (Winter Formula):

$$\text{Expected Paco}_2 = 1.5 * [\text{Actual HCO}_3] + 8 \pm 2 \text{ (in mm Hg)}$$
$$= (1.5 * 5) + 8 = 7.5 + 8 = 15.5 \pm 2 = \textbf{(14 to 18) mm Hg.}$$

This patient's Paco_2 of 20 mm Hg is **higher** than the expected range, and therefore a concomitant **respiratory acidosis** exists.

Q48-5: D
Serum beta-hydroxybutyrate (BHA) and acetone.

Rationale: The patient's presentation is most consistent with DKA. Acute coronary syndrome is a known precipitator of DKA and is the likely cause here. The normal BP with a warm and dry patient is not consistent with heart failure that would cause a lactic acidosis (nor is it entirely consistent with sepsis as a cause). There is nothing in the vignette to suggest drug toxicity, and the serum osmolal gap is normal at +2 mOsm/L. The urine osmolality and the urine anion gap are not helpful here.

$$\text{Calculated Serum Osmolality} = 2 * [\text{Na}^+] + \frac{[\text{Glucose}]}{18} + \frac{[\text{BUN}]}{2.8} + \frac{[\text{EtOH}]}{3.7}$$
$$= 2 * [131] + [688/18] + [22/2.8] + [0/3.7]$$
$$= 308 \text{ mOsm/L.}$$

$$\text{Serum Osmolal Gap (SOG)} = \text{Measured Serum Osmolality}$$
$$- \text{Calculated Serum Osmolality}$$
$$\text{SOG} = 310 - 308 \text{ mOsm/L} = (+2) \text{ mOsm/L,}$$
which is < 10 Osm/L, so this is normal.

Q48-6: A
Hyperemesis.

Rationale: The urine Cl is less than 10, consistent with a chloride-responsive metabolic alkalosis (hyperemesis, post-hypercapnic diuresis, diuretic therapy, contraction). The remaining answers are associated with a chloride-resistant metabolic alkalosis.

Causes of metabolic alkalosis.
History: Rule Out the Following as Causes
• Alkali load ("milk-alkali" or calcium-alkali syndrome, oral sodium bicarbonate, IV sodium bicarbonate)   • Genetic causes (CF)   • Presence of hypercalcemia   • IV β-lactam antibiotics   • Laxative abuse (may also cause a metabolic acidosis depending on diarrheal HCO_3 losses)
If None of the Above, Then. . .
Urine Chloride < 20 mEq/L (Chloride-Responsive Causes)   • Loss of gastric acid (hyperemesis, NGT suctioning)   • Prior diuretic use (in hours to days following discontinuation)   • Post-hypercapnia   • Villous adenoma   • Congenital chloridorrhea   • Chronic laxative abuse (may also cause a metabolic acidosis depending on diarrheal HCO_3 losses)   • CF
OR
Urine Chloride > 20 mEq/L (Chloride-Resistant Causes)
Urine Chloride > 20 mEq/L, Lack of HTN, Urine Potassium < 30 mEq/L
• Hypokalemia or hypomagnesemia   • Laxative abuse (if dominated by hypokalemia)   • Bartter syndrome   • Gitelman syndrome
Urine Chloride > 20 mEq/L, Lack of HTN, Urine Potassium > 30 mEq/L
• Current diuretic use

(Continued)

Causes of metabolic alkalosis. (*continued*)
Urine Chloride > 20 mEq/L, Presence of HTN, Urine Potassium Variable but Usually > 30 mEq/L
Elevated plasma renin level: • Renal artery stenosis   • Renin-secreting tumor   • Renovascular disease
Low plasma renin, low plasma aldosterone: • Cushing syndrome   • Exogenous mineralocorticoid use   • Genetic disorder (11-hydoxylase or 17-hydrolyase deficiency, 11β-HSD deficiency)   • Liddle syndrome   • Licorice toxicity
Low plasma renin, high plasma aldosterone: • Primary hyperaldosteronism   • Adrenal adenoma   • Bilateral adrenal hyperplasia

References

Abreo K, Adlakha A, Kilpatrick S, et al. The milk-alkali syndrome. A reversible form of acute renal failure. Arch Intern Med. 1993;153:1005.

Arroliga AC, Shehab N, McCarthy K, Gonzales JP. Relationship of continuous infusion lorazepam to serum propylene glycol concentration in critically ill adults. Crit Care Med. 2004;32:1709.

Barton CH, Vaziri ND, Ness RL, et al. Cimetidine in the management of metabolic alkalosis induced by nasogastric drainage. Arch Surg. 1979;114:70.

Bear R, Goldstein M, Phillipson E, et al. Effect of metabolic alkalosis on respiratory function in patients with chronic obstructive lung disease. Can Med Assoc J. 1977;117:900.

Braden GL, Strayhorn CH, Germain MJ, et al. Increased osmolal gap in alcoholic acidosis. Arch Intern Med. 1993;153:2377.

DeFronzo RA, Matzuda M, Barret E. Diabetic ketoacidosis: a combined metabolic-nephrologic approach to therapy. Diabetes Rev. 1994;2:209.

Fulop M, Murthy V, Michilli A, et al. Serum beta-hydroxybutyrate measurement in patients with uncontrolled diabetes mellitus. Arch Intern Med. 1999;159:381.

Gabow PA. Ethylene glycol intoxication. Am J Kidney Dis. 1988;11:277.

Galla JH, Gifford JD, Luke RG, Rome L. Adaptations to chloride-depletion alkalosis. Am J Physiol. 1991;261:R771.

Garella S, Chang BS, Kahn SI. Dilution acidosis and contraction alkalosis: review of a concept. Kidney Int. 1975;8:279.

Gennari FJ. Current concepts. Serum osmolality. Uses and limitations. N Engl J Med. 1984;310:102.

Gennari FJ, Weise WJ. Acid-base disturbances in gastrointestinal disease. Clin J Am Soc Nephrol. 2008;3:1861.

Glasser L, Sternglanz PD, Combie J, Robinson A. Serum osmolality and its applicability to drug overdose. Am J Clin Pathol. 1973;60:695.

Hamm LL, Nakhoul N, Hering-Smith KS. Acid-base homeostasis. Clin J Am Soc Nephrol. 2015;10:2232.

Hulter HN, Sebastian A, Toto RD, et al. Renal and systemic acid-base effects of the chronic administration of hypercalcemia-producing agents: calcitriol, PTH, and intravenous calcium. Kidney Int. 1982;21:445.

Khanna A, Kurtzman NA. Metabolic alkalosis. J Nephrol. 2006;19(suppl 9):S86.

Kraut JA, Kurtz I. Toxic alcohol ingestions: clinical features, diagnosis, and management. Clin J Am Soc Nephrol. 2008; 3:208.

Kraut JA, Xing SX. Approach to the evaluation of a patient with an increased serum osmolal gap and high-anion-gap metabolic acidosis. Am J Kidney Dis. 2011;58:480.

Laski ME, Sabatini S. Metabolic alkalosis, bedside and bench. Semin Nephrol. 2006;26:404.

Luke RG, Galla JH. It is chloride depletion alkalosis, not contraction alkalosis. J Am Soc Nephrol. 2012;23:204.

Lynd LD, Richardson KJ, Purssell RA, et al. An evaluation of the osmole gap as a screening test for toxic alcohol poisoning. BMC Emerg Med. 2008;8:5.

Marraffa JM, Holland MG, Stork CM, et al. Diethylene glycol: widely used solvent presents serious poisoning potential. J Emerg Med. 2008;35:401.

Miller PD, Berns AS. Acute metabolic alkalosis perpetuating hypercarbia. A role for acetazolamide in chronic obstructive pulmonary disease. JAMA. 1977;238:2400.

Oster JR, Materson BJ, Rogers AI. Laxative abuse syndrome. Am J Gastroenterol. 1980;74:451.

Patel AM, Goldfarb S. Got calcium? Welcome to the calcium-alkali syndrome. J Am Soc Nephrol. 2010; 21:1440.

Porter WH, Yao HH, Karounos DG. Laboratory and clinical evaluation of assays for beta-hydroxybutyrate. Am J Clin Pathol. 1997;107:353.

Purssell RA, Pudek M, Brubacher J, Abu-Laban RB. Derivation and validation of a formula to calculate the contribution of ethanol to the osmolal gap. Ann Emerg Med. 2001;38:653.

Robinson AG, Loeb JN. Ethanol ingestion–commonest cause of elevated plasma osmolality? N Engl J Med. 1971;284:1253.

Rose BD, Post TW. Clinical Physiology of Acid-Base and Electrolyte Disorders. 5e. New York, NY: McGraw Hill; 2001:559, 809–815.

Schelling JR, Howard RL, Winter SD, Linas SL. Increased osmolal gap in alcoholic ketoacidosis and lactic acidosis. Ann Intern Med. 1990;113:580.

Schwartz WB, Van Ypersele de Strihou, Kassirer JP. Role of anions in metabolic alkalosis and potassium deficiency. N Engl J Med. 1968;279:630.

Shen T, Braude S. Changes in serum phosphate during treatment of diabetic ketoacidosis: predictive significance of severity of acidosis on presentation. Intern Med J. 2012;42:1347.

Sweetser LJ, Douglas JA, Riha RL, Bell SC. Clinical presentation of metabolic alkalosis in an adult patient with cystic fibrosis. Respirology. 2005;10:254.

Taki K, Mizuno K, Takahashi N, Wakusawa R. Disturbance of CO2 elimination in the lungs by carbonic anhydrase inhibition. Jpn J Physiol. 1986;36:523.

Turban S, Beutler KT, Morris RG, et al. Long-term regulation of proximal tubule acid-base transporter abundance by angiotensin II. Kidney Int. 2006;70:660.

Wachtel TJ, Tetu-Mouradjian LM, Goldman DL, et al. Hyperosmolarity and acidosis in diabetes mellitus: a three-year experience in Rhode Island. J Gen Intern Med. 1991;6:495.

CASE 49

A 60-year-old man who has COPD that requires use of multiple inhalers, HTN, GERD, peptic ulcer disease, HTN (for which he takes hydrochlorothiazide), and CKD is brought to the clinic by his son because of altered mental status. The patient is taking amlodipine at home. He is supposed to take omeprazole for GERD, but his son notes that he often takes OTC antacids instead because they provide "instant relief" of his symptoms and the other medication takes several days to take effect. The patient's vital signs are T 37.9°C, RR 9, HR 88, BP 129/77, and Sao$_2$ 100% on room air. The patient is self-sufficient at baseline, drives, performs his own shopping, and cooks for himself 4 to 5 nights a week. At his last primary care visit, 2 months ago, his serum HCO$_3$ was 24 mEq/L on a basic metabolic panel.

Laboratory data.			
ABGs		**Basic Metabolic Panel**	
pH	7.63	Na	139 mEq/L
Paco$_2$	48 mm Hg	K	4.4 mEq/L
Pao$_2$	100 mm Hg	Cl	87 mEq/L
HCO$_3$	48 mEq/L	CO$_2$	49 mEq/L
		BUN	108 mg/dL
		Cr	5.5 mg/dL
		Glucose	88 mg/dL
		Albumin	4.0 g/dL
		EtOH	0 mg/dL

QUESTIONS

Q49-1: Define the patient's baseline acid-base status: Does this patient have an underlying chronic acid-base disorder that we need to account for in order to appropriately interpret the acute acid-base disorders?

A. There is no evidence for an underlying chronic respiratory or metabolic acid-base disorder in this patient, so we would assume a baseline $Paco_2$ of 40 mm Hg and an HCO_3 of 24 mEq/L.

B. While the patient has a condition predisposing him to a chronic acid-base disorder, there is insufficient information to estimate the patient's baseline $Paco_2$ and HCO_3 values; therefore, we will assume a baseline $Paco_2$ of 40 mm Hg and a baseline HCO_3 of 24 mEq/L.

C. The patient has an underlying acid-base condition, and we have sufficient information to estimate the patient's baseline $Paco_2$ and HCO_3 values.

Q49-2: What is/are the primary acid-base disturbance(s) occurring in this case?

A. Metabolic acidosis only
B. Respiratory acidosis only
C. Metabolic acidosis and a respiratory acidosis
D. Metabolic alkalosis and a respiratory alkalosis
E. Metabolic alkalosis only
F. Respiratory alkalosis only

Q49-3: Does the patient in this case demonstrate appropriate respiratory or metabolic compensation? (For this question, assume an acute metabolic alkalosis.)

A. Yes, the respiratory compensation is appropriate.
B. No, a concomitant respiratory alkalosis is present.
C. No, a concomitant respiratory acidosis is present.
D. Yes, the metabolic compensation is appropriate.
E. No, a concomitant metabolic acidosis is present.
F. No, a concomitant metabolic alkalosis is present.

Q49-4: Laboratory testing returns the following results:

Urine Na	20 mEq/L
Urine K	5 mEq/L
Urine Cl	33 mEq/L
Serum calcium	13.4 mg/dL(ULN 10.0 mg/dL)
Serum cortisol	23 mcg/dL (normal range: 7–28)
Serum PTH	< 5 pg/mL (normal range: 10–65)
Serum TSH	Normal

What is the most likely cause of the patient's acid-base disorder?

A. Diuretic therapy
B. Contraction alkalosis
C. Hyperemesis
D. Aspirin overdose
E. Amphotericin exposure
F. Milk-alkali syndrome

ANSWERS

Q49-1: B

While the patient has a condition predisposing him to a chronic acid-base disorder, there is insufficient information to estimate the patient's baseline $Paco_2$ and HCO_3 values; therefore, we will assume a baseline $Paco_2$ of 40 mm Hg and a baseline HCO_3 of 24 mEq/L. This patient has COPD and CKD, which can both be associated with chronic acid-base disorders. The only collateral history that is provided is that a recent serum HCO_3 is 24 mEq/L. Therefore, we will assume that at baseline this patient has a serum HCO_3 of 24 mEq/L. Without a recent blood gas to further define the patient's "baseline," we are therefore left to assume that the patient has a $Paco_2$ of 40 mm Hg as well.

Rationale: Ignoring these underlying chronic acid-base disorders can significantly alter the interpretation of a patient's acute acid-base status. This was demonstrated in the first case of the series. However, often, we do not have the necessary information (eg, prior ABG or VBG, or prior serum chemistry with an HCO_3) and are forced to assume the ongoing processes are all acute in nature. We are primarily concerned about chronic respiratory acid-base disorders, as these can significantly alter the patient's baseline or expected values for the serum HCO_3 and $Paco_2$, and we have reliable equations to predict the expected baseline values. The respiratory compensation for both chronic metabolic acidosis and alkalosis is generally poor, so there are no equations or rules to predict what the $Paco_2$ should be in these cases. While the baseline serum HCO_3 may be significantly off from our standard value of 24 mEq/L in these patients, we would assume a baseline $Paco_2$ of 40 mm Hg in patients with chronic metabolic processes. Once we identify the patient's baseline $Paco_2$ and HCO_3 values, we will need to use these values in the appropriate equations to identify the ongoing acute processes.

Q49-2: E

Metabolic alkalosis only.

Rationale:

1. The pH is 7.63; therefore, the primary disorder is an **alkalosis.**
2. The $Paco_2$ of 48 mm Hg is greater than 40 mm Hg, so **no respiratory alkalosis is present.**
3. The HCO_3 of 49 mEq/L is greater than 24 mEq/L, so there is a **metabolic alkalosis.**

Q49-3: B

No, a concomitant respiratory alkalosis is also present.

Rationale: For an acute metabolic alkalosis, the expected $Paco_2$ is calculated as follows:

Respiratory Compensation for Acute Metabolic Alkalosis:

$$\text{Expected } Paco_2 = \text{Baseline } Paco_2 - (0.7) [\text{Actual } HCO_3 - \text{Baseline } HCO_3]$$
$$= 40 + [0.7 * (49 - 24)] = 40 + 0.7 * 25 = \textbf{58 mm Hg.}$$

This patient's $Paco_2$ of 48 mm Hg is **lower** than the expected range and therefore a concomitant **respiratory alkalosis** also exists.

Q49-4: F
Milk-alkali syndrome.

Rationale: The most important factor to consider here is the patient's history, coupled with the hypercalcemia, metabolic alkalosis, and renal impairment. The patient's history includes that he takes many OTC antacids, which commonly contain calcium carbonate. The resultant hypercalcemia is associated with renal artery vasoconstriction, natriuresis, and inhibition of antidiuretic hormone activity, leading to overall volume depletion. This volume depletion stimulates HCO_3 resorption in the proximal tubules. As these solutions/antacids also contain alkali, there is a significant increase in the serum HCO_3. The urine chloride level is not as helpful diagnostically in these cases as it may depend on what other medications the patient is taking or the composition of the antacids themselves. This patient is actively taking a diuretic so the elevated urine chloride is not surprising.

Classically, acute milk-alkali syndrome presents with nausea, emesis, encephalopathy, seizures, and acute renal failure. However, chronic and subacute forms of the syndrome present primarily as renal failure and pruritus. Modern presentations of the disease tend to be more asymptomatic. A significantly elevated serum calcium and undetectable serum PTH are common laboratory findings.

While the patient does have a respiratory alkalosis, there is no concomitant metabolic acidosis to suggest aspirin toxicity as the primary cause of the disorder. The respiratory alkalosis is likely due to complications of acute hypercalcemia

Causes of metabolic alkalosis.
History: Rule Out the Following as Causes
• Alkali load (**"milk-alkali" or calcium-alkali syndrome**, oral sodium bicarbonate, IV sodium bicarbonate) • Genetic causes (CF) • Presence of hypercalcemia • IV β-lactam antibiotics • Laxative abuse (may also cause a metabolic acidosis depending on diarrheal HCO_3 losses)
If None of the Above, Then. . .
Urine Chloride < 20 mEq/L (Chloride-Responsive Causes) • Loss of gastric acid (hyperemesis, NGT suctioning) • Prior diuretic use (in hours to days following discontinuation) • Post-hypercapnia • Villous adenoma • Congenital chloridorrhea • Chronic laxative abuse (may also cause a metabolic acidosis depending on diarrheal HCO_3 losses) • CF

(Continued)

Causes of metabolic alkalosis. (*continued*)
OR
Urine Chloride > 20 mEq/L (Chloride-Resistant Causes)
Urine Chloride > 20 mEq/L, Lack of HTN, Urine Potassium < 30 mEq/L
• Hypokalemia or hypomagnesemia • Laxative abuse (if dominated by hypokalemia) • Bartter syndrome • Gitelman syndrome
Urine Chloride > 20 mEq/L, Lack of HTN, Urine Potassium > 30 mEq/L
• Current diuretic use
Urine Chloride > 20 mEq/L, Presence of HTN, Urine Potassium Variable but Usually > 30 mEq/L
Elevated plasma renin level: • Renal artery stenosis • Renin-secreting tumor • Renovascular disease
Low plasma renin, low plasma aldosterone: • Cushing syndrome • Exogenous mineralocorticoid use • Genetic disorder (11-hydoxylase or 17-hydrolyase deficiency, 11β-HSD deficiency) • Liddle syndrome • Licorice toxicity
Low plasma renin, high plasma aldosterone: • Primary hyperaldosteronism • Adrenal adenoma • Bilateral adrenal hyperplasia

References

Abreo K, Adlakha A, Kilpatrick S, et al. The milk-alkali syndrome. A reversible form of acute renal failure. Arch Intern Med. 1993;153:1005.

Burnett CH, Commons RR. Hypercalcemia without hypercalcuria or hypophosphatemia, calcinosis and renal insufficiency; a syndrome following prolonged intake of milk and alkali. N Engl J Med. 1949;240:787.

Felsenfeld AJ, Levine BS. Milk alkali syndrome and the dynamics of calcium homeostasis. Clin J Am Soc Nephrol. 2006;1:641.

Medarov BI. Milk-alkali syndrome. Mayo Clin Proc. 2009;84:261.

Orwoll ES. The milk-alkali syndrome: current concepts. Ann Intern Med. 1982;97:242.

Patel AM, Goldfarb S. Got calcium? Welcome to the calcium-alkali syndrome. J Am Soc Nephrol. 2010;21:1440.

Picolos MK, Lavis VR, Orlander PR. Milk-alkali syndrome is a major cause of hypercalcaemia among non-end-stage renal disease (non-ESRD) inpatients. Clin Endocrinol (Oxf). 2005;63:566.

CASE 50

A 22-year-old man presents to the emergency department (ED) with encephalopathy and acute renal failure. He has a history of HTN, for which he takes hydrochlorothiazide, and depression and anxiety, for which he was prescribed citalopram and alprazolam (PRN only, for panic attacks). His parents found him unresponsive at home the morning after an unsuccessful job interview. He is tachycardic with T 37.9°C, RR 22, HR 110, BP 90/70 and Sao$_2$ 99% on room air. He is warm and dry on examination. His examination is unremarkable aside from sinus tachycardia and tachypnea. His parents have brought the citalopram and the alprazolam bottles to the ED. The citalopram bottle contains all 30 tablets, but the alprazolam bottle is empty.

Laboratory data.			
ABGs		Basic Metabolic Panel	
pH	6.99	Na	139 mEq/L
Paco$_2$	34 mm Hg	K	3.2 mEq/L
Pao$_2$	100 mm Hg	Cl	79 mEq/L
HCO$_3$	8 mEq/L	CO$_2$	8 mEq/L
		BUN	66 mg/dL
		Cr	3.4 mg/dL
		Glucose	76 mg/dL
		Albumin	4.0 g/dL
		EtOH	0 mg/dL

QUESTIONS

Q50-1: Define the patient's baseline acid-base status: Does this patient have an underlying chronic acid-base disorder that we need to account for in order to appropriately interpret the acute acid-base disorders?

A. There is no evidence for an underlying chronic respiratory or metabolic acid-base disorder in this patient, so we would assume a baseline $Paco_2$ of 40 mm Hg and an HCO_3 of 24 mEq/L.

B. While the patient has a condition predisposing him to a chronic acid-base disorder, there is insufficient information to estimate the patient's baseline $Paco_2$ and HCO_3 values; therefore, we will assume a baseline $Paco_2$ of 40 mm Hg and a baseline HCO_3 of 24 mEq/L.

C. The patient has an underlying acid-base condition, and we have sufficient information to estimate the patient's baseline $Paco_2$ and HCO_3 values.

Q50-2: What is/are the primary acid-base disturbance(s) occurring in this case?

A. Metabolic acidosis only
B. Respiratory acidosis only
C. Metabolic acidosis and a respiratory acidosis
D. Metabolic alkalosis and a respiratory alkalosis
E. Metabolic alkalosis only
F. Respiratory alkalosis only

Q50-3: How would the metabolic acidosis component be classified in this case?

A. Anion gap acidosis
B. Non-anion gap acidosis
C. Anion and non-anion gap acidosis
D. Anion gap acidosis and a metabolic alkalosis

Q50-4: Does the patient in this case demonstrate appropriate respiratory or metabolic compensation?

A. Yes, the respiratory compensation is appropriate.
B. No, a concomitant respiratory alkalosis is present.
C. No, a concomitant respiratory acidosis is present.
D. Yes, the metabolic compensation is appropriate.
E. No, a concomitant metabolic acidosis is present.
F. No, a concomitant metabolic alkalosis is present.

Q50-5: Laboratory testing returns the following results:

Serum EtOH	< 3 mg/dL
Serum acetaminophen level	< 5 mg/dL (ULN for therapeutic use 20 mg/dL)
Serum salicylates level	< 5 mg/dL (ULN for therapeutic use 30 mg/dL)
Serum osmolality	334 mOsm/kg
Serum L-lactate	2.2 mmol/L (ULN 2.0 mmol/L venous)
Beta-hydroxybutyrate (acetone)	< 0.18 mmol/L (ULN 0.18 mmol/L)
Serum glucose	76 mg/dL
Serum phosphorus	5.6 mg/dL (ULN 4.5 mg/dL)
Urine drug screen	Positive for opioids, benzodiazepines

What is the likely cause of the patient's anion gap acidosis?

A. Lactic acidosis
B. Organic alcohol intoxication
C. Acetaminophen toxicity
D. Aspirin toxicity
E. Opioid overdose
F. Benzodiazepine overdose
G. Alcoholic ketoacidosis

Q50-6: The patient's ICU care nurse reports she is finding precipitates in the patient's Foley catheter bag and examination shows these are consistent with crystal formation. Which organic alcohol did this patient most likely consume?

A. Ethylene glycol
B. Isopropyl alcohol
C. Methyl alcohol (methanol)
D. Ethanol

Q50-7: What is the likely cause of the respiratory acidosis?

A. Citalopram overdose
B. Aspirin overdose
C. Acetaminophen overdose
D. Illicit drug (benzodiazepine, opioid) overdose

Q50-8: You suspect the patient's metabolic alkalosis is related to hyperemesis. Which of the following would you suspect is true of the patient's laboratory studies?

A. Urine sodium less than 10 mEq/L
B. Urine chloride less than 20 mEq/L
C. Urine anion gap less than −20 mEq/L
D. Urine anion gap greater than 10 mEq/L
E. Fractional excretion of HCO_3 greater than 15%
F. Fractional excretion of urea greater than 50%

ANSWERS

Q50-1: A

There is no evidence for an underlying chronic respiratory or metabolic acid-base disorder in this patient, so we would assume a baseline $Paco_2$ of 40 mm Hg and an HCO_3 of 24 mEq/L.

Rationale: Ignoring these underlying chronic acid-base disorders can significantly alter the interpretation of a patient's acute acid-base status. This was demonstrated in the first case of the series. However, often, we do not have the necessary information (eg, prior ABG or VBG, or prior serum chemistry with an HCO_3) and are forced to assume the ongoing processes are all acute in nature. We are primarily concerned about chronic respiratory acid-base disorders, as these can significantly alter the patient's baseline or expected values for the serum HCO_3 and $Paco_2$, and we have reliable equations to predict the expected baseline values. The respiratory compensation for both chronic metabolic acidosis and alkalosis is generally poor, so there are no equations or rules to predict what the $Paco_2$ should be in these cases. While the baseline serum HCO_3 may be significantly off from our standard value of 24 mEq/L in these patients, we would assume a baseline $Paco_2$ of 40 mm Hg in patients with chronic metabolic processes. Once we identify the patient's baseline $Paco_2$ and HCO_3 values, we will need to use these values in the appropriate equations to identify the ongoing acute processes.

Q50-2: A

Metabolic acidosis only.

Rationale:

1. The pH is 6.99; therefore, the primary disorder is an **acidosis.**
2. The $Paco_2$ of 34 mm Hg is less than 40 mm Hg, so a **primary respiratory issue is not likely.**
3. The HCO_3 of 8 mEq/L is less than 24 mEq/L, so there is **a metabolic acidosis.**

Q50-3: D

Anion gap acidosis and a metabolic alkalosis.

Rationale:

1. Is there evidence for a chronic acid-base disorder that requires adjustment of the patient's "normal" HCO_3? No, there is no evidence for a chronic acid-base disorder, so we would assume a baseline $Paco_2$ of 40 mm Hg and an HCO_3 of 24 mEq/L.
2. Expected anion gap:

$$\text{Expected Anion Gap} = 12 - (2.5) * \left[4.0 \frac{g}{dL} - \text{Actual Serum Albumin} \right]$$
$$= 12 - (2.5 * [4.0 - 4.0])$$
$$= 12 - (2.5 * [0]) = \mathbf{12\ mEq/L.}$$

3. Anion gap calculation:

$$Serum\ Anion\ Gap = [Na^+] - [HCO_3^-] - [Cl^-]$$
$$= 139 - (79 + 8) = \textbf{52 mEq/L,}\ which\ is > 12\ mEq/L$$
$$\rightarrow \textbf{anion gap acidosis is present.}$$

4. Delta-delta calculation:

$$\Delta\Delta = \frac{(Actual\ Anion\ Gap - Expected\ Anion\ Gap)}{(Baseline\ HCO_3 - Actual\ HCO_3)}$$
$$= (52 - 12)/(24 - 8) = \textbf{40/16 = 2.5.}$$

Delta-delta interpretation.	
Delta-Delta Value	Condition Present
< 0.4	Non-anion gap only
0.4–0.9	Anion gap AND non-anion gap acidosis
1.0–2.0	Anion gap acidosis only
> 2.0	**Anion gap acidosis and metabolic alkalosis**

Q50-4: C
No, a concomitant respiratory acidosis is present.

Rationale: Using the Winter formula, one can calculate what the expected arterial $Paco_2$ should be for a given serum HCO_3 if the patient were completely compensated.

Respiratory Compensation for Acute Metabolic Acidosis (Winter Formula):

$$Expected\ Paco_2 = 1.5 * [Actual\ HCO_3] + 8 \pm 2\ (in\ mm\ Hg)$$
$$= (1.5 * 8) + 8 = 12 + 8 = 20 \pm 2 = \textbf{(18 to 22) mm Hg.}$$

This patient's $Paco_2$ of 34 mm Hg is **higher** than the expected range and therefore a concomitant **respiratory acidosis** exists.

Q50-5: B
Organic alcohol intoxication.

Rationale: This patient has an elevated anion gap acidosis with an elevated serum osmolal gap. The calculated osmolality is as follows:

$$Calculated\ Serum\ Osmolality = 2 * [Na^+] + \frac{[Glucose]}{18} + \frac{[BUN]}{2.8} + \frac{[EtOH]}{3.7}$$
$$= (139 * 2) + (66/3.4) + (0/3.7) + (76/18)$$
$$= 311\ mOsm/L.$$

The serum osmolal gap is 23, which is greater than 10. Therefore the patient has a positive serum osmolal gap. The following conditions are potential causes of an elevated serum osmolality.

Conditions association with elevated serum osmolality.
With an Elevated Serum Anion Gap
1. Ethanol ingestion with alcohol ketoacidosis (acetone is an unmeasured osmole, in addition to ethanol)—the osmolality is usually elevated more so by the increased ethanol concentration, so the osmolal "gap" depends on whether the term for ethanol is included in the osmolality calculation*
2. Organic alcohol ingestions (methanol, ethylene glycol, diethylene glycol, propylene glycol)
3. DKA—similar to ethanol ingestion, glucose and acetone contribute to the osmolality since the glucose terms is always included in the calculation
4. Salicylate toxicity
5. Renal failure—the BUN is nearly always included in the osmolality, so this is usually accounted for in the equation; however, if one does not include the BUN in the equation for calculated serum osmolality then it would be a potential cause
Without an Elevated Serum Anion Gap
1. Hyperosmolar therapy (mannitol, glycerol)
2. Other organic solvent ingestion (eg, acetone)
3. Isopropyl alcohol ingestion (produces only acetone rather than an organic acid, so no anion gap is seen)
4. Hypertriglyceridemia
5. Hyperproteinemia
*A mildly elevated osmolal gap has been reported in the literature in patients with lactic acidosis in critical illness, particularly severe distributive shock. The pathology is not quite clear, although is likely related to multiorgan failure—particularly the liver and kidneys—and the release of cellular components known to contribute to the osmolal gap). The elevated serum osmolal gap in severe lactic acidosis is typically around 10, although may be as high as 20 to 25 mOsm/L.

This patient also has an anion gap acidosis. Looking through the differential for causes of an elevated serum anion gap with an elevated serum osmolal gap, we can rule out ethanol ingestion, DKA, and salicylate toxicity. Although the patient does have evidence of acute renal failure, we included the term for the BUN in the calculated serum osmolal gap, so this is not likely to be the cause of the osmolal gap (although it is potentially contributing to the serum anion gap). Therefore, an organic alcohol ingestion is most likely, with particular concern for methanol or ethylene glycol. However, it is also possible that the patient has two ongoing processes—one causing an anion gap acidosis (such as renal failure; other ingestion, such as a toluene; or carbon monoxide poisoning) and one causing an isolated serum osmolal gap (such as hypertriglyceridemia or isopropyl alcohol ingestion). Of the possible answers in this case, the most likely culprit (and one of the most morbid if not treated early) would be organic alcohol ingestion. Opioids and benzodiazepine overdose are usually associated with other acid-base disorders.

Q50-6: A
Ethylene glycol.

Rationale: The presentation with an elevated osmolar gap, anion gap acidosis with negative EtOH, and renal failure is most consistent with ethylene glycol. Isopropyl alcohol does not cause an anion gap acidosis. The negative EtOH level rules out ethanol as the primary cause. Methanol is possible, although less likely given the presence of renal failure, which results from crystal formation in the urine, obstructing the collecting system of the nephron. Crystal can often be found in the urine of such patients. Recall that ingestion of methanol is commonly associated with vision changes, whereas isopropyl alcohol ingestion is typically associated with a positive serum ketone study.

Although it would be important to rule out other potential causes or co-ingestions, in this case, immediate treatment for possible ethylene glycol or methanol ingestion should be initiated, including fomepizole and renal replacement therapy.

Q50-7: D
Illicit drug overdose.

Rationale: The patient has a respiratory acidosis, as previously discussed. His drug screen was positive for opioids and benzodiazepines. He is taking a benzodiazepine for his anxiety, but it is still possible he has taken an overdose of his prescribed medication and this has led to his respiratory acidosis. Although benzodiazepine overdose is suspected, we would not use flumazenil here as its use can be associated with acute benzodiazepine withdrawal and seizures, which would further complicate the clinical picture in a patient with suspected organic alcohol ingestion. Opioid use is also associated with suppression of respiratory centers; therefore, appropriate therapy (ie, naloxone) should be initiated.

Q50-8: B
Urine chloride less than 20 mEq/L.

Rationale: Hyperemesis is chloride-responsive form of metabolic alkalosis, so we would expect the urine chloride to be less than 20 mEq/L. However, the patient's diuretic use (hydrochlorothiazide) at baseline could complicate this, and the laboratory result would depend on the patient's last use of the diuretic. A urine sodium of less than 10 mEq/L is used in the evaluation of hepatorenal syndrome. The urine anion gap is useful for the evaluation of a non-anion gap metabolic acidosis. The fractional excretion of HCO_3 is useful for confirming a diagnosis of a proximal (type 2) RTA. The fractional excretion of urea is used in the evaluation of acute renal failure in patients currently using diuretics.

References

Abreo K, Adlakha A, Kilpatrick S, et al. The milk-alkali syndrome. A reversible form of acute renal failure. Arch Intern Med. 1993;153:1005.

Arroliga AC, Shehab N, McCarthy K, Gonzales JP. Relationship of continuous infusion lorazepam to serum propylene glycol concentration in critically ill adults. Crit Care Med. 2004;32:1709.

Barton CH, Vaziri ND, Ness RL, et al. Cimetidine in the management of metabolic alkalosis induced by nasogastric drainage. Arch Surg. 1979;114:70.

Bear R, Goldstein M, Phillipson E, et al. Effect of metabolic alkalosis on respiratory function in patients with chronic obstructive lung disease. Can Med Assoc J. 1977;117:900.

Braden GL, Strayhorn CH, Germain MJ, et al. Increased osmolal gap in alcoholic acidosis. Arch Intern Med. 1993;153:2377.

Carlisle EJ, Donnelly SM, Vasuvattakul S, et al. Glue-sniffing and distal renal tubular acidosis: sticking to the facts. J Am Soc Nephrol. 1991;1:1019.

Church AS, Witting MD. Laboratory testing in ethanol, methanol, ethylene glycol, and isopropanol toxicities. J Emerg Med. 1997;15:687.

Eder AF, Dowdy YG, Gardiner JA, et al. Serum lactate and lactate dehydrogenase in high concentrations interfere in enzymatic assay of ethylene glycol. Clin Chem. 1996;42:1489.

Gabow PA. Ethylene glycol intoxication. Am J Kidney Dis. 1988;11:277.

Galla JH, Gifford JD, Luke RG, Rome L. Adaptations to chloride-depletion alkalosis. Am J Physiol. 1991;261:R771.

Garella S, Chang BS, Kahn SI. Dilution acidosis and contraction alkalosis: review of a concept. Kidney Int. 1975;8:279.

Gennari FJ. Current concepts. Serum osmolality. Uses and limitations. N Engl J Med. 1984;310:102.

Gennari FJ, Weise WJ. Acid-base disturbances in gastrointestinal disease. Clin J Am Soc Nephrol. 2008;3:1861.

Glasser L, Sternglanz PD, Combie J, Robinson A. Serum osmolality and its applicability to drug overdose. Am J Clin Pathol. 1973; 60:695.

Hamm LL, Nakhoul N, Hering-Smith KS. Acid-base homeostasis. Clin J Am Soc Nephrol. 2015;10:2232.

Hoffman RS, Smilkstein MJ, Howland MA, Goldfrank LR. Osmol gaps revisited: normal values and limitations. J Toxicol Clin Toxicol. 1993;31:81.

Höjer J. Severe metabolic acidosis in the alcoholic: differential diagnosis and management. Hum Exp Toxicol. 1996;15:482.

Hulter HN, Sebastian A, Toto RD, et al. Renal and systemic acid-base effects of the chronic administration of hypercalcemia-producing agents: calcitriol, PTH, and intravenous calcium. Kidney Int. 1982;21:445.

Khanna A, Kurtzman NA. Metabolic alkalosis. J Nephrol. 2006;19(suppl 9):S86.

Kraut JA, Kurtz I. Toxic alcohol ingestions: clinical features, diagnosis, and management. Clin J Am Soc Nephrol. 2008;3:208.

Kraut JA, Xing SX. Approach to the evaluation of a patient with an increased serum osmolal gap and high-anion-gap metabolic acidosis. Am J Kidney Dis. 2011;58:480.

Laski ME, Sabatini S. Metabolic alkalosis, bedside and bench. Semin Nephrol. 2006;26:404.

Liesivuori J, Savolainen H. Methanol and formic acid toxicity: biochemical mechanisms. Pharmacol Toxicol. 1991;69:157.

Luke RG, Galla JH. It is chloride depletion alkalosis, not contraction alkalosis. J Am Soc Nephrol. 2012;23:204.

Lynd LD, Richardson KJ, Purssell RA, et al. An evaluation of the osmole gap as a screening test for toxic alcohol poisoning. BMC Emerg Med. 2008;8:5.

Malandain H, Cano Y. Interferences of glycerol, propylene glycol, and other diols in the enzymatic assay of ethylene glycol. Eur J Clin Chem Clin Biochem. 1996;34:651.

Marraffa JM, Holland MG, Stork CM, et al. Diethylene glycol: widely used solvent presents serious poisoning potential. J Emerg Med. 2008;35:401.

Miller PD, Berns AS. Acute metabolic alkalosis perpetuating hypercarbia. A role for acetazolamide in chronic obstructive pulmonary disease. JAMA. 1977;238:2400.

Oster JR, Materson BJ, Rogers AI. Laxative abuse syndrome. Am J Gastroenterol. 1980;74:451.

Patel AM, Goldfarb S. Got calcium? Welcome to the calcium-alkali syndrome. J Am Soc Nephrol. 2010;21:1440.

Purssell RA, Pudek M, Brubacher J, Abu-Laban RB. Derivation and validation of a formula to calculate the contribution of ethanol to the osmolal gap. Ann Emerg Med. 2001;38:653.

Robinson AG, Loeb JN. Ethanol ingestion–commonest cause of elevated plasma osmolality? N Engl J Med. 1971;284:1253.

Rose BD, Post TW. Clinical Physiology of Acid-Base and Electrolyte Disorders. 5e. New York, NY: McGraw Hill; 2001:559

Schelling JR, Howard RL, Winter SD, Linas SL. Increased osmolal gap in alcoholic ketoacidosis and lactic acidosis. Ann Intern Med. 1990;113:580.

Schwartz WB, Van Ypersele de Strihou, Kassirer JP. Role of anions in metabolic alkalosis and potassium deficiency. N Engl J Med. 1968;279:630.

Shirey T, Sivilotti M. Reaction of lactate electrodes to glycolate. Crit Care Med. 1999;27:2305.

Sivilotti ML. Methanol intoxication. Ann Emerg Med. 2000;35:313.

Streicher HZ, Gabow PA, Moss AH, et al. Syndromes of toluene sniffing in adults. Ann Intern Med. 1981;94:758.

Sweetser LJ, Douglas JA, Riha RL, Bell SC. Clinical presentation of metabolic alkalosis in an adult patient with cystic fibrosis. Respirology. 2005;10:254.

Taher SM, Anderson RJ, McCartney R, et al. Renal tubular acidosis associated with toluene "sniffing." N Engl J Med. 1974;290:765.

Taki K, Mizuno K, Takahashi N, Wakusawa R. Disturbance of CO_2 elimination in the lungs by carbonic anhydrase inhibition. Jpn J Physiol. 1986;36:523.

Turban S, Beutler KT, Morris RG, et al. Long-term regulation of proximal tubule acid-base transporter abundance by angiotensin II. Kidney Int. 2006;70:660.

CASE 51

An 18-year-old male college student presents to student health clinic with confusion and blurry vision. He has a history of brittle IDDM and gastroparesis. His roommate reports that the patient was at a party the night before and returned very confused this AM after someone found him on the side of the road. The patient states that he never drinks alcohol, although he reportedly did so at the party last night. He is tachycardic with T 37.3°C, RR 23, HR 121, BP 144/75 Sao$_2$ 100% on room air. He is warm and dry on examination. He is only able to differentiate light and dark on examination and does not cooperate with retinal examination.

Laboratory data.			
ABGs		Basic Metabolic Panel	
pH	7.15	Na	139 mEq/L
Paco$_2$	30 mm Hg	K	6.8 mEq/L
Pao$_2$	100 mm Hg	Cl	110 mEq/L
HCO$_3$	10 mEq/L	CO$_2$	10 mEq/L
		BUN	32 mg/dL
		Cr	1.6 mg/dL
		Glucose	88 mg/dL
		Albumin	4.0 g/dL
		EtOH	10 mg/dL

QUESTIONS

Q51-1: Define the patient's baseline acid-base status: Does this patient have an underlying chronic acid-base disorder that we need to account for in order to appropriately interpret the acute acid-base disorders?

A. There is no evidence for an underlying chronic respiratory or metabolic acid-base disorder in this patient, so we would assume a baseline $Paco_2$ of 40 mm Hg and an HCO_3 of 24 mEq/L.

B. While the patient has a condition predisposing him to a chronic acid-base disorder, there is insufficient information to estimate the patient's baseline $Paco_2$ and HCO_3 values; therefore, we will assume a baseline $Paco_2$ of 40 mm Hg and a baseline HCO_3 of 24 mEq/L.

C. The patient has an underlying acid-base condition, and we have sufficient information to estimate the patient's baseline $Paco_2$ and HCO_3 values.

Q51-2: What is/are the primary acid-base disturbance(s) occurring in this case?

A. Metabolic acidosis only
B. Respiratory acidosis only
C. Metabolic acidosis and a respiratory acidosis
D. Metabolic alkalosis and a respiratory alkalosis
E. Metabolic alkalosis only
F. Respiratory alkalosis only

Q51-3: How would the metabolic acidosis component be classified in this case?

A. Anion gap acidosis
B. Non-anion gap acidosis
C. Anion and non-anion gap acidosis
D. Anion gap acidosis and a metabolic alkalosis

Q51-4: Does the patient in this case demonstrate appropriate respiratory or metabolic compensation?

A. Yes, the respiratory compensation is appropriate.
B. No, a concomitant respiratory alkalosis is present.
C. No, a concomitant respiratory acidosis is present.
D. Yes, the metabolic compensation is appropriate.
E. No, a concomitant metabolic acidosis is present.
F. No, a concomitant metabolic alkalosis is present.

Q51-5: Laboratory testing returns the following results:

Serum EtOH	< 3 mg/dL
Serum acetaminophen level	< 5 mg/dL (ULN for therapeutic use 20 mg/dL)
Serum salicylates level	< 5 mg/dL (ULN for therapeutic use 30 mg/dL)
Serum osmolality	321 mOsm/kg
Serum L-lactate	1.9 mmol/L (ULN 2.0 mmol/L venous)
Beta-hydroxybutyrate (acetone)	< 0.18 mmol/L (ULN 0.18 mmol/L)
Serum glucose	89 mg/dL
Urine drug screen	Positive for THC, opioids
Serum ohosphorus	2.9 mg/dL

What is the likely cause of the patient's anion gap acidosis?

A. Lactic acidosis
B. Acute renal failure
C. Organic alcohol intoxication
D. Acetaminophen toxicity
E. DKA
F. Starvation ketoacidosis
G. Alcoholic ketoacidosis

Q51-6: Which organic alcohol did this patient most likely consume?

A. Ethylene glycol
B. Isopropyl alcohol
C. Methyl alcohol (methanol)
D. Ethanol

Q51-7: The urine pH is less than 5.5 with an elevated serum K. The urine osmolal gap is 90 mOsm/L. What is the likely cause of the patient's non-anion gap acidosis?

A. Diarrhea
B. Type 1 (distal) RTA
C. Type 2 (proximal) RTA
D. Type 4 (collecting duct) RTA

ANSWERS

Q51-1: B

While the patient has a condition (diabetes mellitus) predisposing him to a chronic acid-base disorder, there is insufficient information to estimate the patient's baseline P_{aCO_2} and HCO_3 values; therefore, we will assume a baseline P_{aCO_2} of 40 mm Hg and a baseline HCO_3 of 24 mEq/L.

Rationale: Ignoring these underlying chronic acid-base disorders can significantly alter the interpretation of a patient's acute acid-base status. This was demonstrated in the first case of the series. However, often, we do not have the necessary information (eg, prior ABG or VBG, or prior serum chemistry with an HCO_3) and are forced to assume the ongoing processes are all acute in nature. We are primarily concerned about chronic respiratory acid-base disorders, as these can significantly alter the patient's baseline or expected values for the serum HCO_3 and P_{aCO_2}, and we have reliable equations to predict the expected baseline values. The respiratory compensation for both chronic metabolic acidosis and alkalosis is generally poor, so there are no equations or rules to predict what the P_{aCO_2} should be in these cases. While the baseline serum HCO_3 may be significantly off from our standard value of 24 mEq/L in these patients, we would assume a baseline P_{aCO_2} of 40 mm Hg in patients with chronic metabolic processes. Once we identify the patient's baseline P_{aCO_2} and HCO_3 values, we will need to use these values in the appropriate equations to identify the ongoing acute processes.

Q51-2: A

Metabolic acidosis only.

Rationale:

1. The pH is 7.15; therefore, the primary disorder is an **acidosis.**
2. The P_{aCO_2} of 30 mm Hg is less than 40 mm Hg, so this is **not a primary respiratory issue.**
3. The HCO_3 of 10 mEq/L is less than 24 mEq/L, so there is **a metabolic acidosis.**

Q51-3: C

Anion and non-anion gap acidosis.

Rationale:

1. Is there evidence for a chronic acid-base disorder that requires adjustment of the patient's "normal" HCO_3? No, there is no evidence for a chronic acid-base disorder, so we would assume a baseline P_{aCO_2} of 40 mm Hg and an HCO_3 of 24 mEq/L.
2. Expected anion gap:

$$\text{Expected Anion Gap} = 12 - (2.5) * \left[4.0 \, \frac{\text{g}}{\text{dL}} - \text{Actual Serum Albumin} \right]$$
$$= 12 - (2.5 * [4.0 - 4.0])$$
$$= 12 - (2.5 * [0]) = \textbf{12 mEq/L.}$$

3. Anion gap calculation:

$$\text{Serum Anion Gap} = [Na^+] - [HCO_3^-] - [Cl^-]$$
$$= 139 - (110 + 10) = \textbf{19 mEq/L,} \text{ which is} > 12 \text{ mEq/L}$$
$$\rightarrow \textbf{anion gap acidosis is present.}$$

4. Delta-delta calculation:

$$\Delta\Delta = \frac{(\text{Actual Anion Gap} - \text{Expected Anion Gap})}{(\text{Baseline } HCO_3 - \text{Actual } HCO_3)}$$

$$= (19 - 12)/(24 - 10) = \textbf{7/14 = 0.5.}$$

Delta-delta interpretation.	
Delta-Delta Value	Condition Present
< 0.4	Non-anion gap only
0.4–0.9	**Anion gap *and* non-anion gap acidosis**
1.0–2.0	Anion gap acidosis only
> 2.0	Anion gap acidosis and metabolic alkalosis

Q51-4: C
No, a concomitant respiratory acidosis is present.

Rationale: Using the Winter formula, one can calculate what the expected arterial $Paco_2$ should be for a given serum HCO_3 if the patient were completely compensated.

Respiratory Compensation for Acute Metabolic Acidosis (Winter Formula):

$$\text{Expected } Paco_2 = 1.5 * [\text{Actual } HCO_3] + 8 \pm 2 \text{ (in mm Hg)}$$
$$= (1.5 * 10) + 8 = 15 + 8 = 23 \pm 2 = \textbf{(21 to 25) mm Hg.}$$

This patient's $Paco_2$ of 30 mm Hg is higher than the expected range, and therefore a concomitant **respiratory acidosis** is present.

Q51-5: C
Organic alcohol intoxication.

Rationale: This patient has an elevated anion gap acidosis with an elevated serum osmolal gap. Similar to the serum anion gap, the serum osmolal gap is determined by the difference between the "calculated" serum osmolality and the true, measured serum osmolality. The equation for the serum osmolal gap typically includes factors for sodium, glucose, BUN, and ethanol, as these are readily measurable in most laboratories. Therefore, the serum osmolal gap will represent the osmolality of those "unmeasured" osmoles, including organic alcohols and acetone. The most common form is shown as follows:

$$\text{Calculated Serum Osmolality} = 2 * [Na^+] + \frac{[\text{Glucose}]}{18} + \frac{[\text{BUN}]}{2.8} + \frac{[\text{EtOH}]}{3.7};$$

In which the units of measure are as follows: Na, mEq/L; glucose, mg/dL; BUN, mg/dL; and EtOH, mg/dL. The conversion factors are shown in the preceding equation as well. A normal serum osmolal gap is around −10 to +10 mOsm/L (or mOsm/kg).

Therefore, for this patient,

$$\text{Calculated Osmolality} = (Na * 2) + (BUN/2.8) + (EtOH/3.7) + (Glucose/18)$$
$$= (139 * 2) + (32/3.4) + (10/3.7) + (88/18)$$
$$= 297 \text{ mOsm/L.}$$

The serum osmolal gap is therefore 24 mOsm/L, which is greater than 10. The patient also has an anion gap acidosis with no evidence of a lactic acidosis, ketoacidosis, acetaminophen or salicylate toxicity, or acute renal failure to account for the elevated anion gap.

The differential for an elevated serum osmolal gap is reviewed as follows:

Conditions associated with an elevated serum osmolal gap.
With an Elevated Serum Anion Gap
1. Ethanol ingestion with alcoholic ketoacidosis (acetone is an unmeasured osmole, in addition to ethanol)—the osmolality is usually elevated more so by the increased ethanol concentration, so the osmolal "gap" depends on whether the term for ethanol is included in the osmolality calculation*
2. Organic alcohol ingestions (methanol, ethylene glycol, diethylene glycol, propylene glycol)
3. DKA—similar to ethanol ingestion above, glucose and acetone contribute to the osmolality, since the glucose term is always included in the calculation
4. Salicylate toxicity
5. Renal failure—the BUN is nearly always included in the osmolality
Without an Elevated Serum Anion Gap
1. Hyperosmolar therapy (mannitol, glycerol)
2. Other organic solvent ingestion (eg, acetone)
3. Isopropyl alcohol ingestion (produces only acetone rather than an organic acid, so no anion gap is seen).
4. Hypertriglyceridemia
5. Hyperproteinemia
*A mildly elevated osmolal gap has been reported in the literature in patients with lactic acidosis in critical illness, particularly severe distributive shock. The pathology is not quite clear, although it is likely related to multiorgan failure—particularly the liver and kidneys—and the release of cellular components known to contribute to the osmolal gap). This is typically around 10 mOsm/L, although may be as high as 20 to 25 mOsm/L.

Here, we would be most concerned about a toxic organic alcohol ingestion, particularly given the vignette.

Q51-6: C
Methyl alcohol (methanol).

Rationale: The presentation with an elevated osmolar gap, anion gap acidosis with negative EtOH and blurred vision/blindness is consistent with methanol toxicity. Methanol blood levels reach their peak approximately 60 minutes after an ingestion, although the severity of symptoms does not often correlate with blood levels. Neurologic complications are most common (ataxia, disinhibition, headache, seizures, encephalopathy, coma), followed by vision loss and conduction abnormalities. Formic acid, produced from the metabolism of methanol, accumulates in the optic nerve. Patients will often complain initially of blurred vision, followed by flashing light. Complete vision loss is a common complication.

Q51-7: D
Type 4 RTA.

Rationale: The abnormally low urine osmolal gap points to an issue with urine acidification, most consistent with a type 1 or type 4 RTA. The low urine pH and high serum K are most consistent with a type 4 RTA, which is common in patients with diabetic nephropathy.

Causes of RTA.
Causes of Type 1 (Distal) RTA
Primary • Idiopathic or familial (may be recessive or dominant)
Secondary • Medications: Lithium, amphotericin, ifosfamide, NSAIDs • Rheumatologic disorders: Sjögren syndrome, SLE, RA • Hypercalciuria (idiopathic) or associated with vitamin D deficiency or hyperparathyroidism • Sarcoidosis • Obstructive uropathy • Wilson disease • Rejection of renal transplant allograft
Causes of Type 2 (proximal) RTA
Primary • Idiopathic • Familial (primarily recessive disorders) • Genetic: Fanconi syndrome, cystinosis, glycogen storage disease (type 1), Wilson disease, galactosemia
Secondary • Medications: Acetazolamide, topiramate, aminoglycoside antibiotics, ifosfamide, reverse transcriptase inhibitors (tenofovir) • Heavy metal poisoning: Lead, mercury, copper • Multiple myeloma or amyloidosis (secondary to light chain toxicity) • Sjögren syndrome • Vitamin D deficiency • Rejection of renal transplant allograft

(Continued)

Causes of RTA. (*continued*)
Causes of Type 4 RTA (Hypoaldosteronism or Aldosterone Resistance)
Primary • Primary adrenal insufficiency • Inherited disorders associated with hypoaldosteronism • Pseudohypoaldosteronism (types 1 and 2)
Secondary • Causes of hyporeninemic hypoaldosteronism such as renal disease (diabetic nephropathy), NSAID use, calcineurin inhibitors, volume expansion/volume overload • Causes of distal tubule voltage defects such as sickle cell disease, obstructive uropathy, SLE • Severe illness/septic shock • Angiotensin II–associated medications: ACE inhibitors, ARBs, direct renin inhibitors • Potassium-sparing diuretics: Spironolactone, amiloride, triamterene • Antibiotics: Trimethoprim, pentamidine

References

Arroliga AC, Shehab N, McCarthy K, Gonzales JP. Relationship of continuous infusion lorazepam to serum propylene glycol concentration in critically ill adults. Crit Care Med. 2004;32:1709.

Batlle D, Chin-Theodorou J, Tucker BM. Metabolic acidosis or respiratory alkalosis? Evaluation of a low plasma bicarbonate using the urine anion gap. Am J Kidney Dis. 2017;70:440.

Batlle D, Grupp M, Gaviria M, Kurtzman NA. Distal renal tubular acidosis with intact capacity to lower urinary pH. Am J Med. 1982;72:751.

Batlle D, Haque SK. Genetic causes and mechanisms of distal renal tubular acidosis. Nephrol Dial Transplant. 2012;27:3691.

Batlle DC, Hizon M, Cohen E, et al. The use of the urinary anion gap in the diagnosis of hyperchloremic metabolic acidosis. N Engl J Med. 1988;318:594.

Batlle DC, von Riotte A, Schlueter W. Urinary sodium in the evaluation of hyperchloremic metabolic acidosis. N Engl J Med. 1987;316:140.

Braden GL, Strayhorn CH, Germain MJ, et al. Increased osmolal gap in alcoholic acidosis. Arch Intern Med. 1993;153:2377.

Buckalew VM Jr, McCurdy DK, Ludwig GD, et al. Incomplete renal tubular acidosis. Physiologic studies in three patients with a defect in lowering urine pH. Am J Med. 1968;45:32.

Church AS, Witting MD. Laboratory testing in ethanol, methanol, ethylene glycol, and isopropanol toxicities. J Emerg Med. 1997;15:687.

Eder AF, Dowdy YG, Gardiner JA, et al. Serum lactate and lactate dehydrogenase in high concentrations interfere in enzymatic assay of ethylene glycol. Clin Chem. 1996;42:1489.

Gabow PA. Ethylene glycol intoxication. Am J Kidney Dis. 1988;11:277.

Gennari FJ. Current concepts. Serum osmolality. Uses and limitations. N Engl J Med. 1984;310:102.

Glasser L, Sternglanz PD, Combie J, Robinson A. Serum osmolality and its applicability to drug overdose. Am J Clin Pathol. 1973;60:695.

Hoffman RS, Smilkstein MJ, Howland MA, Goldfrank LR. Osmol gaps revisited: normal values and limitations. J Toxicol Clin Toxicol. 1993;31:81.

Höjer J. Severe metabolic acidosis in the alcoholic: differential diagnosis and management. Hum Exp Toxicol. 1996;15:482.

Karet FE. Mechanisms in hyperkalemic renal tubular acidosis. J Am Soc Nephrol. 2009;20:251.

Kraut JA, Kurtz I. Toxic alcohol ingestions: clinical features, diagnosis, and management. Clin J Am Soc Nephrol. 2008;3:208.

Kraut JA, Madias NE. Differential diagnosis of nongap metabolic acidosis: value of a systematic approach. Clin J Am Soc Nephrol. 2012;7:671.

Kraut JA, Xing SX. Approach to the evaluation of a patient with an increased serum osmolal gap and high-anion-gap metabolic acidosis. Am J Kidney Dis. 2011;58:480.

Liesivuori J, Savolainen H. Methanol and formic acid toxicity: biochemical mechanisms. Pharmacol Toxicol. 1991;69:157.

Lynd LD, Richardson KJ, Purssell RA, et al. An evaluation of the osmole gap as a screening test for toxic alcohol poisoning. BMC Emerg Med. 2008;8:5.

Malandain H, Cano Y. Interferences of glycerol, propylene glycol, and other diols in the enzymatic assay of ethylene glycol. Eur J Clin Chem Clin Biochem. 1996;34:651.

Marraffa JM, Holland MG, Stork CM, et al. Diethylene glycol: widely used solvent presents serious poisoning potential. J Emerg Med. 2008;35:401.

Purssell RA, Pudek M, Brubacher J, Abu-Laban RB. Derivation and validation of a formula to calculate the contribution of ethanol to the osmolal gap. Ann Emerg Med. 2001;38:653.

Rastegar M, Nagami GT. Non-anion gap metabolic acidosis: a clinical approach to evaluation. Am J Kidney Dis. 2017;69:296..

Robinson AG, Loeb JN. Ethanol ingestion–commonest cause of elevated plasma osmolality? N Engl J Med. 1971;284:1253.

Rodríguez Soriano J. Renal tubular acidosis: the clinical entity. J Am Soc Nephrol. 2002;13:2160.

Schelling JR, Howard RL, Winter SD, Linas SL. Increased osmolal gap in alcoholic ketoacidosis and lactic acidosis. Ann Intern Med. 1990;113:580.

Shirey T, Sivilotti M. Reaction of lactate electrodes to glycolate. Crit Care Med. 1999;27:2305.

Sivilotti ML. Methanol intoxication. Ann Emerg Med. 2000;35:313.

Carlisle EJ, Donnelly SM, Vasuvattakul S, et al. Glue-sniffing and distal renal tubular acidosis: sticking to the facts. J Am Soc Nephrol. 1991;1:1019.

Streicher HZ, Gabow PA, Moss AH, et al. Syndromes of toluene sniffing in adults. Ann Intern Med. 1981;94:758.

Taher SM, Anderson RJ, McCartney R, et al. Renal tubular acidosis associated with toluene "sniffing". N Engl J Med. 1974; 290:765.

CASE 52

A 26-year-old man with a history of alcoholism presents with weakness and confusion. He was at a secured inpatient rehabilitation facility and was found in the basement. He has not been out of the facility in the past 4 weeks and has no access to alcohol. He was last seen, appearing normal, about 2 days ago. His vital signs are T 36.3°C, RR 16, HR 90, BP 80/40 Sao$_2$ 96% on room air. He is dry on examination and has no complaints on presentation, other than feeling lightheaded when standing and walking. His WBC count is 4.2, BG is 121, and his breath has a sweet odor. His vision is intact. His BMI is 22, and he has a normal albumin level. He takes no medications regularly.

Laboratory data.			
ABGs		Basic Metabolic Panel	
pH	7.31	Na	135 mEq/L
Paco$_2$	35 mm Hg	K	3.3 mEq/L
Pao$_2$	100 mm Hg	Cl	88 mEq/L
HCO$_3$	17 mEq/L	CO$_2$	17 mEq/L
		BUN	45 mg/dL
		Cr	1.1 mg/dL
		Glucose	121 mg/dL
		Albumin	4.0 g/dL
		EtOH	0 mg/dL

QUESTIONS

Q52-1: Define the patient's baseline acid-base status: Does this patient have an underlying chronic acid-base disorder that we need to account for in order to appropriately interpret the acute acid-base disorders?

A. There is no evidence for an underlying chronic respiratory or metabolic acid-base disorder in this patient, so we would assume a baseline $Paco_2$ of 40 mm Hg and an HCO_3 of 24 mEq/L.
B. While the patient has a condition predisposing him to a chronic acid-base disorder, there is insufficient information to estimate the patient's baseline $Paco_2$ and HCO_3 values; therefore, we will assume a baseline $Paco_2$ of 40 mm Hg and a baseline HCO_3 of 24 mEq/L.
C. The patient has an underlying acid-base condition, and we have sufficient information to estimate the patient's baseline $Paco_2$ and HCO_3 values.

Q53-2: What is/are the primary acid-base disturbance(s) occurring in this case?

A. Metabolic acidosis only
B. Respiratory acidosis only
C. Metabolic acidosis and a respiratory acidosis
D. Metabolic alkalosis and a respiratory alkalosis
E. Metabolic alkalosis only
F. Respiratory alkalosis only

Q52-3: How would the metabolic acidosis component be classified in this case?

A. Anion gap acidosis
B. Non-anion gap acidosis
C. Anion and non-anion gap acidosis
D. Anion gap acidosis and a metabolic alkalosis

Q52-4: Does the patient in this case demonstrate appropriate respiratory or metabolic compensation?

A. Yes, the respiratory compensation is appropriate.
B. No, a concomitant respiratory alkalosis is present.
C. No, a concomitant respiratory acidosis is present.
D. Yes, the metabolic compensation is appropriate.
E. No, a concomitant metabolic acidosis is present.
F. No, a concomitant metabolic alkalosis is present.

Q52-5: Laboratory testing returns the following results:

Serum EtOH	< 3 mg/dL
Serum acetaminophen level	< 5 mg/dL (ULN for therapeutic use 20 mg/dL)
Serum salicylates level	< 5 mg/dL (ULN for therapeutic use 30 mg/dL)
Serum osmolality	333 mOsm/kg
Serum L-lactate	6.7 mmol/L (ULN 2.0 mmol/L venous)
Beta-hydroxybutyrate (acetone)	4.41 mmol/L (ULN 0.18 mmol/L)
Serum glucose	121 mg/dL
Urine drug screen	Negative

What is the likely cause of the patient's anion gap acidosis?

A. Lactic acidosis
B. Acute renal failure
C. Organic alcohol intoxication
D. Diabetic ketoacidosis
E. Starvation ketoacidosis
F. Cyanide poisoning
G. Alcoholic ketoacidosis

Q52-6: Which organic alcohol could produce the constellation of laboratory findings in this patient?

A. Ethylene glycol
B. Methanol
C. Ethanol
D. Propylene glycol
E. Isopropyl alcohol

Q52-7: What is the likely source of the patient's metabolic alkalosis, assuming a urine chloride of 5 mEq/L?

A. Contraction alkalosis
B. Ongoing diuretic use
C. Hyperaldosteronism
D. Diarrhea

ANSWERS

Q52-1: B

While the patient has a condition (alcoholism) predisposing him to a chronic acid-base disorder, there is insufficient information to estimate the patient's baseline $Paco_2$ and HCO_3 values; therefore, we will assume a baseline $Paco_2$ of 40 mm Hg and a baseline HCO_3 of 24 mEq/L.

Rationale: Ignoring these underlying chronic acid-base disorders can significantly alter the interpretation of a patient's acute acid-base status. This was demonstrated in the first case of the series. However, often, we do not have the necessary information (eg, prior ABG or VBG, or prior serum chemistry with an HCO_3) and are forced to assume the ongoing processes are all acute in nature. We are primarily concerned about chronic respiratory acid-base disorders, as these can significantly alter the patient's baseline or expected values for the serum HCO_3 and $Paco_2$, and we have reliable equations to predict the expected baseline values. The respiratory compensation for both chronic metabolic acidosis and alkalosis is generally poor, so there are no equations or rules to predict what the $Paco_2$ should be in these cases. While the baseline serum HCO_3 may be significantly off from our standard value 24 mEq/L in these patients, we would assume a baseline $Paco_2$ of 40 mm Hg in patients with chronic metabolic processes. Once we identify the patient's baseline $Paco_2$ and HCO_3 values, we will need to use these values in the appropriate equations to identify the ongoing acute processes.

Q52-2: A

Metabolic acidosis only.

Rationale:

1. The pH is 7.31; therefore, the primary disorder is an **acidosis.**
2. The $Paco_2$ of 35 mm Hg is less than 40 mm Hg, so a **primary respiratory issue is not likely.**
3. The HCO_3 of 17 mEq/L is less than 24 mEq/L, so there is a **metabolic acidosis.**

Q52-3: D

Anion gap acidosis and a metabolic alkalosis.

Rationale:

1. Is there evidence for a chronic acid-base disorder that requires adjustment of the patient's "normal" HCO_3? No, there is no evidence for a chronic acid-base disorder, so we would assume a baseline $Paco_2$ of 40 mm Hg and an HCO_3 of 24 mEq/L.
2. Expected anion gap:

$$\text{Expected Anion Gap} = 12 - (2.5) * \left[4.0\,\frac{g}{dL} - \text{Actual Serum Albumin} \right]$$
$$= 12 - (2.5 * [4.0 - 4.0])$$
$$= 12 - (2.5 * [0]) = \textbf{12 mEq/L.}$$

3. Anion gap calculation:

$$\text{Serum Anion Gap} = [Na^+] - [HCO_3^-] - [Cl^-]$$
$$= 135 - (88 + 17) = \textbf{30 mEq/L,} \text{ which is} > 12 \text{ mEq/L}$$
$$\rightarrow \textbf{anion gap acidosis is present.}$$

4. Delta-delta calculation:

$$\Delta\Delta = \frac{(\text{Actual Anion Gap} - \text{Expected Anion Gap})}{(\text{Baseline HCO}_3 - \text{Actual HCO}_3)}$$
$$= (30 - 12)/(24 - 17) = \textbf{18/7 = 2.6.}$$

Delta-delta interpretation.	
Delta-Delta Value	Condition Present
< 0.4	Non-anion gap only
0.4–0.9	**Anion gap *and* non-anion gap acidosis**
1.0–2.0	Anion gap acidosis only
> 2.0	**Anion gap acidosis and metabolic alkalosis**

Q52-4: A
Yes, the respiratory compensation is appropriate.

Rationale: Using the Winter formula, one can calculate what the expected arterial $Paco_2$ should be for a given serum HCO_3 if the patient were completely compensated.

Respiratory Compensation for Acute Metabolic Acidosis (Winter Formula):

$$\text{Expected Paco}_2 = 1.5 * [\text{Actual HCO}_3] + 8 \pm 2 \text{ (in mm Hg)}$$
$$= (1.5 * 17) + 8 = 25.5 + 8 = 33.5 +/- 2 = \textbf{(31 to 35) mm Hg.}$$

This patient's $Paco_2$ of 35 mm Hg is within the expected range, and therefore the **respiratory compensation is appropriate**.

Q52-5: A
Lactic acidosis.

Rationale: This is a difficult question overall. The patient has relatively normal renal function, a negative serum ethanol level, and no evidence of acetaminophen or salicylate toxicity. The patient does have an elevated serum lactate level, so a lactic acidosis is possible, as is a ketoacidosis (elevated serum ketone level). The next step is to determine if the patient has a serum osmolal gap. Similar to the serum anion gap, the serum osmolal gap is determined by the difference between the "calculated" serum osmolality and the true, measured serum osmolality. The equation for the serum osmolal gap typically includes factors for sodium, glucose, BUN, and ethanol, as these are readily measurable in most laboratories. Therefore, the serum osmolal gap will represent the osmolality of those "unmeasured" osmoles, including organic alcohols and acetone. The most common form is shown as follows:

$$\text{Calculated Serum Osmolality} = 2 * [\text{Na}^+] + \frac{[\text{Glucose}]}{18} + \frac{[\text{BUN}]}{2.8} + \frac{[\text{EtOH}]}{3.7};$$

In which the units of measure are as follows: Na, mEq/L; glucose, mg/dL; BUN, mg/dL; and EtOH, mg/dL. The conversion factors are shown in the preceding equation as well. A normal serum osmolal gap is around −10 to +10 mOsm/L (or mOsm/kg).

Therefore, for this patient,

$$\text{Calculated Serum Osmolality} = 2 * [135] + [121/18] + [45/2.8] = 293 \text{ mOsm/L}$$
$$\text{Serum Osmolal Gap} = 333 \text{ mOsm/L} - 293 \text{ mOsm/L} = 40 \text{ mOsm/L}.$$

This patient has an elevated anion gap acidosis with an elevated serum osmolal gap, so the initial concern would be for a unifying cause such as methanol or ethylene glycol poisoning. These disorders can be associated with a falsely elevated lactate due to interference with the lactate assay, or can result in distributive shock and resultant lactic acidosis secondary to the acidemia. However, we must also consider the possibility that the patient has two separate ongoing processes, one contributing to the anion gap acidosis and the other to the osmolal gap (recall that *not all organic alcohol ingestions* cause an anion gap acidosis). We should not lose sight of the fact that the patient is hypotensive and likely in distributive shock. The positive serum beta-hydroxybutyrate is consistent with a possible ketoacidosis; however, the patient's glucose is normal, the patient has no history of DKA, and there is no evidence of starvation. Although he is alcoholic, he has not had access to alcohol at the inpatient rehabilitation facility, and his EtOH level is zero, so alcoholic ketoacidosis is unlikely. He has no significant renal failure to account for the acidosis. However, this combination of laboratory findings is consistent with a specific type of organic alcohol ingestion (as discussed in the next answer).

Q52-6: E
Isopropyl alcohol.

Rationale: The finding of the positive serum acetone with positive beta-hydroxybutyrate (BHB) is consistent with isopropyl alcohol poisoning. Isopropyl alcohol is a secondary alcohol that is converted to acetoacetone rather than being converted to aldehydes and subsequent carboxylic acids that lead to an anion gap acidosis. The ketones cause a sweet odor on the breath. The positive ketones could also be seen in high-carbohydrate diets (not present), DKA, pregnancy, salicylate poisoning (negative drug screen), and alcoholism; however, the patient has been in a facility for the past 4 weeks, with a negative EtOH level and normal BMI and albumin, arguing against alcoholic ketoacidosis as the source of the serum acetone and BHB. His history of alcoholism places him at high risk of ingesting an alcohol substitute. Additionally, the lack of vision issues characteristic of renal failure argues against ethylene glycol and methanol as the cause. Propylene glycol toxicity is usually seen in hospitalized patients receiving infusions in which propylene glycol is the carrier, which is not the case here.

Causes of an elevated serum osmolal gap.
With an Elevated Serum Anion Gap
1. Ethanol ingestion with alcoholic ketoacidosis (acetone is an unmeasured osmole, in addition to ethanol)—the osmolality is usually elevated more so by the increased ethanol concentration, so the osmolal "gap" depends on whether the term for ethanol is included in the osmolality calculation*
2. Organic alcohol ingestions (methanol, ethylene glycol, diethylene glycol, propylene glycol)
3. DKA—similar to ethanol ingestion, earlier, glucose and acetone contribute to the osmolality, since the glucose term is always included in the calculation
4. Salicylate toxicity
5. Renal failure—the BUN is nearly always included in the osmolality
Without an Elevated Serum Anion Gap
1. Hyperosmolar therapy (mannitol, glycerol)
2. Other organic solvent ingestion (eg, acetone)
3. Isopropyl alcohol ingestion (**produces only acetone rather than an organic acid, so no anion gap is seen**)
4. Hypertriglyceridemia
5. Hyperproteinemia
*A mildly elevated osmolal gap has been reported in the literature in patients with lactic acidosis in critical illness, particularly severe distributive shock. The pathology is not quite clear, although it likely is related to multiorgan failure—particularly involving the liver and kidneys—and the release of cellular components known to contribute to the osmolal gap. This is typically around 10 mOsm/L, although it may be as high as 20–25 mOsm/L.

In terms of the actual management of such a patient, it would be entirely appropriate to assume an ingestion of a more toxic organic alcohol (eg, ethylene glycol, methanol) until such time as confirmatory testing returned with the actual ingestion. In fact, in this case the patient was treated with fomepizole and intermittent dialysis (in addition to volume resuscitation and temporary vasopressor support) as the confirmatory chromatography test result was not obtained until nearly 24 hours after admission.

Q52-7: A
Contraction alkalosis.

Rationale: The patient presented with a dry appearance on physical examination (skin turgor, etc), with an elevated BUN/Cr ratio of ~40, and symptoms concerning for orthostasis. The low urine chloride is consistent with a chloride-responsive cause, so option A is the likely answer. As the patient has been receiving no medications, diuretic use is unlikely. Hyperaldosteronism is associated with a chloride-resistant metabolic alkalosis, while diarrhea is associated with a metabolic acidosis.

Causes of metabolic alkalosis.
History: Rule Out the Following as Causes
• Alkali load ("milk-alkali" or calcium-alkali syndrome, oral sodium bicarbonate, IV sodium bicarbonate); • Genetic causes (CF) • Presence of hypercalcemia • Intravenous β-lactam antibiotics • Laxative abuse (may also cause a metabolic acidosis depending on diarrheal HCO_3 losses)
If None of the Above, Then…
Urine Chloride < 20 mEq/L (Chloride-Responsive Causes) • Loss of gastric acid (hyperemesis, NGT suctioning) • Prior diuretic use (in hours to days following discontinuation) • Post-hypercapnia • Villous adenoma • Congenital chloridorrhea • Chronic laxative abuse (may also cause a metabolic acidosis depending on diarrheal HCO_3 losses) • CF
OR
Urine Chloride > 20 mEq/L (Chloride-Resistant Causes)
Urine Chloride > 20 mEq/L, Lack of HTN, Urine Potassium < 30 mEq/L
• Hypokalemia or hypomagnesemia • Laxative abuse (if dominated by hypokalemia) • Bartter syndrome • Gitelman syndrome
Urine Chloride > 20 mEq/L, Lack of HTN, Urine Potassium > 30 mEq/L
• Current diuretic use
Urine Chloride > 20 mEq/L, Presence of HTN, Urine Potassium Variable but Usually > 30 mEq/L
Elevated plasma renin level: • Renal artery stenosis • Renin-secreting tumor • Renovascular disease
Low plasma renin, low plasma aldosterone • Cushing syndrome • Exogenous mineralocorticoid use • Genetic disorder (11-hydoxylase or 17-hydrolyase deficiency, 11β-HSD deficiency) • Liddle syndrome • Licorice toxicity
Low plasma renin, high plasma aldosterone • Primary hyperaldosteronism • Adrenal adenoma • Bilateral adrenal hyperplasia

References

Abramson S, Singh AK. Treatment of the alcohol intoxications: ethylene glycol, methanol and iso-propanol. Curr Opin Nephrol Hypertens. 2000;9:695.

Abreo K, Adlakha A, Kilpatrick S, et al. The milk-alkali syndrome. A reversible form of acute renal failure. Arch Intern Med. 1993;153:1005.

Adeva-Andany M, López-Ojén M, Funcasta-Calderón R, et al. Comprehensive review on lactate metabolism in human health. Mitochondrion. 2014;17:76.

Arroliga AC, Shehab N, McCarthy K, Gonzales JP. Relationship of continuous infusion lorazepam to serum propylene glycol concentration in critically ill adults. Crit Care Med. 2004;32:1709.

Barton CH, Vaziri ND, Ness RL, et al. Cimetidine in the management of metabolic alkalosis induced by nasogastric drainage. Arch Surg. 1979;114:70.

Bear R, Goldstein M, Phillipson E, et al. Effect of metabolic alkalosis on respiratory function in patients with chronic obstructive lung disease. Can Med Assoc J. 1977;117:900.

Bekka R, Borron SW, Astier A, et al. Treatment of methanol and isopropanol poisoning with intravenous fomepizole. J Toxicol Clin Toxicol. 2001;39:59.

Braden GL, Strayhorn CH, Germain MJ, et al. Increased osmolal gap in alcoholic acidosis. Arch Intern Med. 1993;153:2377.

Gabow PA. Ethylene glycol intoxication. Am J Kidney Dis. 1988;11:277.

Galla JH, Gifford JD, Luke RG, Rome L. Adaptations to chloride-depletion alkalosis. Am J Physiol. 1991;261:R771.

Garella S, Chang BS, Kahn SI. Dilution acidosis and contraction alkalosis: review of a concept. Kidney Int. 1975;8:279.

Gaudet MP, Fraser GL. Isopropanol ingestion: case report with pharmacokinetic analysis. Am J Emerg Med. 1989;7:297.

Gaulier JM, Lamballais F, Yazdani F, Lachâtre G. Isopropyl alcohol concentrations in postmortem tissues to document fatal intoxication. J Anal Toxicol. 2011;35:254.

Gennari FJ. Current concepts. Serum osmolality. Uses and limitations. N Engl J Med. 1984;310:102.

Gennari FJ, Weise WJ. Acid-base disturbances in gastrointestinal disease. Clin J Am Soc Nephrol. 2008;3:1861.

Glasser L, Ssternglanz PD, Combie J, Robinson A. Serum osmolality and its applicability to drug overdose. Am J Clin Pathol. 1973;60:695.

Hamm LL, Nakhoul N, Hering-Smith KS. Acid-base homeostasis. Clin J Am Soc Nephrol. 2015;10:2232.

Hulter HN, Sebastian A, Toto RD, et al. Renal and systemic acid-base effects of the chronic administration of hypercalcemia-producing agents: calcitriol, PTH, and intravenous calcium. Kidney Int. 1982;21:445.

Jenkins DW, Eckle RE, Craig JW. Alcoholic ketoacidosis. JAMA. 1971;217:177.

Khanna A, Kurtzman NA. Metabolic alkalosis. J Nephrol. 2006;19(suppl 9):S86.

Kraut JA, Kurtz I. Toxic alcohol ingestions: clinical features, diagnosis, and management. Clin J Am Soc Nephrol. 2008;3:208.

Kraut JA, Xing SX. Approach to the evaluation of a patient with an increased serum osmolal gap and high-anion-gap metabolic acidosis. Am J Kidney Dis. 2011;58:480.

Laski ME, Sabatini S. Metabolic alkalosis, bedside and bench. Semin Nephrol. 2006;26:404.

Levy B. Lactate and shock state: the metabolic view. Curr Opin Crit Care. 2006;12:315.

Levy LJ, Duga J, Girgis M, Gordon EE. Ketoacidosis associated with alcoholism in nondiabetic subjects. Ann Intern Med. 1973;78:213.

Luke RG, Galla JH. It is chloride depletion alkalosis, not contraction alkalosis. J Am Soc Nephrol. 2012;23:204.

Lynd LD, Richardson KJ, Purssell RA, et al. An evaluation of the osmole gap as a screening test for toxic alcohol poisoning. BMC Emerg Med. 2008;8:5.

Madias NE. Lactic acidosis. Kidney Int. 1986;29:752.

Marraffa JM, Holland MG, Stork CM, et al. Diethylene glycol: widely used solvent presents serious poisoning potential. J Emerg Med. 2008;35:401.

Mikkelsen ME, Miltiades AN, Gaieski DF, et al. Serum lactate is associated with mortality in severe sepsis independent of organ failure and shock. Crit Care Med. 2009;37:1670.

Miller PD, Berns AS. Acute metabolic alkalosis perpetuating hypercarbia. A role for acetazolamide in chronic obstructive pulmonary disease. JAMA. 1977;238:2400.

Monaghan MS, Ackerman BH, Olsen KM, et al. The use of delta osmolality to predict serum isopropanol and acetone concentrations. Pharmacotherapy. 1993;13:60.

Oster JR, Materson BJ, Rogers AI. Laxative abuse syndrome. Am J Gastroenterol. 1980;74:451.

Palmer BF, Clegg DJ. Electrolyte disturbances in patients with chronic alcohol-use disorder. N Engl J Med. 2017;377:1368.

Pappas AA, Ackerman BH, Olsen KM, Taylor EH. Isopropanol ingestion: a report of six episodes with isopropanol and acetone serum concentration time data. J Toxicol Clin Toxicol. 1991;29:11.

Patel AM, Goldfarb S. Got calcium? Welcome to the calcium-alkali syndrome. J Am Soc Nephrol. 2010;21:1440.

Purssell RA, Pudek M, Brubacher J, Abu-Laban RB. Derivation and validation of a formula to calculate the contribution of ethanol to the osmolal gap. Ann Emerg Med. 2001;38:653.

Reichard GA Jr, Owen OE, Haff AC, et al. Ketone-body production and oxidation in fasting obese humans. J Clin Invest. 1974;53:508.

Robinson AG, Loeb JN. Ethanol ingestion—commonest cause of elevated plasma osmolality? N Engl J Med. 1971;284:1253.

Rose BD, Post TW. Clinical Physiology of Acid-Base and Electrolyte Disorders. 5e. New York, NY: McGraw Hill; 2001:559.

Schelling JR, Howard RL, Winter SD, Linas SL. Increased osmolal gap in alcoholic ketoacidosis and lactic acidosis. Ann Intern Med. 1990;113:580.

Schwartz WB, Van Ypersele de Strihou, Kassirer JP. Role of anions in metabolic alkalosis and potassium deficiency. N Engl J Med. 1968;279:630.

Sweetser LJ, Douglas JA, Riha RL, Bell SC. Clinical presentation of metabolic alkalosis in an adult patient with cystic fibrosis. Respirology. 2005;10:254.

Taki K, Mizuno K, Takahashi N, Wakusawa R. Disturbance of CO2 elimination in the lungs by carbonic anhydrase inhibition. Jpn J Physiol. 1986;36:523.

Toth HL, Greenbaum LA. Severe acidosis caused by starvation and stress. Am J Kidney Dis. 2003;42:E16.

Trullas JC, Aguilo S, Castro P, Nogue S. Life-threatening isopropyl alcohol intoxication: is hemodialysis really necessary? Vet Hum Toxicol. 2004;46:282.

Turban S, Beutler KT, Morris RG, et al. Long-term regulation of proximal tubule acid-base transporter abundance by angiotensin II. Kidney Int 2006;70:660.

Zaman F, Pervez A, Abreo K. Isopropyl alcohol intoxication: a diagnostic challenge. Am J Kidney Dis. 2002;40:E12.

CASE 53

A 66-year-old man with COPD presents to the emergency department (ED) with dyspnea and increased cough over the past 2 to 3 days that is not relieved with his home medications. He is febrile to 39.4°C, and a CXR shows an infiltrate in the right middle and lower lobes. He is hypotensive with RR 21, HR 120, BP 70/40, and Sao_2 92% on 4L/min supplemental oxygen. His other medical problems include HTN, coronary artery disease, and HIV on HAART therapy. He is obtunded on arrival to the ED. His examination is remarkable for rhonchorous breath sounds throughout, sinus tachycardia, and intact cranial nerve reflexes.

Laboratory data.			
ABGs		Basic Metabolic Panel	
pH	7.01	Na	139 mEq/L
$Paco_2$	78 mm Hg	K	5.5 mEq/L
Pao_2	70 mm Hg	Cl	106 mEq/L
HCO_3	18 mEq/L	CO_2	19 mEq/L
		BUN	22 mg/dL
		Cr	0.6 mg/dL
		Glucose	141 mg/dL
		Albumin	4.0 g/dL
		EtOH	0 mg/dL

QUESTIONS

Q53-1: Define the patient's baseline acid-base status: Does this patient have an underlying chronic acid-base disorder that we need to account for in order to appropriately interpret the acute acid-base disorders?

A. There is no evidence for an underlying chronic respiratory or metabolic acid-base disorder in this patient, so we would assume a baseline $Paco_2$ of 40 mm Hg and an HCO_3 of 24 mEq/L.

B. While the patient has a condition predisposing him to a chronic acid-base disorder, there is insufficient information to estimate the patient's baseline $Paco_2$ and HCO_3 values; therefore, we will assume a baseline $Paco_2$ of 40 mm Hg and a baseline HCO_3 of 24 mEq/L.

C. The patient has an underlying acid-base condition, and we have sufficient information to estimate the patient's baseline $Paco_2$ and HCO_3 values.

Q53-2: What is/are the primary acid-base disturbance(s) occurring in this case?

A. Metabolic acidosis only
B. Respiratory acidosis only
C. Metabolic acidosis and a respiratory acidosis
D. Metabolic alkalosis and a respiratory alkalosis
E. Metabolic alkalosis only
F. Respiratory alkalosis only

Q53-3: How would the metabolic acidosis component be classified in this case?

A. Anion gap acidosis
B. Non-anion gap acidosis
C. Anion and non-anion gap acidosis
D. Anion gap acidosis and a metabolic alkalosis

Q53-4: The patient has a negative serum acetone study and negative serum and urine drug screens. The measured serum osmolality is 300 mOsm/L. The serum phosphorus level is 3.4 mg/dL. What is the likely cause of the patient's anion gap acidosis?

A. Lactic acidosis
B. Acute renal failure
C. Organic alcohol intoxication
D. Diabetic ketoacidosis
E. Alcoholic ketoacidosis

Q53-5: The urine anion gap is +33 mEq/L. The patient's urine pH is low. Laboratory testing returns the following additional results:

Urine Na	29 mEq/L
Urine K	33 mEq/L
Urine Cl	28 mEq/L
Urine urea	191 mg/dL
Urine glucose	0 mg/dL
Urine osmolality	288 mOsm/L
Urine pH	5.3
Urine RBCs	None
Urine WBCs	None
Urine protein	Trace
Urine microscopic	None

What is the likely cause of the patient's non-anion gap acidosis?

A. Type 1 RTA
B. Type 4 RTA
C. Diarrhea
D. Hyperemesis
E. Type 2 RTA

Q53-6: What is the likely cause of the patient's type 4 RTA?

A. Acetazolamide use
B. Sjögren syndrome
C. Fanconi syndrome
D. HIV

Q53-7: What is the likely source of the patient's respiratory acidosis?

A. COPD
B. Asthma
C. Compensation for a metabolic alkalosis
D. Neuromuscular disease

ANSWERS

Q53-1: B

While the patient has a condition (COPD) predisposing him to a chronic acid-base disorder, there is insufficient information to estimate the patient's baseline $Paco_2$ and HCO_3 values; therefore, we will assume a baseline $Paco_2$ of 40 mm Hg and a baseline HCO_3 of 24 mEq/L.

Rationale: Ignoring these underlying chronic acid-base disorders can significantly alter the interpretation of a patient's acute acid-base status. This was demonstrated in the first case of the series. However, often, we do not have the necessary information (eg, prior ABG or VBG, or prior serum chemistry with an HCO_3) and are forced to assume the ongoing processes are all acute in nature. We are primarily concerned about chronic respiratory acid-base disorders, as these can significantly alter the patient's baseline or expected values for the serum HCO_3 and $Paco_2$, and we have reliable equations to predict the expected baseline values. The respiratory compensation for both chronic metabolic acidosis and alkalosis is generally poor, so there are no equations or rules to predict what the $Paco_2$ should be in these cases. While the baseline serum HCO_3 may be significantly off from our standard value of 24 mEq/L in these patients, we would assume a baseline $Paco_2$ of 40 mm Hg in patients with chronic metabolic processes. Once we identify the patient's baseline $Paco_2$ and HCO_3 values, we will need to use these values in the appropriate equations to identify the ongoing acute processes.

Q53-2: C

Metabolic acidosis and a respiratory acidosis.

Rationale:

1. The pH is 7.01; therefore, the primary disorder is an **acidosis.**
2. The $Paco_2$ of 78 mm Hg is greater than 40 mm Hg, so there is a **respiratory acidosis.**
3. The HCO_3 of 19 mEq/L is less than 24 mEq/L, so there is also a **metabolic acidosis.**

Q53-3: C

Anion and non-anion gap acidosis.

Rationale:

1. Is there evidence for a chronic acid-base disorder that requires adjustment of the patient's "normal" HCO_3? No, there is no evidence for a chronic acid-base disorder, so we would assume a baseline $Paco_2$ of 40 mm Hg and an HCO_3 of 24 mEq/L.

2. Expected anion gap:

$$\text{Expected Anion Gap} = 12 - (2.5) * \left[4.0 \frac{g}{dL} - \text{Actual Serum Albumin} \right]$$
$$= 12 - (2.5 * [4.0 - 4.0])$$
$$= 12 - (2.5 * [0]) = \textbf{12 mEq/L.}$$

3. Anion gap calculation:

$$\text{Serum Anion Gap} = [Na^+] - [HCO_3^-] - [Cl^-]$$
$$= 139 - (106 + 19) = \textbf{14 mEq/L,} \text{ which is} > 12 \text{ mEq/L}$$
$$\rightarrow \textbf{anion gap acidosis is present.}$$

4. Delta-delta calculation:

$$\Delta\Delta = \frac{(\text{Actual Anion Gap} - \text{Expected Anion Gap})}{(\text{Baseline } HCO_3 - \text{Actual } HCO_3)}$$

$(14 - 12)/(24 - 19) = \textbf{2/5 = 0.4.}$

Delta-delta interpretation.	
Delta-Delta Value	**Condition Present**
< 0.4	Non-anion gap only
0.4–0.9	**Anion gap _and_ non-anion gap acidosis**
1.0–2.0	Anion gap acidosis only
> 2.0	Anion gap acidosis and metabolic alkalosis

Q53-4: A
Lactic acidosis.

Rationale: This patient presented with severe sepsis with hypotension secondary to pneumonia. The most likely etiology of his anion gap acidosis is a lactic acidosis. The negative serum acetone study makes a ketoacidosis unlikely. The negative serum drug screen makes acute acetaminophen and acute salicylate toxicity unlikely. The serum creatinine is normal, and the serum BUN and phosphorus are not significantly elevated, making renal failure less likely. The serum osmolal gap is +6 mOsm/L, which is normal (see further). Therefore, the only likely option is a lactic acidosis. The lactate in this case was 8.7 mmol/L.

$$\text{Calculated Serum Osmolality} = 2 * [Na^+] + \frac{[Glucose]}{18} + \frac{[BUN]}{2.8} + \frac{[EtOH]}{3.7}$$
$$= 294 \text{ mOsm/L}$$

$$\text{Serum Osmolal Gap (SOG)} = \text{Measured Serum Osmolality}$$
$$- \text{Calculated Serum Osmolality}$$
$$\text{SOG} = 300 \text{ mOsm/L} - 294 \text{ mOsm/L} = (+6) \text{ mOsm/L.}$$

Q53-5: B
Type 4 RTA.

Rationale: Recall that we can use either the urine anion gap (UAG) or urine osmolar gap (UOG) to qualitatively estimate urinary ammonium excretion. This is a case where the urine anion gap alone is inconclusive. The patient's urine anion gap is as follows:

$$UAG = [U_{Na}] + [U_{K}] - [U_{Cl}].$$

Therefore, for this patient,

$$UAG = (29 + 33) - (29) = (+34) \text{ mEq/L}.$$

A UAG gap that is greater than 20 mEq/L is associated with reduced renal acid excretion (a type 1 or 4 RTA), while a UAG that is less than −20 mEq/L is most commonly associated with GI loss of HCO_3 (eg, diarrhea), although type 2 RTA is possible. A UAG between −20 and +10 mEq/L is generally considered inconclusive. The UAG can be inappropriately elevated in anion gap acidosis, a situation in which multiple unmeasured anions may be present in the urine (beta-hydroxybutyrate/acetoacetate [ketoacidosis], hippurate [toluene], bicarbonate [proximal RTA], D-lactate [D-lactic acidosis], L-lactate, 5-oxoproline [acetaminophen toxicity]). Therefore, in patients with a significant anion gap, the urine osmolar gap is typically more useful.

$$\text{Calculated Urine Osmolality} = 2*([Na^+]+[K^+])+\frac{[Urea]}{2.8}+\frac{[Glucose]}{18}$$
$$= 191 \text{ mOsm/L}$$
$$UOG = \text{Measured Urine Osmolality}$$
$$- \text{Measured Urine Osmolality} = 97 \text{ mOsm/L}.$$

Similar to the UAG, the UOG is used as a surrogate for the urine ammonium concentration. Therefore, a larger gap indicates increased urinary NH_4 excretion. In normal acid-base conditions, the UOG is between 10 and 100 mOsm/L; this will be less than about 20 to 40 mOsm/L in all forms of RTA. During a significant metabolic acidosis, patients with impaired renal tubular acidification (ie, type 1 and type 4 RTA) are unable to excrete additional acid (NH_4), and therefore the osmolar gap does not change significantly (usually < 150 mOsm/L). Patients with an intact renal response to acidemia (ie, GI losses) should have a significant urine osmolar gap (> 300 to 400 mOsm/L) as a result of increased NH_4 excretion. The primary limitation is its use in conditions with a high osmolar gap, where non-ammonium solutes not included in the calculation may be present in the urine (particularly mannitol). The presence of these unmeasured solutes will increase the osmolal gap inappropriately. Also, the UOG should not be used in patients with a urinary tract infection caused by a urease-producing organism, as urea is metabolized to HCO_3 and ammonium in urine.

Therefore, this patient has an elevated urine anion gap and a reduced urine osmolal gap, indicating a type 1 or type 4 RTA is likely present. The low urine pH and the high serum potassium support the diagnosis of a type 4 RTA.

Evaluation of RTA			
	Type 1 RTA	Type 2 RTA	Type 4 RTA
Severity of metabolic acidosis, (HCO$_3$)	Severe (< 10–12 mEq/L typically)	Intermediate (12–20 mEq/L)	Mild (15–20 mEq/L)
Associated urine abnormalities	Urinary phosphate, calcium are increased; bone disease often present	Urine glucose, amino acids, phosphate, calcium may be elevated	
Urine pH	HIGH (> 5.5)	Low (acidic), until serum HCO$_3$ level exceeds the resorptive ability of the proximal tubule; then becomes alkalotic once reabsorptive threshold is crossed	Low (acidic)
Serum K$^+$	Low to normal; should correct with oral HCO$_3$ therapy	Classically low, although may be normal or even high with rare genetic defects; worsens with oral HCO$_3$ therapy	HIGH
Renal stones	Often	No	No
Renal tubular defect	Reduced NH$_4$ secretion in distal tubule	Reduced HCO$_3$ resorption in proximal tubule	Reduced H$^+$/K$^+$ exchange in distal and collecting tubule due to decreased aldosterone or aldosterone resistance
Urine anion gap	> 10	Negative initially, then positive when receiving serum HCO$_3$, then negative after therapy	> 10
Urine osmolal gap	Reduced (< 150 mOsm/L) during acute acidosis	At baseline is < 100 mEq/L; unreliable during acidosis	Reduced (< 150 mOsm/L) during acute acidosis

Q53-6: D
HIV.

Rationale: Common causes of type 4 RTA include medications (diuretics such as spironolactone; trimethoprim; pentamidine; heparin; NSAIDs; tacrolimus), diabetic nephropathy, HIV/AIDS (HIV-associated nephropathy), Addison disease, sickle cell disease, urinary tract obstruction, autoimmune disease (lupus, etc), amyloidosis, and kidney transplant rejection. This patient's vignette only provides one possible answer here. HIV can lead directly to tubular dysfunction and can also lead to hyporeninemic hypoaldosteronism (also associated with a type 4 RTA). HIV has also been associated with type 1 (distal) and type 2 (proximal) RTA, and renal tubular acidosis can also develop from medications associated with the treatment of HIV (particularly tenofovir, leading to a proximal RTA). These patients are also often treated with pentamidine and trimethoprim, which can further exacerbate the type 4 RTA picture. Renal disease associated with HIV is a complex subject.

Causes of renal tubular acidosis.
Causes of Type 1 (Distal) RTA
Primary • Idiopathic or familial (may be recessive or dominant)
Secondary • Medications: Lithium, amphotericin, ifosfamide, NSAIDs • Rheumatologic disorders: Sjögren syndrome, SLE, RA • Hypercalciuria (idiopathic) or associated with vitamin D deficiency or hyperparathyroidism • Sarcoidosis • Obstructive uropathy • Wilson disease • Rejection of renal transplant allograft • Toluene toxicity
Causes of Type 2 (Proximal) RTA
Primary • Idiopathic • Familial (primarily recessive disorders) • Genetic: Fanconi syndrome, cystinosis, glycogen storage disease (type 1), Wilson disease, galactosemia
Secondary • Medications: Acetazolamide, topiramate, aminoglycoside antibiotics, ifosfamide, reverse transcriptase inhibitors (tenofovir) • Heavy metal poisoning: Lead, mercury, copper • Multiple myeloma or amyloidosis (secondary to light chain toxicity) • Sjögren syndrome • Vitamin D deficiency • Rejection of renal transplant allograft
Causes of Type 4 RTA (Hypoaldosteronism or Aldosterone Resistance)
Primary • Primary adrenal insufficiency • Inherited disorders associated with hypoaldosteronism • Pseudohypoaldosteronism (types 1 and 2)
Secondary • Causes of hyporeninemic hypoaldosteronism such as renal disease (diabetic nephropathy), NSAID use, calcineurin inhibitors, volume expansion/volume overload • Causes of distal tubule voltage defects such as sickle cell disease, obstructive uropathy, SLE • Severe illness/septic shock • Angiotensin II–associated medications: ACE inhibitors, ARBs, direct renin inhibitors • Potassium-sparing diuretics: Spironolactone, amiloride, triamterene • Antibiotics: Trimethoprim, pentamidine

Q53-7: A
COPD.

Rationale: The patient has a significant respiratory acidosis most likely due to his underlying COPD with an acute exacerbation. Patients with advanced COPD often have trouble compensating for a metabolic acidosis and can tire out easily, leading to a concomitant respiratory acidosis. This patient does not have a metabolic alkalosis, but rather a metabolic acidosis.

References

Balow JE. Nephropathy in the context of HIV infection. Kidney Int. 2005;67:1632.

Chattha G, Arieff AI, Cummings C, Tierney LM Jr. Lactic acidosis complicating the acquired immunodeficiency syndrome. Ann Intern Med. 1993;118:37.

Guy RJ, Turberg Y, Davidson RN, et al. Mineralocorticoid deficiency in HIV infection. BMJ. 1989;298:496.

Hall AM, Hendry BM, Nitsch D, Connolly JO. Tenofovir-associated kidney toxicity in HIV-infected patients: a review of the evidence. Am J Kidney Dis. 2011;57:773.

Kalin MF, Poretsky L, Seres DS, Zumoff B. Hyporeninemic hypoaldosteronism associated with acquired immune deficiency syndrome. Am J Med. 1987;82:1035.

Lucas GM, Ross MJ, Stock PG, et al. Clinical practice guideline for the management of chronic kidney disease in patients infected with HIV: 2014 update by the HIV Medicine Association of the Infectious Diseases Society of America. Clin Infect Dis. 2014;59:e96.

Musso CG, Belloso WH, Glassock RJ. Water, electrolytes, and acid-base alterations in human immunodeficiency virus infected patients. World J Nephrol. 2016;5:33.

Peters L, Grint D, Lundgren JD, et al. Hepatitis C virus viremia increases the incidence of chronic kidney disease in HIV-infected patients. AIDS. 2012;26:1917.

Razzak Chaudhary S, Workeneh BT, Montez-Rath ME, et al. Trends in the outcomes of end-stage renal disease secondary to human immunodeficiency virus-associated nephropathy. Nephrol Dial Transplant. 2015;30:1734.

Schwartz EJ, Szczech LA, Ross MJ, et al. Highly active antiretroviral therapy and the epidemic of HIV+ end-stage renal disease. J Am Soc Nephrol 2005;16:2412.

Tourret J, Deray G, Isnard-Bagnis C. Tenofovir effect on the kidneys of HIV-infected patients: a double-edged sword? J Am Soc Nephrol 2013;24:1519.

Velázquez H, Perazella MA, Wright FS, Ellison DH. Renal mechanism of trimethoprim-induced hyperkalemia. Ann Intern Med. 1993;119:296.

Venkatesan EP, Pranesh MB, Gnanashanmugam G, Balasubramaniam J. Tenofovir induced Fanconi syndrome: A rare cause of hypokalemic paralysis. Indian J Nephrol. 2014;24:108.

CASE 54

A 78-year-old man with systolic congestive heart failure (EF 25% to 30%), coronary artery disease, and CKD stage 2 (baseline Cr 1.4) presents with decompensated congestive heart failure. He noted increased weight gain over the past 3 days and increased his use of both furosemide and metolazone considerably in an attempt to remove fluid at home, but this was unsuccessful. He is tachpneic on examination, and is hypoxemic requiring 4L NC. His vitals signs are T 35.9C, BP 100/45, HR 90, RR 25, Sao$_2$ 96% on the 4L/min of supplemental oxygen. He has inspiratory crackles throughout his lung fields. He is warm and edematous on examination.

Laboratory data.			
ABGs		Basic Metabolic Panel	
pH	7.58	Na	134 mEq/L
Paco$_2$	34 mm Hg	K	2.9 mEq/L
Pao$_2$	75 mm Hg	Cl	102 mEq/L
HCO$_3$	32 mEq/L	CO$_2$	31 mEq/L
		BUN	55 mg/dL
		Cr	1.6 mg/dL
		Glucose	89 mg/dL
		Albumin	2.5 g/dL
		EtOH	0 mg/dL

QUESTIONS

Q54-1: Define the patient's baseline acid-base status: Does this patient have an underlying chronic acid-base disorder that we need to account for in order to appropriately interpret the acute acid-base disorders?

A. There is no evidence for an underlying chronic respiratory or metabolic acid-base disorder in this patient, so we would assume a baseline $Paco_2$ of 40 mm Hg and an HCO_3 of 24 mEq/L.

B. While the patient has a condition predisposing him to a chronic acid-base disorder, there is insufficient information to estimate the patient's baseline $Paco_2$ and HCO_3 values; therefore, we will assume a baseline $Paco_2$ of 40 mm Hg and a baseline HCO_3 of 24 mEq/L.

C. The patient has an underlying acid-base condition, and we have sufficient information to estimate the patient's baseline $Paco_2$ and HCO_3 values.

Q54-2: What is/are the primary acid-base disturbance(s) occurring in this case?

A. Metabolic acidosis only
B. Respiratory acidosis only
C. Metabolic acidosis and a respiratory acidosis
D. Metabolic alkalosis and a respiratory alkalosis
E. Metabolic alkalosis only
F. Respiratory alkalosis only

Q54-3: What is the likely source of the patient's respiratory alkalosis?

A. Aspirin overdose
B. Cirrhosis
C. Hypoxemia
D. CNS injury

Q54-4: The patient has a urine chloride value of 33 mEq/L. What is the likely cause of the patient's metabolic alkalosis?

A. Metolazone and furosemide use for volume overload
B. Spironolactone use for congestive heart failure
C. Trimethoprim use for a UTI
D. Acetazolamide use for volume overload
E. Aminoglycoside use for UTI
F. Hyperemesis due to edema

Q54-5: The patient is treated aggressively with IV diuretics over the next 24 hours, and his most recent metabolic panel shows a serum HCO_3 of 37 mEq/L. He is no longer tachypneic, no longer requiring supplemental oxygen, and his CXR is clear. What would you expect the patient's $Paco_2$ to be now if he were compensating appropriately *and* now assuming the metabolic alkalosis is *entirely acute*?

A. 40 mm Hg
B. 45 mm Hg
C. 50 mm Hg
D. 60 mm Hg
E. 65 mm Hg

ANSWERS

Q54-1: B

While the patient has a condition predisposing him to a chronic acid-base disorder, there is insufficient information to estimate the patient's baseline $Paco_2$ and HCO_3 values; therefore, we will assume a baseline $Paco_2$ of 40 mm Hg and a baseline HCO_3 of 24 mEq/L. The patient has congestive heart failure, which can be associated with chronic acid-base disorders. However, we have no evidence to define a new baseline for this patient.

Rationale: Ignoring these underlying chronic acid-base disorders can significantly alter the interpretation of a patient's acute acid-base status. This was demonstrated in the first case of the series. However, often, we do not have the necessary information (eg, prior ABG or VBG, or prior serum chemistry with an HCO_3) and are forced to assume the ongoing processes are all acute in nature. We are primarily concerned about chronic respiratory acid-base disorders, as these can significantly alter the patient's baseline or expected values for the serum HCO_3 and $Paco_2$, and we have reliable equations to predict the expected baseline values. The respiratory compensation for both chronic metabolic acidosis and alkalosis is generally poor, so there are no equations or rules to predict what the $Paco_2$ should be in these cases. While the baseline serum HCO_3 may be significantly off from our standard value of 24 mEq/L in these patients, we would assume a baseline $Paco_2$ of 40 mm Hg in patients with chronic metabolic processes. Once we identify the patient's baseline $Paco_2$ and HCO_3 values, we will need to use these values in the appropriate equations to identify the ongoing acute processes.

Q54-2: D

Metabolic alkalosis and a respiratory alkalosis.

Rationale:

1. The pH is 7.58; therefore, the primary disorder is an **alkalosis**.
2. The $Paco_2$ of 34 mm Hg is less than 40 mm Hg, so there is a **respiratory alkalosis**.
3. The HCO_3 of 31 mEq/L is greater than 24 mEq/L, so there is also a **metabolic alkalosis**.

Q54-3: C

Hypoxemia.

Rationale: This patient has presented with hypoxemia secondary to pulmonary edema from decompensated congestive heart failure. This leads to tachypnea and will decrease the $Paco_2$, leading to respiratory alkalosis. We would expect an anion gap acidosis if aspirin toxicity were the cause. While some patients with congestive heart failure (particularly right-sided) can develop portal hypertension over time, there is no indication that the patient has liver disease, nor is there an indication of CNS injury leading to alterations in respiratory centers.

Q54-4: A
Metolazone and furosemide use for volume overload.

Rationale: The patient has a chloride-resistant metabolic alkalosis ($U_{Cl} > 20$ mEq/L). Prior diuretic use is associated with a chloride-responsive metabolic alkalosis; however, ongoing diuretic use is associated with a chloride-resistant metabolic alkalosis. Spironolactone is usually associated with a type 4 RTA, as is trimethoprim. Acetazolamides are usually associated with a type 2 RTA (proximal). Aminoglycosides can be associated with either a metabolic alkalosis or a non-anion gap metabolic acidosis; however, there is no evidence for use of an aminoglycoside in this patient. Hyperemesis is associated with a chloride-responsive metabolic alkalosis.

Causes of metabolic alkalosis.
History: Rule Out the Following as Causes
• Alkali load ("milk-alkali" or calcium-alkali syndrome, oral sodium bicarbonate, IV sodium bicarbonate) • Genetic causes (CF) • Presence of hypercalcemia • Intravenous β-lactam antibiotics • Laxative abuse (may also cause a metabolic acidosis depending on diarrheal HCO_3 losses)
If None of the Above, Then…
Urine Chloride < 20 mEq/L (Chloride-Responsive Causes) • Loss of gastric acid (hyperemesis, NGT suctioning) • Prior diuretic use (in hours to days following discontinuation) • Post-hypercapnia • Villous adenoma • Congenital chloridorrhea • Chronic laxative abuse (may also cause a metabolic acidosis depending on diarrheal HCO_3 losses) • CF
OR
Urine Chloride > 20 mEq/L (Chloride-Resistant Causes)
Urine Chloride > 20 mEq/L, Lack of HTN, Urine Potassium < 30 mEq/L
• Hypokalemia or hypomagnesemia • Laxative abuse (if dominated by hypokalemia) • Bartter syndrome • Gitelman syndrome
Urine Chloride > 20 mEq/L, Lack of HTN, Urine Potassium > 30 mEq/L
• Current diuretic use
Urine Chloride > 20 mEq/L, Presence of HTN, Urine Potassium Variable but Usually > 30 mEq/L
Elevated plasma renin level: • Renal artery stenosis • Renin-secreting tumor • Renovascular disease

(Continued)

Causes of metabolic alkalosis. (*continued*)
Low plasma renin, low plasma aldosterone
• Cushing syndrome
• Exogenous mineralocorticoid use
• Genetic disorder (11-hydoxylase or 17-hydrolyase deficiency, 11β-HSD deficiency)
• Liddle syndrome
• Licorice toxicity
Low plasma renin, high plasma aldosterone
• Primary hyperaldosteronism
• Adrenal adenoma
• Bilateral adrenal hyperplasia

Q54-5: C
50 mm Hg.

Rationale: The expected compensatory $Paco_2$ for an acute metabolic alkalosis is calculated as follows:

$$\text{Expected } Paco_2 = \text{Baseline } Paco_2 - (0.7)\ [\text{Actual } HCO_3 - \text{Baseline } HCO_3]$$
$$\text{Expected } Paco_2 = 40 + (0.7) * (37 - 24) = 40 + (0.7) * (13) = \sim\textbf{50 mm Hg.}$$

References

Abreo K, Adlakha A, Kilpatrick S, et al. The milk-alkali syndrome. A reversible form of acute renal failure. Arch Intern Med. 1993;153:1005.

Barton CH, Vaziri ND, Ness RL, et al. Cimetidine in the management of metabolic alkalosis induced by nasogastric drainage. Arch Surg. 1979;114:70.

Bear R, Goldstein M, Phillipson E, et al. Effect of metabolic alkalosis on respiratory function in patients with chronic obstructive lung disease. Can Med Assoc J. 1977;117:900.

Galla JH, Gifford JD, Luke RG, Rome L. Adaptations to chloride-depletion alkalosis. Am J Physiol. 1991;261:R771.

Garella S, Chang BS, Kahn SI. Dilution acidosis and contraction alkalosis: review of a concept. Kidney Int. 1975;8:279.

Gennari FJ, Weise WJ. Acid-base disturbances in gastrointestinal disease. Clin J Am Soc Nephrol. 2008;3:1861.

Hamm LL, Nakhoul N, Hering-Smith KS. Acid-base homeostasis. Clin J Am Soc Nephrol. 2015;10:2232.

Hulter HN, Sebastian A, Toto RD, et al. Renal and systemic acid-base effects of the chronic administration of hypercalcemia-producing agents: calcitriol, PTH, and intravenous calcium. Kidney Int. 1982;21:445.

Khanna A, Kurtzman NA. Metabolic alkalosis. J Nephrol. 2006;19(suppl 9):S86.

Laski ME, Sabatini S. Metabolic alkalosis, bedside and bench. Semin Nephrol. 2006;26:404.

Luke RG, Galla JH. It is chloride depletion alkalosis, not contraction alkalosis. J Am Soc Nephrol. 2012;23:204.

CASE 55

A 64-year old male patient with bladder cancer, status post-bladder resection, and ureteroenterostomy presents with altered mental status. He has been experiencing issues with back pain recently and was taking an OTC pain relief powder frequently over the past few days. He is tachypneic on presentation with T 36.7°C, BP 110/70, HR 110, RR 30, with Sao$_2$ 94% on 2L NC. A head CT scan is negative. His CXR demonstrates bilateral infiltrates or edema, and he is hypoxemic requiring 4 L NC.

Laboratory data.			
ABGs		Basic Metabolic Panel	
pH	7.52	Na	139 mEq/L
Paco$_2$	19 mm Hg	K	2.8 mEq/L
Paco$_2$	80 mm Hg	Cl	112 mEq/L
HCO$_3$	15 mEq/L	CO$_2$	15 mEq/L
		BUN	22 mg/dL
		Cr	0.5 mg/dL
		Glucose	89 mg/dL
		Albumin	2.5 g/dL
		EtOH	0 mg/dL

QUESTIONS

Q55-1: Define the patient's baseline acid-base status: Does this patient have an underlying chronic acid-base disorder that we need to account for in order to appropriately interpret the acute acid-base disorders?

A. There is no evidence for an underlying chronic respiratory or metabolic acid-base disorder in this patient, so we would assume a baseline $Paco_2$ of 40 mm Hg and an HCO_3 of 24 mEq/L.

B. While the patient has a condition predisposing him to a chronic acid-base disorder, there is insufficient information to estimate the patient's baseline $Paco_2$ and HCO_3 values; therefore, we will assume a baseline $Paco_2$ of 40 mm Hg and a baseline HCO_3 of 24 mEq/L.

C. The patient has an underlying acid-base condition, and we have sufficient information to estimate the patient's baseline $Paco_2$ and HCO_3 values.

Q55-2: What is/are the primary acid-base disturbance(s) occurring in this case?

A. Metabolic acidosis only
B. Respiratory acidosis only
C. Metabolic acidosis and a respiratory acidosis
D. Metabolic alkalosis and a respiratory alkalosis
E. Metabolic alkalosis only
F. Respiratory alkalosis only

Q55-3: How would the metabolic acidosis component be classified in this case?

A. Anion gap acidosis
B. Non-anion gap acidosis
C. Anion and non-anion gap acidosis
D. Anion gap acidosis and a metabolic alkalosis
E. The reduction in HCO_3 represents appropriate metabolic compensation

Q55-4: Laboratory testing returns the following results:

Serum EtOH	< 3 mg/dL
Serum osmolality	312 mOsm/kg
Serum L-lactate	0.9 mmol/L (ULN 2.0 mmol/L venous)
Beta-hydroxybutyrate (acetone)	< 0.18 mmol/L (ULN 0.18 mmol/L)
Serum glucose	89 mg/dL
Serum phosphorus	2.9 mg/dL

What is the likely etiology for the patient's primary acid-base disorder?

A. Lactic acidosis
B. Acute renal failure
C. Heart failure
D. Organic alcohol intoxication
E. CNS injury
F. Aspirin overdose
G. Acetaminophen overdose

Q55-5: The urine anion gap is −55. The urine pH is 5.6. There is no evidence of glucose or protein in the urine. What is the most likely cause of the patient's non-anion gap acidosis?

A. Type 1 RTA (distal)
B. Diarrhea
C. Carbonic anhydrase inhibitor use
D. Total parenteral nutrition (TPN)
E. Ureteroenterostomy
F. Addison disease

ANSWERS

Q55-1: B

While the patient has a condition predisposing him to a chronic acid-base disorder, there is insufficient information to estimate the patient's baseline $Paco_2$ and HCO_3 values; therefore, we will assume a baseline $Paco_2$ of 40 mm Hg and a baseline HCO_3 of 24 mEq/L. The patient has a ureteroenterostomy, which can be associated with chronic acid-base disorders if the ostomy becomes obstructed or dysfunctional. However, at present no evidence supports that etiology.

Rationale: Ignoring these underlying chronic acid-base disorders can significantly alter the interpretation of a patient's acute acid-base status. This was demonstrated in the first case of the series. However, often, we do not have the necessary information (eg, prior ABG or VBG, or prior serum chemistry with an HCO_3) and are forced to assume the ongoing processes are all acute in nature. We are primarily concerned about chronic respiratory acid-base disorders, as these can significantly alter the patient's baseline or expected values for the serum HCO_3 and $Paco_2$, and we have reliable equations to predict the expected baseline values. The respiratory compensation for both chronic metabolic acidosis and alkalosis is generally poor, so there are no equations or rules to predict what the $Paco_2$ should be in these cases. While the baseline serum HCO_3 may be significantly off from our standard value of 24 mEq/L in these patients, we would assume a baseline $Paco_2$ of 40 mm Hg in patients with chronic metabolic processes. Once we identify the patient's baseline $Paco_2$ and HCO_3 values, we will need to use these values in the appropriate equations to identify the ongoing acute processes.

Q55-2: F

Respiratory alkalosis only.

Rationale:

1. The pH is 7.52; therefore, the primary disorder is an **alkalosis.**
2. The $Paco_2$ of 19 mm Hg is less than 40 mmHg, so there is a **respiratory alkalosis.**
3. The HCO_3 of 15 mEq/L is less than 24 mEq/L, so a **primary metabolic alkalosis is not present.**

Q55-3: C

Anion and non-anion gap acidosis.

Rationale:

1. Is there evidence for a chronic acid-base disorder that requires adjustment of the patient's "normal" HCO_3? No, there is no evidence for a chronic acid-base disorder, so we would assume a baseline $Paco_2$ of 40 mm Hg and an HCO_3 of 24 mEq/L.
2. Does the reduction in the patient's serum HCO_3 represent an appropriate metabolic compensation for acute respiratory alkalosis?

Expected HCO_3 = Baseline HCO_3 – (0.20) [Actual $Paco_2$ – Baseline $Paco_2$]
Expected HCO_3 = 24 mEq/L – (0.20) * [40 mmHg – 19 mm Hg] = 19.8 mEq/L.

Since the patient's actual HCO_3 is less than the expected 20 mEq/L, there is also a concomitant metabolic acidosis.

3. Is the patient's serum albumin 4.0? No, so the expected anion gap is as follows:

$$\text{Expected Anion Gap} = 12 - (2.5) * \left[4.0 \frac{g}{dL} - \text{Actual Serum Albumin} \right]$$

$$\text{Expected Gap} = 12 - (2.5) * (4.0 - 2.5) = 12 - (2.5) * (1.5)$$
$$= 8.25 \sim \textbf{8 mEq/L.}$$

4. Anion gap calculation:

$$\text{Serum Anion Gap} = [Na^+] - [HCO_3^-] - [Cl^-]$$
$$139 - (112 + 15) = \textbf{12 mEq/L, which is} > 8 \text{ mEq/L}$$
$$\rightarrow \text{anion gap acidosis is present.}$$

We would have missed this anion gap acidosis if we did not take into account the reduced albumin in this patient.

5. Delta-Delta calculation:

$$\Delta\Delta = \frac{(\text{Actual Anion Gap} - \text{Expected Anion Gap})}{(\text{Baseline } HCO_3 - \text{Actual } HCO_3)}$$

$$= (12 - 8)/(24 - 15) = \textbf{4/9} = \textbf{0.4.}$$

Delta-delta interpretation	
Delta-Delta Value	Condition Present
< 0.4	Non-anion gap only
0.4–0.9	**Anion gap *and* non-anion gap acidosis**
1.0–2.0	Anion gap acidosis only
> 2.0	Anion gap acidosis and metabolic alkalosis

Q55-4: D
Aspirin overdose.

Rationale: This patient's primary presenting acid-base disorder is a respiratory alkalosis. Coupled with the anion gap metabolic acidosis, this is a classic presentation of aspirin overdose. While the patient is hypoxemic with infiltrates on CXR, there is no information that he has a history of heart disease. Additionally, aspirin toxicity can lead to the development of pulmonary edema, which is non-cardiogenic. The lactate result is negative, so there is no lactic acidosis. The serum acetone is also negative, so there is no DKA, alcoholic ketoacidosis, or starvation ketoacidosis (although note that aspirin can actually cause ketosis via blockade of oxidative phosphorylation).

The serum osmolality is 312, so the osmolar gap is 5 (calculated using Na, BUN, and EtOH), and glucose is 307, which is normal, ruling out an organic acid ingestion.

$$\text{Calculated Serum Osmolality} = 2*[Na^+] + \frac{[\text{Glucose}]}{18} + \frac{[\text{BUN}]}{2.8} + \frac{[\text{EtOH}]}{3.7}$$

$$= [2*139] + [89/18] + [22/2.8] + [0/3.7] = 307\ \text{mOsm/L}$$

$$\text{Serum Osmolal Gap (SOG)} = \text{Measured Serum Osmolality}$$
$$- \text{Calculated Serum Osmolality}$$
$$= 312\ \text{mOsm/L} - 307 = (+5)\ \text{mOsm/L}.$$

Additionally, the BUN is not significantly elevated nor is the serum phosphorus, and his renal function is likely close to baseline, so renal failure is not likely.

The patient's presentation with back pain and frequent use of OTC pain relief powders is most consistent with a salicylate or ASA overdose. Although the patient has a detectable acetaminophen level, acetaminophen overdose is not associated with respiratory alkalosis (unless the patient is in florid liver failure), and is associated most commonly with a lactic acidosis. Pain relief powder medications often come in combinations, including aspirin and acetaminophen, so these will often been seen together in such cases. Therefore the ASA overdose accounts for both the respiratory alkalosis as well as the anion gap acidosis.

Acute overdoses of ASA or salicylates initially may yield hyperactivity, respiratory alkalosis, fever, seizures, and delirium, but may quickly progress to respiratory failure, rhabdomyolysis, and lethargy/obtundation. Symptoms of chronic toxicity are usually more subtle in nature.

Q55-5: E
Ureteroenterostomy.

Rationale: This patient has a uteroenterostomy, which is a conduit from the ureters to the small bowel as a replacement for the bladder. Urine contains large amounts of chloride. Rather than being excreted during urination, the chloride is resorbed in the sigmoid colon via a Cl/HCO$_3$ transported in the sigmoid colon. Patients with bladder resection often develop a non-anion gap acidosis as a result of HCO$_3$ loss in the stool. This is further supported by the low serum potassium. The prompt does not include evidence that the patient has diarrhea, so this etiology is unlikely (although if present it would also be associated with a significantly reduced urine anion gap and hypokalemia). There is likewise no evidence that the patient was given TPN or a carbonic anhydrase inhibitor. Addison disease is typically associated with a type 4 RTA. TPN is more commonly associated with an anion gap acidosis. A type 1 RTA would be associated with a high urine pH, an elevated urine anion gap, and a low serum potassium level.

References

Batlle D, Chin-Theodorou J, Tucker BM. Metabolic acidosis or respiratory alkalosis? Evaluation of a low plasma bicarbonate using the urine anion gap. Am J Kidney Dis. 2017;70:440.

Batlle D, Grupp M, Gaviria M, Kurtzman NA. Distal renal tubular acidosis with intact capacity to lower urinary pH. Am J Med. 1982;72:751.

Batlle D, Haque SK. Genetic causes and mechanisms of distal renal tubular acidosis. Nephrol Dial Transplant. 2012;27:3691.

Batlle DC, Hizon M, Cohen E, et al. The use of the urinary anion gap in the diagnosis of hyperchloremic metabolic acidosis. N Engl J Med. 1988;318:594.

Batlle DC, von Riotte A, Schlueter W. Urinary sodium in the evaluation of hyperchloremic metabolic acidosis. N Engl J Med. 1987;316:140.

Buckalew VM Jr, McCurdy DK, Ludwig GD, et al. Incomplete renal tubular acidosis. Physiologic studies in three patients with a defect in lowering urine pH. Am J Med. 1968;45:32.

Eichenholz A, Mulhausen RO, Redleaf PS. Nature of acid-base disturbance in salicylate intoxication. Metabolism. 1963;12:164.

Gabow PA, Anderson RJ, Potts DE, Schrier RW. Acid-base disturbances in the salicylate-intoxicated adult. Arch Intern Med. 1978;138:1481.

Hill JB. Salicylate intoxication. N Engl J Med. 1973;288:1110.

Karet FE. Mechanisms in hyperkalemic renal tubular acidosis. J Am Soc Nephrol. 2009;20:251.

Kraut JA, Madias NE. Differential diagnosis of nongap metabolic acidosis: value of a systematic approach. Clin J Am Soc Nephrol. 2012;7:671.

Rastegar M, Nagami GT. Non-anion gap metabolic acidosis: a clinical approach to evaluation. Am J Kidney Dis. 2017;69:296.

Rodríguez Soriano J. Renal tubular acidosis: the clinical entity. J Am Soc Nephrol. 2002;13:2160.

Temple AR. Acute and chronic effects of aspirin toxicity and their treatment. Arch Intern Med. 1981;141:364.

Thisted B, Krantz T, Strøom J, Sørensen MB. Acute salicylate self-poisoning in 177 consecutive patients treated in ICU. Acta Anaesthesiol Scand. 1987;31:312.

CASE 56

A 44-year-old man with a history of alcoholism and IV drug abuse presents to the clinic from home with encephalopathy. He has been taking OTC anti-inflammatory medications for a pinched nerve over the past few days. His vital signs are T 39.1°C, RR 28, HR 123, BP 100/60, and Sao_2 95% on RA. He takes spironolactone, furosemide, propranolol, and rifaximin at home. A CT scan of the head is negative. Lumbar puncture is also negative. His examination is unremarkable aside from the previously noted tachypnea and sinus tachycardia.

Laboratory data.				
ABGs		Basic Metabolic Panel		
pH	7.22	Na	131 mEq/L	
$Paco_2$	20 mm Hg	K	5.5 mEq/L	
Pao_2	100 mm Hg	Cl	112 mEq/L	
HCO_3	8 mEq/L	CO_2	8 mEq/L	
		BUN	29	mg/dL
		Cr	2.3	mg/dL
		Glucose	89	mg/dL
		Albumin	1.5	g/dL
		EtOH	0	mg/dL

QUESTIONS

Q56-1: Define the patient's baseline acid-base status: Does this patient have an underlying chronic acid-base disorder that we need to account for in order to appropriately interpret the acute acid-base disorders?

A. There is no evidence for an underlying chronic respiratory or metabolic acid-base disorder in this patient, so we would assume a baseline $Paco_2$ of 40 mm Hg and an HCO_3 of 24 mEq/L.

B. While the patient has a condition predisposing him to a chronic acid-base disorder, there is insufficient information to estimate the patient's baseline $Paco_2$ and HCO_3 values; therefore, we will assume a baseline $Paco_2$ of 40 mm Hg and a baseline HCO_3 of 24 mEq/L.

C. The patient has an underlying acid-base condition, and we have sufficient information to estimate the patient's baseline $Paco_2$ and HCO_3 values.

Q56-2: What is/are the primary acid-base disturbance(s) occurring in this case?

A. Metabolic acidosis only
B. Respiratory acidosis only
C. Metabolic acidosis and a respiratory acidosis
D. Metabolic alkalosis and a respiratory alkalosis
E. Metabolic alkalosis only
F. Respiratory alkalosis only

Q56-3: For a perfectly healthy patient, a normal anion gap is assumed to be 12 mEq/L. What should be considered a normal anion gap in this patient?

A. 12 mEq/L
B. 10 mEq/L
C. 6 mEq/L
D. 4 mEq/L

Q56-4: How would the metabolic acidosis component be classified in this case?

A. Anion gap acidosis
B. Non-anion gap acidosis
C. Anion and non-anion gap acidosis
D. Anion gap acidosis and a metabolic alkalosis

Q56-5: Does the patient in this case demonstrate appropriate respiratory or metabolic compensation?

A. Yes, the respiratory compensation is appropriate.
B. No, a concomitant respiratory alkalosis is present.
C. No, a concomitant respiratory acidosis is present.
D. Yes, the metabolic compensation is appropriate.
E. No, a concomitant metabolic acidosis is present.
F. No, a concomitant metabolic alkalosis is present.

Q56-6: Some of the patient's remaining test results are as follows:

Serum EtOH	< 3 mg/dL
Serum osmolality	284 mOsm/kg
Serum L-Lactate	3.5 mmol/L (ULN 2.0 mmol/L venous)
Beta-hydroxybutyrate (acetone)	< 0.18 mmol/L (ULN 0.18 mmol/L)
Serum glucose	89 mg/dL
Serum phosphorus	1.9 mg/dL
Serum total bilirubin	14.7 mg/dL
AST	29,000 IU/mL
CK	213 IU/mL
Troponin	0.21 ng/mL
Urine drug screen	Negative
INR	3.1 (unitless) (ULN 1.3)

What is the likely cause of the patient's anion gap acidosis?

A. Aspirin toxicity
B. Lactic acidosis secondary to sepsis
C. Ethylene glycol toxicity
D. Methanol toxicity
E. Opioid overdose
F. Acetaminophen overdose
G. DKA
H. Alcoholic ketoacidosis

Q56-7: What organic acid is responsible for the anion gap acidosis in acetaminophen toxicity?

A. Pyroglutamic acid (5-oxoproline)
B. Oxalic acid
C. Lactic acid
D. Hippuric acid

Q56-8: The patient's urine results, including electrolytes, are shown as follows:

Urine Na	28 mEq/L
Urine K	34 mEq/L
Urine Cl	31 mEq/L
Urine urea	334 mg/dL
Urine glucose:	0 mg/dL
Urine osmolality	310 mOsm/L
Urine pH	5.3
Urine RBCs	None
Urine WBCs	None
Urine protein	Mild
Urine microscopic	None

What is the likely cause of the non-anion gap acidosis?

A. Acetazolamide

B. Spironolactone

C. Propranolol

D. Amphotericin

ANSWERS

Q56-1: B

While the patient has a condition predisposing him to a chronic acid-base disorder, there is insufficient information to estimate the patient's baseline $Paco_2$ and HCO_3 values; therefore, we will assume a baseline $Paco_2$ of 40 mm Hg and a baseline HCO_3 of 24 mEq/L. The patient has a history of alcoholism, which can be associated with chronic acid-base disorders. However, we lack sufficient evidence to make any assumptions at this point.

Rationale: Ignoring these underlying chronic acid-base disorders can significantly alter the interpretation of a patient's acute acid-base status. This was demonstrated in the first case of the series. However, often, we do not have the necessary information (eg, prior ABG or VBG, or prior serum chemistry with an HCO_3) and are forced to assume the ongoing processes are all acute in nature. We are primarily concerned about chronic respiratory acid-base disorders, as these can significantly alter the patient's baseline or expected values for the serum HCO_3 and $Paco_2$, and we have reliable equations to predict the expected baseline values. The respiratory compensation for both chronic metabolic acidosis and alkalosis is generally poor, so there are no equations or rules to predict what the $Paco_2$ should be in these cases. While the baseline serum HCO_3 may be significantly off from our standard value 24 mEq/L in these patients, we would assume a baseline $Paco_2$ of 40 mm Hg in patients with chronic metabolic processes. Once we identify the patient's baseline $Paco_2$ and HCO_3 values, we will need to use these values in the appropriate equations to identify the ongoing acute processes.

Q56-2: A

Metabolic acidosis only.

Rationale:

1. The pH is 7.22; therefore, the primary disorder is an **acidosis.**
2. The $Paco_2$ of 20 mm Hg is less than 40 mm Hg, so a **primary respiratory process is unlikely.**
3. The HCO_3 of 8 mEq/L is less than 24 mEq/L, so there is a **primary metabolic acidosis.**

Q56-3: C

6 mEq/L.

Rationale: The normal anion gap is 12 mEq/L. The term *anion gap* refers to those ions (negatively charged molecules) in the bloodstream that we do not routinely measure, including phosphates, sulfates, organic acids, and negatively charged plasma proteins. One of the most abundant negatively charged ions in the blood is serum albumin. A normal serum albumin is 4.0 g/dL. For patients with hypoalbuminemia (low serum albumin), the normal or expected anion gap is smaller.

$$\text{Expected Anion Gap} = 12 - (2.5) * \left[4.0 \frac{g}{dL} - \text{Actual Serum Albumin} \right].$$

Therefore, for this patient,

$$\text{Expected Anion Gap} = 12 - [2.5 * (4 - 1.5)] = 12 - (2.5 * 2.5) = 6 \text{ mEq/L}.$$

This is an important concept, as patients with hypoalbuminemia may "hide" an anion gap acidosis if this correction is not performed.

Q56-4: A
Anion gap acidosis.

Rationale:

1. Is there evidence for a chronic acid-base disorder that requires adjustment of the patient's "normal" HCO_3? No, there is no evidence for a chronic acid-base disorder, so we would assume a baseline $Paco_2$ of 40 mm Hg and an HCO_3 of 24 mEq/L.
2. Expected anion gap:

$$\text{Expected Anion Gap} = 12 - (2.5) * \left[4.0 \frac{g}{dL} - \text{Actual Serum Albumin} \right]$$
$$= 12 - (2.5 * [4.0 - 1.5])$$
$$= 12 - (2.5 * [2.5]) = 5.75 \sim \mathbf{6 \text{ mEq/L}}.$$

3. Anion gap calculation:

$$\text{Serum Anion Gap} = [Na^+] - [HCO_3^-] - [Cl^-]$$
$$= 131 - (112 + 8) = \mathbf{11 \text{ mEq/L}}, \text{ which is} > 6 \text{ mEq/L}$$
$$\rightarrow \textbf{anion gap acidosis is present.}$$

Note: If we did not adjust the expected anion gap for the low albumin, we would have missed this anion gap acidosis.

4. Delta-Delta calculation:

$$\Delta\Delta = \frac{(\text{Actual Anion Gap} - \text{Expected Anion Gap})}{(\text{Baseline HCO}_3 - \text{Actual HCO}_3)}$$
$$= (11 - 6)/(24 - 8) = \mathbf{5/16, \text{ which is} \sim 0.4.}$$

Delta-delta interpretation.	
Delta-Delta Value	**Condition Present**
< 0.4	Non-anion gap only
0.4–0.9	**Anion gap and non-anion gap acidosis**
1.0–2.0	Anion gap acidosis only
> 2.0	Anion gap acidosis and metabolic alkalosis

Q56-5: A
Yes, the respiratory compensation is appropriate.

Rationale: Using the Winter formula, one can calculate what the expected arterial $Paco_2$ should be for a given serum HCO_3 if the patient were completely compensated.

$$\text{Expected Paco}_2 = 1.5 * (\text{Actual HCO}_3) + 8 \ (\pm 2)$$
$$= (1.5 * 8) + 8 = 12 + 8 = 20 \pm 2 = (18 \text{ to } 22) \text{ mm Hg.}$$

The patient's $Paco_2$ of **20 mm Hg** is within the expected range, so this represents *appropriate compensation*.

Q56-6: F
Acetaminophen overdose.

Rationale: This patient has evidence of acute liver failure in the setting of an anion gap acidosis. He has a mild elevation in lactate, which is not enough to account for the anion gap present, he is normotensive, and this may be related to the liver failure. There is no evidence of ketones in the serum, so DKA and alcoholic ketoacidosis are unlikely. The serum osmolal gap is normal, so ethylene glycol and methanol toxicity are unlikely. The urine drug screen is negative, so an opioid overdose is not present. ASA toxicity is not commonly associated with liver failure and patients often have an associated respiratory alkalosis. Acetaminophen overdose is commonly associated with liver failure.

Q56-7: A
Pyroglutamic acid (5-oxoproline).

Rationale: 5-Oxoproline is the organic acid that is the cause of anion gap acidosis in acetaminophen overdose.

Q56-8: B
Spironolactone.

Rationale: The patient's urine anion gap is elevated and the serum osmolal gap is inappropriately reduced, suggesting dysfunction in urinary acidification.

$$\text{Urine Anion Gap} = [U_{Na}] + [U_K] - [U_{Cl}]$$
$$= (28 + 34) - (31) = (+31) \text{ mEq/L.}$$

This is consistent with either a type 1 or a type 4 RTA (or chronic renal insufficiency). The serum osmolal gap is as follows:

$$\text{Calculated Urine Osmolality} = 2 * ([Na^+] + [K^+]) + \frac{[\text{Urea}]}{2.8} + \frac{[\text{Glucose}]}{18}$$
$$= 243 \text{ mOsm/L}$$

$$\text{Urine Osmolal Gap} = \text{Measured Urine Osmolality}$$
$$- \text{Measured Urine Osmolality} = 91 \text{ mOsm/L.}$$

Similar to the urine anion gap, the urine osmolar gap is used as a surrogate for the urine ammonium concentration. Therefore, a larger gap indicates increased urinary NH_4 excretion. In normal acid-base conditions, the urine osmolar gap is between 10 and 100 mOsm/L. During a significant metabolic acidosis, patients with impaired renal tubular acidification (type 1 and type 4 RTA) are unable to excrete additional acid (NH_4), and therefore the osmolar gap does not change. Patients with an intact renal response to acidemia (ie, GI losses) should have a significant urine osmolar gap ($\sim > 300$ to 400 mOsm/L) as a result of increased NH_4 excretion.

Evaluation of RTA:			
	Type 1 RTA	Type 2 RTA	Type 4 RTA
Severity of metabolic acidosis, (HCO_3)	Severe (< 10–12 mEq/L typically)	Intermediate (12–20 mEq/L)	Mild (15–20 mEq/L)
Associated urine abnormalities	Urinary phosphate, calcium are increased; bone disease often present	Urine glucose, amino acids, phosphate, calcium may be elevated	
Urine pH	HIGH (> 5.5)	Low (acidic), until serum HCO_3 level exceeds the resorptive ability of the proximal tubule; then becomes alkalotic once reabsorptive threshold is crossed	Low (acidic)
Serum K^+	Low to normal; should correct with oral HCO_3 therapy	Classically low, although may be normal or even high with rare genetic defects; worsens with oral HCO_3 therapy	HIGH
Renal stones	Often	No	No
Renal tubular defect	Reduced NH_4 secretion in distal tubule	Reduced HCO_3 resorption in proximal tubule	Reduced H^+/K^+ exchange in distal and collecting tubule due to decreased aldosterone or aldosterone resistance
Urine anion gap	> 10	Negative initially, then positive when receiving serum HCO_3, then negative after therapy	> 10
Urine osmolal gap	Reduced (< 150 mOsm/L) during acute acidosis	At baseline is < 100 mEq/L; unreliable during acidosis	Reduced (< 150 mOsm/L) during acute acidosis

Here, the patient's urine pH is normal, with an elevated serum potassium, suggestive of a type 4 RTA. The only medication listed that is consistent with a type 4 RTA is spironolactone.

Causes of renal tubular acidosis.
Causes of Type 1 (Distal) RTA
Primary
• Idiopathic or familial (may be recessive or dominant)
Secondary
• Medications: Lithium, amphotericin, ifosfamide, NSAIDs
• Rheumatologic disorders: Sjögren syndrome, SLE, RA
• Hypercalciuria (idiopathic) or associated with vitamin D deficiency or hyperparathyroidism
• Sarcoidosis
• Obstructive uropathy
• Wilson disease
• Rejection of renal transplant allograft
• Toluene toxicity
Causes of Type 2 (Proximal) RTA
Primary
• Idiopathic
• Familial (primarily recessive disorders)
• Genetic: Fanconi syndrome, cystinosis, glycogen storage disease (type 1), Wilson disease, galactosemia
Secondary
• Medications: Acetazolamide, topiramate, aminoglycoside antibiotics, ifosfamide, reverse transcriptase inhibitors (tenofovir)
• Heavy metal poisoning: Lead, mercury, copper
• Multiple myeloma or amyloidosis (secondary to light chain toxicity)
• Sjögren syndrome
• Vitamin D deficiency
• Rejection of renal transplant allograft
Causes of Type 4 RTA (Hypoaldosteronism or Aldosterone Resistance)
Primary
• Primary adrenal insufficiency
• Inherited disorders associated with hypoaldosteronism
• Pseudohypoaldosteronism (types 1 and 2)
Secondary
• Causes of hyporeninemic hypoaldosteronism such as renal disease (diabetic nephropathy), NSAID use, calcineurin inhibitors, volume expansion/volume overload
• Causes of distal tubule voltage defects such as sickle cell disease, obstructive uropathy, SLE
• Severe illness/septic shock
• Angiotensin II–associated medications: ACE inhibitors, ARBs, direct renin inhibitors
• Potassium-sparing diuretics: Spironolactone, amiloride, triamterene
• Antibiotics: Trimethoprim, pentamidine

References

Adrogué HJ, Madias NE. Secondary responses to altered acid-base status: the rules of engagement. J Am Soc Nephrol. 2010;21:920.

Batlle D, Chin-Theodorou J, Tucker BM. Metabolic acidosis or respiratory alkalosis? Evaluation of a low plasma bicarbonate using the urine anion gap. Am J Kidney Dis. 2017;70:440.

Batlle D, Grupp M, Gaviria M, Kurtzman NA. Distal renal tubular acidosis with intact capacity to lower urinary pH. Am J Med. 1982;72:751.

Batlle D, Haque SK. Genetic causes and mechanisms of distal renal tubular acidosis. Nephrol Dial Transplant. 2012;27:3691.

Batlle DC, Hizon M, Cohen E, et al. The use of the urinary anion gap in the diagnosis of hyperchloremic metabolic acidosis. N Engl J Med. 1988;318:594.

Batlle DC, von Riotte A, Schlueter W. Urinary sodium in the evaluation of hyperchloremic metabolic acidosis. N Engl J Med. 1987;316:140.

Berend K, de Vries AP, Gans RO. Physiological approach to assessment of acid-base disturbances. N Engl J Med. 2014;371:1434.

Buckalew VM Jr, McCurdy DK, Ludwig GD, et al. Incomplete renal tubular acidosis. Physiologic studies in three patients with a defect in lowering urine pH. Am J Med. 1968;45:32.

Farwell WR, Taylor EN. Serum anion gap, bicarbonate and biomarkers of inflammation in healthy individuals in a national survey. CMAJ. 2010;182:137.

Feldman M, Soni N, Dickson B. Influence of hypoalbuminemia or hyperalbuminemia on the serum anion gap. J Lab Clin Med. 2005;146:317.

Karet FE. Mechanisms in hyperkalemic renal tubular acidosis. J Am Soc Nephrol. 2009;20:251.

Kraut JA, Madias NE. Differential diagnosis of nongap metabolic acidosis: value of a systematic approach. Clin J Am Soc Nephrol. 2012;7:671.

Kraut JA, Nagami GT. The serum anion gap in the evaluation of acid-base disorders: what are its limitations and can its effectiveness be improved? Clin J Am Soc Nephrol. 2013;8:2018.

Rastegar M, Nagami GT. Non-anion gap metabolic acidosis: a clinical approach to evaluation. Am J Kidney Dis. 2017;69:296.

Rodríguez Soriano J. Renal tubular acidosis: the clinical entity. J Am Soc Nephrol. 2002;13:2160.

CASE 57

A 55-year-old man with chronic alcohol abuse disorder presents to the emergency department after wandering out in traffic and being struck by a motorcyclist. His roommate notes he has been on a "bender" for the past 3 days and has not been eating, working, or "doing much of anything" except drinking alcohol. His vital signs are T 37.2°C, HR 130, BP 17/70, RR 8, Sao$_2$ 89% on 4L/min NC. CXR shows numerous contiguous rib fractures on the left and some pulmonary contusion versus pulmonary edema. The patient is obtunded and is intubated on arrival. He apparently takes no medications on a regular basis. He has no known history of cirrhosis or complicated alcohol withdrawal.

Laboratory data.			
ABGs		Basic Metabolic Panel	
pH	6.97	Na	117 mEq/L
Paco$_2$	46 mm Hg	K	2.1 mEq/L
Pao$_2$	100 mm Hg	Cl	70 mEq/L
HCO$_3$	10 mEq/L	CO$_2$	10 mEq/L
		BUN	35 mg/dL
		Cr	0.5 mg/dL
		Glucose	59 mg/dL
		Albumin	2.0 g/dL
		EtOH	375 mg/dL

QUESTIONS

Q57-1: Define the patient's baseline acid-base status: Does this patient have an underlying chronic acid-base disorder that we need to account for in order to appropriately interpret the acute acid-base disorders?

A. There is no evidence for an underlying chronic respiratory or metabolic acid-base disorder in this patient, so we would assume a baseline $Paco_2$ of 40 mm Hg and an HCO_3 of 24 mEq/L.

B. While the patient has a condition predisposing him to a chronic acid-base disorder, there is insufficient information to estimate the patient's baseline $Paco_2$ and HCO_3 values; therefore, we will assume a baseline $Paco_2$ of 40 mm Hg and a baseline HCO_3 of 24 mEq/L.

C. The patient has an underlying acid-base condition, and we have sufficient information to estimate the patient's baseline $Paco_2$ and HCO_3 values.

Q57-2: What is/are the primary acid-base disturbance(s) occurring in this case?

A. Metabolic acidosis only
B. Respiratory acidosis only
C. Metabolic acidosis and a respiratory acidosis
D. Metabolic alkalosis and a respiratory alkalosis
E. Metabolic alkalosis only
F. Respiratory alkalosis only

Q57-3: For a perfectly healthy patient, a normal anion gap is assumed to be 12 mEq/L. What should be considered a normal anion gap in this patient?

A. 12 mEq/L
B. 10 mEq/L
C. 7 mEq/L
D. 4 mEq/L

Q57-4: How would the metabolic acidosis component be classified in this case?

A. Anion gap acidosis
B. Non-anion gap acidosis
C. Anion and non-anion gap acidosis
D. Anion gap acidosis and a metabolic alkalosis

Q57-5: What is the likely cause of the patient's respiratory acidosis?

A. Hypoxemia
B. Neuromuscular disorder
C. Reactive airway disease (eg, asthma)
D. Chest wall injury (eg, flail chest)
E. Pulmonary fibrosis

Q57-6: The serum osmolality is reported as 360 mOsm/L. What is the patient's serum osmolal gap?

A. 6 mOsm/L
B. 14 mOsm/L
C. 22 mOsm/L
D. 31 mOsm/L

Q57-7: The patient's remaining tests are as follows:

Serum EtOH	375 mg/dL
Serum acetaminophen level	< 5 mg/dL (ULN for therapeutic use 20 mg/dL)
Serum salicylates level	< 5 mg/dL (ULN for therapeutic use 30 mg/dL)
Serum osmolality	360 mOsm/kg
Serum L-lactate	2.4 mmol/L (ULN 2.0 mmol/L venous)
Beta-hydroxybutyrate (acetone)	4.81 mmol/L (ULN 0.18 mmol/L)
Serum glucose	59 mg/dL
Serum phosphorus	0.8 mg/dL
Serum uric acid	2.3 mg/dL
Serum calcium	6.7 mg/dL

What is the likely cause of the patient's anion gap acidosis?

A. Aspirin toxicity
B. Lactic acidosis secondary to sepsis
C. Ethylene glycol toxicity
D. Methanol toxicity
E. Opioid overdose
F. Acetaminophen overdose
G. Diabetic ketoacidosis
H. Alcoholic ketoacidosis

Q57-8: The urine electrolyte values are as follows:

Urine Na	12 mEq/L
Urine K	59 mEq/L
Urine Cl	7 mEq/L
Urine pH	5.5

What is the most likely cause of the patient's metabolic alkalosis?

A. Ongoing diuretic use
B. Addison disease
C. Milk-alkali ingestion
D. Contraction alkalosis/volume depletion
E. Fanconi syndrome

ANSWERS

Q57-1: B

While the patient has a condition predisposing him to a chronic acid-base disorder, there is insufficient information to estimate the patient's baseline $Paco_2$ and HCO_3 values; therefore, we will assume a baseline $Paco_2$ of 40 mm Hg and a baseline HCO_3 of 24 mEq/L. The patient has a chronic alcohol abuse disorder, and this can be associated with additional chronic acid-base disorders. However, we lack sufficient information to make such an assumption.

Rationale: Ignoring these underlying chronic acid-base disorders can significantly alter the interpretation of a patient's acute acid-base status. This was demonstrated in the first case of the series. However, often, we do not have the necessary information (eg, prior ABG or VBG, or prior serum chemistry with an HCO_3) and are forced to assume the ongoing processes are all acute in nature. We are primarily concerned about chronic respiratory acid-base disorders, as these can significantly alter the patient's baseline or expected values for the serum HCO_3 and $Paco_2$, and we have reliable equations to predict the expected baseline values. The respiratory compensation for both chronic metabolic acidosis and alkalosis is generally poor, so there are no equations or rules to predict what the $Paco_2$ should be in these cases. While the baseline serum HCO_3 may be significantly off from our standard value of 24 mEq/L in these patients, we would assume a baseline $Paco_2$ of 40 mm Hg in patients with chronic metabolic processes. Once we identify the patient's baseline $Paco_2$ and HCO_3 values, we will need to use these values in the appropriate equations to identify the ongoing acute processes.

Q57-2: C

Metabolic acidosis and a respiratory acidosis.

Rationale:

1. The pH is 6.97; therefore, the primary disorder is an **acidosis.**
2. The $Paco_2$ of 46 mm Hg is greater than 40 mm Hg, so there is a **primary respiratory acidosis.**
3. The HCO_3 of 10 mEq/L is less than 24 mEq/L, so there is also a **primary metabolic acidosis.**

Q57-3: C

7 mEq/L.

Rationale: The normal anion gap is 12 mEq/L. The term *anion gap* refers to those ions (negatively charged molecules) in the bloodstream that we do not routinely measure, including phosphates, sulfates, organic acids, and negatively charged plasma proteins. One of the most abundant negatively charged ions in the blood is serum albumin. A normal serum albumin is 4.0 g/dL. For patients with hypoalbuminemia (low serum albumin), the normal or expected anion gap is smaller.

$$\text{Expected Anion Gap} = 12 - (2.5) * \left[4.0\frac{g}{dL} - \text{Actual Serum Albumin} \right].$$

Therefore, for this patient,

$$\text{Expected Anion Gap} = 12 - [2.5 * (4 - 2)] = 12 - (2.5 * 2) = 7 \text{ mEq/L}.$$

This is an important concept, as patients with hypoalbuminemia may "hide" an anion gap acidosis if this correction is not performed.

Q57-4: D
Anion gap acidosis and metabolic alkalosis.

Rationale:

1. Is there evidence for a chronic acid-base disorder that requires adjustment of the patient's "normal" HCO_3? No, there is no evidence for a chronic acid-base disorder, so we would assume a baseline $Paco_2$ of 40 mm Hg and an HCO_3 of 24 mEq/L.

2. Expected anion gap:

$$\text{Expected Anion Gap} = 12 - (2.5) * \left[4.0 \frac{g}{dL} - \text{Actual Serum Albumin} \right]$$
$$= 12 - (2.5 * [4.0 - 2.0])$$
$$= 12 - (2.5 * [2.0]) = \textbf{7 mEq/L}.$$

3. Anion gap calculation:

$$\text{Serum Anion Gap} = [Na^+] - [HCO_3^-] - [Cl^-]$$
$$= 117 - (70 + 10) = \textbf{37}, \text{ which is} > 7$$
$$\rightarrow \textbf{anion gap acidosis is present.}$$

4. Delta-delta calculation:

$$(\text{Measured AG} - \text{Normal AG})/(\text{Normal } HCO_3 - \text{Measured } HCO_3)$$
$$(37 - 7)/(24 - 10) = \textbf{30/14, which is ~2.15.}$$

Delta-delta interpretation.	
Delta-Delta Value	Condition Present
< 0.4	Non-anion gap only
0.4–0.9	**Anion gap *and* non-anion gap acidosis**
1.0–2.0	Anion gap acidosis only
> 2.0	**Anion gap acidosis and metabolic alkalosis**

Q57-5: D
Chest wall injury (eg, flail chest).

Rationale: This patient has multiple rib fractures on the left side of the chest, noted as contiguous in the prompt. This is indicative of flail chest, a condition in which the chest wall does not function properly during inspiration due to deformity of the rib cage. In addition to pain, which leads to splinting, patients can develop a respiratory acidosis, and it prevents them from compensating appropriately for a metabolic acidosis, as well. Hypoxemia generally causes a respiratory alkalosis, although in the long term this can lead to respiratory acidosis as respiratory muscles fatigue. This patient has no evidence of asthma, COPD, or pulmonary fibrosis, and no history of a neuromuscular disorder.

Q57-6: A
6 mOsm/L.

Rationale: Similar to the serum anion gap, the serum osmolal gap is determined by the difference between the "calculated" serum osmolality and the true, measured serum osmolality. The equation for the serum osmolal gap typically includes factors for sodium, glucose, BUN, and ethanol, as these are readily measurable in most laboratories. Therefore, the serum osmolal gap will represent the osmolality of those "unmeasured" osmoles, including organic alcohols and acetone. The most common form is as follows:

$$\text{Calculated Serum Osmolality} = 2*[Na^+] + \frac{[\text{Glucose}]}{18} + \frac{[\text{BUN}]}{2.8} + \frac{[\text{EtOH}]}{3.7};$$

In which the units of measure are as follows: Na, mEq/L; glucose, mg/dL; BUN, mg/dL; and EtOH, mg/dL. The conversion factors are shown in the preceding equation as well. A normal serum osmolal gap is around -10 to $+10$ mOsm/L (or mOsm/kg).

Therefore, for this patient,

$$\text{Calculated Serum Osmolality} = 2*[Na^+] + \frac{[\text{Glucose}]}{18} + \frac{[\text{BUN}]}{2.8} + \frac{[\text{EtOH}]}{3.7}$$
$$= (2*117) + (59/18) + (35/2.8) + (375/3.7)$$
$$= 354 \text{ mOsm/L,}$$

$$\text{Serum Osmolal Gap (SOG)} = \text{Measured Serum Osmolality}$$
$$- \text{Calculated Serum Osmolality}$$
$$= (360 - 354) = 6 \text{ mOsm/L} < 10 \text{ mOsm/L}$$
$$\rightarrow \textit{no} \text{ serum osmolal gap exists.}$$

Note what a significant contribution the patient's serum ethanol level makes to the overall serum osmolality.

Q57-7: H
Alcoholic ketoacidosis.

Rationale: This is a patient with alcoholism, who has been drinking regularly and avoiding food intake. He has a negative serum drug screen, making acetaminophen and aspirin overdose unlikely. (Chronic ingestion can result in normal levels, but not zero generally.) There is no significant lactate present. The normal osmolar gap would be unusual for ethylene glycol and methanol ingestion. (Although very late after ingestion, once the alcohols have been converted to organic acids, the osmolar gap does approach normal.) There is no opioid overdose present, and this generally only leads to respiratory acidosis unless severe hypotension has been present as a result of use. The positive urine ketones could be consistent with either option G or H here, but the low glucose and the alcohol history are consistent with alcoholic ketoacidosis. This is further supported by the hyponatremia and other electrolyte abnormalities.

Q57-8: D
Contraction alkalosis/volume depletion.

Rationale: The patient has a chloride-responsive metabolic alkalosis ($U_{Cl} < 10$). Possible causes include contraction, diuretic use (usually distal tubule and/or loop diuretics), post-hypercapnia, and hyperemesis. HCO_3 infusion, Addison disease, and milk-alkali syndrome are most often associated with a chloride-resistant metabolic alkalosis. The patient is likely dehydrated from the hyperosmolar state and lack of PO intake. He has an elevated BUN:Cr ratio (70) as well.

Causes of metabolic alkalosis.
History: Rule Out the Following as Causes
• Alkali load ("milk-alkali" or calcium-alkali syndrome, oral sodium bicarbonate, IV sodium bicarbonate) • Genetic causes (CF) • Presence of hypercalcemia • Intravenous β-lactam antibiotics • Laxative abuse (may also cause a metabolic acidosis depending on diarrheal HCO_3 losses)
If None of the Above, Then…
Urine Chloride < 20 mEq/L (Chloride-Responsive Causes)
• Loss of gastric acid (hyperemesis, NGT suctioning) • Prior diuretic use (in hours to days following discontinuation) • Post-hypercapnia • Villous adenoma • Congenital chloridorrhea • Chronic laxative abuse (may also cause a metabolic acidosis depending on diarrheal HCO_3 losses) • CF

(Continued)

Causes of metabolic alkalosis. (*continued*)
OR
Urine Chloride > 20 mEq/L (Chloride-Resistant Causes)
Urine Chloride > 20 mEq/L, Lack of HTN, Urine Potassium < 30 mEq/L
• Hypokalemia or hypomagnesemia • Laxative abuse (if dominated by hypokalemia) • Bartter syndrome • Gitelman syndrome
Urine Chloride > 20 mEq/L, Lack of HTN, Urine Potassium > 30 mEq/L
• Current diuretic use
Urine Chloride > 20 mEq/L, Presence of HTN, Urine Potassium Variable but Usually > 30 mEq/L
Elevated plasma renin level: • Renal artery stenosis • Renin-secreting tumor • Renovascular disease
Low plasma renin, low plasma aldosterone: • Cushing syndrome • Exogenous mineralocorticoid use • Genetic disorder (11-hydoxylase or 17-hydrolyase deficiency, 11β-HSD deficiency) • Liddle syndrome • Licorice toxicity
Low plasma renin, high plasma aldosterone: • Primary hyperaldosteronism • Adrenal adenoma • Bilateral adrenal hyperplasia

References

Abreo K, Adlakha A, Kilpatrick S, et al. The milk-alkali syndrome. A reversible form of acute renal failure. Arch Intern Med. 1993;153:1005.

Arroliga AC, Shehab N, McCarthy K, Gonzales JP. Relationship of continuous infusion lorazepam to serum propylene glycol concentration in critically ill adults. Crit Care Med. 2004;32:1709.

Barton CH, Vaziri ND, Ness RL, et al. Cimetidine in the management of metabolic alkalosis induced by nasogastric drainage. Arch Surg. 1979;114:70.

Bear R, Goldstein M, Phillipson E, et al. Effect of metabolic alkalosis on respiratory function in patients with chronic obstructive lung disease. Can Med Assoc J. 1977;117:900.

Braden GL, Strayhorn CH, Germain MJ, et al. Increased osmolal gap in alcoholic acidosis. Arch Intern Med. 1993;153:2377.

Gabow PA. Ethylene glycol intoxication. Am J Kidney Dis. 1988;11:277.

Galla JH, Gifford JD, Luke RG, Rome L. Adaptations to chloride-depletion alkalosis. Am J Physiol. 1991;261:R771.

Garella S, Chang BS, Kahn SI. Dilution acidosis and contraction alkalosis: review of a concept. Kidney Int. 1975;8:279.

Gennari FJ. Current concepts. Serum osmolality. Uses and limitations. N Engl J Med. 1984;310:102.

Gennari FJ, Weise WJ. Acid-base disturbances in gastrointestinal disease. Clin J Am Soc Nephrol. 2008;3:1861.

Glasser L, Sternglanz PD, Combie J, Robinson A. Serum osmolality and its applicability to drug overdose. Am J Clin Pathol. 1973;60:695.

Hamm LL, Nakhoul N, Hering-Smith KS. Acid-base homeostasis. Clin J Am Soc Nephrol. 2015;10:2232.

Hulter HN, Sebastian A, Toto RD, et al. Renal and systemic acid-base effects of the chronic administration of hypercalcemia-producing agents: calcitriol, PTH, and intravenous calcium. Kidney Int. 1982;21:445.

Khanna A, Kurtzman NA. Metabolic alkalosis. J Nephrol. 2006;19(suppl 9):S86.

Kraut JA, Kurtz I. Toxic alcohol ingestions: clinical features, diagnosis, and management. Clin J Am Soc Nephrol. 2008;3:208.

Kraut JA, Xing SX. Approach to the evaluation of a patient with an increased serum osmolal gap and high-anion-gap metabolic acidosis. Am J Kidney Dis. 2011;58:480.

Jenkins DW, Eckle RE, Craig JW. Alcoholic ketoacidosis. JAMA. 1971;217:177.

Laski ME, Sabatini S. Metabolic alkalosis, bedside and bench. Semin Nephrol. 2006;26:404.

Levy LJ, Duga J, Girgis M, Gordon EE. Ketoacidosis associated with alcoholism in nondiabetic subjects. Ann Intern Med. 1973;78:213.

Luke RG, Galla JH. It is chloride depletion alkalosis, not contraction alkalosis. J Am Soc Nephrol. 2012;23:204.

Lynd LD, Richardson KJ, Purssell RA, et al. An evaluation of the osmole gap as a screening test for toxic alcohol poisoning. BMC Emerg Med. 2008;8:5.

Marraffa JM, Holland MG, Stork CM, et al. Diethylene glycol: widely used solvent presents serious poisoning potential. J Emerg Med. 2008;35:401.

Miller PD, Berns AS. Acute metabolic alkalosis perpetuating hypercarbia. A role for acetazolamide in chronic obstructive pulmonary disease. JAMA. 1977;238:2400.

Oster JR, Materson BJ, Rogers AI. Laxative abuse syndrome. Am J Gastroenterol. 1980;74:451.

Palmer BF, Clegg DJ. Electrolyte disturbances in patients with chronic alcohol-use disorder. N Engl J Med. 2017;377:1368.

Patel AM, Goldfarb S. Got calcium? Welcome to the calcium-alkali syndrome. J Am Soc Nephrol. 2010;21:1440.

Purssell RA, Pudek M, Brubacher J, Abu-Laban RB. Derivation and validation of a formula to calculate the contribution of ethanol to the osmolal gap. Ann Emerg Med. 2001;38 :653.

Reichard GA Jr, Owen OE, Haff AC, et al. Ketone-body production and oxidation in fasting obese humans. J Clin Invest. 1974;53:508.

Robinson AG, Loeb JN. Ethanol ingestion--commonest cause of elevated plasma osmolality? N Engl J Med. 1971;284:1253.

Rose BD, Post TW. Clinical Physiology of Acid-Base and Electrolyte Disorders. 5e. New York, NY: McGraw Hill; 559.

Schelling JR, Howard RL, Winter SD, Linas SL. Increased osmolal gap in alcoholic ketoacidosis and lactic acidosis. Ann Intern Med. 1990;113:580.

Schwartz WB, Van Ypersele de Strihou, Kassirer JP. Role of anions in metabolic alkalosis and potassium deficiency. N Engl J Med. 1968;279:630.

Sweetser LJ, Douglas JA, Riha RL, Bell SC. Clinical presentation of metabolic alkalosis in an adult patient with cystic fibrosis. Respirology. 2005;10:254.

Taki K, Mizuno K, Takahashi N, Wakusawa R. Disturbance of CO2 elimination in the lungs by carbonic anhydrase inhibition. Jpn J Physiol. 1986;36:523.

Toth HL, Greenbaum LA. Severe acidosis caused by starvation and stress. Am J Kidney Dis. 2003;42:E16.

Turban S, Beutler KT, Morris RG, et al. Long-term regulation of proximal tubule acid-base transporter abundance by angiotensin II. Kidney Int. 2006;70:660.

CASE 58

An inpatient is found in her room in the morning with signs of altered mental status. There is an empty bottle of birth control pills in her room, the bedside table has been knocked over, the hand sanitizer device in the room has been broken open, and the device is empty. She was last seen appearing normal approximately 12 hours ago. The patient was admitted for bipolar disorder with mania 2 weeks ago. She has hypertension, hyperlipidemia, and IDDM. Her vital signs are T 37.0C, HR 83, BP 123/75, RR 21, Sao$_2$ 98% on room air. Physical examination demonstrates some slight bruising on her right hand and arm, and a mental status examination consistent with delirium/encephalopathy. She had therapeutic lithium level on admission and has been receiving the medication as scheduled. She is also receiving amlodipine, insulin, and atorvastatin. A set of laboratory studies is requested immediately, with the following results:

Laboratory data.			
ABGs		Basic Metabolic Panel	
pH	7.52	Na	144 mEq/L
Paco$_2$	23 mm Hg	K	5.5 mEq/L
Pao$_2$	100 mm Hg	Cl	117 mEq/L
HCO$_3$	18 mEq/L	CO$_2$	18 mEq/L
		BUN	22 mg/dL
		Cr	1.5 mg/dL
		Glucose	90 mg/dL
		Albumin	4.0 g/dL
		EtOH	0 mg/dL

QUESTIONS

Q58-1: Define the patient's baseline acid-base status: Does this patient have an underlying chronic acid-base disorder that we need to account for in order to appropriately interpret the acute acid-base disorders?

A. There is no evidence for an underlying chronic respiratory or metabolic acid-base disorder in this patient, so we would assume a baseline $Paco_2$ of 40 mm Hg and an HCO_3 of 24 mEq/L.

B. While the patient has a condition predisposing her to a chronic acid-base disorder, there is insufficient information to estimate the patient's baseline $Paco_2$ and HCO_3 values; therefore, we will assume a baseline $Paco_2$ of 40 mm Hg and a baseline HCO_3 of 24 mEq/L.

C. The patient has an underlying acid-base condition, and we have sufficient information to estimate the patient's baseline $Paco_2$ and HCO_3 values.

Q58-2: What is/are the primary acid-base disturbance(s) occurring in this case?

A. Metabolic acidosis only
B. Respiratory acidosis only
C. Metabolic acidosis and a respiratory acidosis
D. Metabolic alkalosis and a respiratory alkalosis
E. Metabolic alkalosis only
F. Respiratory alkalosis only

Q58-3: How would the reduction in the patient's serum HCO_3 be classified in this case?

A. Anion gap acidosis.
B. Non-anion gap acidosis.
C. Anion and non-anion gap acidosis.
D. Anion gap acidosis and a metabolic alkalosis.
E. The reduction in serum HCO_3 represents an appropriate compensation for the respiratory alkalosis; therefore, there is no metabolic acidosis.

Q58-4: What is the likely cause of the patient's respiratory alkalosis?

A. Aspirin overdose
B. Cirrhosis
C. Hypoxemia
D. CNS injury
E. Progesterone overdose/toxicity

Q58-5: The serum osmolality is determined to be 333 mOsm/L. What is the patient's serum osmolal gap?

A. 5 mOsm/L
B. 10 mOsm/L
C. 20 mOsm/L
D. 30 mOsm/L

Q58-6: What is the likely cause of the patient's elevated osmolar gap?

A. Ethanol ingestion
B. Methanol ingestion
C. Ethylene glycol ingestion
D. Propylene glycol ingestion
E. Isopropyl alcohol ingestion

Q58-7: What other laboratory abnormality would you expect with isopropyl alcohol ingestion?

A. Positive for lactate
B. Elevated serum calcium
C. Elevated serum potassium
D. Elevated serum phosphorus
E. Positive for urine ketones

ANSWERS

Q58-1: B

While the patient has a condition predisposing her to a chronic acid-base disorder, there is insufficient information to estimate the patient's baseline $Paco_2$ and HCO_3 values; therefore, we will assume a baseline $Paco_2$ of 40 mm Hg and a baseline HCO_3 of 24 mEq/L. The patient has diabetes and an elevated serum Cr, which could indicate a baseline chronic acid-base disorder. However, we lack sufficient information to make any conclusions.

Rationale: Ignoring these underlying chronic acid-base disorders can significantly alter the interpretation of a patient's acute acid-base status. This was demonstrated in the first case of the series. However, often, we do not have the necessary information (eg, prior ABG or VBG, or prior serum chemistry with an HCO_3) and are forced to assume the ongoing processes are all acute in nature. We are primarily concerned about chronic respiratory acid-base disorders, as these can significantly alter the patient's baseline or expected values for the serum HCO_3 and $Paco_2$, and we have reliable equations to predict the expected baseline values. The respiratory compensation for both chronic metabolic acidosis and alkalosis is generally poor, so there are no equations or rules to predict what the $Paco_2$ should be in these cases. While the baseline serum HCO_3 may be significantly off from our standard value of 24 mEq/L in these patients, we would assume a baseline $Paco_2$ of 40 mm Hg in patients with chronic metabolic processes. Once we identify the patient's baseline $Paco_2$ and HCO_3 values, we will need to use these values in the appropriate equations to identify the ongoing acute processes.

Q58-2: B

Respiratory acidosis only.

Rationale:

1. The pH is 7.52; therefore, the primary disorder is an **alkalosis**.
2. The $Paco_2$ of 23 mm Hg is less than 40 mm Hg, so there is a **respiratory alkalosis**.
3. The HCO_3 of 18 mEq/L is less than 24 mEq/L, so there is **no metabolic alkalosis**.

This patient has a respiratory alkalosis as the primary condition.

Q58-3: B

Non-anion gap acidosis.

Rationale: First, we have to determine if the reduction in the patient' serum HCO_3 represents appropriate compensation for the respiratory alkalosis present, or if there is a separate metabolic acid-base disorder ongoing. Since we are assuming an acute respiratory alkalosis, we can use the following equation:

Metabolic Compensation for Acute Respiratory Alkalosis:

$$\text{Expected HCO}_3 = \text{Baseline HCO}_3 - (0.20)[\text{Actual Paco}_2 - \text{Baseline Paco}_2]$$
$$= (24 \text{ mEq/L}) - (0.20)[40 - 23] = 24 \text{ mEq/L} - 3.4 = 20.6 \text{ mEq/L}.$$

Since the patient serum HCO_3 is 18 mEq/L, which is less than the expected ~21 mEq/L, we would assume there is also a metabolic acidosis present. Therefore, we will undertake our standard approach:

1. Is there evidence for a chronic acid-base disorder that requires adjustment of the patient's "normal" HCO_3? No, there is no evidence for a chronic acid-base disorder, so we would assume a baseline $Paco_2$ of 40 mm Hg and an HCO_3 of 24 mEq/L.
2. Expected anion gap:

$$\text{Expected Anion Gap} = 12 - (2.5) * \left[4.0 \, \frac{g}{dL} - \text{Actual Serum Albumin} \right].$$

3. The expected anion gap is 12, given the patient has a normal albumin.
4. Anion gap calculation:

$$\text{Serum Anion Gap} = [Na^+] - [HCO_3^-] - [Cl^-]$$
$$= (144) - (117 + 18) = 9 \rightarrow \textbf{no anion gap acidosis exists.}$$

We do not need the delta-delta equation in this situation. The patient has non-anion gap metabolic alkalosis. Because the patient has a primary alkalosis, the interpretation of urine studies may not be helpful at this point in identifying the etiology of the patient's non-anion gap acidosis. In a compensatory response to the respiratory alkalosis, bicarbonate will be wasted. Additionally, as there isn't a primary acidosis, the serum osmolal gap becomes more difficult to interpret.

Cause of NAGMA
Low Serum Potassium
GI: Diarrhea, pancreaticoduodenal fistula, urinary intestinal diversion Renal: Type 1 RTA (distal), type 2 RTA (proximal) Medications/exposures: Carbonic anhydrase inhibitors, toluene Other: D-Lactic acidosis
High (or Normal) Serum Potassium
GI: Elevated ileostomy output Renal: Type 4 RTA or CKD Medications: NSAIDs; antibiotics (trimethoprim, pentamidine); heparin; ACE inhibitors, ARBs, aldosterone antagonists (spironolactone); acid administration (TPN)

Given the patient's serum potassium is mildly elevated, we might expect that a type 4 RTA or stage 2 CKD secondary to diabetic nephropathy is the likely cause.

Q58-4: E
Progesterone overdose/toxicity.

Rationale: The patient has an empty bottle of birth control pills in her room. No aspirin bottle is noted, she has no history of cirrhosis or CNS injury, and there is no mention of hypoxemia. Progesterone stimulates the respiratory center and leads to hyperventilation and reduced $Paco_2$.

Q58-5: D
30 mOsm/L.

Rationale: Similar to the serum anion gap, the serum osmolal gap is determined by the difference between the "calculated" serum osmolality and the true, measured serum osmolality. The equation for the serum osmolal gap typically includes factors for sodium, glucose, BUN, and ethanol, as these are readily measurable in most laboratories. Therefore, the serum osmolal gap will represent the osmolality of those "unmeasured" osmoles, including organic alcohols and acetone. The most common form is as follows:

$$\text{Calculated Serum Osmolality} = 2*[Na^+] + \frac{[Glucose]}{18} + \frac{[BUN]}{2.8} + \frac{[EtOH]}{3.7}$$

$$\text{Serum Osmolal Gap (SOG)} = \text{Measured Serum Osmolality} - \text{Calculated Serum Osmolality;}$$

In which the units of measure are as follows: Na, mEq/L; glucose, mg/dL; BUN, mg/dL; and EtOH, mg/dL. The conversion factors are shown in the preceding equation as well. A normal serum osmolal gap is around -10 to $+10$ mOsm/L (or mOsm/kg).

Therefore, for this patient,

$$\text{Calculated Serum Osmolality} = (2*144) + (90/18) + (22/2.8) + (0/3.7)$$
$$= 303 \text{ mOsm/L}$$
$$SOG = (333 - 303) = 30, \text{ which is} > 10$$
$$\rightarrow \textbf{a serum osmolal gap is present.}$$

Q58-6: E
Isopropyl alcohol ingestion.

Rationale: Isopropyl alcohol can cause an osmolar gap but no anion gap acidosis, as it is not converted into an organic acid. Testing for ethanol was negative in this patient, and the remaining options are associated with an anion gap acidosis. Isopropyl alcohol is the main ingredient in most hand sanitizers, and this patient is believed to have ingested the hand sanitizer from the dispenser in her room. Supportive care is the appropriate treatment.

Causes of an elevated serum osmolar gap.
With an Elevated Serum Anion Gap
1. Ethanol ingestion with alcoholic ketoacidosis (acetone is an unmeasured osmole, in addition to ethanol)—the osmolality is usually elevated more so by the increased ethanol concentration, so the osmolal "gap" depends on whether the term for ethanol is included in the osmolality calculation*
2. Organic alcohol ingestions (methanol, ethylene glycol, diethylene glycol, propylene glycol)
3. Diabetic ketoacidosis—similar to ethanol ingestion, earlier, glucose and acetone contribute to the osmolality, since the glucose terms is always included in the calculation
4. Salicylate toxicity
5. Renal failure—the BUN is nearly always included in the osmolality
Without an Elevated Serum Anion Gap
1. Hyperosmolar therapy (mannitol, glycerol)
2. Other organic solvent ingestion (eg, acetone)
3. Isopropyl alcohol ingestion (produces only acetone rather than an organic acid, so no anion gap is seen)
4. Hypertriglyceridemia
5. Hyperproteinemia
A mildly elevated osmolal gap has been reported in the literature in patients with lactic acidosis in critical illness, particularly severe distributive shock. The pathology is not quite clear, although it likely is related to multiorgan failure—particularly involving the liver and kidneys—and the release of cellular components known to contribute to the osmolal gap. This is typically around 10 mOsm/L, although it may be as high as 20 to 25 mOsm/L.

Q58-7: E
Positive urine ketones.

Rationale: The patient's lab results would be expected to be positive for serum ketones. Isopropyl alcohol is a secondary organic alcohol and is converted to an aldehyde and subsequently to ketones, rather than to an organic acid, and thus is not associated with anion gap acidosis but with an increase in serum osmolality.

Isopropyl alcohol ingestions are typically self-limited, although if massive amounts of isopropyl alcohol are ingested, patients can develop hemodynamic instability secondary to vasodilation. Isopropyl alcohol is converted to acetoacetone rather than more toxic organic acid/anions. While fomepizole and renal replacement therapy are effective, they are rarely warranted. Supportive care is generally all that is required, including isotonic fluids and respiratory support in patients with severe encephalopathy. Co-ingestions are common.

References

Abramson S, Singh AK. Treatment of the alcohol intoxications: ethylene glycol, methanol and isopropanol. Curr Opin Nephrol Hypertens. 2000;9:695.

Bekka R, Borron SW, Astier A, et al. Treatment of methanol and isopropanol poisoning with intravenous fomepizole. J Toxicol Clin Toxicol. 2001;39:59.

Gaudet MP, Fraser GL. Isopropanol ingestion: case report with pharmacokinetic analysis. Am J Emerg Med. 1989;7:297.

Gaulier JM, Lamballais F, Yazdani F, Lachâtre G. Isopropyl alcohol concentrations in postmortem tissues to document fatal intoxication. J Anal Toxicol. 2011;35:254.

Monaghan MS, Ackerman BH, Olsen KM, et al. The use of delta osmolality to predict serum isopropanol and acetone concentrations. Pharmacotherapy. 1993;13:60.

Pappas AA, Ackerman BH, Olsen KM, Taylor EH. Isopropanol ingestion: a report of six episodes with isopropanol and acetone serum concentration time data. J Toxicol Clin Toxicol. 1991;29:11.

Trullas JC, Aguilo S, Castro P, Nogue S. Life-threatening isopropyl alcohol intoxication: is hemodialysis really necessary? Vet Hum Toxicol. 2004;46:282.

Zaman F, Pervez A, Abreo K. Isopropyl alcohol intoxication: a diagnostic challenge. Am J Kidney Dis. 2002;40:E12.

CASE 59

A 24-year-old IV drug user is brought to the emergency department by his roommate. The patient is obtunded and intubated, and neither he nor the roommate is able to provide any history. The patient's medical record shows that he works as a painter and has a long history of alcohol and drug abuse, but no use of prescribed or OTC medications. His vital signs are T 36.5°C, HR 133, BP 110/80, RR 4, Sao$_2$ 97% on room air. On exam, the patient demonstrates an agonal breathing pattern. His roommate states that the patient had been vomiting all night. The physical examination is benign except for obtundation and some perioral and perinasal irritation and skin discoloration.

Laboratory data.			
ABGs		Basic Metabolic Panel	
pH	6.92	Na	140 mEq/L
Paco$_2$	66 mm Hg	K	2.3 mEq/L
Pao$_2$	100 mm Hg	Cl	87 mEq/L
HCO$_3$	13 mEq/L	CO$_2$	13 mEq/L
		BUN	33 mg/dL
		Cr	1.6 mg/dL
		Glucose	70 mg/dL
		Albumin	4.0 g/dL
		EtOH	0 mg/dL

QUESTIONS

Q59-1: Define the patient's baseline acid-base status: Does this patient have an underlying chronic acid-base disorder that we need to account for in order to appropriately interpret the acute acid-base disorders?

A. There is no evidence for an underlying chronic respiratory or metabolic acid-base disorder in this patient, so we would assume a baseline P_{aCO_2} of 40 mm Hg and an HCO_3 of 24 mEq/L.

B. While the patient has a condition predisposing him to a chronic acid-base disorder, there is insufficient information to estimate the patient's baseline P_{aCO_2} and HCO_3 values; therefore, we will assume a baseline P_{aCO_2} of 40 mm Hg and a baseline HCO_3 of 24 mEq/L.

C. The patient has an underlying acid-base condition, and we have sufficient information to estimate the patient's baseline P_{aCO_2} and HCO_3 values.

Q59-2: What is/are the primary acid-base disturbance(s) occurring in this case?

A. Metabolic acidosis only
B. Respiratory acidosis only
C. Metabolic acidosis and a respiratory acidosis
D. Metabolic alkalosis and a respiratory alkalosis
E. Metabolic alkalosis only
F. Respiratory alkalosis only

Q59-3: How would the metabolic acidosis component be classified in this case?

A. Anion gap acidosis
B. Non-anion gap acidosis
C. Anion and non-anion gap acidosis
D. Anion gap acidosis and a metabolic alkalosis

Q59-4: The patient's urine electrolyte values are as follows:

Urine Na	23 mEq/L
Urine K	30 mEq/L
Urine C:	6 mEq/L
Urine pH	5.5

What is the most likely cause of the patient's metabolic alkalosis?

A. Bicarbonate infusion
B. Addison disease
C. Milk-alkali ingestion
D. Hyperemesis
E. Diarrhea
F. Bactrim use
G. Acetazolamide use
H. Aminoglycoside use
I. Ifosfamide chemotherapy

Q59-5: The patient's remaining test results are as follows:

Serum EtOH	< 3 mg/dL
Serum acetaminophen level	< 5 mg/dL (ULN for therapeutic use 20 mg/dL)
Serum salicylates level	< 5 mg/dL (ULN for therapeutic use 30 mg/dL)
Serum osmolality	302 mOsm/kg
Serum L-lactate	1.8 mmol/L (ULN 2.0 mmol/L venous)
Beta-hydroxybutyrate (acetone)	< 018 mmol/L (ULN 0.18 mmol/L)
Serum glucose	70 mg/dL
Serum phosphorus	5.5 mg/dL (ULN 4.5 mg/dL)
Serum ALT	2355 IU/mL (ULN 70 IU/mL)
Urine drug screen	Positive for opioids

Which of the following is the most likely cause of the patient's anion gap acidosis?

A. Aspirin toxicity
B. Lactic acidosis secondary to sepsis
C. Ethylene glycol toxicity
D. Methanol toxicity
E. Toluene toxicity
F. Acetaminophen overdose
G. Diabetic ketoacidosis
H. Alcoholic ketoacidosis

Q59-6: What is the likely cause of the patient's respiratory acidosis?

A. Hypoxemia
B. Neuromuscular disorder
C. Asthma
D. COPD
E. Chest wall injury or deformity
F. Pulmonary fibrosis
G. Opioid overdose
H. Benzodiazepine overdose
I. Iatrogenic cause

ANSWERS

Q59-1: A

There is no evidence for an underlying chronic respiratory or metabolic acid-base disorder in this patient, so we would assume a baseline P_{aCO_2} of 40 mm Hg and an HCO_3 of 24 mEq/L.

Rationale: Ignoring these underlying chronic acid-base disorders can significantly alter the interpretation of a patient's acute acid-base status. This was demonstrated in the first case of the series. However, often, we do not have the necessary information (eg, prior ABG or VBG, or prior serum chemistry with an HCO_3) and are forced to assume the ongoing processes are all acute in nature. We are primarily concerned about chronic respiratory acid-base disorders, as these can significantly alter the patient's baseline or expected values for the serum HCO_3 and P_{aCO_2}, and we have reliable equations to predict the expected baseline values. The respiratory compensation for both chronic metabolic acidosis and alkalosis is generally poor, so there are no equations or rules to predict what the P_{aCO_2} should be in these cases. While the baseline serum HCO_3 may be significantly off from our standard value of 24 mEq/L in these patients, we would assume a baseline P_{aCO_2} of 40 mm Hg in patients with chronic metabolic processes. Once we identify the patient's baseline P_{aCO_2} and HCO_3 values, we will need to use these values in the appropriate equations to identify the ongoing acute processes.

Q59-2: C

Metabolic acidosis and a respiratory acidosis.

Rationale:

1. The pH is 6.92; therefore, the primary disorder is an **acidosis.**
2. The P_{aCO_2} of 66 mm Hg is greater than 40 mm Hg, so there is a **respiratory acidosis.**
3. The HCO_3 of 13 mEq/L is less than 24 mEq/L, so there is also a **metabolic acidosis.**

Q59-3: D

Anion gap acidosis and metabolic alkalosis.

Rationale:

1. Is there evidence for a chronic respiratory acid-base disorder that requires adjustment of the patient's "normal" HCO_3? No, there is no evidence for a chronic respiratory acid-base disorder, so we would assume a baseline P_{aCO_2} of 40 mm Hg and an HCO_3 of 24 mEq/L.
2. Expected anion gap:

$$\text{Expected Anion Gap} = 12 - (2.5) * \left[4.0 \frac{g}{dL} - \text{Actual Serum Albumin} \right]$$
$$= 12 - (2.5 * [4.0 - 4.0])$$
$$= 12 - (2.5 * [0]) = \textbf{12 mEq/L.}$$

3. Anion gap calculation:

$$\text{Serum Anion Gap} = [Na^+] - [HCO_3^-] - [Cl^-]$$
$$= 140 - (87 + 13) = 40 \text{ mEq/L, which is} > 12 \text{ mEq/L}$$
$$\rightarrow \textbf{anion gap acidosis is present.}$$

4. Delta-delta calculation:

$$\Delta\Delta = \frac{(\text{Actual Anion Gap} - \text{Expected Anion Gap})}{(\text{Baseline HCO}_3 - \text{Actual HCO}_3)}$$
$$= (40 - 12)/(24 - 13) = \textbf{28/9, which is \textasciitilde2.6.}$$

Delta-delta interpretation.	
Delta-Delta Value	Condition Present
< 0.4	Non-anion gap only
0.4–0.9	Anion gap *and* non-anion gap acidosis
1.0–2.0	Anion gap acidosis only
> 2.0	**Anion gap acidosis and metabolic alkalosis**

Q59-4: D
Hyperemesis.

Rationale: The patient has a chloride-responsive ($U_{Cl} < 10$) metabolic alkalosis. Based on the differential (hyperemesis, diuretic use, contraction, post-hypercapnia), hyperemesis is listed in the vignette as a possible cause. The remaining causes are associated with non-anion gap acidosis or chloride-resistant causes of metabolic alkalosis.

Causes of metabolic alkalosis.
History: Rule Out the Following as Causes
• Alkali load ("milk-alkali" or calcium-alkali syndrome, oral sodium bicarbonate, IV sodium bicarbonate)   • Genetic causes (CF)   • Presence of hypercalcemia   • IV β-lactam antibiotics   • Laxative abuse (may also cause a metabolic acidosis depending on diarrheal HCO_3 losses)
If None of the Above, Then...
Urine Chloride < 20 mEq/L (Chloride-Responsive Causes)
• Loss of gastric acid (hyperemesis, NGT suctioning)   • Prior diuretic use (in hours to days following discontinuation)   • Post-hypercapnia   • Villous adenoma   • Congenital chloridorrhea   • Chronic laxative abuse (may also cause a metabolic acidosis depending on diarrheal HCO_3 losses)   • CF
OR
Urine Chloride > 20 mEq/L (Chloride-Resistant Causes)

(Continued)

Causes of metabolic alkalosis. (*continued*)
Urine Chloride > 20 mEq/L, Lack of HTN, Urine Potassium < 30 mEq/L
• Hypokalemia or hypomagnesemia • Laxative abuse (if dominated by hypokalemia) • Bartter syndrome • Gitelman syndrome
Urine Chloride > 20 mEq/L, Lack of HTN, Urine Potassium > 30 mEq/L
• Current diuretic use
Urine Chloride > 20 mEq/L, Presence of HTN, Urine Potassium Variable but Usually > 30 mEq/L
Elevated plasma renin level: • Renal artery stenosis • Renin-secreting tumor • Renovascular disease
Low plasma renin, low plasma aldosterone: • Cushing syndrome • Exogenous mineralocorticoid use • Genetic disorder (11-hydoxylase or 17-hydrolyase deficiency, 11β-HSD deficiency) • Liddle syndrome • Licorice toxicity
Low plasma renin, high plasma aldosterone: • Primary hyperaldosteronism • Adrenal adenoma • Bilateral adrenal hyperplasia

Q59-5: E
Toluene toxicity.

Rationale: The patient has a large anion gap acidosis with associated hypokalemia, hypocalcemia, and hypophosphatemia. He has no osmolar gap (see further) and his laboratory results are negative for urine ketones, ASA, and acetaminophen. His lactate level is within normal limits. He has liver injury based on the ALT. He is at risk for toluene exposure based on his occupation (painter) and drug use history (which places him at risk for toluene abuse). Toluene and benzene are common organic compounds associated with inhalation drug use termed *huffing*. Painters, textile workers, oil refinery/gasoline plant workers, and rubber plant workers are at risk for occupational exposure. Toluene is also present in model glue and certain furniture finishes/varnishes. Toluene exposure is associated with tachypnea, tachycardia, inhalation drug injury leading to mucosal injury (burns, etc), as well as lung injury (hypoxemia), "huffer's eczema," nystagmus, encephalopathy, seizures, hypotension, fever, rhabdomyolysis, and severe liver injury.

$$\text{Calculated Serum Osmolality} = 2*[\text{Na}^+] + \frac{[\text{Glucose}]}{18} + \frac{[\text{BUN}]}{2.8} + \frac{[\text{EtOH}]}{3.7}$$
$$= 296 \text{ mOsm/L}$$

$$\text{Serum Osmolal Gap (SOG)} = \text{Measured Serum Osmolality}$$
$$- \text{Calculated Serum Osmolality}$$
$$= 302 - 296 = (+6) \text{ mOsm/L (normal)}.$$

While the patient has an opioid-positive toxicology screen, this does not cause an anion gap acidosis directly. Patients can, however, develop lactic acidosis as a result of complications from opioid use, including hypotension, respiratory acidosis, or hypoxemia.

Toluene toxicity more commonly causes a non-anion gap metabolic acidosis with marked hypokalemia and urine studies consistent with a distal RTA. Toluene is metabolized to hippuric acid and then to hippurate. Hippurate is an anion, which combines with sodium and potassium, and is actively filtered at the glomerulus but is also actively secreted in the tubules. The hippurate replaces chloride in the urine, raising the urine anion gap. However, in cases in which the kidneys are not functioning properly (in this case the patient's Cr is 1.6), the hippurate is not secreted and accumulates in the bloodstream, causing an anion gap acidosis.

Q59-6: G
Opioid overdose.

Rationale: The patient has a respiratory acidosis, with a positive opioid screen. Hypoxemia is commonly associated with a respiratory alkalosis due to tachypnea. The remaining causes are unlikely in this patient outside of benzodiazepine overdose, although the urine drug screen was negative for benzodiazepines. **Co-ingestions are very common in drug overdose cases.**

References

Abreo K, Adlakha A, Kilpatrick S, et al. The milk-alkali syndrome. A reversible form of acute renal failure. Arch Intern Med. 1993;153:1005.

Arroliga AC, Shehab N, McCarthy K, Gonzales JP. Relationship of continuous infusion lorazepam to serum propylene glycol concentration in critically ill adults. Crit Care Med. 2004;32:1709.

Barton CH, Vaziri ND, Ness RL, et al. Cimetidine in the management of metabolic alkalosis induced by nasogastric drainage. Arch Surg. 1979;114:70.

Batlle D, Chin-Theodorou J, Tucker BM. Metabolic acidosis or respiratory alkalosis? Evaluation of a low plasma bicarbonate using the urine anion gap. Am J Kidney Dis. 2017;70:440.

Batlle D, Grupp M, Gaviria M, Kurtzman NA. Distal renal tubular acidosis with intact capacity to lower urinary pH. Am J Med. 1982;72:751.

Batlle D, Haque SK. Genetic causes and mechanisms of distal renal tubular acidosis. Nephrol Dial Transplant. 2012;27:3691.

Batlle DC, Hizon M, Cohen E, et al. The use of the urinary anion gap in the diagnosis of hyperchloremic metabolic acidosis. N Engl J Med. 1988;318:594.

Batlle DC, von Riotte A, Schlueter W. Urinary sodium in the evaluation of hyperchloremic metabolic acidosis. N Engl J Med. 1987;316:140.

Bear R, Goldstein M, Phillipson E, et al. Effect of metabolic alkalosis on respiratory function in patients with chronic obstructive lung disease. Can Med Assoc J. 1977;117:900.

Braden GL, Strayhorn CH, Germain MJ, et al. Increased osmolal gap in alcoholic acidosis. Arch Intern Med. 1993;153:2377.

Buckalew VM Jr, McCurdy DK, Ludwig GD, et al. Incomplete renal tubular acidosis. Physiologic studies in three patients with a defect in lowering urine pH. Am J Med 1968;45:32.

Cámara-Lemarroy CR, Gónzalez-Moreno EI, Rodriguez-Gutierrez R, González-González JG. Clinical presentation and management in acute toluene intoxication: a case series. Inhal Toxicol. 2012;24:434.

Gabow PA. Ethylene glycol intoxication. Am J Kidney Dis. 1988;11:277.

Galla JH, Gifford JD, Luke RG, Rome L. Adaptations to chloride-depletion alkalosis. Am J Physiol. 1991;261:R771.

Garella S, Chang BS, Kahn SI. Dilution acidosis and contraction alkalosis: review of a concept. Kidney Int. 1975;8:279.

Gennari FJ. Current concepts. Serum osmolality. Uses and limitations. N Engl J Med. 1984;310:102.

Gennari FJ, Weise WJ. Acid-base disturbances in gastrointestinal disease. Clin J Am Soc Nephrol. 2008;3:1861.

Glasser L, Sternglanz PD, Combie J, Robinson A. Serum osmolality and its applicability to drug overdose. Am J Clin Pathol. 1973;60:695.

Hamm LL, Nakhoul N, Hering-Smith KS. Acid-base homeostasis. Clin J Am Soc Nephrol. 2015;10:2232.

Hulter HN, Sebastian A, Toto RD, et al. Renal and systemic acid-base effects of the chronic administration of hypercalcemia-producing agents: calcitriol, PTH, and intravenous calcium. Kidney Int. 1982;21:445.

Karet FE. Mechanisms in hyperkalemic renal tubular acidosis. J Am Soc Nephrol. 2009;20:251.

Khanna A, Kurtzman NA. Metabolic alkalosis. J Nephrol. 2006;19(suppl 9):S86.

Kraut JA, Kurtz I. Toxic alcohol ingestions: clinical features, diagnosis, and management. Clin J Am Soc Nephrol. 2008;3:208.

Kraut JA, Madias NE. Differential diagnosis of nongap metabolic acidosis: value of a systematic approach. Clin J Am Soc Nephrol. 2012;7:671.

Kraut JA, Xing SX. Approach to the evaluation of a patient with an increased serum osmolal gap and high-anion-gap metabolic acidosis. Am J Kidney Dis. 2011;58:480.

Laski ME, Sabatini S. Metabolic alkalosis, bedside and bench. Semin Nephrol. 2006;26:404.

Luke RG, Galla JH. It is chloride depletion alkalosis, not contraction alkalosis. J Am Soc Nephrol. 2012;23:204.

Lynd LD, Richardson KJ, Purssell RA, et al. An evaluation of the osmole gap as a screening test for toxic alcohol poisoning. BMC Emerg Med. 2008;8:5.

Marraffa JM, Holland MG, Stork CM, et al. Diethylene glycol: widely used solvent presents serious poisoning potential. J Emerg Med. 2008;35:401.

Miller PD, Berns AS. Acute metabolic alkalosis perpetuating hypercarbia. A role for acetazolamide in chronic obstructive pulmonary disease. JAMA. 1977;238:2400.

Oster JR, Materson BJ, Rogers AI. Laxative abuse syndrome. Am J Gastroenterol. 1980;74:451.

Patel AM, Goldfarb S. Got calcium? Welcome to the calcium-alkali syndrome. J Am Soc Nephrol. 2010;21:1440.

Purssell RA, Pudek M, Brubacher J, Abu-Laban RB. Derivation and validation of a formula to calculate the contribution of ethanol to the osmolal gap. Ann Emerg Med. 2001;38:653.

Rastegar M, Nagami GT. Non-anion gap metabolic acidosis: a clinical approach to evaluation. Am J Kidney Dis. 2017;69:296.

Robinson AG, Loeb JN. Ethanol ingestion–commonest cause of elevated plasma osmolality? N Engl J Med. 1971;284:1253.

Rodríguez Soriano J. Renal tubular acidosis: the clinical entity. J Am Soc Nephrol. 2002;13:2160.

Rose BD, Post TW. Clinical Physiology of Acid-Base and Electrolyte Disorders, 5e. New York, NY: McGraw Hill; 2001:559

Schelling JR, Howard RL, Winter SD, Linas SL. Increased osmolal gap in alcoholic ketoacidosis and lactic acidosis. Ann Intern Med 1990; 113:580.

Schwartz WB, Van Ypersele de Strihou, Kassirer JP. Role of anions in metabolic alkalosis and potassium deficiency. N Engl J Med. 1968;279:630.

Streicher HZ, Gabow PA, Moss AH, et al. Syndromes of toluene sniffing in adults. Ann Intern Med. 1981;94:758.

Sweetser LJ, Douglas JA, Riha RL, Bell SC. Clinical presentation of metabolic alkalosis in an adult patient with cystic fibrosis. Respirology. 2005;10:254.

Taher SM, Anderson RJ, McCartney R, et al. Renal tubular acidosis associated with toluene "sniffing". N Engl J Med. 1974;290:765.

Taki K, Mizuno K, Takahashi N, Wakusawa R. Disturbance of CO2 elimination in the lungs by carbonic anhydrase inhibition. Jpn J Physiol. 1986;36:523.

Turban S, Beutler KT, Morris RG, et al. Long-term regulation of proximal tubule acid-base transporter abundance by angiotensin II. Kidney Int. 2006;70:660.

Yücel M, Takagi M, Walterfang M, Lubman DI. Toluene misuse and long-term harms: a systematic review of the neuropsychological and neuroimaging literature. Neurosci Biobehav Rev. 2008;32:910.

CASE 60

A 55-year-old man is transferred to the ICU from the PACU following surgery for a benign skin tumor. He required general anesthesia due to the location of the tumor. The procedure required only 20 minutes, and the patient returned to the PACU, where he was noted to develop hypertension, tachypnea, and muscle rigidity. He was transferred emergently to the ICU for further management. His vital signs are T 36.5°C, HR 133, BP 110/80, RR 4, Sao$_2$ 97% on room air. On exam, the patient demonstrates an agonal breathing pattern. He has no significant medical conditions outside of glaucoma.

Laboratory data.			
ABGs		Basic Metabolic Panel	
pH	6.92	Na	139 mEq/L
Paco$_2$	50 mm Hg	K	6.5 mEq/L
Pao$_2$	100 mm Hg	Cl	99 mEq/L
HCO$_3$	10 mEq/L	CO$_2$	10 mEq/L
		BUN	44 mg/dL
		Cr	1.9 mg/dL
		Glucose	67 mg/dL
		Albumin	4.0 g/dL
		EtOH	0 mg/dL

QUESTIONS

Q60-1: Define the patient's baseline acid-base status: Does this patient have an underlying chronic acid-base disorder that we need to account for in order to appropriately interpret the acute acid-base disorders?

A. There is no evidence for an underlying chronic respiratory or metabolic acid-base disorder in this patient, so we would assume a baseline $Paco_2$ of 40 mm Hg and an HCO_3 of 24 mEq/L.

B. While the patient has a condition predisposing him to a chronic acid-base disorder, there is insufficient information to estimate the patient's baseline $Paco_2$ and HCO_3 values; therefore, we will assume a baseline $Paco_2$ of 40 mm Hg and a baseline HCO_3 of 24 mEq/L.

C. The patient has an underlying acid-base condition, and we have sufficient information to estimate the patient's baseline $Paco_2$ and HCO_3 values.

Q60-2: What is/are the primary acid-base disturbance(s) occurring in this case?

A. Metabolic acidosis only
B. Respiratory acidosis only
C. Metabolic acidosis and a respiratory acidosis
D. Metabolic alkalosis and a respiratory alkalosis
E. Metabolic alkalosis only
F. Respiratory alkalosis only

Q60-3: How would the metabolic acidosis component be classified in this case?

A. Anion gap acidosis
B. Non-anion gap acidosis
C. Anion and non-anion gap acidosis
D. Anion gap acidosis and a metabolic alkalosis

Q60-4: This patient also has a respiratory acidosis. If the patient only had a metabolic acidosis, as described previously, and was compensating appropriately, what would you expect the $Paco_2$ to be in this case?

A. 12 mm Hg
B. 17 mm Hg
C. 23 mm Hg
D. 27 mm Hg
E. 33 mm Hg
F. 42 mm Hg

Q60-5: The serum osmolality is 304 mOsm/L. What is the patient's serum osmolal gap?

A. 5 mOsm/L
B. 10 mOsm/L
C. 15 mOsm/L
D. 20 mOsm/L

Q60-6: The patient's remaining test results are as follows:

Serum EtOH	< 3 mg/dL
Serum acetaminophen level	< 3 mg/dL (ULN for therapeutic use 20 mg/dL)
Serum salicylates level	2.3 mg/dL (ULN for therapeutic use 30 mg/dL)
Serum osmolality	304 mOsm/kg
Serum L-lactate	7.0 mmol/L (ULN 2.0 mmol/L venous)
Beta-hydroxybutyrate (acetone)	< 0.18 mmol/L (ULN 0.18 mmol/L)
Serum creatinine kinase	23,000 IU/mL
Serum calcium	10.6 mg/dL
Serum troponin	1.11 ng/mL
Serum phosphorus	12.0 mg/dL

What is the likely cause of the patient's anion gap acidosis?

A. Aspirin toxicity

B. Propylene glycol toxicity

C. Ethylene glycol toxicity

D. Methanol toxicity

E. Lactic acidosis due to sepsis

F. Lactic acidosis due to malignant hyperthermia

G. Lactic acidosis due to metformin use

Q60-7: The patient's RR is 34 with a minute ventilation of 14 L/min. What is the cause of the respiratory acidosis?

A. Reduced gas diffusion

B. Reduced cardiac output

C. Hypermetabolic state

D. Reduced oxygen utilization

Q60-8: Besides supportive care, what is the appropriate medical therapy for malignant hyperthermia?

A. Dilaudid

B. Dantrolene

C. Methylene blue

D. Hyperbaric oxygen therapy

E. Dimercaprol

F. Flumazenil

G. Naloxone

H. DigiFAB

I. Atropine

J. Acetylcysteine

ANSWERS

Q60-1: A

There is no evidence for an underlying chronic respiratory or metabolic acid-base disorder in this patient, so we would assume a baseline $Paco_2$ of 40 mm Hg and an HCO_3 of 24 mEq/L.

Rationale: Ignoring these underlying chronic acid-base disorders can significantly alter the interpretation of a patient's acute acid-base status. This was demonstrated in the first case of the series. However, often, we do not have the necessary information (eg, prior ABG or VBG, or prior serum chemistry with an HCO_3) and are forced to assume the ongoing processes are all acute in nature. We are primarily concerned about chronic respiratory acid-base disorders, as these can significantly alter the patient's baseline or expected values for the serum HCO_3 and $Paco_2$, and we have reliable equations to predict the expected baseline values. The respiratory compensation for both chronic metabolic acidosis and alkalosis is generally poor, so there are no equations or rules to predict what the $Paco_2$ should be in these cases. While the baseline serum HCO_3 may be significantly off from our standard value of 24 mEq/L in these patients, we would assume a baseline $Paco_2$ of 40 mm Hg in patients with chronic metabolic processes. Once we identify the patient's baseline $Paco_2$ and HCO_3 values, we will need to use these values in the appropriate equations to identify the ongoing acute processes.

Q60-2: C

Metabolic acidosis and respiratory acidosis.

Rationale:

1. The pH is 6.92; therefore, the primary disorder is an **acidosis.**
2. The $Paco_2$ of 50 mm Hg is greater than 40 mm Hg, so there is a **respiratory acidosis.**
3. The HCO_3 of 10 mEq/L is less than 24 mEq/L, so there is also a **metabolic acidosis.**

Q60-3: A

Anion gap acidosis.

Rationale:

1. Is there evidence for a chronic respiratory acid-base disorder that requires adjustment of the patient's "normal" HCO_3? No, there is no evidence for a chronic respiratory acid-base disorder, so we would assume a baseline $Paco_2$ of 40 mm Hg and an HCO_3 of 24 mEq/L.
2. Expected anion gap:

$$\text{Expected Anion Gap} = 12 - (2.5) * \left[4.0 \frac{g}{dL} - \text{Actual Serum Albumin} \right]$$
$$= 12 - (2.5 * [4.0 - 4.0])$$
$$= 12 - (2.5 * [0]) = \textbf{12 mEq/L.}$$

3. Anion gap calculation:

$$\text{Serum Anion Gap} = [Na^+] - [HCO_3^-] - [Cl^-]$$
$$= 139 - (99 + 10) = \textbf{30 mEq/L,} \text{ which is} > 12 \text{ mEq/L}$$
$$\rightarrow \textbf{anion gap acidosis is present.}$$

4. Delta-delta calculation:

$$\Delta\Delta = \frac{(\text{Actual Anion Gap} - \text{Expected Anion Gap})}{(\text{Baseline HCO}_3 - \text{Actual HCO}_3)}$$
$$= (30 - 12)/(24 - 10) = \textbf{18/14, which is} \sim \textbf{1.3.}$$

Delta-delta interpretation.	
Delta-Delta Value	Condition Present
< 0.4	Non-anion gap only
0.4–0.9	Anion gap *and* non-anion gap acidosis
1.0–2.0	**Anion gap acidosis only**
> 2.0	Anion gap acidosis and metabolic alkalosis

Q60-4: C
23 mm Hg.

Rationale: Using the Winter formula, one can calculate what the expected arterial $Paco_2$ should be for a given serum HCO_3 if the patient were appropriately compensated.

Respiratory Compensation for Acute Metabolic Acidosis (Winter Formula):

$$\text{Expected Paco}_2 = 1.5 * [\text{Actual HCO}_3] + 8 \pm 2 \text{ (in mm Hg)}$$
$$= (1.5 * 10) + 8 = 15 + 8 = 23 \pm 2 = (21 \text{ to } 25) \text{ mm Hg.}$$

Q60-5: A
5 mOsm/L.

Rationale: Similar to the serum anion gap, the serum osmolal gap is determined by the difference between the "calculated" serum osmolality and the true, measured serum osmolality. The equation for the serum osmolal gap typically includes factors for sodium, glucose, BUN, and ethanol, as these are readily measurable in most laboratories. Therefore, the serum osmolal gap will represent the osmolality of those "unmeasured" osmoles, including organic alcohols and acetone. The most common form is as follows:

$$\text{Calculated Serum Osmolality} = 2 * [Na^+] + \frac{[\text{Glucose}]}{18} + \frac{[\text{BUN}]}{2.8} + \frac{[\text{EtOH}]}{3.7};$$

In which the units of measure are as follows: Na, mEq/L; glucose, mg/dL; BUN, mg/dL; and EtOH, mg/dL. The conversion factors are shown in the preceding equation as well. A normal serum osmolal gap is around −10 to +10 mOsm/L (or mOsm/kg).

Therefore, for this patient:

$$\text{Calculated Serum Osmolality} = (2 * 139) + (67/18) + (44/2.8) + (0/3.7)$$
$$= 299 \text{ mOsm/L.}$$

$$\text{Serum Osmolal Gap} = \text{Measured Serum Osmolality}$$
$$- \text{Calculated Osmolality}$$
$$= (304 - 299) = \textbf{5, which is} < 10 \text{ mOsm/L}$$
$$\rightarrow \textbf{no serum osmolal gap exists.}$$

Q60-6: F
Lactic acidosis due to malignant hyperthermia.

Rationale: The patient presented with malignant hyperthermia. He has fever, rhabdomyolysis, muscle rigidity, hyperkalemia, hyperphosphatemia, hypercalcemia, and renal failure following the use of general anesthetics. The metabolic acidosis is caused by a hypermetabolic state, outstripping the oxygen supply and leading to an anaerobic state and lactic acidosis. Acute renal failure can also contribute to the anion gap acidosis. There is no evidence of sepsis. Metformin can lead to a type B lactic acidosis, but there is no mention of metformin use in the vignette. The normal serum osmolal gap makes ethylene glycol and methanol toxicity unlikely.

Q60-7: C
Hypermetabolic state.

Rationale: The patient has a hypermetabolic state, with increased CO_2 production in peripheral tissues that the body is unable to clear, despite the presence of intact gas diffusion, increased cardiac output, and increased ventilation. This is a classic presentation of malignant hyperthermia.

Malignant hyperthermia is a rare but life-threatening clinical condition of subclinical myopathy caused by genetic mutations in a calcium release channel (most commonly RYR-1 or CACNA1S). Massive calcium release from the sarcoplasmic reticulum of skeletal muscle occurs as a result of exposure to anesthetics. The calcium release results in stimulation of aerobic and anaerobic metabolism, yielding muscle rigidity, metabolic and respiratory acidosis, hyperkalemia, and renal failure. The lactate can often reach levels above the threshold of most clinical labs (> 20 mmol/L). Tachycardia, tachypnea, dysrhythmia, hyperthermia (resulting from the massive increase in exothermic metabolic reactions), rhabdomyolysis, hyperkalemia, hyperphosphatemia, hypercalcemia, and edema are common complications. If not treated appropriately, this metabolic response will lead to seizures, DIC, multiple organ failure, and death.

Other conditions to consider in the differential diagnosis of malignant hyperthermia include thyroid storm, neuroleptic malignant syndrome, hemophagocytic lympho-histiocytosis (HLH), and severe sepsis/septic shock.

Q60-8: B
Dantrolene.

Rationale: Dantrolene inhibits calcium release from the sarcoplasmic reticulum. Methylene blue is an antidote for methemoglobinemia, Hypercarbic oxygen therapy is used for carboxyhemoglobinemia. Dimercaprol is used in heavy metal poisoning. Flumazenil is used for benzodiazepine reversal, while naloxone is used for opioid reversal. DigiFAB is used in digoxin toxicity, atropine for organophosphate toxicity, and acetylcysteine for acetaminophen toxicity. Dialudid (hydromorphone) is an opioid and is not an antedote for malignant hyperthermia.

References

Ali SZ, Taguchi A, Rosenberg H. Malignant hyperthermia. Best Pract Res Clin Anaesthesiol. 2003;17:519.

Harrison GG. Control of the malignant hyperpyrexic syndrome in MHS swine by dantrolene sodium. Br J Anaesth. 1975;47:62

Hopkins PM. Malignant hyperthermia: pharmacology of triggering. Br J Anaesth. 2011;107:48.

Kolb ME, Horne ML, Martz R. Dantrolene in human malignant hyperthermia. Anesthesiology. 1982;56:254.

Larach MG, Brandom BW, Allen GC, et al. Cardiac arrests and deaths associated with malignant hyperthermia in North America from 1987 to 2006: a report from the North American malignant hyperthermia registry of the Malignant Hyperthermia Association of the United States. Anesthesiology. 2008;108:603.

Larach MG, Localio AR, Allen GC, et al. A clinical grading scale to predict malignant hyperthermia susceptibility. Anesthesiology. 1994;80:771.

Litman RS, Rosenberg H. Malignant hyperthermia: update on susceptibility testing. JAMA. 2005;293:2918.

Rosenberg H, Pollock N, Schiemann A, et al. Malignant hyperthermia: a review. Orphanet J Rare Dis. 2015;10:93.

Schneiderbanger D, Johannsen S, Roewer N, Schuster F. Management of malignant hyperthermia: diagnosis and treatment. Ther Clin Risk Manag. 2014;10:355.

CASE 61

A 77-year-old male patient with chronic respiratory failure (both hypoxemic and hypercarbic) presents to the emergency department with respiratory distress. His vital signs are T 39.1°C, HR 120, BP 80/40, RR 9, and Sao$_2$ 97% on room air. The patient's WBC is 22,300 per microliter, with 72% mature neutrophils 20% bands. CXR shows a large infiltrate in the right lower lobe. A month ago, during an outpatient pulmonary appointment, the patient's ABGs were as follows: pH 7.35, Paco$_2$ 65 mm Hg, and HCO$_3$ 33 mEq/L. The patient's medication list is at home with his wife, who is on her way to the hospital. The patient also has a history of bipolar disorder and PTSD. He does not take illicit drugs or use alcohol. His examination demonstrates mild encephalopathy and focal rhonchi in the right lower lung field with diminished breath sounds at the apices bilaterally.

Laboratory data.			
ABGs		Basic Metabolic Panel	
pH	7.22	Na	140 mEq/L
Paco$_2$	60 mm Hg	K	3.1 mEq/L
Pao$_2$	100 mm Hg	Cl	100 mEq/L
HCO$_3$	24 mEq/L	CO$_2$	24 mEq/L
		BUN	20 mg/dL
		Cr	0.7 mg/dL
		Glucose	100 mg/dL
		Albumin	4.0 g/dL
		EtOH	0 mg/dL

QUESTIONS

Q61-1: Define the patient's baseline acid-base status: Does this patient have an underlying chronic acid-base disorder that we need to account for in order to appropriately interpret the acute acid-base disorders?

A. There is no evidence for an underlying chronic respiratory or metabolic acid-base disorder in this patient, so we would assume a baseline $Paco_2$ of 40 mm Hg and an HCO_3 of 24 mEq/L.

B. While the patient has a condition predisposing him to a chronic acid-base disorder, there is insufficient information to estimate the patient's baseline $Paco_2$ and HCO_3 values; therefore, we will assume a baseline $Paco_2$ of 40 mm Hg and a baseline HCO_3 of 24 mEq/L.

C. The patient has an underlying acid-base condition, and we have sufficient information to estimate the patient's baseline $Paco_2$ and HCO_3 values.

Q61-2: The vignette lists the patient's baseline $Paco_2$ as 65 mm Hg and the baseline HCO_3 as 33 mEq/L. What is/are the primary acid-base disturbance(s) occurring in this case?

A. Metabolic acidosis only
B. Respiratory acidosis only
C. Metabolic acidosis and a respiratory acidosis
D. Metabolic alkalosis and a respiratory alkalosis
E. Metabolic alkalosis only
F. Respiratory alkalosis only

Q61-3: How would the metabolic acidosis component be classified in this case?

A. Anion gap acidosis
B. Non-anion gap acidosis
C. Anion and non-anion gap acidosis
D. Anion gap acidosis and a metabolic alkalosis

Q61-4: Does the patient in this case demonstrate appropriate respiratory or metabolic compensation?

A. Yes, the respiratory compensation is appropriate.
B. No, a concomitant respiratory alkalosis is present.
C. No, a concomitant respiratory acidosis is present.
D. Yes, the metabolic compensation is appropriate.
E. No, a concomitant metabolic acidosis is present.
F. No, a concomitant metabolic alkalosis is present.

Q61-5: What is the likely cause of the patient's respiratory acidosis?

A. Hypoxemia
B. Neuromuscular disorder
C. COPD
D. Chest wall injury (eg, flail chest)
E. Pulmonary fibrosis

Q61-6: The patient's remaining test results are as follows:

Serum EtOH	< 3 mg/dL
Serum acetaminophen level	< 5 mg/dL (ULN for therapeutic use 20 mg/dL)
Serum salicylates level	< 5 mg/dL (ULN for therapeutic use 30 mg/dL)
Serum osmolality	298 mOsm/kg
Beta-hydroxybutyrate (acetone)	< 0.18 mmol/L (ULN 0.18 mmol/L)
Serum glucose	100 mg/dL
Serum phosphorus	2.3 mg/dL

What is the likely cause of the patient's anion gap acidosis?

A. Aspirin toxicity
B. Lactic acidosis secondary to sepsis
C. Ethylene glycol toxicity
D. Methanol toxicity
E. Opioid overdose
F. Acetaminophen overdose
G. Diabetic ketoacidosis
H. Alcoholic ketoacidosis

Q61-7: The patient's urine electrolyte values are as follows:

Urine Na	20 mEq/L
Urine K	80 mEq/L
Urine Cl	60 mEq/L
Urine urea	234 mg/dL
Urine glucose	0 mg/dL
Urine osmolality	354 mOsm/L
Urine pH	7.9
Urine RBCs	None
Urine WBCs	None
Urine protein	None
Urine microscopic	None

What is the most likely type of non-anion gap acidosis present?

A. Diarrhea
B. Type 1 RTA (distal tubule)
C. Type 2 RTA (proximal tubule)
D. Type 4 RTA (distal tubule/collecting duct)

Q61-8: Which of these medications is most commonly associated with a type 1 RTA?

A. Trimethoprim
B. Lisinopril
C. Lithium
D. Tacrolimus

ANSWERS

Q61-1: C

The patient has an underlying acid-base condition, and we have sufficient information to estimate the patient's baseline $Paco_2$ and HCO_3 values. This patient has a chronic respiratory acidosis with a baseline HCO_3 of 33 mEq/L and $Paco_2$ of 65 mm Hg.

Rationale: Ignoring these underlying chronic acid-base disorders can significantly alter the interpretation of a patient's acute acid-base status. This was demonstrated in the first case of the series. However, often, we do not have the necessary information (eg, prior ABG or VBG, or prior serum chemistry with an HCO_3) and are forced to assume the ongoing processes are all acute in nature. We are primarily concerned about chronic respiratory acid-base disorders, as these can significantly alter the patient's baseline or expected values for the serum HCO_3 and $Paco_2$, and we have reliable equations to predict the expected baseline values. The respiratory compensation for both chronic metabolic acidosis and alkalosis is generally poor, so there are no equations or rules to predict what the $Paco_2$ should be in these cases. While the baseline serum HCO_3 may be significantly off from our standard value of 24 mEq/L in these patients, we would assume a baseline $Paco_2$ of 40 mm Hg in patients with chronic metabolic processes. Once we identify the patient's baseline $Paco_2$ and HCO_3 values, we will need to use these values in the appropriate equations to identify the ongoing acute processes.

Q61-2: A

Metabolic acidosis only.

Rationale: The patient has chronic respiratory failure (chronic respiratory acidosis), and at baseline (with appropriate compensation), he has a compensatory metabolic alkalosis. We need to adjust our criteria to his chronic baseline when examining the case for acute changes:

1. The pH is 7.22; therefore, the primary disorder is an **acidosis.**
2. The $Paco_2$ is 60 mm Hg, which is less than his baseline of 65 mm Hg, so this is *not* an acute respiratory acidosis.
3. The HCO_3 is 24 mEq/L; despite being "normal," this is substantially lower than this patient's chronic baseline HCO_3 of 33 mEq/L, so there is an **acute metabolic acidosis.**

Q61-3: D

Anion gap acidosis and metabolic alkalosis.

Rationale:

1. Is there evidence for a chronic respiratory acid-base disorder that requires adjustment of the patient's "normal" HCO_3? Yes, the patient has a chronic respiratory acidosis with an appropriate metabolic compensation, with a baseline HCO_3 of 33 mEq/L.

2. Expected anion gap:

$$\text{Expected Anion Gap} = 12 - (2.5) * \left[4.0 \frac{g}{dL} - \text{Actual Serum Albumin} \right]$$
$$= 12 - (2.5 * [4.0 - 4.0])$$
$$= 12 - (2.5 * [0]) = \textbf{12 mEq/L.}$$

3. Anion gap calculation: This equation does not change (the expected anion gap is still only 12).

$$\text{Serum Anion Gap} = [Na^+] - [HCO_3^-] - [Cl^-]$$
$$= 140 - (100 + 24) = 16 \text{ mEq/L, which is} > 12 \text{ mEq/L}$$
$$\rightarrow \textbf{anion gap acidosis is present.}$$

4. Delta-delta calculation: **Remember to correct for normal HCO$_3$ here.**

$$\Delta\Delta = \frac{(\text{Actual Anion Gap} - \text{Expected Anion Gap})}{(\text{Baseline HCO}_3 - \text{Actual HCO}_3)}$$
$$= (16 - 12)/(33 - 24) = \textbf{4/9, which is ~0.44.}$$

Delta-delta interpretation.	
Delta-Delta Value	Condition Present
< 0.4	Non-anion gap only
0.4–0.9	**Anion gap *and* non-anion gap acidosis**
1.0–2.0	Anion gap acidosis only
> 2.0	Anion gap acidosis and metabolic alkalosis

Q61-4: C
No, a concomitant respiratory acidosis is present.

Rationale: Using the Winter formula, one can calculate what the expected arterial Paco$_2$ should be for a given serum HCO$_3$ if the patient were completely compensated. This equation does not change in this case, as it does not contain a term for his baseline HCO$_3$.

Respiratory Compensation for Acute Metabolic Acidosis (Winter Formula):

$$\text{Expected Paco}_2 = 1.5 * [\text{Actual HCO}_3] + 8 \pm 2 \text{ (in mm Hg)}$$
$$= (1.5 * 24) + 8 = 36 + 8 = 44 \pm 2 = (42 \text{ to } 46) \text{ mm Hg.}$$

This patient has a concomitant respiratory acidosis, with **Paco$_2$ of 60 mm Hg**, well above the expected range (42 to 46 mm Hg). Therefore a respiratory acidosis is also present.

Q61-5: C
COPD.

Rationale: The patient has baseline COPD with chronic respiratory acidosis. Compared to his baseline $Paco_2$ of 65 mm Hg, his current $Paco_2$ of 60 mm Hg shows his body is attempting to compensate for the new metabolic acidosis but is unable to mount what we consider appropriate compensation ($Paco_2$ of 42 to 46 mm Hg), so there is an acute respiratory acidosis present as well. COPD is associated with reduced respiratory reserve and patients with this disorder are often unable to compensate appropriately for a severe metabolic acidosis.

Q61-6: B
Lactic acidosis secondary to sepsis.

Rationale: The patient presented with a new pneumonia, hypotension, and a metabolic acidosis. This is most consistent with lactic acidosis due to sepsis. The patient has a negative serum ketone study indicating that a ketoacidosis is unlikely. The serum aspirin and acetaminophen levels are negative, so toxicity from either is unlikely. The patient has a normal serum creatinine with a normal BUN and serum phosphorus, so acute renal failure is not likely present. The calculated serum osmolality is 293 mOsm/L:

$$Calculated\ Serum\ Osmolality = 2*[Na^+] + \frac{[Glucose]}{18} + \frac{[BUN]}{2.8} + \frac{[EtOH]}{3.7}$$
$$= 2*[140] + [100/18] + [20/2.8] + [0/3.7]$$
$$= 293\ mOsm/L.$$

Therefore, the serum osmolal gap is +5 mOsm/L, which is normal. This indicates that toxicity with an organic alcohol is unlikely. A lactic acidosis secondary to sepsis is the most likely cause. In this case, the patient's lactate test returned an elevated result at 6.7 mmol/L, consistent with this diagnosis.

Q61-7: B
Type 1 RTA (distal).

Rationale: Recall that we can use either the urine anion gap (UAG) or the urine osmolal gap (UOG) to qualitatively estimate urinary ammonium excretion. This is a case in which the UAG alone is inconclusive. The patient's UAG is calculated as follows:

Urine Anion Gap:

$$UAG = [U_{Na}] + [U_K] - [U_{Cl}].$$

Therefore, for this patient,

$$UAG = U_{Na} + U_K - U_{Cl} = (20 + 80) - 60 = (+40).$$

The UAG is elevated, consistent with a likely type 1 or type 4 RTA in this patient. However, the UAG can be inappropriately elevated in anion gap acidosis, a situation in which multiple unmeasured anions may be present in the urine (beta-hydroxybutyrate/acetoacetate [ketoacidosis], hippurate [toluene], HCO_3 [proximal RTA], D-lactate [D-lactic acidosis], L-lactate, 5-oxoproline [acetaminophen toxicity]). Therefore, in patients with a significant anion gap, the UOG is typically more useful. First, we calculate the urine osmolality:

$$\text{Calculated Urine Osmolality} = 2 * ([Na^+] + [K^+]) + \frac{[Urea]}{2.8} + \frac{[Glucose]}{18}$$
$$= 2 * [20 + 80] + [20/2.8] + [20/18] = 284 \text{ mOsm/L}.$$

The UOG is then calculated:

$$\text{Urine Osmolal Gap} = \text{Measured Urine Osmolality} - \text{Measured Urine Osmolality}$$
$$UOG = 334 - 184 \text{ mOsm/L} = 50 \text{ mOsm/L}.$$

Here, the UOG is inappropriately low urinary acidification, most consistent with a type 1 or 4 RTA. Again, this is not particularly useful for the diagnosis of a type 2 (proximal) RTA, where other serum or urine lab abnormalities are more helpful. The primary limitation is its use in conditions with a high osmolar gap, where non-ammonium solutes not included in the calculation may be present in the urine (particularly mannitol). The presence of these unmeasured solutes will increase the osmolal gap inappropriately. Also, the UOG should not be used in patients with a urinary tract infection caused by a urease-producing organism, as urea is metabolized to HCO_3 and ammonium in urine.

Similar to the UAG, the urine UOG is used as a surrogate for the urine ammonium concentration. Therefore, a larger gap indicates increased urinary NH_4 excretion. In normal acid-base conditions, the UOG is between 10 and 100 mOsm/L. During a significant metabolic acidosis, patients with impaired renal tubular acidification (type 1 and type 4 RTA) are unable to excrete additional acid (NH_4), and therefore the osmolar gap does not change. Patients with an intact renal response to acidemia (ie, GI losses) should have a significant urine osmolar gap ($\sim > 300$ to 400 mOsm/L) as a result of increased NH_4 excretion.

Therefore, this patient likely has a type 1 or type 4 RTA. We can use the remaining information to determine which type of RTA is present. The low serum potassium and the elevated urine pH are highly suggestive of a distal RTA.

Evaluation of RTA.			
	Type 1 RTA	Type 2 RTA	Type 4 RTA
Severity of metabolic acidosis, (HCO$_3$)	Severe (< 10–12 mEq/L typically)	Intermediate (12–20 mEq/L)	Mild (15–20 mEq/L)
Associated urine abnormalities	Urinary phosphate, calcium are increased; bone disease often present	Urine glucose, amino acids, phosphate, calcium may be elevated	
Urine pH	HIGH (> 5.5)	Low (acidic), until serum HCO$_3$ level exceeds the resorptive ability of the proximal tubule; then becomes alkalotic once reabsorptive threshold is crossed	Low (acidic)
Serum K$^+$	Low to normal; should correct with oral HCO$_3$ therapy	Classically low, although may be normal or even high with rare genetic defects; worsens with oral HCO$_3$ therapy	HIGH
Renal stones	Often	No	No
Renal tubular defect	Reduced NH$_4$ secretion in distal tubule	Reduced HCO$_3$ resorption in proximal tubule	Reduced H$^+$/K$^+$ exchange in distal and collecting tubule due to decreased aldosterone or aldosterone resistance
UAG	> 10	Negative initially, then positive when receiving serum bicarbonate, then negative after therapy.	> 10
UOG	Reduced (< 150 mOsm/L) during acute acidosis	At baseline < 100 mEq/L; unreliable during acidosis	Reduced (< 150 mOsm/L) during acute acidosis

Q61-8: C
Lithium.

Rationale: Type 1 RTA is commonly associated with lithium, amphotericin B, aminoglycoside use, and ifosfamide. NSAIDs have also been associated with a type 1 RTA. The remaining medications are associated with a type 4 RTA.

Causes of RTA.
Causes of Type 1 (Distal) RTA
Primary • Idiopathic or familial (may be recessive or dominant)
Secondary • Medications: Lithium, amphotericin, ifosfamide, NSAIDs • Rheumatologic disorders: Sjögren syndrome, SLE, RA • Hypercalciuria (idiopathic) or associated with vitamin D deficiency or hyperparathyroidism • Sarcoidosis • Obstructive uropathy • Wilson disease • Rejection of renal transplant allograft
Causes of Type 2 (Proximal) RTA
Primary • Idiopathic • Familial (primarily recessive disorders) • Genetic: Fanconi syndrome, cystinosis, glycogen storage disease (type 1), Wilson disease, galactosemia
Secondary • Medications: Acetazolamide, topiramate, aminoglycoside antibiotics, ifosfamide, reverse transcriptase inhibitors (tenofovir) • Heavy metal poisoning: Lead, mercury, copper • Multiple myeloma or amyloidosis (secondary to light chain toxicity) • Sjögren syndrome • Vitamin D deficiency • Rejection of renal transplant allograft
Causes of Type 4 RTA (Hypoaldosteronism or Aldosterone Resistance)
Primary • Primary adrenal insufficiency • Inherited disorders associated with hypoaldosteronism • Pseudohypoaldosteronism (types 1 and 2)
Secondary • Causes of hyporeninemic hypoaldosteronism such as renal disease (diabetic nephropathy), NSAID use, calcineurin inhibitors, volume expansion/volume overload • Causes of distal tubule voltage defects such as sickle cell disease, obstructive uropathy, SLE • Severe illness/septic shock • Angiotensin II–associated medications: ACE inhibitors, ARBs, direct renin inhibitors • Potassium-sparing diuretics: Spironolactone, amiloride, triamterene • Antibiotics: Trimethoprim, pentamidine

References

Adeva-Andany M, López-Ojén M, Funcasta-Calderón R, et al. Comprehensive review on lactate metabolism in human health. Mitochondrion. 2014;17:76.

Arbus GS, Herbert LA, Levesque PR, et al. Characterization and clinical application of the "significance band" for acute respiratory alkalosis. N Engl J Med. 1969;280:117.

Arroliga AC, Shehab N, McCarthy K, Gonzales JP. Relationship of continuous infusion lorazepam to serum propylene glycol concentration in critically ill adults. Crit Care Med. 2004;32:1709.

Batlle D, Chin-Theodorou J, Tucker BM. Metabolic acidosis or respiratory alkalosis? Evaluation of a low plasma bicarbonate using the urine anion gap. Am J Kidney Dis. 2017;70:440.

Batlle D, Grupp M, Gaviria M, Kurtzman NA. Distal renal tubular acidosis with intact capacity to lower urinary pH. Am J Med. 1982;72:751.

Batlle D, Haque SK. Genetic causes and mechanisms of distal renal tubular acidosis. Nephrol Dial Transplant. 2012;27:3691.

Batlle DC, Hizon M, Cohen E, et al. The use of the urinary anion gap in the diagnosis of hyperchloremic metabolic acidosis. N Engl J Med. 1988;318:594.

Batlle DC, von Riotte A, Schlueter W. Urinary sodium in the evaluation of hyperchloremic metabolic acidosis. N Engl J Med. 1987;316:140.

Braden GL, Strayhorn CH, Germain MJ, et al. Increased osmolal gap in alcoholic acidosis. Arch Intern Med. 1993;153:2377.

Buckalew VM Jr, McCurdy DK, Ludwig GD, et al. Incomplete renal tubular acidosis. Physiologic studies in three patients with a defect in lowering urine pH. Am J Med. 1968;45:32.

Daniel SR, Morita SY, Yu M, Dzierba A. Uncompensated metabolic acidosis: an underrecognized risk factor for subsequent intubation requirement. J Trauma. 2004;57:993.

Dyck RF, Asthana S, Kalra J, et al. A modification of the urine osmolal gap: an improved method for estimating urine ammonium. Am J Nephrol. 1990;10:359.

Fulop M. A guide for predicting arterial CO2 tension in metabolic acidosis. Am J Nephrol. 1997;17:421.

Gabow PA. Ethylene glycol intoxication. Am J Kidney Dis. 1988;11:277.

Gennari FJ. Current concepts. Serum osmolality. Uses and limitations. N Engl J Med. 1984;310:102.

Glasser L, Sternglanz PD, Combie J, Robinson A. Serum osmolality and its applicability to drug overdose. Am J Clin Pathol. 1973;60:695.

Gledhill N, Beirne GJ, Dempsey JA. Renal response to short-term hypocapnia in man. Kidney Int. 1975;8:376.

Howard RS, Rudd AG, Wolfe CD, Williams AJ. Pathophysiological and clinical aspects of breathing after stroke. Postgrad Med J. 2001;77:700.

Karet FE. Mechanisms in hyperkalemic renal tubular acidosis. J Am Soc Nephrol. 2009;20:251.

Kim GH, Han JS, Kim YS, et al. Evaluation of urine acidification by urine anion gap and urine osmolal gap in chronic metabolic acidosis. Am J Kidney Dis. 1996;27:42.

Krapf R, Beeler I, Hertner D, Hulter HN. Chronic respiratory alkalosis. The effect of sustained hyperventilation on renal regulation of acid-base equilibrium. N Engl J Med. 1991;324:1394.

Kraut JA, Kurtz I. Toxic alcohol ingestions: clinical features, diagnosis, and management. Clin J Am Soc Nephrol. 2008;3:208.

Kraut JA, Madias NE. Differential diagnosis of nongap metabolic acidosis: value of a systematic approach. Clin J Am Soc Nephrol. 2012;7:671.

Kraut JA, Xing SX. Approach to the evaluation of a patient with an increased serum osmolal gap and high-anion-gap metabolic acidosis. Am J Kidney Dis. 2011;58:480.

Lee MC, Klassen AC, Heaney LM, Resch JA. Respiratory rate and pattern disturbances in acute brain stem infarction. Stroke. 1976;7:382.

Levy B. Lactate and shock state: the metabolic view. Curr Opin Crit Care. 2006;12:315.

Lynd LD, Richardson KJ, Purssell RA, et al. An evaluation of the osmole gap as a screening test for toxic alcohol poisoning. BMC Emerg Med. 2008;8:5.

Madias NE. Lactic acidosis. Kidney Int. 1986;29:752.

Marraffa JM, Holland MG, Stork CM, et al. Diethylene glycol: widely used solvent presents serious poisoning potential. J Emerg Med. 2008;35:401.

Martinu T, Menzies D, Dial S. Re-evaluation of acid-base prediction rules in patients with chronic respiratory acidosis. Can Respir J. 2003;10:311.

Meregalli P, Lüthy C, Oetliker OH, Bianchetti MG. Modified urine osmolal gap: an accurate method for estimating the urinary ammonium concentration? Nephron. 1995;69:98.

Mikkelsen ME, Miltiades AN, Gaieski DF, et al. Serum lactate is associated with mortality in severe sepsis independent of organ failure and shock. Crit Care Med. 2009;37:1670.

Pierce NF, Fedson DS, Brigham KL, et al. The ventilatory response to acute base deficit in humans. Time course during development and correction of metabolic acidosis. Ann Intern Med. 1970;72:633.

Purssell RA, Pudek M, Brubacher J, Abu-Laban RB. Derivation and validation of a formula to calculate the contribution of ethanol to the osmolal gap. Ann Emerg Med. 2001;38:653.

Rastegar M, Nagami GT. Non-anion gap metabolic acidosis: a clinical approach to evaluation. Am J Kidney Dis. 2017;69:296.

Robinson AG, Loeb JN. Ethanol ingestion–commonest cause of elevated plasma osmolality? N Engl J Med. 1971;284:1253.

Rodríguez Soriano J. Renal tubular acidosis: the clinical entity. J Am Soc Nephrol. 2002;13:2160.

Schelling JR, Howard RL, Winter SD, Linas SL. Increased osmolal gap in alcoholic ketoacidosis and lactic acidosis. Ann Intern Med. 1990;113:580.

Wiederseiner JM, Muser J, Lutz T, et al. Acute metabolic acidosis: characterization and diagnosis of the disorder and the plasma potassium response. J Am Soc Nephrol. 2004;15:1589.

CASE 62

A 68-year-old man with multiple myeloma presents to the emergency department from his skilled nursing facility with weakness, fatigue, and tachypnea. His functional status has been declining for the past 2 to 3 days, and he is somewhat lethargic. He has a history of GERD, diabetes mellitus, and HTN, and is taking no medications other than ondansetron for nausea. His vital signs are T 36.9°C, HR 105, BP 110/70, RR 14, and Sao$_2$ 95% on room air. His examination is otherwise unremarkable aside from cachexia.

Laboratory data.			
ABGs		Basic Metabolic Panel	
pH	7.22	Na	140 mEq/L
Paco$_2$	35 mm Hg	K	3.1 mEq/L
Pao$_2$	100 mm Hg	Cl	110 mEq/L
HCO$_3$	14 mEq/L	CO$_2$	14 mEq/L
		BUN	33 mg/dL
		Cr	1.3 mg/dL
		Glucose	55 mg/dL
		Albumin	2.5 g/dL
		EtOH	0 mg/dL
		Total protein	11.1 g/dL

QUESTIONS

Q62-1: Define the patient's baseline acid-base status: Does this patient have an underlying chronic acid-base disorder that we need to account for in order to appropriately interpret the acute acid-base disorders?

A. There is no evidence for an underlying chronic respiratory or metabolic acid-base disorder in this patient, so we would assume a baseline $Paco_2$ of 40 mm Hg and an HCO_3 of 24 mEq/L.

B. While the patient has a condition predisposing him to a chronic acid-base disorder, there is insufficient information to estimate the patient's baseline $Paco_2$ and HCO_3 values; therefore, we will assume a baseline $Paco_2$ of 40 mm Hg and a baseline HCO_3 of 24 mEq/L.

C. The patient has an underlying acid-base condition, and we have sufficient information to estimate the patient's baseline $Paco_2$ and HCO_3 values.

Q62-2: What is/are the primary acid-base disturbance(s) occurring in this case?

A. Metabolic acidosis only
B. Respiratory acidosis only
C. Metabolic acidosis and a respiratory acidosis
D. Metabolic alkalosis and a respiratory alkalosis
E. Metabolic alkalosis only
F. Respiratory alkalosis only

Q62-3: For a perfectly healthy patient, a normal anion gap is assumed to be 12 mEq/L. What should be considered a normal anion gap in this patient?

A. 12 mEq/L
B. 10 mEq/L
C. 8 mEq/L
D. 4 mEq/L

Q62-4: How would the metabolic acidosis component be classified in this case?

A. Anion gap acidosis
B. Non-anion gap acidosis
C. Anion and non-anion gap acidosis
D. Anion gap acidosis and a metabolic alkalosis

Q62-5: Does the patient in this case demonstrate appropriate respiratory or metabolic compensation?

A. Yes, the respiratory compensation is appropriate.
B. No, a concomitant respiratory alkalosis is present.
C. No, a concomitant respiratory acidosis is present.
D. Yes, the metabolic compensation is appropriate.
E. No, a concomitant metabolic acidosis is present.
F. No, a concomitant metabolic alkalosis is present.

Q62-6: The measured serum osmolality is 337. What is the patient's serum osmolal gap?

A. 5 mOsm/L
B. 10 mOsm/L
C. 20 mOsm/L
D. 40 mOsm/L

Q62-7: The patient's remaining test results are as follows:

Serum EtOH	< 3 mg/dL
Serum acetaminophen level	< 5 mg/dL (ULN for therapeutic use 20 mg/dL)
Serum salicylates level	< 5 mg/dL (ULN for therapeutic use 30 mg/dL)
Serum osmolality	337 mOsm/kg
Serum L-lactate	7.8 mmol/L (ULN 2.0 mmol/L venous)
Beta-hydroxybutyrate (acetone)	< 0.18 mmol/L (ULN 0.18 mmol/L)
Serum glucose	55 mg/dL
Serum phosphorus	5.9 mg/dL
Serum calcium	7.8 mg/dL
Serum uric acids	9.1 mg/dL
Peripheral blood smear	Numerous blast forms present
Urine drug screen	Negative

What is the likely cause of the patient's anion gap acidosis?

A. Renal failure
B. Lactic acidosis due to sepsis
C. Lactic acidosis due to malignancy
D. Lactic acidosis due to metformin toxicity
E. Lactic acidosis due to bowel ischemia
F. Acetaminophen overdose
G. Diabetic ketoacidosis
H. Alcoholic ketoacidosis

Q62-8: What is the likely cause of the patient's elevated osmolal gap?

A. Ethanol ingestion
B. Methanol ingestion
C. Ethylene glycol ingestion
D. Mannitol infusion
E. Hypertriglyceridemia
F. Hypergammaglobulinemia
G. Isopropyl alcohol ingestion

Q62-9: The patient's urine electrolyte values are as follows:

Urine Na	20 mEq/L
Urine K	40 mEq/L
Urine Cl	70 mEq/L
Urine pH	5.5

What is the likely cause of the patient's non-anion gap acidosis?

A. Sjögren syndrome
B. Diabetes mellitus
C. Sickle cell disease
D. Human immunodeficiency virus (HIV)
E. Multiple myeloma
F. ACE inhibitor use
G. Systemic corticosteroid use

Q62-10: What is the most appropriate study to determine if the non-anion gap is due to a type 2 RTA?

A. Fractional excretion of urea
B. Fractional excretion of potassium
C. Trans-tubular potassium gradient
D. Fractional excretion of HCO_3
E. Urine osmolal gap

ANSWERS

Q62-1: B

While the patient has a condition predisposing him to a chronic acid-base disorder, there is insufficient information to estimate the patient's baseline $Paco_2$ and HCO_3 values; therefore, we will assume a baseline $Paco_2$ of 40 mm Hg and a baseline HCO_3 of 24 mEq/L. The patient does have a particular malignancy, which can be associated with a chronic acid-base disorder; however, we lack the necessary information to make an inference.

Rationale: Ignoring these underlying chronic acid-base disorders can significantly alter the interpretation of a patient's acute acid-base status. This was demonstrated in the first case of the series. However, often, we do not have the necessary information (eg, prior ABG or VBG, or prior serum chemistry with an HCO_3) and are forced to assume the ongoing processes are all acute in nature. We are primarily concerned about chronic respiratory acid-base disorders, as these can significantly alter the patient's baseline or expected values for the serum HCO_3 and $Paco_2$, and we have reliable equations to predict the expected baseline values. The respiratory compensation for both chronic metabolic acidosis and alkalosis is generally poor, so there are no equations or rules to predict what the $Paco_2$ should be in these cases. While the baseline serum HCO_3 may be significantly off from our standard value of 24 mEq/L in these patients, we would assume a baseline $Paco_2$ of 40 mm Hg in patients with chronic metabolic processes. Once we identify the patient's baseline $Paco_2$ and HCO_3 values, we will need to use these values in the appropriate equations to identify the ongoing acute processes.

Q62-2: A

Metabolic acidosis only.

Rationale:

1. The pH is 7.22; therefore, the primary disorder is an **acidosis.**
2. The $Paco_2$ of 35 mm Hg is less than 40 mm Hg, so it is *not* a primary respiratory issue.
3. The HCO_3 of 14 mEq/L is less than 24 mEq/L, so a there is a **metabolic acidosis.**

Q62-3: C

8 mEq/L.

Rationale: The normal anion gap is 12 mEq/L. The term *anion gap* refers to those ions (negatively charged molecules) in the bloodstream that we do not routinely measure, including phosphates, sulfates, organic acids, and negatively charged plasma proteins. One of the most abundant negatively charged ions in the blood is serum albumin. A normal serum albumin is 4.0 g/dL. For patients with hypoalbuminemia (low serum albumin), the normal or expected anion gap is smaller.

$$\text{Expected Anion Gap} = 12 - (2.5) * \left[4.0 \frac{g}{dL} - \text{Actual Serum Albumin} \right].$$

Therefore, for this patient,

$$\text{Expected Anion Gap} = 12 - [2.5 * (4 - 2.5)] = 12 - (2.5 * 1.5) = \sim 8 \text{ mEq/L}.$$

This is an important concept, as patients with hypoalbuminemia may "hide" an anion gap acidosis if this correction is not performed.

Q62-4: C
Anion and non-anion gap acidosis.

Rationale:

1. Is there evidence for a chronic acid-base disorder that requires adjustment of the patient's "normal" HCO_3? No, there is no evidence for a chronic acid-base disorder, so we would assume a baseline $Paco_2$ of 40 mm Hg and an HCO_3 of 24 mEq/L.

2. Expected anion gap:

$$\text{Expected Anion Gap} = 12 - (2.5) * \left[4.0 \frac{g}{dL} - \text{Actual Serum Albumin} \right]$$
$$= 12 - (2.5 * [4.0 - 2.5])$$
$$= 12 - (2.5 * [1.5]) = \sim\textbf{8 mEq/L.}$$

3. Anion gap calculation:

$$\text{Serum Anion Gap} = [Na^+] - [HCO_3^-] - [Cl^-]$$
$$= 140 - (110 + 14) = \textbf{16 mEq/L,} \text{ which is} > 8 \text{ mEq/L}$$
$$\rightarrow \textbf{anion gap acidosis is present.}$$

4. Delta-delta calculation:

$$\Delta\Delta = \frac{(\text{Actual Anion Gap} - \text{Expected Anion Gap})}{(\text{Baseline HCO}_3 - \text{Actual HCO}_3)}$$
$$= (16 - 8)/(24 - 14) = \textbf{8/10, which is 0.8.}$$

Delta-delta interpretation.	
Delta-Delta Value	Condition Present
< 0.4	Non-anion gap only
0.4–0.9	**Anion gap *and* non-anion gap acidosis**
1.0–2.0	Anion gap acidosis only
> 2.0	Anion gap acidosis and metabolic alkalosis

Q62-5: C
No, a concomitant respiratory acidosis is present.

Rationale: Using the Winter formula, one can calculate what the expected arterial $Paco_2$ should be for a given serum HCO_3 if the patient were completely compensated.

Respiratory Compensation for Acute Metabolic Acidosis (Winter Formula):

$$\text{Expected Paco}_2 = 1.5 * [\text{Actual HCO}_3] + 8 \pm 2 \text{ (in mm Hg)}$$
$$= (1.5 * 14) + 8 = 21 + 8 = 29 \pm 2 = (27 \text{ to } 31) \text{ mm Hg.}$$

This patient has a concomitant respiratory acidosis, with **Paco$_2$ of 35 mm Hg**, above the expected range (27 to 31 mm Hg).

Q62-6: D
40.

Rationale: Similar to the serum anion gap, the serum osmolal gap is determined by the difference between the "calculated" serum osmolality and the true, measured serum osmolality. The equation for the serum osmolal gap typically includes factors for sodium, glucose, BUN, and ethanol, as these are readily measurable in most laboratories. Therefore, the serum osmolal gap will represent the osmolality of those "unmeasured" osmoles, including organic alcohols and acetone. The most common form is as follows:

$$\text{Calculated Serum Osmolality} = 2 * [\text{Na}^+] + \frac{[\text{Glucose}]}{18} + \frac{[\text{BUN}]}{2.8} + \frac{[\text{EtOH}]}{3.7},$$

In which the units of measure are as follows: Na, mEq/L; glucose, mg/dL; BUN, mg/dL; and EtOH, mg/dL. The conversion factors are shown in the preceding equation as well. A normal serum osmolal gap is around -10 to $+10$ mOsm/L (or mOsm/kg). The serum osmolal gap is the difference between the laboratory measured ("true") serum osmolality, and a "calculated" osmolality based on commonly measured compounds that are known to contribute to the serum osmolality.

$$\text{Serum Osmolal Gap (SOG)} = \text{Measured Serum Osmolality}$$
$$- \text{Calculated Serum Osmolality.}$$

Therefore, similar to the serum anion gap, the SOG represents the "unmeasured" compounds also contributing to the serum osmolality. The SOG can be helpful in determining whether an organic alcohol ingestion has occurred recently. The following are potential causes of an elevated serum osmolality.

Conditions associated with elevated serum osmolality.
With an Elevated Serum Anion Gap
1. Ethanol ingestion with alcoholic ketoacidosis (acetone is an unmeasured osmole, in addition to ethanol)—the osmolality is usually elevated more so by the increased ethanol concentration, so the osmolal "gap" depends on whether the term for ethanol is included in the osmolality calculation*
2. Organic alcohol ingestions (methanol, ethylene glycol, diethylene glycol, propylene glycol)
3. Diabetic ketoacidosis—similar to ethanol ingestion earlier, glucose and acetone contribute to the osmolality, since the glucose term is always included in the calculation
4. Salicylate toxicity
5. Renal failure—the BUN is nearly always included in the osmolality
Without an Elevated Serum Anion Gap
1. Hyperosmolar therapy (mannitol, glycerol)
2. Other organic solvent ingestion (eg, acetone)
3. Isopropyl alcohol ingestion (produces only acetone rather than an organic acid, so no anion gap is seen)
4. Hypertriglyceridemia
5. Hyperproteinemia
*A mildly elevated osmolal gap has been reported in the literature in patients with lactic acidosis in critical illness, particularly severe distributive shock. The pathology is not quite clear, although it likely is related to multiorgan failure—particularly involving the liver and kidneys—and the release of cellular components known to contribute to the osmolal gap. This is typically around 10 mOsm/L, although it may be as high as 20 to 25 mOsm/L.

The expected serum osmolality is calculated using the patients Na, BUN, glucose, and EtOH (also sometimes K). The SOG is calculated as the difference between the patient's measured serum osmolarity (or osmolality) and the calculated serum osmolality based on laboratory data. The calculated osmolality equation is:

$$\text{Calculated Osmolality} = (2 * 140) + (55/18) + (33/2.8) + (0/3.7)$$
$$= 297 \text{ mOsm/L}$$
$$\text{SOG} = (337 - 297) = 40 \text{ mOsm/L} < 10 \text{ mOsm/L}$$
$$\rightarrow \textbf{positive serum osmolal gap.}$$

Therefore, this patient has a positive serum osmolal gap.

Q62-7: C
Lactic acidosis due malignancy.

Rationale: This patient has a lactic acidosis without evidence of hypotension. This is referred to "type B" lactic acidosis; that is, an acidosis in which the issue is not with oxygen delivery to the tissue. This type of acidosis can occur in a number of settings, including metformin toxicity and in hematologic malignancies, where the cancer cells activate both oxidative phosphorylation as well as glycolysis despite the presence of oxygen—a process referred to as aerobic glycolysis, or the "Warburg effect." This process is often accelerated by the overwhelming energy demand of these highly proliferating cells. Additionally, hematologic malignancies tend to impact liver function, reducing the ability of the body to utilize lactate. This patient has blasts on his peripheral blood smear, as well elevated phosphorus and uric acid levels, consistent with a blast crisis. In patients with bowel ischemia and sepsis, lactic acidosis primarily results from reduced oxygen delivery to the tissue (although it is truly a mixed picture). The remaining causes are unlikely based on the laboratory values reported. Renal failure, although common in multiple myeloma, is not severe enough to cause this level of an anion gap acidosis.

Q62-8: F
Hypergammaglobulinema.

Rationale: The patient has multiple myeloma with an elevated total protein level and a low albumin level (difference ~ 8.5 g/dL, normal ~3 g/dL), consistent with hypergammaglobulinemia. The patient has an anion gap acidosis and an SOG; therefore, as in Q62-6, we would be particularly concerned about one of the causes identified for an elevated SOG "With an Elevated Serum Anion Gap."

However, as in Q62-6, we have ruled the majority of those conditions out. The patient is a nursing home resident who is debilitated, so it is highly unlikely that he has been ingesting methanol or ethylene glycol (although possible). Given that we have identified a type B lactic acidosis as the cause of the patient's anion gap acidosis, it is reasonable to consider that the anion gap acidosis and the osmolal gap represent distinct processes. Therefore, we can consider the causes identified earlier for an elevated SOG "Without an Elevated Anion Gap."

The patient has not received mannitol, per the prompt. However, the patient does have multiple myeloma, with a significantly elevated serum protein level. This results from malignant plasma cells producing an overabundance of paraprotein/immunoglobulin. This is a reasonable and well-known cause for an elevated SOG.

Q62-9: E
Multiple myeloma.

Rationale: This is a case in which the history ends up being more helpful than the objective laboratory data. The patient has a urine anion gap of −10 mEq/L:

$$\text{Urine Anion Gap (UAG)} = [U_{Na}] + [U_K] - [U_{Cl}]$$
$$\text{UAG} = (20 + 40) - (70) = (-10) \text{ mEq/L.}$$

Interpretation:

- A urine anion gap that is greater than +20 mEq/L → reduced renal acid excretion (RTA).
- A urine anion gap that is less than −20) mEq/L → GI loss of bicarbonate (eg, diarrhea), although type 2 RTA is possible.
- **A urine anion gap between −20 and +10 mEq/L is generally considered inconclusive.**

Additionally, the urine anion gap can be *inappropriately elevated* in anion gap acidosis, a situation in which multiple unmeasured anions may be present in the urine (beta-hydroxybutyrate/acetoacetate [ketoacidosis], hippurate [toluene], HCO_3 [proximal RTA], D-lactate [D-lactic acidosis], L-lactate, 5-oxoproline [acetaminophen toxicity]).

However, here we have a slightly negative urine anion gap, with a normal urine pH and low serum potassium. There is no evidence of GI loss of HCO_3, such as diarrhea, to explain this. Additionally, since the urine anion gap is negative, there is no evidence of a type 1 or type 4 RTA. (Recall that the urine anion gap can be inappropriate elevated by a serum anion gap acidosis but is typically not inappropriately reduced.) Therefore, one must consider a type 2 (proximal) RTA. Multiple myeloma is a known cause of type 2 RTA, in which the paraproteins are toxic to the proximal tubules. Autoimmune diseases are associated with type 1 RTAs, although they can also be associated with type 2 RTAs. This patient has no history of Sjögren syndrome. The remaining disorders listed are associated with a type 4 RTA.

Causes of RTA.
Causes of Type 1 (Distal) RTA
Primary • Idiopathic or familial (may be recessive or dominant)
Secondary • Medications: Lithium, amphotericin, ifosfamide, NSAIDs • Rheumatologic disorders: Sjögren syndrome, SLE, RA • Hypercalciuria (idiopathic) or associated with vitamin D deficiency or hyperparathyroidism • Sarcoidosis • Obstructive uropathy • Wilson disease • Rejection of renal transplant allograft
Causes of Type 2 (Proximal) RTA
Primary • Idiopathic • Familial (primarily recessive disorders) • Genetic: Fanconi syndrome, cystinosis, glycogen storage disease (type 1), Wilson disease, galactosemia
Secondary • Medications: Acetazolamide, topiramate, aminoglycoside antibiotics, ifosfamide, reverse transcriptase inhibitors (tenofovir) • Heavy metal poisoning: Lead, mercury, copper • **Multiple myeloma or amyloidosis (secondary to light chain toxicity)** • Sjögren syndrome • Vitamin D deficiency • Rejection of renal transplant allograft
Causes of Type 4 RTA (Hypoaldosteronism or Aldosterone Resistance)
Primary • Primary adrenal insufficiency • Inherited disorders associated with hypoaldosteronism • Pseudohypoaldosteronism (types 1 and 2)
Secondary • Causes of hyporeninemic hypoaldosteronism such as renal disease (diabetic nephropathy), NSAID use, calcineurin inhibitors, volume expansion/volume overload • Causes of distal tubule voltage defects such as sickle cell disease, obstructive uropathy, SLE • Severe illness/septic shock • Angiotensin II–associated medications: ACE inhibitors, ARBs, direct renin inhibitors • Potassium-sparing diuretics: Spironolactone, amiloride, triamterene • Antibiotics: Trimethoprim, pentamidine

Q62-10: D
Fractional excretion of HCO$_3$.

Rationale: The fractional excretion of HCO$_3$ is the next most appropriate study in this patient. In bicarbonaturia, the fractional excretion should be greater than 15%. Additionally, one could administer HCO$_3$ to the patient and monitor for an increase in the urine pH as well as an increase in the urine anion gap with this therapy.

Fractional Excretion of HCO$_3$ for RTA:

$$FE_{HCO_3^-} = \frac{[Urine\ HCO_3^-] * Serum\ Cr}{[Serum\ HCO_3^-] * Urine\ Cr}$$

References

Adrogué HJ, Madias NE. Secondary responses to altered acid-base status: the rules of engagement. J Am Soc Nephrol. 2010;21:920.

Batlle D, Chin-Theodorou J, Tucker BM. Metabolic acidosis or respiratory alkalosis? Evaluation of a low plasma bicarbonate using the urine anion gap. Am J Kidney Dis. 2017;70:440.

Batlle D, Grupp M, Gaviria M, Kurtzman NA. Distal renal tubular acidosis with intact capacity to lower urinary pH. Am J Med. 1982;72:751.

Batlle D, Haque SK. Genetic causes and mechanisms of distal renal tubular acidosis. Nephrol Dial Transplant. 2012;27:3691.

Batlle DC, Hizon M, Cohen E, et al. The use of the urinary anion gap in the diagnosis of hyperchloremic metabolic acidosis. N Engl J Med. 1988;318:594.

Batlle DC, von Riotte A, Schlueter W. Urinary sodium in the evaluation of hyperchloremic metabolic acidosis. N Engl J Med. 1987;316:140.

Berend K, de Vries AP, Gans RO. Physiological approach to assessment of acid-base disturbances. N Engl J Med. 2014;371:1434.

Buckalew VM Jr, McCurdy DK, Ludwig GD, et al. Incomplete renal tubular acidosis. Physiologic studies in three patients with a defect in lowering urine pH. Am J Med. 1968;45:32.

Farwell WR, Taylor EN. Serum anion gap, bicarbonate and biomarkers of inflammation in healthy individuals in a national survey. CMAJ. 2010;182:137.

Feldman M, Soni N, Dickson B. Influence of hypoalbuminemia or hyperalbuminemia on the serum anion gap. J Lab Clin Med. 2005;146:317.

Fernandez PC, Cohen RM, Feldman GM. The concept of bicarbonate distribution space: the crucial role of body buffers. Kidney Int. 1989;36:747.

Karet FE. Mechanisms in hyperkalemic renal tubular acidosis. J Am Soc Nephrol. 2009;20:251.

Kraut JA, Madias NE. Differential diagnosis of nongap metabolic acidosis: value of a systematic approach. Clin J Am Soc Nephrol. 2012;7:671.

Kraut JA, Nagami GT. The serum anion gap in the evaluation of acid-base disorders: what are its limitations and can its effectiveness be improved? Clin J Am Soc Nephrol. 2013;8:2018.

Rastegar M, Nagami GT. Non-anion gap metabolic acidosis: a clinical approach to evaluation. Am J Kidney Dis. 2017;69:296.

Rodríguez Soriano J. Renal tubular acidosis: the clinical entity. J Am Soc Nephrol. 2002;13:2160.

A 34-year-old white female patient presents with muscle weakness and reported paralysis of her limbs. She is alert and oriented. She denies any other symptoms recently but notes that she had muscle cramps frequently over the past week. The review of systems is notable only for dry mouth and occasional joint aches. Her vital signs are as follows: T 37.4°C, HR 110, BP 100/70, RR 21, and Sao$_2$ 97% on room air. She denies any drug use, alcohol use, tobacco use, or environmental or social exposures. She also states that she has not had any recent illnesses. Her examination is notable for profound weakness in the distal extremities throughout, bilaterally. The remaining examination is normal.

Laboratory data.			
ABGs		Basic Metabolic Panel	
pH	7.31	Na	140 mEq/L
Paco$_2$	35 mm Hg	K	1.8 mEq/L
Pao$_2$	100 mm Hg	Cl	107 mEq/L
HCO$_3$	13 mEq/L	CO$_2$	13 mEq/L
		BUN	44 mg/dL
		Cr	1.8 mg/dL
		Glucose	55 mg/dL
		Albumin	4.0 g/dL
		EtOH	0 mg/dL

QUESTIONS

Q63-1: Define the patient's baseline acid-base status: Does this patient have an underlying chronic acid-base disorder that we need to account for in order to appropriately interpret the acute acid-base disorders?

A. There is no evidence for an underlying chronic respiratory or metabolic acid-base disorder in this patient, so we would assume a baseline $Paco_2$ of 40 mm Hg and an HCO_3 of 24 mEq/L.

B. While the patient has a condition predisposing her to a chronic acid-base disorder, there is insufficient information to estimate the patient's baseline $Paco_2$ and HCO_3 values; therefore, we will assume a baseline $Paco_2$ of 40 mm Hg and a baseline HCO_3 of 24 mEq/L.

C. The patient has an underlying acid-base condition, and we have sufficient information to estimate the patient's baseline $Paco_2$ and HCO_3 values.

Q63-2: What is/are the primary acid-base disturbance(s) occurring in this case?

A. Metabolic acidosis only
B. Respiratory acidosis only
C. Metabolic acidosis and a respiratory acidosis
D. Metabolic alkalosis and a respiratory alkalosis
E. Metabolic alkalosis only
F. Respiratory alkalosis only

Q63-3: How would the metabolic acidosis component be classified in this case?

A. Anion gap acidosis
B. Non-anion gap acidosis
C. Anion and non-anion gap acidosis
D. Anion gap acidosis and a metabolic alkalosis

Q63-4: Does the patient in this case demonstrate appropriate respiratory or metabolic compensation?

A. Yes, the respiratory compensation is appropriate.
B. No, a concomitant respiratory alkalosis is present.
C. No, a concomitant respiratory acidosis is present.
D. Yes, the metabolic compensation is appropriate.
E. No, a concomitant metabolic acidosis is present.
F. No, a concomitant metabolic alkalosis is present.

Q63-5: Results from the patient's remaining tests are as follows:

Serum EtOH	< 3 mg/dL
Serum acetaminophen level	< 5 mg/dL (ULN for therapeutic use 20 mg/dL)
Serum salicylates level	< 5 mg/dL (ULN for therapeutic use 30 mg/dL)
Serum osmolality	306 mOsm/kg
Serum L-lactate	3.5 mmol/L (ULN 2.0 mmol/L venous)
Beta-hydroxybutyrate (acetone)	< 0.18 mmol/L (ULN 0.18 mmol/L)
Serum glucose	55 mg/dL
Serum phosphorus	9.8 mg/dL (ULN 4.5 mg/dL)
Serum calcium	5.7 mg/dL (LLN 8.5 mg/dL)
Serum creatinine kinase (CK)	9000 IU/mL (ULN 275 IU/mL)
Urine drug screen	Negative (THC, cocaine, opioids, amphetamines, benzodiazepines)

What is the likely cause of the patient's anion gap acidosis?

A. Aspirin toxicity
B. Starvation ketoacidosis
C. Ethylene glycol ingestion
D. Lactic acidosis due to sepsis
E. Rhabdomyolysis
F. Diabetic ketoacidosis

Q63-6: What is the cause of the patient's rhabdomyolysis?

A. Trauma
B. Thrombosis
C. Hypokalemia
D. Hyperthermia

Q63-7: The patient's urine electrolyte values are as follows:

Urine Na	34 mEq/L
Urine K	114 mEq/L
Urine Cl	60 mEq/L
Urine urea	214 mg/dL
Urine glucose	0 mg/dL
Urine osmolality	430 mOsm/L
Urine pH	7.8
Urine myoglobin	Positive

What is the most likely type of non-anion gap acidosis present?

A. Diarrhea
B. Type 1 RTA (distal tubule)
C. Type 2 RTA (proximal tubule)
D. Type 4 RTA (distal tubule/collecting duct)

Q63-8: What is the likely cause of the non-anion gap acidosis mentioned in Q63-7?

A. Sjögren syndrome
B. Acetazolamide use
C. Diabetes mellitus
D. Spironolactone use
E. Sickle cell disease

Q63-9: Which of the following laboratory tests would you suspect would be positive in this patient?

A. Anti-cyclic citrullinated peptide (anti-CCP)
B. Antineutrophil cytoplasmic antibodies (ANCA)
C. Anti-Ro/La antibodies (SSA/SSB)
D. Anti-Jo1 antibodies
E. Anti-Scl70 antibodies

ANSWERS

Q63-1: B

While the patient has a condition predisposing her to a chronic acid-base disorder, there is insufficient information to estimate the patient's baseline $Paco_2$ and HCO_3 values; therefore, we will assume a baseline $Paco_2$ of 40 mm Hg and a baseline HCO_3 of 24 mEq/L. The patient has a constellation of symptoms that have been evolving over the past week, so it is possible there is a chronic component to her acid-base disorder. However, we have no evidence to support a baseline acid-base disorder, and we will therefore assume the standard values.

Rationale: Ignoring these underlying chronic acid-base disorders can significantly alter the interpretation of a patient's acute acid-base status. This was demonstrated in the first case of the series. However, often, we do not have the necessary information (eg, prior ABG or VBG, or prior serum chemistry with an HCO_3) and are forced to assume the ongoing processes are all acute in nature. We are primarily concerned about chronic respiratory acid-base disorders, as these can significantly alter the patient's baseline or expected values for the serum HCO_3 and $Paco_2$, and we have reliable equations to predict the expected baseline values. The respiratory compensation for both chronic metabolic acidosis and alkalosis is generally poor, so there are no equations or rules to predict what the $Paco_2$ should be in these cases. While the baseline serum HCO_3 may be significantly off from our standard value of 24 mEq/L in these patients, we would assume a baseline $Paco_2$ of 40 mm Hg in patients with chronic metabolic processes. Once we identify the patient's baseline $Paco_2$ and HCO_3 values, we will need to use these values in the appropriate equations to identify the ongoing acute processes.

Q63-2: A

Metabolic acidosis only.

Rationale:

1. The pH is 7.31; therefore, the primary disorder is an **acidosis.**
2. The $Paco_2$ of 35 mm Hg is less than 40 mm Hg, so this is *not* a primary respiratory acidosis.
3. The HCO_3 of 17 mEq/L is less than 24 mEq/L, so this is a **metabolic acidosis.**

Q63-3: C

Anion and non-anion gap acidosis.

Rationale:

1. Is there evidence for a chronic acid-base disorder that requires adjustment of the patient's "normal" HCO_3? No, there is no evidence for a chronic acid-base disorder, so we would assume a baseline $Paco_2$ of 40 mm Hg and an HCO_3 of 24 mEq/L.

2. Expected anion gap:

$$\text{Expected Anion Gap} = 12 - (2.5) * \left[4.0 \, \frac{g}{dL} - \text{Actual Serum Albumin} \right]$$
$$= 12 - (2.5 * [4.0 - 4.0])$$
$$= 12 - (2.5 * [0]) = \mathbf{12 \ mEq/L}.$$

3. Anion gap calculation:

$$\text{Serum Anion Gap} = [Na^+] - [HCO_3^-] - [Cl^-]$$
$$= 140 - (107 + 13) = 20 \ \text{mEq/L, which is} > 12 \ \text{mEq/L}$$
$$\rightarrow \textbf{anion gap acidosis is present.}$$

4. Delta-delta calculation:

$$\Delta\Delta = \frac{(\text{Actual Anion Gap} - \text{Expected Anion Gap})}{(\text{Baseline HCO}_3 - \text{Actual HCO}_3)}$$
$$= (20 - 12)/(24 - 13) = \mathbf{8/9, \ which \ is \sim 0.88.}$$

Delta-delta interpretation.	
Delta-Delta Value	**Condition Present**
< 0.4	Non-anion gap only
0.4–0.9	**Anion gap *and* non-anion gap acidosis**
1.0–2.0	Anion gap acidosis only
> 2.0	Anion gap acidosis and metabolic alkalosis

Q63-4: A
Yes, the respiratory compensation is appropriate.

Rationale: Using the Winter formula, one can calculate what the expected arterial $Paco_2$ should be for a given serum HCO_3 if the patient were completely compensated.

$$\text{Expected Paco}_2 = 1.5 * [\text{Actual HCO}_3] + 8 \pm 2 \ \text{(in mm Hg)}$$
$$= (1.5 * 17) + 8 = 25.5 + 8 = 33.5 \pm 2 = (31 \ \text{to} \ 35) \ \text{mm Hg}.$$

This patient has an appropriate compensation, with **Paco$_2$ of 35 mm Hg**, within the expected range (31 to 35 mm Hg).

Q63-5: E
Rhabdomyolysis.

Rationale: The patient has a negative serum acetaminophen and salicylate level, and the serum ketones are negative as well. The lactate is mildly elevated, but there is no evidence of sepsis. The patient has no serum osmolal gap.

$$\text{Calculated Serum Osmolality} = 2*[Na^+] + \frac{[Glucose]}{18} + \frac{[BUN]}{2.8} + \frac{[EtOH]}{3.7}$$
$$= 2*[140] + [55/18] + [44/2.8] + [0/3.7]$$
$$= 299 \text{ mOsm/L.}$$
$$\text{Serum Osmolal Gap (SOG)} = \text{Measured Serum Osmolality}$$
$$- \text{Calculated Serum Osmolality}$$
$$\text{SOG} = 306 - 300 \text{ mOsm/L} = (+6) \text{ mOsm/L.}$$

Therefore, of the possible options, rhabdomyolysis is the most likely. The patient has a significantly elevated serum CK as well as an elevated BUN and Cr overall, indicating some likely renal dysfunction potentially related to the rhabdomyolysis. Rhabdomyolysis is associated with the generation of an anion gap acidosis due to muscle breakdown and release of lactate and organic acids. Myoglobin release and accumulation of heme degradation products can lead to renal failure, reduced clearance of organic acids, and the development of hyperphosphatemia and hypocalcemia as well. Patients can also develop hyperkalemia, which is a major cause of mortality in rhabdomyolysis. Alternatively, this patient has hypokalemia, which is related to another process.

Q63-6: C
Hypokalemia.

Rationale: Severe hypokalemia, such as that encountered here, can lead to muscle ischemia and rhabdomyolysis. The patient has no evidence of trauma, thrombosis, or hyperthermia, although all three may cause rhabdomyolysis.

Q63-7: A
Type 1 RTA (distal tubule).

Rationale: The patient has a positive urine anion gap with an abnormally low urine osmolal gap, as follows:

Urine Anion Gap:

$$\text{Urine Anion Gap} = [U_{Na}] + [U_K] - [U_{Cl}].$$

Therefore, for this patient,

$$\text{Urine Anion Gap} = U_{Na} + U_K - U_{Cl} = (34 + 114) - 60 = (+84).$$

Interpretation:

- A urine anion gap that is greater than +20 mEq/L → reduced renal acid excretion (RTA).
- A urine anion gap that is less than −20 mEq/L → GI loss of HCO_3 (eg, diarrhea), although type 2 RTA is possible.
- A urine anion gap between −20 and +10 mEq/L is generally considered inconclusive.

Limitation: The urine anion gap can be inappropriately elevated in anion gap acidosis, a situation in which multiple unmeasured anions may be present in the urine (beta-hydroxybutyrate/acetoacetate [ketoacidosis], hippurate [toluene], HCO_3 [proximal RTA], D-lactate [D-lactic acidosis], L-lactate, 5-oxoproline [acetaminophen toxicity]). Therefore, in patients with a significant anion gap, the urine osmolal gap (UOG) is typically more useful. Here the UOG is as follows:

$$\text{Calculated Urine Osmolality} = 2*([Na^+]+[K^+]) + \frac{[Urea]}{2.8} + \frac{[Glucose]}{18}$$
$$\text{Calculated Urine Osmolarity} = 372 \text{ mOsm/L.}$$

The UOG is then calculated:

$$\text{Urine Osmolal Gap} = \text{Measured Urine Osmolality} - \text{Measured Urine Osmolality}$$
$$\text{UOG} = 430 - 372 \text{ mOsm/L} = 57 \text{ mOsm/L.}$$

Interpretation (in setting of a metabolic acidosis):

- UOG greater than 400 mOsm/L (or kg)—there is appropriate urinary acidification, consistent with a GI source and normal renal acidification.
- UOG less than 100 to 150 mOsm/L (of kg)—there is inappropriately low urinary acidification, most consistent with a type 1 or 4 RTA.
- Again, this is not particularly useful for the diagnosis of a type 2 (proximal) RTA, where other serum or urine lab abnormalities are more helpful.

Limitations: The primary limitation of the UOG is its use in conditions with a high osmolar gap, where non-ammonium solutes not included in the calculation may be present in the urine (particularly mannitol). The presence of these unmeasured solutes will increase the osmolal gap inappropriately. Also, the UOG should not be used in patients with a urinary tract infection caused by a urease-producing organism, as urea is metabolized to HCO_3 and ammonium in urine.

Therefore, we would suspect either a type 1 RTA or a type 4 RTA in this situation. Additionally, the patient has an elevated urine pH and a low serum K. This is consistent with a type 1 RTA. This is the source of the patient's hypokalemia, which led to the acid-base disorder.

Evaluation of RTA.			
	Type 1 RTA	Type 2 RTA	Type 4 RTA
Severity of metabolic acidosis, (HCO_3)	Severe (< 10–12 mEq/L typically)	Intermediate (12–20 mEq/L)	Mild (15–20 mEq/L)
Associated urine abnormalities	Urinary phosphate, calcium are increased; bone disease often present	Urine glucose, amino acids, phosphate, calcium may be elevated	
Urine pH	HIGH (> 5.5)	Low (acidic), until serum HCO_3 level exceeds the resorptive ability of the proximal tubule; then becomes alkalotic once reabsorptive threshold is crossed	Low (acidic)
Serum K^+	Low to normal; should correct with oral HCO_3 therapy	Classically low, although may be normal or even high with rare genetic defects; worsens with oral HCO_3 therapy	HIGH
Renal stones	Often	No	No
Renal tubular defect	Reduced NH_4 secretion in distal tubule	Reduced HCO_3 resorption in proximal tubule	Reduced H^+/K^+ exchange in distal and collecting tubule due to decreased aldosterone or aldosterone resistance
Urine anion gap	> 10	Negative initially, then positive when receiving serum HCO_3, then negative after therapy	> 10
Urine osmolal gap	Reduced (< 150 mOsm/L) during acute acidosis	At baseline < 100 mEq/L; unreliable during acidosis	Reduced (< 150 mOsm/L) during acute acidosis

Nephrogenic diabetes insipidus, hypokalemic paralysis, renal calculi, and osteomalacia are the main complications of distal renal tubular acidosis, while the main manifestations of hypokalemic rhabdomyolysis include muscle pain, cramps, fatigability and generalized weakness.

Q63-8: A
Sjögren syndrome.

Rationale: Sjögren syndrome is an autoimmune disease commonly associated with the development of type 1 RTA. Acetazolamide use is associated with a type 2 RTA, while options C, D, and E are associated with a type 4 RTA. The treatment for this patient would include immunosuppression for treatment of the underlying cause of the disorder, potassium repletion for the hypokalemia (and likely magnesium and calcium supplementation), fluid resuscitation for the rhabdomyolysis, and alkali therapy for the acidosis.

Q63-9: C
Anti-Ro/La antibodies (SSA/SSB).

Rationale: Ant-Ro/La autoantibodies are the most common antibodies found to be positive in patients with Sjögren syndrome, aside from the standard anti-nuclear antibody (ANA) test. Anti-CCP is associated with rheumatoid arthritis, while ANCA antibodies are associated with vasculitis. Anti Jo1 antibodies are associated with polymyositis, while anti-Scl70 antibodies are most commonly associated with scleroderma.

References

Agrawal S, Bharti V, Jain MN, et al. Sjogren's syndrome presenting with hypokalemic periodic paralysis. J Assoc Physicians India. 2012;60:55.

Cherif E, Ben Hassine L, Kechaou I, Khalfallah N. Hypokalemic rhabdomyolysis: an unusual presentation of Sjogren's syndrome. BMJ Case Rep. 2013;2013. pii: bcr2013201345.

Comer DM, Droogan AG, Young IS, Maxwell AP. Hypokalaemic paralysis precipitated by distal renal tubular acidosis secondary to Sjögren's syndrome. Ann Clin Biochem. 2008;45(pt 2):221.

Jung YL, Kang JY. Rhabdomyolysis following severe hypokalemia caused by familial hypokalemic periodic paralysis. World J Clin Cases. 2017;5:56.

Poux JM, Peyronnet P, Le Meur Y, et al. Hypokalemic quadriplegia and respiratory arrest revealing primary Sjögren's syndrome. Clin Nephrol. 1992;37:189.

Prakash EB, Fernando ME, Sathiyasekaran M, et al. Primary Sjö-gren's syndrome presenting with distal, renal tubular acidosis and rhabdomyolysis. J Assoc Physicians India. 2006;54:949.

Rastegar A. Attending rounds: patient with hypokalemia and metabolic acidosis. Clin J Am Soc Nephrol. 2011;6:2516.

Sedhain A, Acharya K, Sharma A, et al. Renal tubular acidosis and hypokalemic paralysis as a first presentation of primary Sjögren's syndrome. Case Rep Nephrol. 2018;2018:9847826.

Taylor I, Parsons M. Hypokalemic paralysis revealing Sjögren's syndrome. J Clin Neurosci. 2004;11:319.

Yılmaz H, Kaya M, Özbek M, Üreten K, et al. Hypokalemic periodic paralysis in Sjogren's syndrome secondary to distal renal tubular acidosis. Rheumatol Int. 2013;33:1879.

CASE 64

A 23-year-old man is brought to the emergency department with refractory seizures. His roommate found him at home with tonic-clonic seizure activity and called EMS. The seizures did not respond to benzodiazepines and phenytoin, but eventually subsided. The patient is obtunded and was intubated by EMS before arrival. Vital signs are as follows: T 37.6°C, RR 20, HR 110, BP 120/80, and Sao_2 95% on RA. The patient's medical history shows he has been taking loperamide for diarrhea associated with a stomach virus and was recently prescribed isoniazid after a positive PPD test at work. He had a negative HIV and hepatitis C screening test 2 months ago. His family history is notable for a grandfather with osteoarthritis and early-onset dementia. He recently traveled to the northwestern United States for a camping trip but had no issues while away. His roommate reports that the patient drinks no alcohol, does not use illicit drugs, and does not smoke. His last seizure activity was approximately 3 minutes before his laboratory studies were drawn.

Laboratory data.			
ABGs		Basic Metabolic Panel	
pH	7.02	Na	140 mEq/L
$Paco_2$	48 mm Hg	K	2.9 mEq/L
Pao_2	100 mm Hg	Cl	107 mEq/L
HCO_3	12 mEq/L	CO_2	12 mEq/L
		BUN	22 mg/dL
		Cr	0.9 mg/dL
		Glucose	100 mg/dL
		Albumin	4.0 g/dL
		EtOH	0 mg/dL

QUESTIONS

Q64-1: Define the patient's baseline acid-base status: Does this patient have an underlying chronic acid-base disorder that we need to account for in order to appropriately interpret the acute acid-base disorders?

A. There is no evidence for an underlying chronic respiratory or metabolic acid-base disorder in this patient, so we would assume a baseline $Paco_2$ of 40 mm Hg and an HCO_3 of 24 mEq/L.

B. While the patient has a condition predisposing him to a chronic acid-base disorder, there is insufficient information to estimate the patient's baseline $Paco_2$ and HCO_3 values; therefore, we will assume a baseline $Paco_2$ of 40 mm Hg and a baseline HCO_3 of 24 mEq/L.

C. The patient has an underlying acid-base condition, and we have sufficient information to estimate the patient's baseline $Paco_2$ and HCO_3 values.

Q64-2: What is/are the primary acid-base disturbance(s) occurring in this case?

A. Metabolic acidosis only
B. Respiratory acidosis only
C. Metabolic acidosis and a respiratory acidosis
D. Metabolic alkalosis and a respiratory alkalosis
E. Metabolic alkalosis only
F. Respiratory alkalosis only

Q64-3: How would the metabolic acidosis component be classified in this case?

A. Anion gap acidosis
B. Non-anion gap acidosis
C. Anion and non-anion gap acidosis
D. Anion gap acidosis and a metabolic alkalosis

Q64-4: The serum osmolality is 301 mOsm/L. What is the patient's serum osmolal gap?

A. 6 mOsm/L
B. 14 mOsm/L
C. 22 mOsm/L
D. 31 mOsm/L

Q64-5: Results of the patient's remaining laboratory tests are as follows:

Serum EtOH	< 3 mg/dL
Serum acetaminophen level	< 5 mg/dL (ULN for therapeutic use 20 mg/dL)
Serum salicylates level	< 5 mg/dL (ULN for therapeutic use 30 mg/dL)
Serum osmolality	301 mOsm/kg
Serum L-lactate	6.7 mmol/L (ULN 2.0 mmol/L venous)
Beta-hydroxybutyrate (acetone)	0.29 mmol/L (ULN 0.18 mmol/L)
Serum glucose	100 mg/dL
Urine drug screen	Negative

What is the likely cause of the patient's anion gap acidosis?

A. Aspirin toxicity
B. Lactic acidosis secondary to sepsis
C. Ethylene glycol toxicity
D. Isoniazid (INH) overdose
E. Starvation ketosis
F. Acetaminophen overdose
G. Diabetic ketoacidosis
H. Alcoholic ketoacidosis

Q64-6: What is the likely cause of the patient's respiratory acidosis?

A. Hypoxemia
B. Neuromuscular disorder
C. Asthma
D. COPD
E. Chest wall injury or deformity
F. Pulmonary fibrosis
G. Seizure
H. Benzodiazepine overdose
I. Iatrogenic cause

Q64-7: The patient's urine electrolyte values are as follows:

Urine Na	20 mEq/L
Urine K	30 mEq/L
Urine Cl	70 mEq/L
Urine pH	5.5
Serum osmolal gap	484 mOsm/L

What is the most likely type of non-anion gap acidosis present?

A. Diarrhea
B. Type 1 RTA (distal tubule)
C. Type 2 RTA (proximal tubule)
D. Type 4 RTA (distal tubule/collecting duct)

Q64-8: **What is the next most appropriate step in the management of this patient with INH toxicity?**

A. Thiamine supplementation
B. Fosphenytoin infusion
C. Pyridoxine (B_6) supplementation
D. Folate supplementation
E. Fomepizole infusion
F. Methylene blue treatment

ANSWERS

Q64-1: A

There is no evidence for an underlying chronic respiratory or metabolic acid-base disorder in this patient, so we would assume a baseline $Paco_2$ of 40 mm Hg and an HCO_3 of 24 mEq/L.

Rationale: Ignoring these underlying chronic acid-base disorders can significantly alter the interpretation of a patient's acute acid-base status. This was demonstrated in the first case of the series. However, often, we do not have the necessary information (eg, prior ABG or VBG, or prior serum chemistry with an HCO_3) and are forced to assume the ongoing processes are all acute in nature. We are primarily concerned about chronic respiratory acid-base disorders, as these can significantly alter the patient's baseline or expected values for the serum HCO_3 and $Paco_2$, and we have reliable equations to predict the expected baseline values. The respiratory compensation for both chronic metabolic acidosis and alkalosis is generally poor, so there are no equations or rules to predict what the $Paco_2$ should be in these cases. While the baseline serum HCO_3 may be significantly off from our standard value of 24 mEq/L in these patients, we would assume a baseline $Paco_2$ of 40 mm Hg in patients with chronic metabolic processes. Once we identify the patient's baseline $Paco_2$ and HCO_3 values, we will need to use these values in the appropriate equations to identify the ongoing acute processes.

Q64-2: C

Metabolic acidosis and a respiratory acidosis.

Rationale:

1. The pH is 7.02; therefore, the primary disorder is an **acidosis.**
2. The $Paco_2$ of 48 mm Hg is greater than 40 mm Hg, so there is a **respiratory acidosis.**
3. The HCO_3 of 12 is less than 24, so there is also a **metabolic acidosis.**

Therefore, this patient has both a primary respiratory acidosis and a metabolic acidosis.

Q64-3: C

Anion and non-anion gap acidosis.

Rationale:

1. Is there evidence for a chronic acid-base disorder that requires adjustment of the patient's "normal" HCO_3? No, there is no evidence for a chronic acid-base disorder, so we would assume a baseline $Paco_2$ of 40 mm Hg and an HCO_3 of 24 mEq/L.

2. Expected anion gap:

$$\text{Expected Anion Gap} = 12 - (2.5) * \left[4.0 \frac{g}{dL} - \text{Actual Serum Albumin} \right]$$
$$= 12 - (2.5 * [4.0 - 4.0])$$
$$= 12 - (2.5 * [0]) = \textbf{12 mEq/L.}$$

3. Anion gap calculation:

$$\text{Serum Anion Gap} = [Na^+] - [HCO_3^-] - [Cl^-]$$
$$= 140 - (107 + 12) = 21 \text{ mEq/L, which is} > 12 \text{ mEq/L}$$
$$\rightarrow \textbf{anion gap acidosis is present.}$$

4. Delta-delta calculation:

$$\Delta\Delta = \frac{(\text{Actual Anion Gap} - \text{Expected Anion Gap})}{(\text{Baseline HCO}_3 - \text{Actual HCO}_3)}$$
$$= (21 - 12)/(24 - 12) = \textbf{9/12, which is ~0.75.}$$

Delta-delta interpretation.	
Delta-Delta Value	**Condition Present**
< 0.4	Non-anion gap only
0.4–0.9	**Anion gap *and* non-anion gap acidosis**
1.0–2.0	Anion gap acidosis only
> 2.0	Anion gap acidosis and metabolic alkalosis

Q64-4: A
6 mOsm/L.

Rationale: Similar to the serum anion gap, the serum osmolal gap is determined by the difference between the "calculated" serum osmolality and the true, measured serum osmolality. The equation for the serum osmolal gap typically includes factors for sodium, glucose, BUN, and ethanol, as these are readily measurable in most laboratories. Therefore, the serum osmolal gap will represent the osmolality of those "unmeasured" osmoles, including organic alcohols and acetone. The most common form is as follows:

$$\text{Calculated Serum Osmolality} = 2 * [Na^+] + \frac{[Glucose]}{18} + \frac{[BUN]}{2.8} + \frac{[EtOH]}{3.7};$$

In which the units of measure are: Na, mEq/L; glucose, mg/dL; BUN, mg/dL; and EtOH, mg/dL. The conversion factors are shown in the preceding equation as well. A normal serum osmolal gap is between −10 and +10 mOsm/L (or mOsm/kg).

Therefore, for this patient,

Calculated Serum Osmolality = $(2 * 140) + (100/18) + (22/2.8) + (0/3.7)$
$= 295$ mOsm/L.
Serum Osmolal Gap (SOG) = Measured Serum Osmolality
$-$ Calculated Serum Osmolality
SAG = $(301 - 295) = 6$ mOsm/L, which is < 10 mOsm/L
→ *no* **serum osmolal gap exists.**

The following are potential causes of an elevated serum osmolality.

Conditions associated with elevated serum osmolarity.
With an Elevated Serum Anion Gap
1. Ethanol ingestion with alcoholic ketoacidosis (acetone is an unmeasured osmole, in addition to ethanol)—the osmolality is usually elevated more so by the increased ethanol concentration, so the osmolal "gap" depends on whether the term for ethanol is included in the osmolality calculation*
2. Organic alcohol ingestions (methanol, ethylene glycol, diethylene glycol, propylene glycol)
3. Diabetic ketoacidosis—similar to ethanol ingestion, earlier, glucose and acetone contribute to the osmolality, since the glucose term is always included in the calculation
4. Salicylate toxicity
5. Renal failure—the BUN is nearly always included in the osmolality
Without an Elevated Serum Anion Gap
1. Hyperosmolar therapy (mannitol, glycerol)
2. Other organic solvent ingestion (eg, acetone)
3. Isopropyl alcohol ingestion (produces only acetone rather than an organic acid, so no anion gap is seen)
4. Hypertriglyceridemia
5. Hyperproteinemia
A mildly elevated osmolal gap has been reported in the literature in patients with lactic acidosis in critical illness, particularly severe distributive shock. The pathology is not quite clear, although it likely is related to multiorgan failure—particularly involving the liver and kidneys—and the release of cellular components known to contribute to the osmolal gap. This is typically around 10 mOsm/L, although it may be as high as 20 to 25 mOsm/L.

Q64-5: D
Isoniazid (INH) overdose.

Rationale: The patient presents with what we presumed to be new-onset seizure disorder, with a significant metabolic acidosis and respiratory acidosis. He has an elevated serum lactate level in the setting of a normal perfusion pressure, and no clear evidence of sepsis. The patient has a mildly elevated serum ketone study but is not diabetic, and there is no clear evidence of chronic alcoholism or starvation (eg, reduced serum albumin) to suggest another cause of ketoacidosis. The serum osmolal gap is negative, which makes an organic alcohol ingestion less likely. The serum acetaminophen and aspirin levels are negative. This leaves us with isoniazid (INH) toxicity as the likely cause of the patient's presentation. Although transient lactic acidosis secondary to seizure activity may also be contributing, the patient has no evidence of sepsis at this point.

INH is commonly prescribed for the treatment of latent TB. However, INH has a narrow therapeutic window: an acute ingestion of as little as 1.5 g (or approximately 5 times the daily dose) can lead to recurrent seizures, profound metabolic acidosis, coma, and death. The seizures are often refractory to standard anticonvulsant therapy. INH inhibits the body's ability to synthesize the neurotransmitter GABA, leading to brain hyperexcitation and seizures (which can lead to a significant albeit transient lactic acidosis due to prolonged muscle contraction). Additionally, it can replace NAD in the tricarboxylic acid cycle, leading to a moderate type B lactic acidosis as well as mild ketosis due to the inability to completely utilize oxidative phosphorylation for cellular metabolism.

Q64-6: G
Seizure.

Rationale: During tonic-clonic seizure activity, normal respiratory center activity can be lost and patients can become completely apneic. This leads to hypercarbia and respiratory acidosis. This state is usually transient and will resolve once the seizures dissipate.

Q64-7: A
Diarrhea.

Rationale: The urine anion gap is negative, with a normal urinary pH (for a patient in acidosis) as well as a low serum potassium. The negative urine anion gap and the appropriately elevated urine osmolal gap indicate that there is appropriate urinary acidification, ruling out a type 1 and type 4 RTA. The information provided in the prompt suggests that the patient has recently been experiencing diarrhea from a recent GI illness, and this is the more likely cause of the patient's current acid-base disorder.

Urine Anion Gap:

$$\text{Urine Anion Gap} = [U_{Na}] + [U_{K}] - [U_{Cl}]$$
$$= (20 + 30 - 70) = (-20) \text{ mEq/L.}$$

Interpretation:

- A urine anion gap that is greater than +20 mEq/L → reduced renal acid excretion (RTA).
- A urine anion gap that is less than −20 mEq/L → GI loss of bicarbonate (eg, diarrhea), although type 2 RTA is possible.
- A urine anion gap between −20 and +10 mEq/L is generally considered inconclusive.

An alternative approach is to consider the urine osmolal gap (UOG).

Urine Osmolal Gap:

$$\text{Calculated Urine Osmolality} = 2 * ([Na^+] + [K^+]) + \frac{[Urea]}{2.8} + \frac{[Glucose]}{18}$$

$$\text{Urine Osmolal Gap (UOG)} = \text{Measured Urine Osmolality} - \text{Measured Urine Osmolality}$$

$$\text{UOG} = 484 \text{ mOsm/L (given in the prompt)}.$$

Interpretation (in setting of a metabolic acidosis):

- UOG greater than 400 mOsm/L (or kg)—appropriate urinary acidification, consistent with a GI source and normal renal acidification.
- UOG less than 100 to 150 mOsm/L (or kg)—inappropriately low urinary acidification, most consistent with a type 1 or 4 RTA.
- Again, this is not particularly useful for the diagnosis of a type 2 (proximal) RTA, where other serum or urine lab abnormalities are more helpful.

Cause of NAGMA.
Low Serum Potassium
GI: Diarrhea, pancreaticoduodenal fistula, urinary intestinal diversion Renal: Type 1 RTA (distal), type 2 RTA (proximal) Medications/exposures: Carbonic anhydrase inhibitors, toluene Other: D-Lactic acidosis
High (or Normal) Serum Potassium:
GI: Elevated ileostomy output Renal: Type 4 RTA or CKD Medications: NSAIDs; antibiotics (trimethoprim, pentamidine); heparin; ACE inhibitors, ARBs, aldosterone antagonists (spironolactone); acid administration (TPN)

Q64-8: C
Pyridoxine (B$_6$) supplementation.

Rationale: INH interferes with the fatty acid synthesis and cell wall synthesis in mycotic organisms; however, it also inhibits pyridoxine phosphokinase, the enzyme necessary for pyridoxine conversion to pyridoxal 5' phosphate. The latter compound is the active cofactor for B$_6$-dependent reactions and is the cause for the many potential side effects of INH therapy. Pyridoxine is often coadministered with INH in the treatment of latent TB to prevent such complications. Pyridoxine should be administered at the dose similar to that of the suspect intoxication (usually 5 g is sufficient). IV administration is preferred, although oral administration is also sufficient.

References

Alvarez FG, Guntupalli KK. Isoniazid overdose: four case reports and review of the literature. Intensive Care Med. 1995;21:641.

Batlle D, Chin-Theodorou J, Tucker BM. Metabolic acidosis or respiratory alkalosis? Evaluation of a low plasma bicarbonate using the urine anion gap. Am J Kidney Dis. 2017;70:440.

Gokhale YA, Vaidya MS, Mehta AD, Rathod NN. Isoniazid toxicity presenting as status epilepticus and severe metabolic acidosis. J Assoc Physicians India. 2009;57:70.

Batlle DC, Hizon M, Cohen E, et al. The use of the urinary anion gap in the diagnosis of hyperchloremic metabolic acidosis. N Engl J Med. 1988;318:594.

Kraut JA, Madias NE. Differential diagnosis of nongap metabolic acidosis: value of a systematic approach. Clin J Am Soc Nephrol. 2012;7:671.

Kraut JA, Nagami GT. The serum anion gap in the evaluation of acid-base disorders: what are its limitations and can its effectiveness be improved? Clin J Am Soc Nephrol. 2013;8:2018.

Madias NE. Lactic acidosis. Kidney Int. 1986;29:752.

Minns AB, Ghafouri N, Clark RF. Isoniazid-induced status epilepticus in a pediatric patient after inadequate pyridoxine therapy. Pediatr Emerg Care. 2010;26:380.

Morrow LE, Wear RE, Schuller D, Malesker M. Acute isoniazid toxicity and the need for adequate pyridoxine supplies. Pharmacotherapy. 2006;26:1529.

Puri MM, Kumar L, Vishwakarma PD, Behera D. Seizures with single therapeutic dose of isoniazid. Indian J Tuberc. 2012;59:100.

Rastegar M, Nagami GT. Non-anion gap metabolic acidosis: a clinical approach to evaluation. Am J Kidney Dis. 2017;69:296.

Romero JA, Kuczler FJ Jr. Isoniazid overdose: recognition and management. Am Fam Physician. 1998;57:749.

Stead DF, Mason CR. Three cases of intentional isoniazid overdose – a life-threatening condition. S Afr Med J. 2016;106:891.

Temmerman W, Dhondt A, Vandewoude K. Acute isoniazid intoxication: seizures, acidosis and coma. Acta Clin Belg. 1999;54:211.

Topcu I, Yentur EA, Kefi A, et al. Seizures, metabolic acidosis and coma resulting from acute isoniazid intoxication. Anaesth Intensive Care. 2005;33:518.

CASE 65

A 44-year-old male patient with early-stage ALS presents with pneumonia. He did not require non-invasive ventilation at baseline but has been experiencing more respiratory symptoms over the past few months, as well as significant diarrhea. On examination today, he is encephalopathic and hypotensive, with BP 80/40. His remaining vitals signs are T 39.8°C, HR 115, RR 14, and Sao_2 84% on room air and improved to 94% on 4L/min supplemental O_2 via nasal cannula. His urine antigen tests are positive for *Legionella* pneumonia. His pulmonary examination is notable for purulent sputum and rhonchorous breath sounds in the right lower lung field. His CXR demonstrates a small pleural effusion on the right and some airspace opacities in the right middle lobe.

Laboratory data.			
ABGs		Basic Metabolic Panel	
pH	6.98	Na	131 mEq/L
$Paco_2$	66 mm Hg	K	3.3 mEq/L
Pao_2	60 mm Hg	Cl	101 mEq/L
HCO_3	15 mEq/L	CO_2	15 mEq/L
		BUN	12 mg/dL
		Cr	0.3 mg/dL
		Glucose	100 mg/dL
		Albumin	3.0 g/dL
		EtOH	0 mg/dL

QUESTIONS

Q65-1: Define the patient's baseline acid-base status: Does this patient have an underlying chronic acid-base disorder that we need to account for in order to appropriately interpret the acute acid-base disorders?

A. There is no evidence for an underlying chronic respiratory or metabolic acid-base disorder in this patient, so we would assume a baseline $Paco_2$ of 40 mm Hg and an HCO_3 of 24 mEq/L.

B. While the patient has a condition predisposing him to a chronic acid-base disorder, there is insufficient information to estimate the patient's baseline $Paco_2$ and HCO_3 values; therefore, we will assume a baseline $Paco_2$ of 40 mm Hg and a baseline HCO_3 of 24 mEq/L.

C. The patient has an underlying acid-base condition, and we have sufficient information to estimate the patient's baseline $Paco_2$ and HCO_3 values.

Q65-2: What is/are the primary acid-base disturbance(s) occurring in this case?

A. Metabolic acidosis only
B. Respiratory acidosis only
C. Metabolic acidosis and a respiratory acidosis
D. Metabolic alkalosis and a respiratory alkalosis
E. Metabolic alkalosis only
F. Respiratory alkalosis only

Q65-3: How would the metabolic acidosis component be classified in this case?

A. Anion gap acidosis
B. Non-anion gap acidosis
C. Anion and non-anion gap acidosis
D. Anion gap acidosis and a metabolic alkalosis

Q65-4: Results of the patient's remaining laboratory tests are as follows:

Serum EtOH	< 3 mg/dL
Serum acetaminophen	< 5 mg/dL (ULN for therapeutic use 20 mg/dL)
Serum salicylates	< 5 mg/dL (ULN for therapeutic use 30 mg/dL)
Serum osmolality	277 mOsm/kg
Serum L-lactate	6.8 mmol/L (ULN 2.0 mmol/L venous)
Beta-hydroxybutyrate (acetone)	< 0.18 mmol/L (ULN 0.18 mmol/L)
Serum glucose	100 mg/dL

What is the likely cause of the patient's anion gap acidosis?

A. Aspirin toxicity
B. Lactic acidosis secondary to sepsis
C. Ethylene glycol toxicity
D. Methanol toxicity
E. Opioid overdose
F. Acetaminophen overdose
G. Diabetic ketoacidosis
H. Alcoholic ketoacidosis

Q65-5: What is the likely cause of the patient's respiratory acidosis?

A. Hypoxemia
B. Neuromuscular disorder
C. Asthma
D. COPD
E. Chest wall injury or deformity
F. Pulmonary fibrosis
G. Opioid overdose
H. Benzodiazepine overdose
I. Iatrogenic cause

Q65-6: The urine electrolyte values are as follows:

Urine Na	10 mEq/L
Urine K	40 mEq/L
Urine Cl	70 mEq/L
Urine urea	334 mg/dL
Urine glucose	0 mg/dL
Urine osmolality	789 mOsm/L
Urine pH	5.2
Urine RBCs	None
Urine WBCs	None
Urine protein	None
Urine microscopic	None

What is the most likely type of non-anion gap acidosis present?

A. Diarrhea
B. Type 1 RTA (distal tubule)
C. Type 2 RTA (proximal tubule)
D. Type 4 RTA (distal tubule/collecting duct)

Q65-7: This patient has a respiratory acidosis due to ALS, which prevents him from compensating appropriately for the lactic acidosis from sepsis. What would you expect the patient's $Paco_2$ and arterial pH to be if the patient did not have a respiratory acidosis? (Assume appropriate renal compensation for an acute metabolic acidosis.)

A. pH 7.28, $Paco_2$ 34 mm Hg
B. pH 7.30, $Paco_2$ 30 mm Hg
C. pH 7.52, $Paco_2$ 45 mm Hg
D. pH 6.91, $Paco_2$ 66 mm Hg

ANSWERS

Q65-1: B

While the patient has a condition predisposing him to a chronic acid-base disorder, there is insufficient information to estimate the patient's baseline $Paco_2$ and HCO_3 values; therefore, we will assume a baseline $Paco_2$ of 40 mm Hg and a baseline HCO_3 of 24 mEq/L. The patient has ALS, and therefore we would be concerned about a possible chronic respiratory acidosis. However, the prompt notes that the patient has not required initiation of non-invasive ventilation and provides no evidence for a chronic respiratory acid-base disorder at this point.

Rationale: Ignoring these underlying chronic acid-base disorders can significantly alter the interpretation of a patient's acute acid-base status. This was demonstrated in the first case of the series. However, often, we do not have the necessary information (eg, prior ABG or VBG, or prior serum chemistry with an HCO_3) and are forced to assume the ongoing processes are all acute in nature. We are primarily concerned about chronic respiratory acid-base disorders, as these can significantly alter the patient's baseline or expected values for the serum HCO_3 and $Paco_2$, and we have reliable equations to predict the expected baseline values. The respiratory compensation for both chronic metabolic acidosis and alkalosis is generally poor, so there are no equations or rules to predict what the $Paco_2$ should be in these cases. While the baseline serum HCO_3 may be significantly off from our standard value of 24 mEq/L in these patients, we would assume a baseline $Paco_2$ of 40 mm Hg in patients with chronic metabolic processes. Once we identify the patient's baseline $Paco_2$ and HCO_3 values, we will need to use these values in the appropriate equations to identify the ongoing acute processes.

Q65-2: C

Metabolic acidosis and a respiratory acidosis.

Rationale:

1. The pH is 6.98; therefore, the primary disorder is an **acidosis.**
2. The $Paco_2$ of 66 mm Hg is greater than 40 mm Hg, so there is a **respiratory acidosis.**
3. The HCO_3 of 15 mEq/L is less than 24 mEq/L, so there is also a **metabolic acidosis.**

Q65-3: C

Anion and non-anion gap acidosis.

Rationale:

1. Is there evidence for a chronic acid-base disorder that requires adjustment of the patient's "normal" HCO_3? No, there is no evidence for a chronic acid-base disorder, so we would assume a baseline $Paco_2$ of 40 mm Hg and an HCO_3 of 24 mEq/L.
2. Expected anion gap:

$$\text{Expected Anion Gap} = 12 - (2.5) * \left[4.0 \, \frac{g}{dL} - \text{Actual Serum Albumin} \right]$$
$$= 12 - (2.5 * [4.0 - 3.0])$$
$$= 12 - (2.5 * [1.0]) = \textbf{9.5 mEq/L.}$$

3. Anion gap calculation:

$$\text{Serum Anion Gap} = [Na^+] - [HCO_3^-] - [Cl^-]$$
$$= 117 - (70 + 10) = 15 \text{ mEq/L, which is} > 9.5 \text{ mEq/L}$$
$$\rightarrow \textbf{anion gap acidosis is present.}$$

4. Delta-delta calculation:

$$\Delta\Delta = \frac{(\text{Actual Anion Gap} - \text{Expected Anion Gap})}{(\text{Baseline HCO}_3 - \text{Actual HCO}_3)}$$
$$= (15 - 9.5)/(24 - 15) = \textbf{5.5/9, which is ~0.61.}$$

Delta-delta interpretation.	
Delta-Delta Value	Condition Present
< 0.4	Non-anion gap only
0.4–0.9	**Anion gap *and* non-anion gap acidosis**
1.0–2.0	Anion gap acidosis only
> 2.0	Anion gap acidosis and metabolic alkalosis

Q65-4: B
Lactic acidosis secondary to sepsis.

Rationale: The patient has a new pneumonia and hypotension, and a urine antigen test that is positive for *Legionella*, consistent with pneumonia. The patient has a negative ethanol level, a negative screen for acetaminophen and aspirin, and a negative serum ketone study for ketoacidosis. The calculated serum osmolality is as follows:

$$\text{Calculated Serum Osmolality} = 2*[Na^+] + \frac{[\text{Glucose}]}{18} + \frac{[\text{BUN}]}{2.8} + \frac{[\text{EtOH}]}{3.7}$$
$$= 271 \text{ mOsm/L.}$$

Therefore, the serum osmolal gap is +6 mOsm/L, which is normal. This rules out an organic alcohol ingestion. Given the significantly elevated lactate, a type A lactic acidosis secondary to sepsis is the most likely etiology. Opioid overdose is most commonly associated with a respiratory acidosis, although when patients become significantly acidotic or hypoxemic from the respiratory acidosis, a metabolic acidosis can ensue.

Q65-5: B
Neuromuscular disorder.

Rationale: This patient has ALS, a neuromuscular disorder associated with respiratory failure as the disease progresses. The patient has limited respiratory reserve as a result and is not able to compensate for his metabolic acidosis. Eventually, the respiratory muscles fatigue and the patient developed worsening hypercarbia.

Q65-6: A
Diarrhea.

Rationale: The patient has a negative urine anion gap and an appropriately elevated serum osmolal gap given the overall acidemia. This is consistent with intact renal acidification, eliminating options B and D.

Urine Anion Gap:

$$\text{Urine Anion Gap (UAG)} = [U_{Na}] + [U_K] - [U_{Cl}]$$
$$\text{UAG} = (10 + 40 - 70) = (-20 \text{ mEq/L})$$

Interpretation:

- A UAG that is greater than +20 mEq/L → reduced renal acid excretion (RTA).
- A UAG that is less than −20 mEq/L → GI loss of HCO_3 (eg, diarrhea), although type 2 RTA is possible.
- A UAG between −20 and +10 mEq/L is generally considered inconclusive.

Urine Osmolal Gap:

$$\text{Calculated Urine Osmolality} = 2 * [U_{Na} + U_K] + \frac{[U_{BUN}]}{2.8} + \frac{[U_{glucose}]}{18}$$
$$= 2 * [50] + [334/2.8] + [0/18]$$
$$= 219 \text{ mOsm/L.}$$

$$\text{Urine Osmolal Gap (UOG)} = \text{Measured Urine Osmolality} - \text{Calculated Urine Osmolality}$$
$$\text{UOG} = 789 - 219 = 560 \text{ mOsm/L.}$$

Interpretation (in setting of a metabolic acidosis):

- A UOG that is greater than 400 mOsm/L (or kg) → appropriate urinary acidification, consistent with a GI source and normal renal acidification.
- A UOG that is less than 100 to 150 mOsm/L (or kg) → inappropriately low urinary acidification, most consistent with a type 1 or 4 RTA.
- Again, this is not particularly useful for the diagnosis of a type 2 (proximal) RTA, where other serum or urine lab abnormalities are more helpful.

Now, we are left with either a type 2 RTA (proximal) or diarrhea. The urine pH and serum potassium are not particularly helpful here. However, the lack of glucose in the urine points away from a type 2 RTA caused by Fanconi syndrome, although it does not rule out other potential causes of a type 2 RTA. The patient presented with complaints of diarrhea (*Legionella* pneumonia is commonly associated with diarrhea and hyponatremia, as in this case). Given the constellation of symptoms and the objective evidence, the HCO_3 loss is most likely associated with a GI source, making diarrhea the appropriate answer.

Cause of NAGMA.

Evaluation Strategy

1. History (acute or chronic issues, medications, altered GI anatomy, genetic diseases, etc).
2. Does the patient have chronic renal insufficiency? If so, this alone may be responsible for the non-anion gap acidosis.
3. Calculate UAG and UOG. The UAG may be of limited value in patients with severe serum anion gap acidosis, as it may be falsely elevated. Similarly, the UAG may be inappropriately elevated in patients with a significant serum osmolal gap (particularly due to mannitol).
4. Note the serum potassium as well as the urine pH.
5. If proximal RTA is suspected, look for evidence of other inappropriate compounds In the urine (amino acids, elevated phosphate, glucosuria), and calculate the fractional resorption of sodium bicarbonate (should be > 15%). Also check serum for evidence of dysfunctional of the PTH–vitamin D–calcium axis.

Low Serum Potassium

GI: Diarrhea, pancreaticoduodenal fistula, urinary intestinal diversion

Renal: Type 1 RTA (distal), type 2 RTA (proximal)

Medications/exposures: Carbonic anhydrase inhibitors, toluene

Other: D-Lactic acidosis

High (or Normal) Serum Potassium

GI: Elevated ileostomy output

Renal: Type 4 RTA or CKD

Medications: NSAIDs; antibiotics (trimethoprim, pentamidine); heparin; ACE inhibitors, ARBs, aldosterone antagonists (spironolactone); acid administration (TPN)

Evaluation of RTA.

	Type 1 RTA	Type 2 RTA	Type 4 RTA
Severity of metabolic acidosis, (HCO$_3$)	Severe (< 10–12 mEq/L typically)	Intermediate (12–20 mEq/L)	Mild (15–20 mEq/L)
Associated urine abnormalities	Urinary phosphate, calcium increased; bone disease often present	Urine glucose, amino acids, phosphate, calcium may be elevated	
Urine pH	HIGH (> 5.5)	Low (acidic), until serum HCO$_3$ level exceeds resorptive ability of proximal tubule; then becomes alkalotic once reabsorptive threshold is crossed	Low (acidic)
Serum K$^+$	Low to normal; should correct with oral HCO$_3$ therapy	Classically low, although may be normal or even high with rare genetic defects; worsens with oral HCO$_3$ therapy	HIGH
Renal stones	Often	No	No

(Continued)

Evaluation of RTA. *(continued)*			
Renal tubular defect	Reduced NH_4 secretion in distal tubule	Reduced HCO_3 resorption in proximal tubule	Reduced H^+/K^+ exchange in distal and collecting tubule due to decreased aldosterone or aldosterone resistance
UAG	> 10	Negative initially, then positive when receiving serum HCO_3, then negative after therapy.	> 10
UOG	Reduced (< 150 mOsm/L) during acute acidosis	At baseline is < 100 mEq/L; unreliable during acidosis	Reduced (< 150 mOsm/L) during acute acidosis

Causes of RTA.

Causes of Type 1 (Distal) RTA

Primary
• Idiopathic or familial (may be recessive or dominant)

Secondary
• Medications: Lithium, amphotericin, ifosfamide, NSAIDs
• Rheumatologic disorders: Sjögren syndrome, SLE, RA
• Hypercalciuria (idiopathic) or associated with vitamin D deficiency or hyperparathyroidism
• Sarcoidosis
• Obstructive uropathy
• Wilson disease
• Rejection of renal transplant allograft
• Toluene toxicity

Causes of Type 2 (Proximal) RTA

Primary
• Idiopathic
• Familial (primarily recessive disorders)
• Genetic: Fanconi syndrome, cystinosis, glycogen storage disease (type 1), Wilson disease, galactosemia

Secondary
• Medications: Acetazolamide, topiramate, aminoglycoside antibiotics, ifosfamide, reverse transcriptase inhibitors (tenofovir)
• Heavy metal poisoning: Lead, mercury, copper
• Multiple myeloma or amyloidosis (secondary to light chain toxicity)
• Sjögren syndrome
• Vitamin D deficiency
• Rejection of renal transplant allograft

Causes of Type 4 RTA (Hypoaldosteronism or Aldosterone Resistance)

Primary
• Primary adrenal insufficiency
• Inherited disorders associated with hypoaldosteronism
• Pseudohypoaldosteronism (types 1 and 2)

(Continued)

Causes of RTA. (*continued*)

Secondary
- Causes of hyporeninemic hypoaldosteronism such as renal disease (diabetic nephropathy), NSAID use, calcineurin inhibitors, volume expansion/volume overload
- Causes of distal tubule voltage defects such as sickle cell disease, obstructive uropathy, SLE
- Severe illness/septic shock
- Angiotensin II–associated medications: ACE inhibitors, ARBs, direct renin inhibitors
- Potassium-sparing diuretics: Spironolactone, amiloride, triamterene
- Antibiotics: Trimethoprim, pentamidine

Q65-7: B
pH 7.30, Paco$_2$ 30 mm Hg.

Rationale: First, we need to determine the expected arterial Paco$_2$ if we assume that (1) this is an acute metabolic acidosis, and (2) there is appropriate (complete) compensation. For this, we will use the Winter formula.

Respiratory Compensation for Acute Metabolic Acidosis (Winter Formula):

$$\text{Expected Paco}_2 = 1.5 * [\text{Actual HCO}_3] + 8 \pm 2 \text{ (in mm Hg)}$$
$$\text{Expected Paco}_2 = 1.5 * [15] + 8 \pm 2 = 30.5 \text{ mm Hg} \pm 2.$$

In this patient, for calculation of the pH, we will use the median value of the preceding range (30.5 mm Hg).

Henderson-Hasselbalch Equation:

$$pH = 6.10 + \log\left(\frac{[\text{HCO}_3]}{0.03 * \text{Paco}_2}\right)$$

or,

$$pH = 7.61 + \log_{10}\left(\frac{[\text{HCO}_3]}{\text{Paco}_2}\right).$$

Therefore, the pH is 7.30, with an HCO$_3$ of 15 mEq/L and a Paco$_2$ of 30.5 mm Hg.

References

Adeva-Andany M, López-Ojén M, Funcasta-Calderón R, et al. Comprehensive review on lactate metabolism in human health. Mitochondrion. 2014;17:76.

Batlle D, Chin-Theodorou J, Tucker BM. Metabolic acidosis or respiratory alkalosis? Evaluation of a low plasma bicarbonate using the urine anion gap. Am J Kidney Dis. 2017;70:440.

Batlle D, Grupp M, Gaviria M, Kurtzman NA. Distal renal tubular acidosis with intact capacity to lower urinary pH. Am J Med. 1982;72:751.

Batlle D, Haque SK. Genetic causes and mechanisms of distal renal tubular acidosis. Nephrol Dial Transplant. 2012;27:3691.

Batlle DC, Hizon M, Cohen E, et al. The use of the urinary anion gap in the diagnosis of hyperchloremic metabolic acidosis. N Engl J Med. 1988;318:594.

Batlle DC, von Riotte A, Schlueter W. Urinary sodium in the evaluation of hyperchloremic metabolic acidosis. N Engl J Med. 1987;316:140.

Buckalew VM Jr, McCurdy DK, Ludwig GD, et al. Incomplete renal tubular acidosis. Physiologic studies in three patients with a defect in lowering urine pH. Am J Med. 1968;45:32.

Daniel SR, Morita SY, Yu M, Dzierba A. Uncompensated metabolic acidosis: an underrecognized risk factor for subsequent intubation requirement. J Trauma. 2004;57:993.

Fulop M. A guide for predicting arterial CO2 tension in metabolic acidosis. Am J Nephrol. 1997;17:421.

Karet FE. Mechanisms in hyperkalemic renal tubular acidosis. J Am Soc Nephrol. 2009;20:251.

Kraut JA, Madias NE. Differential diagnosis of nongap metabolic acidosis: value of a systematic approach. Clin J Am Soc Nephrol. 2012;7:671.

Levy B. Lactate and shock state: the metabolic view. Curr Opin Crit Care. 2006;12:315.

Madias NE. Lactic acidosis. Kidney Int. 1986;29:752.

Mikkelsen ME, Miltiades AN, Gaieski DF, et al. Serum lactate is associated with mortality in severe sepsis independent of organ failure and shock. Crit Care Med. 2009;37:1670.

Pierce NF, Fedson DS, Brigham KL, et al. The ventilatory response to acute base deficit in humans. Time course during development and correction of metabolic acidosis. Ann Intern Med. 1970;72:633.

Rastegar M, Nagami GT. Non-anion gap metabolic acidosis: a clinical approach to evaluation. Am J Kidney Dis. 2017;69:296.

Rodríguez Soriano J. Renal tubular acidosis: the clinical entity. J Am Soc Nephrol. 2002;13:2160.

Weinberger SE, Schwartzstein RM, Weiss JW. Hypercapnia. N Engl J Med. 1989;321:1223.

West JB. Causes of carbon dioxide retention in lung disease. N Engl J Med. 1971;284:1232.

Wiederseiner JM, Muser J, Lutz T, et al. Acute metabolic acidosis: characterization and diagnosis of the disorder and the plasma potassium response. J Am Soc Nephrol. 2004;15:1589.

Williams MH Jr, Shim CS. Ventilatory failure. Etiology and clinical forms. Am J Med. 1970;48:477.

CASE 66

A 78-year-old male patient presents with ataxia and tachypnea. He has a history of tobacco use, HTN, coronary artery disease, and hyperlipidemia. His vital signs are T 36.5°C, HR 80, BP 170/90, RR 25, and Sao$_2$ 92% on room air. He is taking very deep and rapid breaths and states that he cannot control his breathing. A review of his home medications indicates that he takes lisinopril, amlodipine, metoprolol, and atorvastatin. A neurologist is consulted and is concerned for a cerebellar/brainstem CVA. Brain CT and MRI scans are ordered. The brain CT shows no hemorrhage, but MRI shows a potential stroke in the brainstem.

Laboratory data.			
ABGs		Basic Metabolic Panel	
pH	7.62	Na	140 mEq/L
Paco$_2$	15 mm Hg	K	5.1 mEq/L
Pao$_2$	60 mm Hg	Cl	120 mEq/L
HCO$_3$	15 mEq/L	CO$_2$	15 mEq/L
		BUN	15 mg/dL
		Cr	0.5 mg/dL
		Glucose	100 mg/dL
		Albumin	4.0 g/dL
		EtOH	0 mg/dL

QUESTIONS

Q66-1: Define the patient's baseline acid-base status: Does this patient have an underlying chronic acid-base disorder that we need to account for in order to appropriately interpret the acute acid-base disorders?

A. There is no evidence for an underlying chronic respiratory or metabolic acid-base disorder in this patient, so we would assume a baseline $Paco_2$ of 40 mm Hg and an HCO_3 of 24 mEq/L.

B. While the patient has a condition predisposing him to a chronic acid-base disorder, there is insufficient information to estimate the patient's baseline $Paco_2$ and HCO_3 values; therefore, we will assume a baseline $Paco_2$ of 40 mm Hg and a baseline HCO_3 of 24 mEq/L.

C. The patient has an underlying acid-base condition, and we have sufficient information to estimate the patient's baseline $Paco_2$ and HCO_3 values.

Q66-2: What is/are the primary acid-base disturbance(s) occurring in this case?

A. Metabolic acidosis only
B. Respiratory acidosis only
C. Metabolic acidosis and a respiratory acidosis
D. Metabolic alkalosis and a respiratory alkalosis
E. Metabolic alkalosis only
F. Respiratory alkalosis only

Q66-3: Does the patient in this case demonstrate appropriate respiratory or metabolic compensation?

A. Yes, the respiratory compensation is appropriate.
B. No, a concomitant respiratory alkalosis is present.
C. No, a concomitant respiratory acidosis is present.
D. Yes, the metabolic compensation is appropriate.
E. No, a concomitant metabolic acidosis is present.
F. No, a concomitant metabolic alkalosis is present.

Q66-4: How would the metabolic acidosis component be classified in this case?

A. Anion gap acidosis
B. Non-anion gap acidosis
C. Anion and non-anion gap acidosis
D. Anion gap acidosis and a metabolic alkalosis

Q66-5: The patient's urine and serum drug screens are negative. Results of his urine studies are as follows:

Urine Na	20 mEq/L
Urine K	22 mEq/L
Urine Cl	10 mEq/L
Urine urea	234 mg/dL
Urine glucose	0 mg/dL
Urine osmolality	225 mOsm/L
Urine pH	5.5

Match the acid-base disorders in this patient to the most likely etiology from the list below. (Choose only one answer per disorder.)

A. COPD
B. CNS injury
C. Aspirin overdose
D. Diuresis
E. Hypoxemia
F. Acetazolamide use
G. Autoimmune disease
H. ACE inhibitor use
— Non-anion gap acidosis
— Respiratory alkalosis

ANSWERS

Q66-1: B

While the patient has a condition predisposing him to a chronic acid-base disorder, there is insufficient information to estimate the patient's baseline $Paco_2$ and HCO_3 values; therefore, we will assume a baseline $Paco_2$ of 40 mm Hg and a baseline HCO_3 of 24 mEq/L. This will be addressed in further questions in this case.

Rationale: Ignoring these underlying chronic acid-base disorders can significantly alter the interpretation of a patient's acute acid-base status. This was demonstrated in the first case of the series. However, often, we do not have the necessary information (eg, prior ABG or VBG, or prior serum chemistry with an HCO_3) and are forced to assume the ongoing processes are all acute in nature. We are primarily concerned about chronic respiratory acid-base disorders, as these can significantly alter the patient's baseline or expected values for the serum HCO_3 and $Paco_2$, and we have reliable equations to predict the expected baseline values. The respiratory compensation for both chronic metabolic acidosis and alkalosis is generally poor, so there are no equations or rules to predict what the $Paco_2$ should be in these cases. While the baseline serum HCO_3 may be significantly off from our standard value of 24 mEq/L in these patients, we would assume a baseline $Paco_2$ of 40 mm Hg in patients with chronic metabolic processes. Once we identify the patient's baseline $Paco_2$ and HCO_3 values, we will need to use these values in the appropriate equations to identify the ongoing acute processes.

Q66-2: F
Respiratory alkalosis only.

Rationale:

1. The pH is 7.54; therefore, the primary disorder is an **acidosis.**
2. The $Paco_2$ of 15 mm Hg is less than 40 mm Hg, so there is a **respiratory alkalosis.**
3. The HCO_3 of 15 mEq/L is less than 24 mEq/L, so this not a primary metabolic alkalosis.

Q66-3: E
No, a concomitant metabolic acidosis is present.

Rationale: Here, the primary issue is a respiratory alkalosis. Recall that metabolic compensation is rather slow. Assuming an acute respiratory alkalosis:

Metabolic Compensation for Acute Respiratory Alkalosis:

$$\text{Expected } HCO_3 = \text{Baseline } HCO_3 - (0.20)[\text{Actual } Paco_2 - \text{Baseline } Paco_2]$$
$$= 24 - (0.20 * [40 - 15]) = 24 - (0.20 * 25) = 19.6 \text{ mEq/L.}$$

The patient has an HCO_3 of 15 mEq/L, which is less than that expected (19.6 mEq/L), so a metabolic acidosis is present as well.

Q66-4: B
Non-anion gap acidosis.

Rationale:

1. Is there evidence for a chronic acid-base disorder that requires adjustment of the patient's "normal" HCO_3? No, there is no evidence for a chronic acid-base disorder, so we would assume a baseline $Paco_2$ of 40 mm Hg and an HCO_3 of 24 mEq/L.
2. Expected anion gap:

$$\text{Expected Anion Gap} = 12 - (2.5) * \left[4.0 \frac{g}{dL} - \text{Actual Serum Albumin} \right]$$
$$= 12 - (2.5 * [4.0 - 4.0])$$
$$= 12 - (2.5 * [0]) = \textbf{12 mEq/L.}$$

3. Anion gap calculation:

$$\text{Serum Anion Gap} = [Na^+] - [HCO_3^-] - [Cl^-]$$
$$140 - (120 + 15) = 5 \text{ mEq/L, which is} < 12 \text{ mEq/L}$$
$$\rightarrow \textbf{no anion gap acidosis is present.}$$

Therefore, this patient has a non-anion gap metabolic acidosis. There is no need for the delta-delta calculation in this case.

Q66-5: H; D.
ACE inhibitor use; CNS injury.

Rationale: The patient has a primary respiratory alkalosis and a non-anion gap acidosis. The respiratory alkalosis is likely due to his cerebellar stroke, with the development of chronic neurogenic hyperventilation. He has no other clear cause of respiratory alkalosis.

As for the non-anion gap acidosis, the patient has a positive urine anion gap (UAG)—an abnormal (low) UAG, indicating reduced urinary acidification and most consistent with either a type 1 (distal) or a type 4 RTA. He also has an elevated serum K, and a low urine pH, indicative of a type 4 RTA. The only cause of type 4 RTA in the options provided is ACE inhibitor use, which is listed among the patient's home medications. This may, in fact, be a chronic condition.

Urine Anion Gap:

$$\text{Urine Anion Gap (UAG)} = [U_{Na}] + [U_K] - [U_{Cl}].$$

Therefore, for this patient,

$$UAG = U_{Na} + U_K - U_{Cl} = (20 + 22) - 10 = (+34).$$

Interpretation:

- A UAG that is greater than +20 mEq/L → reduced renal acid excretion (RTA).
- A UAG that is less than −20 mEq/L → GI loss of HCO_3 (eg, diarrhea), although type 2 RTA is possible.
- A UAG between −20 and +10 mEq/L is generally considered inconclusive.

Limitation: The UAG can be inappropriately elevated in anion gap acidosis, a situation in which multiple unmeasured anions may be present in the urine (beta-hydroxybutyrate/ acetoacetate [ketoacidosis], hippurate [toluene], HCO_3 [proximal RTA], D-lactate [D-lactic acidosis], L-lactate, 5-oxoproline [acetaminophen toxicity]).

Therefore, in patients with a significant anion gap, the urine osmolal gap (UOG) is typically more useful. Here the calculated UOG is as follows:

$$\text{Calculated Urine Osmolality} = 2 * ([Na^+] + [K^+]) + \frac{[Urea]}{2.8} + \frac{[Glucose]}{18}$$
$$\text{Urine Osmolal Gap (UOG)} = \text{Measured Urine Osmolality} - \text{Measured Urine Osmolality}$$
$$\text{Calculated Urine Osmolarity} = 2 * ([U_{Na}] + [U_K]) + (U_{Urea} \, (mg/dL)/2.8]$$
$$+ [U_{glucose} \, (mg/dL)/18]$$
$$= 172 \text{ mOsm/L.}$$

The UOG is then calculated,

$$\text{UOG} = 225 - 172 \text{ Osm/L} = 53 \text{ mOsm/L.}$$

Interpretation (in the setting of a metabolic acidosis):

- A UOG greater than 400 mOsm/L (or kg) → appropriate urinary acidification, consistent with normal renal acidification.
- A UOG less than 100 to 150 mOsm/L (or kg) → inappropriately low urinary acidification, most consistent with a type 1 or 4 RTA.
- Again, this is not particularly useful for the diagnosis of a type 2 (proximal) RTA, where other serum or urine lab abnormalities are more helpful.

Limitations: The primary limitation of the UOG is its use in conditions with a high osmolal gap, where non-ammonium solutes not included in the calculation may be present in the urine (particularly mannitol). The presence of these unmeasured solutes will increase the osmolal gap inappropriately. Also, the UOG should not be used in patients with a urinary tract infection caused by a urease-producing organism, as urea is metabolized to HCO_3 and ammonium in urine.

Evaluation of RTA.

	Type 1 RTA	Type 2 RTA	Type 4 RTA
Severity of metabolic acidosis, (HCO_3)	Severe (< 10–12 mEq/L typically)	Intermediate (12–20 mEq/L)	Mild (15–20 mEq/L)
Associated urine abnormalities	Urinary phosphate, calcium are increased; bone disease often present.	Urine glucose, amino acids, phosphate, calcium may be elevated	
Urine pH	HIGH (> 5.5)	Low (acidic), until serum HCO_3 level exceeds the resorptive ability of the proximal tubule; then becomes alkalotic once reabsorptive threshold is crossed	Low (acidic)
Serum K^+	Low to normal; should correct with oral HCO_3 therapy	Classically low, although may be normal or even high with rare genetic defects; worsens with oral bicarbonate therapy	HIGH
Renal stones	Often	No	No
Renal tubular defect	Reduced NH_4 secretion in distal tubule	Reduced HCO_3 resorption in proximal tubule	Reduced H^+/K^+ exchange in distal and collecting tubule due to decreased aldosterone or aldosterone resistance
UAG	> 10	Negative initially, then positive when receiving serum HCO_3, then negative after therapy	> 10
UOG	Reduced (< 150 mOsm/L) during acute acidosis	At baseline < 100 mEq/L; unreliable during acidosis	Reduced (< 150 mOsm/L) during acute acidosis

Causes of RTA.

Causes of Type 1 (Distal) RTA

Primary
- Idiopathic or familial (may be recessive or dominant)

Secondary
- Medications: Lithium, amphotericin, ifosfamide, NSAIDs
- Rheumatologic disorders: Sjögren syndrome, SLE, RA
- Hypercalciuria (idiopathic) or associated with vitamin D deficiency or hyperparathyroidism
- Sarcoidosis
- Obstructive uropathy
- Wilson disease
- Rejection of renal transplant allograft
- Toluene toxicity

(Continued)

Causes of RTA. (*continued*)
Causes of Type 2 (Proximal) RTA
Primary • Idiopathic • Familial (primarily recessive disorders) • Genetic: Fanconi syndrome, cystinosis, glycogen storage disease (type 1), Wilson disease, galactosemia
Secondary • Medications: Acetazolamide, topiramate, aminoglycoside antibiotics, ifosfamide, reverse transcriptase inhibitors (tenofovir) • Heavy metal poisoning: Lead, mercury, copper • Multiple myeloma or amyloidosis (secondary to light chain toxicity) • Sjögren syndrome • Vitamin D deficiency • Rejection of renal transplant allograft
Causes of Type 4 RTA (Hypoaldosteronism or Aldosterone Resistance)
Primary • Primary adrenal insufficiency • Inherited disorders associated with hypoaldosteronism • Pseudohypoaldosteronism (types 1 and 2)
Secondary • Causes of hyporeninemic hypoaldosteronism such as renal disease (diabetic nephropathy), NSAID use, calcineurin inhibitors, volume expansion/volume overload • Causes of distal tubule voltage defects such as sickle cell disease, obstructive uropathy, SLE • Severe illness/septic shock • Angiotensin II–associated medications: ACE inhibitors, ARBs, direct renin inhibitors • Potassium-sparing diuretics: Spironolactone, amiloride, triamterene • Antibiotics: Trimethoprim, pentamidine

References

Asplund K, Fugl-Meyer AR, Engde M, et al. Respiratory alkalosis early after stroke: its relation to loco-motor function. Scand J Rehabil Med Suppl. 1983;9:103.

Batlle D, Chin-Theodorou J, Tucker BM. Metabolic acidosis or respiratory alkalosis? Evaluation of a low plasma bicarbonate using the urine anion gap. Am J Kidney Dis. 2017;70:440.

Batlle D, Grupp M, Gaviria M, Kurtzman NA. Distal renal tubular acidosis with intact capacity to lower urinary pH. Am J Med. 1982;72:751.

Batlle D, Haque SK. Genetic causes and mechanisms of distal renal tubular acidosis. Nephrol Dial Transplant. 2012;27:3691.

Batlle DC, Hizon M, Cohen E, et al. The use of the urinary anion gap in the diagnosis of hyperchloremic metabolic acidosis. N Engl J Med. 1988;318:594.

Batlle DC, von Riotte A, Schlueter W. Urinary sodium in the evaluation of hyperchloremic metabolic acidosis. N Engl J Med. 1987;316:140.

Bouchama A, De Vol EB. Acid-base alterations in heatstroke. Intensive Care Med. 2001;27:680.

Buckalew VM Jr, McCurdy DK, Ludwig GD, et al. Incomplete renal tubular acidosis. Physiologic studies in three patients with a defect in lowering urine pH. Am J Med. 1968;45:32.

Karet FE. Mechanisms in hyperkalemic renal tubular acidosis. J Am Soc Nephrol. 2009;20:251.

Kraut JA, Madias NE. Differential diagnosis of nongap metabolic acidosis: value of a systematic approach. Clin J Am Soc Nephrol. 2012;7:671.

Lee MC, Klassen AC, Heaney LM, Resch JA. Respiratory rate and pattern disturbances in acute brain stem infarction. Stroke. 1976;7:382.

Rastegar M, Nagami GT. Non-anion gap metabolic acidosis: a clinical Approach to evaluation. Am J Kidney Dis. 2017;69:296.

Rodríguez Soriano J. Renal tubular acidosis: the clinical entity. J Am Soc Nephrol. 2002;13:2160.

CASE 67

A 28-year-old man who is a marathon runner presents the night following a 50-mile ultra-marathon. He states that he is having muscle cramps, palpitations, polyuria, and polydipsia. He feels weak and fatigued overall. His vital signs are T 37.5°C, HR 120, BP 90/60, RR 23, and Sao$_2$ 93% on room air. He takes no other medications and has no other medical problems or history. His examination is grossly unremarkable aside from slight tachypnea.

Laboratory data.			
ABGs		Basic Metabolic Panel	
pH	7.29	Na	140 mEq/L
Paco$_2$	26 mm Hg	K	2.6 mEq/L
Pao$_2$	60 mm Hg	Cl	89 mEq/L
HCO$_3$	12 mEq/L	CO$_2$	12 mEq/L
		BUN	44 mg/dL
		Cr	2.2 mg/dL
		Glucose	80 mg/dL
		Albumin	4.0 g/dL
		EtOH	0 mg/dL

QUESTIONS

Q67-1: Define the patient's baseline acid-base status: Does this patient have an underlying chronic acid-base disorder that we need to account for in order to appropriately interpret the acute acid-base disorders?

A. There is no evidence for an underlying chronic respiratory or metabolic acid-base disorder in this patient, so we would assume a baseline $Paco_2$ of 40 mm Hg and an HCO_3 of 24 mEq/L.

B. While the patient has a condition predisposing him to a chronic acid-base disorder, there is insufficient information to estimate the patient's baseline $Paco_2$ and HCO_3 values; therefore, we will assume a baseline $Paco_2$ of 40 mm Hg and a baseline HCO_3 of 24 mEq/L.

C. The patient has an underlying acid-base condition, and we have sufficient information to estimate the patient's baseline $Paco_2$ and HCO_3 values.

Q67-2: What is/are the primary acid-base disturbance(s) occurring in this case?

A. Metabolic acidosis only
B. Respiratory acidosis only
C. Metabolic acidosis and a respiratory acidosis
D. Metabolic alkalosis and a respiratory alkalosis
E. Metabolic alkalosis only
F. Respiratory alkalosis only

Q67-3: How would the metabolic acidosis component be classified in this case?

A. Anion gap acidosis
B. Non-anion gap acidosis
C. Anion and non-anion gap acidosis
D. Anion gap acidosis and a metabolic alkalosis

Q67-4: Does the patient in this case demonstrate appropriate respiratory or metabolic compensation?

A. Yes, the respiratory compensation is appropriate.
B. No, a concomitant respiratory alkalosis is present.
C. No, a concomitant respiratory acidosis is present.
D. Yes, the metabolic compensation is appropriate.
E. No, a concomitant metabolic acidosis is present.
F. No, a concomitant metabolic alkalosis is present.

Q67-5: The patient's remaining test results are as follows:

Serum EtOH	< 3 mg/dL
Serum acetaminophen	< 5 mg/dL (ULN for therapeutic use 20 mg/dL)
Serum salicylates	< 5 mg/dL (ULN for therapeutic use 30 mg/dL)
Serum osmolality	308 mOsm/kg
Serum L-lactate	4.4 mmol/L (ULN 2.0 mmol/L venous)
Beta-hydroxybutyrate (acetone)	< 0.18 mmol/L (ULN 0.18 mmol/L)
Serum glucose	80 mg/dL
Troponin-T	0.11 ng/mL (ULN 0.05 ng/mL)
Serum phosphorus	8.9 mg/dL (ULN 4.5 mg/dL)
Uric acid	8.2 mg/dL (ULN 7.2 mg/dL)
Urine myoglobin	Positive
Urine ketones	Negative
Urine drug screen	Negative
Serum calcium	6.8 mg/dL (LLN 8.0 mg/dL)

What is the likely cause of the patient's anion gap acidosis?

A. Aspirin toxicity
B. Lactic acidosis secondary to sepsis
C. Ethylene glycol toxicity
D. Methanol toxicity
E. Rhabdomyolysis
F. Acetaminophen overdose
G. Diabetic ketoacidosis
H. Alcoholic ketoacidosis

Q67-6: The urine electrolyte values are as follows:

Urine Na	10 mEq/L
Urine K	65 mEq/L
Urine Cl	9 mEq/L
Urine urea	244 mg/dL
Urine glucose	10 mg/dL
Urine osmolality	243 mOsm/L
Urine pH	5.1
Urine RBCs	0 per HPF
Urine WBCs	< 5 per HPF
Urine protein	Trace
Urine microscopic	No stones

What is most likely cause of the patient's metabolic alkalosis?

A. HCO_3 infusion
B. Addison disease
C. Milk-alkali ingestion
D. Contraction alkalosis
E. Hyperemesis
F. Diarrhea
G. Bactrim use
H. Acetazolamide use
I. Ifosfamide chemotherapy

Q67-7: On examination, the patient has no focal pain and there is no evidence of compartment syndrome. What is the most important step in management of rhabdomyolysis?

A. IV fluid resuscitation
B. Acetazolamide therapy
C. Prophylactic antibiotics
D. Hyperbaric oxygen therapy
E. Continuous bladder irrigation

ANSWERS

Q67-1: A

There is no evidence for an underlying chronic respiratory or metabolic acid-base disorder in this patient, so we would assume a baseline Paco₂ of 40 mm Hg and an HCO₃ of 24 mEq/L.

Rationale: Ignoring these underlying chronic acid-base disorders can significantly alter the interpretation of a patient's acute acid-base status. This was demonstrated in the first case of the series. However, often, we do not have the necessary information (eg, prior ABG or VBG, or prior serum chemistry with an HCO₃) and are forced to assume the ongoing processes are all acute in nature. We are primarily concerned about chronic respiratory acid-base disorders, as these can significantly alter the patient's baseline or expected values for the serum HCO₃ and Paco₂, and we have reliable equations to predict the expected baseline values. The respiratory compensation for both chronic metabolic acidosis and alkalosis is generally poor, so there are no equations or rules to predict what the Paco₂ should be in these cases. While the baseline serum HCO₃ may be significantly off from our standard value of 24 mEq/L in these patients, we would assume a baseline Paco₂ of 40 mm Hg in patients with chronic metabolic processes. Once we identify the patient's baseline Paco₂ and HCO₃ values, we will need to use these values in the appropriate equations to identify the ongoing acute processes.

Q67-2: A

Metabolic acidosis only.

Rationale:

1. The pH is 7.29; therefore, the primary disorder is an **acidosis.**
2. The Paco₂ of 26 mm Hg is less than 40 mm Hg, so a primary respiratory acidosis is not present.
3. The HCO₃ of 12 mEq/L is less than 24 mEq/L, so there is a **metabolic acidosis.**

Q67-3: D

Anion gap acidosis and a metabolic alkalosis.

Rationale:

1. Is there evidence for a chronic acid-base disorder that requires adjustment of the patient's "normal" HCO₃? No, there is no evidence for a chronic acid-base disorder, so we would assume a baseline Paco₂ of 40 mm Hg and an HCO₃ of 24 mEq/L.
2. Expected anion gap:

$$\text{Expected Anion Gap} = 12 - (2.5) * \left[4.0\,\frac{g}{dL} - \text{Actual Serum Albumin} \right]$$
$$= 12 - (2.5 * [4.0 - 4.0])$$
$$= 12 - (2.5 * [0]) = \textbf{12 mEq/L.}$$

3. Anion gap calculation:

$$\text{Serum Anion Gap} = [Na^+] - [HCO_3^-] - [Cl^-]$$
$$= 140 - (89 + 12) = 39 \text{ mEq/L, which is} > 12 \text{ mEq/L}$$
$$\rightarrow \textbf{anion gap acidosis is present.}$$

4. Delta-delta calculation:

$$\Delta\Delta = \frac{(\text{Actual Anion Gap} - \text{Expected Anion Gap})}{(\text{Baseline HCO}_3 - \text{Actual HCO}_3)}$$
$$= (39 - 12)/(24 - 12) = \textbf{27/12, which is ~2.25.}$$

Delta-delta interpretation.	
Delta-Delta Value	Condition Present
< 0.4	Non-anion gap only
0.4–0.9	Anion gap *and* non-anion gap acidosis
1.0–2.0	Anion gap acidosis only
> 2.0	**Anion gap acidosis and metabolic alkalosis**

Q67-4: A
Yes, the respiratory compensation is appropriate.

Rationale: Using the Winter formula, one can calculate what the expected arterial $Paco_2$ should be for a given serum HCO_3 if the patient were completely compensated.

Respiratory Compensation for Acute Metabolic Acidosis (Winters Formula):

$$\text{Expected Paco}_2 = 1.5 * [\text{Actual HCO}_3] + 8 \pm 2 \text{ (in mm Hg)}$$
$$= (1.5 * 12) + 8 = 18 + 8 = 26 \pm 2 = (24 \text{ to } 28) \text{ mm Hg.}$$

The patient's actual $Paco_2$ of 26 mm Hg therefore represents appropriate respiratory compensation, and no additional respiratory acidosis or alkalosis exists.

Q67-5: E
Rhabdomyolysis.

Rationale: The patient has an elevated serum lactate, with normal perfusion pressure. There is no evidence of acetaminophen or salicylate toxicity. The patient's serum osmolal gap is calculated as follows:

Calculated Serum Osmolality:

$$\text{Calculated Serum Osmolality} = 2 * [Na^+] + \frac{[\text{Glucose}]}{18} + \frac{[\text{BUN}]}{2.8} + \frac{[\text{EtOH}]}{3.7}$$
$$= 2 * [140] + [80/18] + [44/2.8] + [0/3.7]$$
$$= 300 \text{ mOsm/L.}$$

The serum osmolal gap is therefore +8 mOsm/L, so there is no osmolal gap. The serum and urine ketone studies are negative, so there is no evidence of a ketoacidosis. The patient has acute renal failure with an elevated BUN and phosphorus, so this is likely contributing; however, this is not an available answer. The patient has exercise-induced rhabdomyolysis, with associated anion gap acidosis, hypokalemia, hypocalcemia, hyperphosphatemia, and a positive urine myoglobin. The anion gap acidosis in rhabdomyolysis is multifactorial, arising from the generation of lactate during anaerobic metabolism and the release of organic acids with muscle breakdown. Additionally, acute renal failure contributes the retention of phosphate and organic acids, and reduced clearance of lactate. The patient's lab values and history demonstrate no other cause consistent with an anion gap acidosis.

Q67-6: D
Contraction alkalosis.

Rationale: Rhabdomyolysis results in diuresis, and is therefore associated with significant volume depletion, and this patient has a contraction alkalosis as a result of net diuresis. The low urine chloride points to a chloride-responsive cause of the alkalosis. The only other cause of chloride-responsive metabolic alkalosis is hyperemesis, and there is no indication of this in the prompt. There is also no evidence from the vignette that the patient ingested significant antacids, and the serum calcium is low, making milk-alkali syndrome unlikely. Nor is there any indication that the patient has received an HCO_3 infusion, although this is commonly used in the treatment of rhabdomyolysis. Ifosfamide chemotherapy, acetazolamide use, trimethoprim (Bactrim) use, Addison disease, and diarrhea are all associated with a non-anion gap metabolic acidosis.

Causes of metabolic alkalosis.
History: Rule Out the Following as Causes
• Alkali load ("milk-alkali" or calcium-alkali syndrome, oral sodium bicarbonate, IV sodium bicarbonate)   • Genetic causes (CF)   • Presence of hypercalcemia   • IV β-lactam antibiotics   • Laxative abuse (may also cause a metabolic acidosis depending on diarrheal HCO_3 losses)
If None of the Above, Then . . .
Urine Chloride < 20 mEq/L (Chloride-Responsive Causes)   • Loss of gastric acid (hyperemesis, NGT suctioning)   • Prior diuretic use (in hours to days following discontinuation)   • Post-hypercapnia   • Villous adenoma   • Congenital chloridorrhea   • Chronic laxative abuse (may also cause a metabolic acidosis depending on diarrheal HCO_3 losses)   • CF

(Continued)

Causes of metabolic alkalosis. (*continued*)
OR
Urine Chloride > 20 mEq/L (Chloride-Resistant Causes)
Urine Chloride > 20 mEq/L, Lack of HTN, Urine Potassium < 30 mEq/L
• Hypokalemia or hypomagnesemia • Laxative abuse (if dominated by hypokalemia) • Bartter syndrome • Gitelman syndrome
Urine Chloride > 20 mEq/L, Lack of HTN, Urine Potassium > 30 mEq/L
• Current diuretic use
Urine Chloride > 20 mEq/L, Presence of HTN, Urine Potassium Variable but Usually > 30 mEq/L
Elevated plasma renin level: • Renal artery stenosis • Renin-secreting tumor • Renovascular disease
Low plasma renin, low plasma aldosterone: • Cushing syndrome • Exogenous mineralocorticoid use • Genetic disorder (11-hydoxylase or 17-hydrolyase deficiency, 11β-HSD deficiency) • Liddle syndrome • Licorice toxicity
Low plasma renin, high plasma aldosterone: • Primary hyperaldosteronism • Adrenal adenoma • Bilateral adrenal hyperplasia

Q67-7: A
IV fluid resuscitation.

Rationale: Aside from identifying any limb trauma and ruling out compartment syndrome, IV fluid resuscitation is the most critical step in the management of rhabdomyolysis. This should be initiated as soon as possible after diagnosis. No randomized controlled trials have been performed to identify the best fluid repletion regimen, with sodium bicarbonate (150 mEq/L in D5), normal saline, and lactate Ringer solution being the most commonly used solutions. Isotonic IV fluid resuscitation, when adequate to maintain urine output above 1 mL/kg/h, is associated with more rapid improvements in renal function. Injured myocytes swell considerably, consuming large volumes of extracellular fluid, and patients may often require more than 60 mL/kg of isotonic fluid. Renal failure results from precipitation of toxins (ferrihemate), formation of uric acid crystals, and reduced glomerular filtration. The use of sodium bicarbonate infusion (150 mEq/L in D5, which is nearly isotonic) allows for alkalinization of the urine, which prevents the formation of nephrotoxic ferrihemate precipitates, which occurs more readily below a urinary pH of ~5.8. Evidence supporting the use of sodium bicarbonate infusion as opposed to other isotonic solutions is based on retrospective reviews and smaller animal studies, with no randomized clinical trials to date. This issue remains highly debated, although sodium bicarbonate infusions are generally used in patients presenting with metabolic acidemia. Diuretics can be used in patients in whom volume status is a concern or in those with urine output below the target of 2 mL/kg/h (or 200 mL/h).The diuretics of choice are generally mannitol (osmotic diuresis) or furosemide. Correction of electrolyte abnormalities is also essential in these patients, particularly management of hyperkalemia. Dialysis (renal replacement therapy) may be required in patients with oliguric failure, severe acid-base or electrolyte abnormalities, or conditions that would prevent administration of large volumes of IV fluid (congestive heart failure, pulmonary hypertension, cirrhosis).

References

Abreo K, Adlakha A, Kilpatrick S, et al. The milk-alkali syndrome. A reversible form of acute renal failure. Arch Intern Med. 1993;153:1005.

Al-Ismaili Z, Piccioni M, Zappitelli M. Rhabdomyolysis: pathogenesis of renal injury and management. Pediatr Nephrol. 2011;26:1781.

Barton CH, Vaziri ND, Ness RL, et al. Cimetidine in the management of metabolic alkalosis induced by nasogastric drainage. Arch Surg. 1979;114:70.

Bear R, Goldstein M, Phillipson E, et al. Effect of metabolic alkalosis on respiratory function in patients with chronic obstructive lung disease. Can Med Assoc J. 1977;117:900.

Bosch X, Poch E, Grau JM. Rhabdomyolysis and acute kidney injury. N Engl J Med. 2009;361:62.

Cervellin G, Comelli I, Benatti M, et al. Non-traumatic rhabdomyolysis: background, laboratory features, and acute clinical management. Clin Biochem. 2017;50:656.

Furman J. When exercise causes exertional rhabdomyolysis. JAAPA. 2015;28:38.

Galla JH, Gifford JD, Luke RG, Rome L. Adaptations to chloride-depletion alkalosis. Am J Physiol. 1991;261:R771.

Garella S, Chang BS, Kahn SI. Dilution acidosis and contraction alkalosis: review of a concept. Kidney Int. 1975;8:279.

Gennari FJ, Weise WJ. Acid-base disturbances in gastrointestinal disease. Clin J Am Soc Nephrol. 2008;3:1861.

Hamm LL, Nakhoul N, Hering-Smith KS. Acid-base homeostasis. Clin J Am Soc Nephrol. 2015;10:2232.

Hohenegger M. Drug induced rhabdomyolysis. Curr Opin Pharmacol. 2012;12:335.

Hulter HN, Sebastian A, Toto RD, et al. Renal and systemic acid-base effects of the chronic administration of hypercalcemia-producing agents: calcitriol, PTH, and intravenous calcium. Kidney Int. 1982;21:445.

Khanna A, Kurtzman NA. Metabolic alkalosis. J Nephrol. 2006;19(suppl 9):S86.

Laski ME, Sabatini S. Metabolic alkalosis, bedside and bench. Semin Nephrol. 2006;26:404.

Luke RG, Galla JH. It is chloride depletion alkalosis, not contraction alkalosis. J Am Soc Nephrol. 2012;23:204.

McKinney B, Gaunder C, Schumer R. Acute exertional compartment syndrome with rhabdomyolysis: case report and review of literature. Am J Case Rep. 2018;19:145.

Miller PD, Berns AS. Acute metabolic alkalosis perpetuating hypercarbia. A role for acetazolamide in chronic obstructive pulmonary disease. JAMA. 1977;238:2400.

Oster JR, Materson BJ, Rogers AI. Laxative abuse syndrome. Am J Gastroenterol. 1980;74:451.

Oster JR, Singer I, Contreras GN, et al. Metabolic acidosis with extreme elevation of anion gap: case report and literature review. Am J Med Sci. 1999;317:38.

Patel AM, Goldfarb S. Got calcium? Welcome to the calcium-alkali syndrome. J Am Soc Nephrol. 2010;21:1440.

Petejova N, Martinek A. Acute kidney injury due to rhabdomyolysis and renal replacement therapy: a critical review. Crit Care. 2014;18:224.

Rose BD, Post TW. Clinical Physiology of Acid-Base and Electrolyte Disorders, 5e. New York, NY: McGraw Hill; 2001:559.

Schwartz WB, Van Ypersele de Strihou, Kassirer JP. Role of anions in metabolic alkalosis and potassium deficiency. N Engl J Med. 1968;279:630.

Singhal PC, Rubin RB, Peters A, et al. Rhabdomyolysis and acute renal failure associated with cocaine abuse. Toxicol Clin Toxicol. 1990;28:321.

Sweetser LJ, Douglas JA, Riha RL, Bell SC. Clinical presentation of metabolic alkalosis in an adult patient with cystic fibrosis. Respirology. 2005;10:254.

Taki K, Mizuno K, Takahashi N, Wakusawa R. Disturbance of CO2 elimination in the lungs by carbonic anhydrase inhibition. Jpn J Physiol. 1986;36:523.

Turban S, Beutler KT, Morris RG, et al. Long-term regulation of proximal tubule acid-base transporter abundance by angiotensin II. Kidney Int. 2006;70:660.

CASE 68

A 34-year-old man from Kenya, on vacation in the United States, presents to the emergency department with diffuse abdominal pain and nausea. He has HIV, is currently on HAART therapy including D4T (stavudine—an HIV nucleoside analog reverse transcriptase inhibitor that is no longer used in the United States). He has a history of multiple prior bouts of pancreatitis at home, states that he does not consume alcohol, and had a cholecystectomy and an appendectomy several years ago. He mentions that his pancreas is "not normal." A CT scan demonstrates peripancreatic stranding consistent with acute pancreatitis. The lipase level is 23,000. His vital signs are T 37.9°C, HR 130, BP 120/60, RR 28, and Sao$_2$ 90% on room air. His abdomen is diffusely tender with guarding but no rebound.

Laboratory data.			
ABGs		Basic Metabolic Panel	
pH	7.57	Na	140 mEq/L
Paco$_2$	19 mm Hg	K	2.9 mEq/L
Pao$_2$	60 mm Hg	Cl	106 mEq/L
HCO$_3$	17 mEq/L	CO$_2$	17 mEq/L
		BUN	54 mg/dL
		Cr	1.8 mg/dL
		Glucose	132 mg/dL
		Albumin	4.0 g/dL
		EtOH	0 mg/dL

QUESTIONS

Q68-1: Define the patient's baseline acid-base status: Does this patient have an underlying chronic acid-base disorder that we need to account for in order to appropriately interpret the acute acid-base disorders?

A. There is no evidence for an underlying chronic respiratory or metabolic acid-base disorder in this patient, so we would assume a baseline $Paco_2$ of 40 mm Hg and an HCO_3 of 24 mEq/L.

B. While the patient has a condition predisposing him to a chronic acid-base disorder, there is insufficient information to estimate the patient's baseline $Paco_2$ and HCO_3 values; therefore, we will assume a baseline $Paco_2$ of 40 mm Hg and a baseline HCO_3 of 24 mEq/L.

C. The patient has an underlying acid-base condition, and we have sufficient information to estimate the patient's baseline $Paco_2$ and HCO_3 values.

Q68-2: What is/are the primary acid-base disturbance(s) occurring in this case?

A. Metabolic acidosis only
B. Respiratory acidosis only
C. Metabolic acidosis and a respiratory acidosis
D. Metabolic alkalosis and a respiratory alkalosis
E. Metabolic alkalosis only
F. Respiratory alkalosis only

Q68-3: Does the patient in this case demonstrate appropriate metabolic compensation?

A. Yes, the respiratory compensation is appropriate.
B. No, a concomitant respiratory alkalosis is present.
C. No, a concomitant respiratory acidosis is present.
D. Yes, the metabolic compensation is appropriate.
E. No, a concomitant metabolic acidosis is present.
F. No, a concomitant metabolic alkalosis is present.

Q68-4: How would the metabolic acidosis component be classified in this case?

A. Anion gap acidosis
B. Non-anion gap acidosis
C. Anion and non-anion gap acidosis
D. Anion gap acidosis and a metabolic alkalosis

Q68-5: The patient receives 3 L of IV isotonic fluid and pain medication. His BP remains within normal limits. His remaining laboratory values are as follows:

Serum EtOH	< 3 mg/dL
Serum acetaminophen	< 5 mg/dL (ULN for therapeutic use 20 mg/dL)
Serum salicylates	< 5 mg/dL (ULN for therapeutic use 30 mg/dL)
Serum osmolality	313 mOsm/kg
Serum L-lactate	4.4 mmol/L (ULN 2.0 mmol/L venous)
Beta-hydroxybutyrate (acetone)	< 0.18 mmol/L (ULN 0.18 mmol/L)
Serum glucose	132 mg/dL
Serum phosphorus	2.3 mg/dL
Serum calcium	5.7 mmol/L

What is the likely cause of the patient's anion gap acidosis?

A. Aspirin toxicity
B. Lactic acidosis
C. Ethylene glycol toxicity
D. Methanol toxicity
E. Opioid overdose
F. Acetaminophen overdose
G. Diabetic ketoacidosis
H. Alcoholic ketoacidosis

Q68-6: The urine electrolyte values are shown as follows. The patient denies any recent diarrhea.

Urine Na	5 mEq/L
Urine K	50 mEq/L
Urine Cl	65 mEq/L
Urine urea	284 mg/dL
Urine glucose	0 mg/dL
Urine osmolality	678 mOsm/L
Urine pH	5.2
Urine RBCs	None
Urine WBCs	None
Urine protein	None
Urine microscopic	None

What is the most likely type of non-anion gap acidosis present?

A. Diarrhea
B. Pancreaticoduodenal fistula
C. Ureteroenteric fistula
D. Type 1 RTA (distal tubule)
E. Type 2 RTA (proximal tubule)
F. Type 4 RTA (distal tubule/collecting duct)

ANSWERS

Q68-1: B

While the patient has a condition predisposing him to a chronic acid-base disorder, there is insufficient information to estimate the patient's baseline $Paco_2$ and HCO_3 values; therefore, we will assume a baseline $Paco_2$ of 40 mm Hg and a baseline HCO_3 of 24 mEq/L. The patient has HIV, which can be associated with chronic metabolic acid-base disorders. However, no information is provided in the prompt to support that scenario at this point.

Rationale: Ignoring these underlying chronic acid-base disorders can significantly alter the interpretation of a patient's acute acid-base status. This was demonstrated in the first case of the series. However, often, we do not have the necessary information (eg, prior ABG or VBG, or prior serum chemistry with an HCO_3) and are forced to assume the ongoing processes are all acute in nature. We are primarily concerned about chronic respiratory acid-base disorders, as these can significantly alter the patient's baseline or expected values for the serum HCO_3 and $Paco_2$, and we have reliable equations to predict the expected baseline values. The respiratory compensation for both chronic metabolic acidosis and alkalosis is generally poor, so there are no equations or rules to predict what the $Paco_2$ should be in these cases. While the baseline serum HCO_3 may be significantly off from our standard value of 24 mEq/L in these patients, we would assume a baseline $Paco_2$ of 40 mm Hg in patients with chronic metabolic processes. Once we identify the patient's baseline $Paco_2$ and HCO_3 values, we will need to use these values in the appropriate equations to identify the ongoing acute processes.

Q68-2: F

Respiratory alkalosis only.

Rationale:

1. The pH is 7.57; therefore, the primary disorder is an **alkalosis**.
2. The $Paco_2$ of 19 mm Hg is less than 40 mm Hg, so there is a **respiratory alkalosis**.
3. The HCO_3 of 17 mEq/L is less than 24 mEq/L, so a primary metabolic alkalosis is not present.

Q68-3: E

No, a concomitant metabolic acidosis is present.

Rationale: Assuming the respiratory alkalosis is acute, the renal compensation can be calculated as follows:

Metabolic Compensation for Acute Respiratory Alkalosis:

$$\text{Expected } HCO_3 = \text{Baseline } HCO_3 - (0.20)[\text{Actual } Paco_2 - \text{Baseline } Paco_2]$$
$$= 24 - (0.20) * [40 - 19]$$
$$= 24 - (0.20) * [21] = 19.8 \text{, which is } \sim\textbf{20 mEq/L.}$$

The patient's HCO_3 of 17 mEq/L is lower than expected, so the patient has a concomitant metabolic acidosis.

Q68-4: C
Anion and non-anion gap acidosis.

Rationale:

1. Is there evidence for a chronic acid-base disorder that requires adjustment of the patient's "normal" HCO_3? No, there is no evidence for a chronic acid-base disorder, so we would assume a baseline $Paco_2$ of 40 mm Hg and an HCO_3 of 24 mEq/L.
2. Expected anion gap:

$$\text{Expected Anion Gap} = 12 - (2.5) * \left[4.0 \frac{g}{dL} - \text{Actual Serum Albumin} \right]$$
$$= 12 - (2.5 * [4.0 - 4.0])$$
$$= 12 - (2.5 * [0]) = \textbf{12 mEq/L.}$$

3. Anion gap calculation:

$$\text{Serum Anion Gap} = [Na^+] - [HCO_3^-] - [Cl^-]$$
$$= 140 - (106 + 17) = 17 \text{ mEq/L, which is} > 12 \text{ mEq/L}$$
$$\rightarrow \textbf{anion gap acidosis is present.}$$

4. Delta-delta calculation:

$$\Delta\Delta = \frac{(\text{Actual Anion Gap} - \text{Expected Anion Gap})}{(\text{Baseline } HCO_3 - \text{Actual } HCO_3)}$$
$$= (17 - 12)/(24 - 17) = \textbf{5/7, which is } \textbf{~0.7.}$$

Delta-delta interpretation.	
Delta-Delta Value	Condition Present
< 0.4	Non-anion gap only
0.4–0.9	**Anion gap *and* non-anion gap acidosis**
1.0–2.0	Anion gap acidosis only
> 2.0	Anion gap acidosis and metabolic alkalosis

Q68-5: B
Lactic acidosis.

Rationale: The patient has a lactic acidosis. The patient has an anion gap acidosis, with a negative ketone study. The calculated serum osmolality is:

$$\text{Calculated Serum Osmolality} = 2 * [Na^+] + \frac{[\text{Glucose}]}{18} + \frac{[\text{BUN}]}{2.8} + \frac{[\text{EtOH}]}{3.7}$$
$$= 2 * [140] + [132/18] + [54/2.8] + [0/3.7]$$
$$= 307 \text{ mOsm/L.}$$

Therefore, the serum osmolal gap is +6 mOsm/L, which is normal, making an organic alcohol ingestion highly unlikely. Additionally, the patient has negative acetaminophen and salicylate levels. Therefore, a lactic acidosis is the most likely etiology of those remaining. The reduced calcium is classically seen in pancreatitis due to saponification.

This is a *type B lactic acidosis*, as the patient currently has no apparent perfusion/oxygen delivery issue. The patient is taking a medication called D4T (stavudine), which is associated with both medication-induced lactic acidosis (via mitochondrial toxicity) and medication-associated pancreatitis. Although this medication is not used in most developed nations, it can still be prescribed in some developing countries. There has been significant effort to replace this medication in all HAART regimens throughout the world due to its serious adverse effects.

Other medications and conditions associated with type B lactic acidosis include metformin (phenformin was much more common but is no longer prescribed in the United States), valproic acid, INH, antiretroviral drugs, severe renal and/or hepatic dysfunction, thiamine deficiency, poisoning or uncoupling of the electron transport chain for oxidative phosphorylation (eg, cyanide), pheochromocytoma, pyruvate dehydrogenase deficiency, glucose-6-phosphate deficiency, malignancies (particularly aggressive lymphomas and leukemias), and hypoglycemia.

Q68-6: B
Pancreaticoduodenal fistula.

Rationale: The patient has a slightly negative urine anion gap, an elevated urine osmolal gap, and a low serum potassium (2.8 mEq/L).

Urine Anion Gap:

$$\text{Urine Anion Gap} = [U_{Na}] + [U_K] - [U_{Cl}]$$
$$= [5] + [50] - [65] = (-10) \text{ mEq/L.}$$

Calculated Urine Osmolality:

$$\text{Urine Osmolality} = 2*[U_{Na} + U_K] + \frac{[U_{BUN}]}{2.8} + \frac{[U_{glucose}]}{18}$$
$$= 2*[5 + 50] + [284/2.8] + [0/18] = 211 \text{ mOsm/L}$$
$$\text{Urine Osmolal Gap} = 678 - 211 \text{ mOsm/L}$$
$$= 467 \text{ mOsm/L } (> 400 \text{ mOsm/L}).$$

The vignette indicates that the patient did not report any diarrhea, but he has a history of chronic pancreatitis and an anatomic abnormality. This is most consistent with a pancreaticoduodenal fistula, which can arise from recurrent episodes of pancreatitis. The low serum potassium is also consistent with this finding.

Cause of NAGMA.
Evaluation Strategy
1. History (acute or chronic issues, medications, altered GI anatomy, genetic diseases, etc).
2. Does the patient have chronic renal insufficiency? If so, this alone may be responsible for the non-anion gap acidosis.
3. Calculate urine anion gap and urine osmolal gap. The urine anion gap may be of limited value in patients with severe serum anion gap acidosis, as it may be falsely elevated. Similarly, the urine osmolal gap may be inappropriately elevated in patients with a significant serum osmolal gap (particularly due to mannitol).
4. Note the serum potassium as well as the urine pH.
5. If proximal RTA is suspected, look for evidence of other inappropriate compounds in the urine (amino acids, elevated phosphate, glucosuria), and calculate the fractional resorption of sodium bicarbonate (should be > 15%). Also check serum for evidence of dysfunctional of the PTH–vitamin D–calcium axis.
Low Serum Potassium
GI: Diarrhea, pancreaticoduodenal fistula, urinary intestinal diversion Renal: Type 1 RTA (distal), type 2 RTA (proximal) Medications/exposures: Carbonic anhydrase inhibitors, toluene Other: D-Lactic acidosis
High (or Normal) Serum Potassium
GI: Elevated ileostomy output Renal: Type 4 RTA or CKD Medications: NSAIDs; antibiotics (trimethoprim, pentamidine); heparin; ACE inhibitors, ARBs, aldosterone antagonists (spironolactone); acid administration (TPN)

References

Adinaro D. Liver failure and pancreatitis. Fluid and electrolyte concerns. Nurs Clin North Am. 1987;22:843.

Calza L, Manfredi R, Chiodo F. Hyperlactataemia and lactic acidosis in HIV-infected patients receiving antiretroviral therapy. Clin Nutr. 2005;24:5.

Claessens YE, Chiche JD, Mira JP, Cariou A. Bench-to-bedside review: severe lactic acidosis in HIV patients treated with nucleoside analogue reverse transcriptase inhibitors. Crit Care. 2003;7:226.

Cornejo-Juárez P, Sierra-Madero J, Volkow-Fernández P. Metabolic acidosis and hepatic steatosis in two HIV-infected patients on stavudine (d4T) treatment. Arch Med Res. 2003;34:64.

Khouri S, Cushing H. Lactic acidosis secondary to nucleoside analogue antiretroviral therapy. AIDS Read. 2000;10:602.

Mokrzycki MH, Harris C, May H, et al. Lactic acidosis associated with stavudine administration: a report of five cases. Clin Infect Dis. 2000;30:198.

CASE 69

A 44-year-old woman is transferred to the ICU. She underwent a bowel resection for ischemia related to abdominal adhesions 14 days ago but has had a slow recovery. She was started on total parenteral nutrition (TPN) 11 days ago because she was unable to take PO nutrition due to frequent nausea, but she has not been experiencing emesis. This morning, she developed fever, hypotension, tachycardia, and respiratory distress necessitating the transfer to the ICU. The patient's vital signs are as follows: T 39.7°C, RR 22, HR 130, BP 70/50, and Sao_2 98% on RA. She is on a PCA pump for abdominal pain, and otherwise was started on broad-spectrum antibiotics (linezolid, ceftazidime) prior to transfer. Results of the patient's blood cultures and urine culture are pending; her UA shows no evidence of infection. Her abdominal wound appears clean, dry, and well-healing, with no discharge. She has mild abdominal tenderness with no rebound tenderness or guarding. At baseline, the patient has no known medical issues, and takes only OTC medications on a PRN basis. She does not smoke or use drugs, and drinks 2 to 3 alcoholic beverages per week.

Laboratory data.			
ABGs		Basic Metabolic Panel	
pH	7.24	Na	140 mEq/L
$Paco_2$	34 mm Hg	K	4 mEq/L
Pao_2	60 mm Hg	Cl	115 mEq/L
HCO_3	16 mEq/L	CO_2	16 mEq/L
		BUN	34 mg/dL
		Cr	1.8 mg/dL
		Glucose	66 mg/dL
		Albumin	1.5 g/dL
		EtOH	0 mg/dL

QUESTIONS

Q69-1: Define the patient's baseline acid-base status: Does this patient have an underlying chronic acid-base disorder that we need to account for in order to appropriately interpret the acute acid-base disorders?

A. There is no evidence for an underlying chronic respiratory or metabolic acid-base disorder in this patient, so we would assume a baseline $Paco_2$ of 40 mm Hg and an HCO_3 of 24 mEq/L.

B. While the patient has a condition predisposing her to a chronic acid-base disorder, there is insufficient information to estimate the patient's baseline $Paco_2$ and HCO_3 values; therefore, we will assume a baseline $Paco_2$ of 40 mm Hg and a baseline HCO_3 of 24 mEq/L.

C. The patient has an underlying acid-base condition, and we have sufficient information to estimate the patient's baseline $Paco_2$ and HCO_3 values.

Q69-2: What is/are the primary acute acid-base disturbance(s) occurring in this case?

A. Metabolic acidosis only
B. Respiratory acidosis only
C. Metabolic acidosis and a respiratory acidosis
D. Metabolic alkalosis and a respiratory alkalosis
E. Metabolic alkalosis only
F. Respiratory alkalosis only

Q69-3: How would the metabolic acidosis component be classified in this case?

A. Anion gap acidosis
B. Non-anion gap acidosis
C. Anion and non-anion gap acidosis
D. Anion gap acidosis and a metabolic alkalosis

Q69-4: Does the patient in this case demonstrate appropriate respiratory or metabolic compensation?

A. Yes, the respiratory compensation is appropriate.
B. No, a concomitant respiratory alkalosis is present.
C. No, a concomitant respiratory acidosis is present.
D. Yes, the metabolic compensation is appropriate.
E. No, a concomitant metabolic acidosis is present.
F. No, a concomitant metabolic alkalosis is present.

Q69-5: Additional laboratory test results are as follows:

Serum EtOH	< 3 mg/dL
Serum acetaminophen	< 5 mg/dL (ULN for therapeutic use 20 mg/dL)
Serum salicylates	< 5 mg/dL (ULN for therapeutic use 30 mg/dL)
Serum osmolality	299 mOsm/kg
Serum L-lactate	5.1 mmol/L (ULN 2.0 mmol/L venous)
Beta-hydroxybutyrate (acetone)	< 0.18 mmol/L (ULN 0.18 mmol/L)
Serum glucose	66 mg/dL
Urine ketones	Negative

What is the likely cause of the patient's anion gap acidosis?

A. Aspirin toxicity
B. Lactic acidosis secondary to sepsis
C. Opioid overdose
D. Acetaminophen overdose
E. Diabetic ketoacidosis
F. Alcoholic ketoacidosis

Q69-6: The patient's urine anion gap is equivocal at +2 mEq/L. The urine osmolar gap is 400 mOsm/L. What is the likely cause of the patient's non-anion gap acidosis?

A. Diarrhea
B. Hyperemesis
C. Ureteroenteric fistula
D. Addison disease
E. Type 1 RTA (distal tubule)
F. Acetazolamide use
G. Parenteral nutrition
H. Type 4 RTA (distal tubule/collecting duct)

ANSWERS

Q69-1: A

There is no evidence for an underlying chronic respiratory or metabolic acid-base disorder in this patient, so we would assume a baseline $Paco_2$ of 40 mm Hg and an HCO_3 of 24 mEq/L.

Rationale: Ignoring these underlying chronic acid-base disorders can significantly alter the interpretation of a patient's acute acid-base status. This was demonstrated in the first case of the series. However, often, we do not have the necessary information (eg, prior ABG or VBG, or prior serum chemistry with an HCO_3) and are forced to assume the ongoing processes are all acute in nature. We are primarily concerned about chronic respiratory acid-base disorders, as these can significantly alter the patient's baseline or expected values for the serum HCO_3 and $Paco_2$, and we have reliable equations to predict the expected baseline values. The respiratory compensation for both chronic metabolic acidosis and alkalosis is generally poor, so there are no equations or rules to predict what the $Paco_2$ should be in these cases. While the baseline serum HCO_3 may be significantly off from our standard value of 24 mEq/L in these patients, we would assume a baseline $Paco_2$ of 40 mm Hg in patients with chronic metabolic processes. Once we identify the patient's baseline $Paco_2$ and HCO_3 values, we will need to use these values in the appropriate equations to identify the ongoing acute processes.

Q69-2: A

Metabolic acidosis only.

Rationale:

1. The pH is 7.24; therefore, the primary disorder is an **acidosis.**
2. The $Paco_2$ of 34 mm Hg is less than 40 mm Hg, so this is not a primary respiratory acidosis.
3. The HCO_3 of 16 mEq/L is less than 24 mEq/L, so there is a **metabolic acidosis.**

Therefore, this patient has a primary metabolic acidosis.

Q69-3: C

Anion and non-anion gap acidosis.

Rationale:

1. Is there evidence for a chronic acid-base disorder that requires adjustment of the patient's "normal" HCO_3? No, there is no evidence for a chronic acid-base disorder, so we would assume a baseline $Paco_2$ of 40 mm Hg and an HCO_3 of 24 mEq/L.

2. Expected anion gap:

$$\text{Expected Anion Gap} = 12 - (2.5) * \left[4.0\frac{g}{dL} - \text{Actual Serum Albumin} \right]$$
$$= 12 - (2.5 * [4.0 - 1.5])$$
$$= 12 - (2.5 * [2.5]) = \textbf{6 mEq/L.}$$

3. Anion gap calculation:

$$\text{Serum Anion Gap} = [Na^+] - [HCO_3^-] - [Cl^-]$$
$$= 140 - (115 + 16) = 9 \text{ mEq/L, which is} > 6 \text{ mEq/L}$$
$$\rightarrow \textbf{anion gap acidosis is present.}$$

4. Delta-delta calculation:

$$\Delta\Delta = \frac{(\text{Actual Anion Gap} - \text{Expected Anion Gap})}{(\text{Baseline HCO}_3 - \text{Actual HCO}_3)}$$
$$= (9 - 6)/(24 - 17) = 3/7, \text{ which is } \sim 0.4.$$

Delta-delta table:	
Delta-Delta Value	**Condition Present**
< 0.4	Non-anion gap only
0.4–0.9	**Anion gap *and* non-anion gap acidosis**
1.0–2.0	Anion gap acidosis only
> 2.0	Anion gap acidosis and metabolic alkalosis

Q69-4: A
Yes, the respiratory compensation is appropriate.

Rationale: Using the Winter formula, one can calculate what the expected arterial $Paco_2$ should be for a given serum HCO_3 if the patient were completely compensated.

Respiratory Compensation for Acute Metabolic Acidosis (Winter Formula):

$$\text{Expected Paco}_2 = 1.5 * [\text{Actual HCO}_3] + 8 \pm 2 \text{ (in mm Hg)}$$
$$= (1.5 * 16) + 8 = 24 + 8 = 32 \pm 2 = (30 \text{ to } 34) \text{ mm Hg.}$$

This patient has an appropriate compensatory response to the metabolic acidosis.

Q69-5: B
Lactic acidosis secondary to sepsis.

Rationale: The patient has severe sepsis with hypotension, fever, tachycardia, and tachypnea. She is on TPN, which is a potential source of infection. Additionally, she had recent abdominal surgery and has been in the hospital for a prolonged period of time. Starvation ketosis is a possible consideration, but the beta-hydroxybutyrate and urine ketones are negative, and therefore the more likely answer is lactic acidosis due to sepsis. The serum osmolal gap is only 3 mOsm/L, so there is no evidence of an organic alcohol ingestion.

$$\text{Calculated Serum Osmolality} = 2*[Na^+] + \frac{[Glucose]}{18} + \frac{[BUN]}{2.8} + \frac{[EtOH]}{3.7}$$
$$= 296 \text{ mOsm/L}$$
$$\text{Serum Osmolal Gap} = 299 \text{ mOsm/kg (or L water)} - 296 \text{ mOsm/L}$$
$$= (+3) \text{ mOsm/L (no osmolal gap)}.$$

Q69-6: G
Parental nutrition.

Rationale: Parenteral nutrition (TPN) is associated with the development of a non-anion gap acidosis, although the use of the urine anion gap is not always straightforward as these patients often have both GI and renal contributions. TPN is associated with excess chloride administration and an increased acid administration. The increased acid load results from cationic amino acids and amino acid formulations containing titratable acids, particularly sulfuric acid. Additionally, these patients often have significantly altered carbohydrate and lipid metabolism and also suffer from thiamine deficiency and hypophosphatemia, which may further contribute to the metabolic acidosis. The non-anion gap acidosis is usually transient during TPN administration.

The equivocal urine anion gap and the elevated urine osmolar gap rules out a renal issue with urinary acidification (eg, a type 1 or type 4 RTA), as well as Addison disease. Diarrhea is usually associated with a significantly negative urine anion gap (−20 to −50 mEq/L). Hyperemesis is usually associated with a metabolic alkalosis. Acetazolamide causes a type 2 proximal RTA, which is possible here, although there is no evidence leading us to think the patient would have received this drug. The normal serum K also argues against a type 2 RTA. There is no reason to suspect a ureteroenteric fistula in this patient. A pancreaticoduodenal fistula would potentially be of concern if the patient had small bowel resection or pancreatitis issues, but that is not an option here.

Cause of NAGMA.
Evaluation Strategy
1. History (acute or chronic issues, medications, altered GI anatomy, genetic diseases, etc).
2. Does the patient have chronic renal insufficiency? If so, this alone may be responsible for the non-anion gap acidosis.
3. Calculate urine anion gap and urine osmolal gap. The urine anion gap may be of limited value in patients with severe serum anion gap acidosis, as it may be falsely elevated. Similarly, the urine osmolal gap may be inappropriately elevated in patients with a significant serum osmolal gap (particularly due to mannitol).
4. Note the serum potassium as well as the urine pH.
5. If proximal RTA is suspected, look for evidence of other inappropriate compounds in the urine (amino acids, elevated phosphate, glucosuria), and calculate the fractional resorption of sodium bicarbonate (should be > 15%). Also check serum for evidence of dysfunctional of the PTH–vitamin D–calcium axis.

(Continued)

Cause of NAGMA. (*continued*)
Low Serum Potassium
GI: Diarrhea, pancreaticoduodenal fistula, urinary intestinal diversion Renal: Type 1 RTA (distal), type 2 RTA (proximal) Medications/exposures: Carbonic anhydrase inhibitors, toluene Other: D-Lactic acidosis
High (or Normal) Serum Potassium
GI: Elevated ileostomy output Renal: Type 4 RTA or CKD Medications: NSAIDs; antibiotics (trimethoprim, pentamidine); heparin; ACE inhibitors, ARBs, aldosterone antagonists (spironolactone); acid administration (TPN)

Evaluation of RTA.			
	Type I RTA	**Type 2 RTA**	**Type 4 RTA**
Severity of metabolic acidosis, (HCO_3)	Severe (< 10–12 mEq/L typically)	Intermediate (12–20 mEq/L)	Mild (15–20 mEq/L)
Associated urine abnormalities	Urinary phosphate, calcium are increased; bone disease often present	Urine glucose, amino acids, phosphate, calcium may be elevated	
Urine pH	HIGH (> 5.5)	Low (acidic), until serum HCO_3 level exceeds the resorptive ability of the proximal tubule; then becomes alkalotic once reabsorptive threshold is crossed	Low (acidic)
Serum K^+	Low to normal; should correct with oral HCO_3 therapy	Classically low, although may be normal or even high with rare genetic defects; worsens with oral HCO_3 therapy	HIGH
Renal stones	Often	No	No
Renal tubular defect	Reduced NH_4 secretion in distal tubule	Reduced HCO_3 resorption in proximal tubule	Reduced H^+/K^+ exchange in distal and collecting tubule due to decreased aldosterone or aldosterone resistance
Urine anion gap	> 10	Negative initially, then positive when receiving serum HCO_3, then negative after therapy	> 10
Urine osmolal gap	Reduced (< 150 mOsm/L) during acute acidosis	At baseline < 100 mEq/L; unreliable during acidosis	Reduced (< 150 mOsm/L) during acute acidosis

Causes of RTA.
Causes of Type 1 (Distal) RTA
Primary   • Idiopathic or familial (may be recessive or dominant)
Secondary   • Medications: Lithium, amphotericin, ifosfamide, NSAIDs   • Rheumatologic disorders: Sjögren syndrome, SLE, RA   • Hypercalciuria (idiopathic) or associated with vitamin D deficiency or hyperparathyroidism   • Sarcoidosis   • Obstructive uropathy   • Wilson disease   • Rejection of renal transplant allograft   • Toluene toxicity
Causes of Type 2 (Proximal) RTA
Primary   • Idiopathic   • Familial (primarily recessive disorders)   • Genetic: Fanconi syndrome, cystinosis, glycogen storage disease (type 1), Wilson disease, galactosemia
Secondary   • Medications: Acetazolamide, topiramate, aminoglycoside antibiotics, ifosfamide, reverse transcriptase inhibitors (tenofovir)   • Heavy metal poisoning: Lead, mercury, copper   • Multiple myeloma or amyloidosis (secondary to light chain toxicity)   • Sjögren syndrome   • Vitamin D deficiency   • Rejection of renal transplant allograft
Causes of Type 4 RTA (Hypoaldosteronism or Aldosterone Resistance)
Primary   • Primary adrenal insufficiency   • Inherited disorders associated with hypoaldosteronism   • Pseudohypoaldosteronism (types 1 and 2)
Secondary   • Causes of hyporeninemic hypoaldosteronism such as renal disease (diabetic nephropathy), NSAID use, calcineurin inhibitors, volume expansion/volume overload   • Causes of distal tubule voltage defects such as sickle cell disease, obstructive uropathy, SLE   • Severe illness/septic shock   • Angiotensin II–associated medications: ACE inhibitors, ARBs, direct renin inhibitors   • Potassium-sparing diuretics: Spironolactone, amiloride, triamterene   • Antibiotics: Trimethoprim, pentamidine

References

Arroliga AC, Shehab N, McCarthy K, Gonzales JP. Relationship of continuous infusion lorazepam to serum propylene glycol concentration in critically ill adults. Crit Care Med. 2004;32:1709.

Batlle D, Grupp M, Gaviria M, Kurtzman NA. Distal renal tubular acidosis with intact capacity to lower urinary pH. Am J Med. 1982;72:751.

Batlle D, Haque SK. Genetic causes and mechanisms of distal renal tubular acidosis. Nephrol Dial Transplant. 2012;27:3691.

Batlle DC, Hizon M, Cohen E, et al. The use of the urinary anion gap in the diagnosis of hyperchloremic metabolic acidosis. N Engl J Med. 1988;318:594.

Batlle DC, von Riotte A, Schlueter W. Urinary sodium in the evaluation of hyperchloremic metabolic acidosis. N Engl J Med. 1987;316:140.

Braden GL, Strayhorn CH, Germain MJ, et al. Increased osmolal gap in alcoholic acidosis. Arch Intern Med. 1993;153:2377.

Buckalew VM Jr, McCurdy DK, Ludwig GD, et al. Incomplete renal tubular acidosis. Physiologic studies in three patients with a defect in lowering urine pH. Am J Med. 1968;45:32.

Dounousi E, Zikou X, Koulouras V, Katopodis K. Metabolic acidosis during parenteral nutrition: pathophysiological mechanisms. Indian J Crit Care Med. 2015;19:270.

Dudrick SJ, Maharaj AR, McKelvey AA. Artificial nutritional support in patients with gastrointestinal fistulas. World J Surg. 1999;23:570.

Dyck RF, Asthana S, Kalra J, et al. A modification of the urine osmolal gap: an improved method for estimating urine ammonium. Am J Nephrol. 1990;10:359.

Gabow PA. Ethylene glycol intoxication. Am J Kidney Dis. 1988;11:277.

Gennari FJ. Current concepts. Serum osmolality. Uses and limitations. N Engl J Med. 1984;310:102.

Glasser L, Sternglanz PD, Combie J, Robinson A. Serum osmolality and its applicability to drug overdose. Am J Clin Pathol. 1973;60:695.

Karet FE. Mechanisms in hyperkalemic renal tubular acidosis. J Am Soc Nephrol. 2009;20:251.

Kim GH, Han JS, Kim YS, et al. Evaluation of urine acidification by urine anion gap and urine osmolal gap in chronic metabolic acidosis. Am J Kidney Dis. 1996;27:42.

Kraut JA, Kurtz I. Toxic alcohol ingestions: clinical features, diagnosis, and management. Clin J Am Soc Nephrol. 2008;3:208.

Kraut JA, Xing SX. Approach to the evaluation of a patient with an increased serum osmolal gap and high-anion-gap metabolic acidosis. Am J Kidney Dis. 2011;58:480.

Lee Hamm L, Hering-Smith KS, Nakhoul NL. Acid-base and potassium homeostasis. Semin Nephrol. 2013;33:257.

Lynd LD, Richardson KJ, Purssell RA, et al. An evaluation of the osmole gap as a screening test for toxic alcohol poisoning. BMC Emerg Med. 2008;8:5.

Marraffa JM, Holland MG, Stork CM, et al. Diethylene glycol: widely used solvent presents serious poisoning potential. J Emerg Med. 2008;35:401.

Meregalli P, Lüthy C, Oetliker OH, Bianchetti MG. Modified urine osmolal gap: an accurate method for estimating the urinary ammonium concentration? Nephron. 1995;69:98.

Oh M, Carroll HJ. Value and determinants of urine anion gap. Nephron. 2002;90:252.

Purssell RA, Pudek M, Brubacher J, Abu-Laban RB. Derivation and validation of a formula to calculate the contribution of ethanol to the osmolal gap. Ann Emerg Med. 2001;38 :653.

Robinson AG, Loeb JN. Ethanol ingestion–commonest cause of elevated plasma osmolality? N Engl J Med. 1971;284:1253.

Rodríguez Soriano J. Renal tubular acidosis: the clinical entity. J Am Soc Nephrol. 2002;13:2160.

Schelling JR, Howard RL, Winter SD, Linas SL. Increased osmolal gap in alcoholic ketoacidosis and lactic acidosis. Ann Intern Med. 1990;113:580.

CASE 70

A 28-year-old male patient with cystic fibrosis (CF) comes to the clinic because of recent lethargy. The patient has IDDM related to CF and pancreatic insufficiency. He takes insulin glargine and lispro, Zenpep pancrelipase tablets, nebulized albuterol, nebulized DNase, inhaled budesonide/formoterol, and dietary supplements. He states that he has not been feeling well for the past 2 to 3 days. Vital signs are as follows: T 38.3°C, RR 22, HR 105, BP 95/65, and Sao_2 94% on RA. His examination is remarkable for crackles at the lung bases bilaterally, and increased accessory muscle usage. The patient has sinus tachycardia without rubs or gallops. The abdominal examination is benign. There is no edema of the lower extremities. His laboratory results are as follows:

Laboratory data.			
ABGs		Basic Metabolic Panel	
pH	7.09	Na	140 mEq/L
$Paco_2$	34 mm Hg	K	4 mEq/L
Pao_2	60 mm Hg	Cl	80 mEq/L
HCO_3	10 mEq/L	CO_2	10 mEq/L
		BUN	21 mg/dL
		Cr	1.1 mg/dL
		Glucose	234 mg/dL
		Albumin	4 g/dL
		EtOH	0 mg/dL

QUESTIONS

Q70-1: Define the patient's baseline acid-base status: Does this patient have an underlying chronic acid-base disorder that we need to account for in order to appropriately interpret the acute acid-base disorders?

A. There is no evidence for an underlying chronic respiratory or metabolic acid-base disorder in this patient, so we would assume a baseline $Paco_2$ of 40 mm Hg and an HCO_3 of 24 mEq/L.

B. While the patient has a condition predisposing him to a chronic acid-base disorder, there is insufficient information to estimate the patient's baseline $Paco_2$ and HCO_3 values; therefore, we will assume a baseline $Paco_2$ of 40 mm Hg and a baseline HCO_3 of 24 mEq/L.

C. The patient has an underlying acid-base condition, and we have sufficient information to estimate the patient's baseline $Paco_2$ and HCO_3 values.

Q70-2: What is/are the primary acid-base disturbance(s) occurring in this case?

A. Metabolic acidosis only
B. Respiratory acidosis only
C. Metabolic acidosis and a respiratory acidosis
D. Metabolic alkalosis and a respiratory alkalosis
E. Metabolic alkalosis only
F. Respiratory alkalosis only

Q70-3: How would the metabolic acidosis component be classified in this case?

A. Anion gap acidosis
B. Non-anion gap acidosis
C. Anion and non-anion gap acidosis
D. Anion gap acidosis and a metabolic alkalosis

Q70-4: Does the patient in this case demonstrate appropriate respiratory or metabolic compensation?

A. Yes, the respiratory compensation is appropriate.
B. No, a concomitant respiratory alkalosis is present.
C. No, a concomitant respiratory acidosis is present.
D. Yes, the metabolic compensation is appropriate.
E. No, a concomitant metabolic acidosis is present.
F. No, a concomitant metabolic alkalosis is present.

Q70-5: Additional laboratory test results are as follows:

Serum EtOH	< 3 mg/dL
Serum acetaminophen	< 5 mg/dL (ULN for therapeutic use 20 mg/dL)
Serum salicylates	< 5 mg/dL (ULN for therapeutic use 30 mg/dL)
Serum osmolar gap	8 mOsm/kg
Serum L-lactate	3.1 mmol/L (ULN 2.0 mmol/L venous)
Beta-hydroxybutyrate (acetone)	2.11 mmol/L (ULN 0.18 mmol/L)
Serum glucose	234 mg/dL

What is the likely cause of the patient's anion gap acidosis?

A. Aspirin toxicity
B. Lactic acidosis secondary to sepsis
C. Ethylene glycol toxicity
D. Methanol toxicity
E. Opioid overdose
F. Acetaminophen overdose
G. DKA
H. Alcoholic ketoacidosis

Q70-6: What is the likely cause of the patient's respiratory acidosis?

A. Hypoxemia
B. Neuromuscular disorder
C. CF-related lung disease
D. Chest wall injury or deformity
E. Opioid overdose
F. Iatrogenic cause

Q70-7: The urine electrolyte values are as follows:

Urine Na	23 mEq/L
Urine K	30 mEq/L
Urine Cl	7 mEq/L
Urine urea	234 mg/dL
Urine glucose	0 mg/dL
Urine osmolality	490 mOsm/L
Urine pH	5.5

What is most likely cause of the patient's metabolic alkalosis?

A. HCO_3 infusion
B. Addison disease
C. Milk-alkali ingestion
D. CF
E. Hyperemesis
F. Diarrhea
G. Bactrim use
H. Acetazolamide use
I. Aminoglycoside use
J. Ifosfamide chemotherapy

ANSWERS

Q70-1: B

While the patient has a condition predisposing him to a chronic acid-base disorder, there is insufficient information to estimate the patient's baseline $Paco_2$ and HCO_3 values; therefore, we will assume a baseline $Paco_2$ of 40 mm Hg and a baseline HCO_3 of 24 mEq/L. CF can be associated with chronic acid-base disorders, both respiratory and metabolic. However, given the information in the prompt, we do not have enough information to suggest an altered baseline acid-base status at this point.

Rationale: Ignoring these underlying chronic acid-base disorders can significantly alter the interpretation of a patient's acute acid-base status. This was demonstrated in the first case of the series. However, often, we do not have the necessary information (eg, prior ABG or VBG, or prior serum chemistry with an HCO_3) and are forced to assume the ongoing processes are all acute in nature. We are primarily concerned about chronic respiratory acid-base disorders, as these can significantly alter the patient's baseline or expected values for the serum HCO_3 and $Paco_2$, and we have reliable equations to predict the expected baseline values. The respiratory compensation for both chronic metabolic acidosis and alkalosis is generally poor, so there are no equations or rules to predict what the $Paco_2$ should be in these cases. While the baseline serum HCO_3 may be significantly off from our standard value of 24 mEq/L in these patients, we would assume a baseline $Paco_2$ of 40 mm Hg in patients with chronic metabolic processes. Once we identify the patient's baseline $Paco_2$ and HCO_3 values, we will need to use these values in the appropriate equations to identify the ongoing acute processes.

Q70-2: A

Metabolic acidosis only.

Rationale:

1. The pH is 7.09; therefore, the primary disorder is an **acidosis.**
2. The $Paco_2$ of 34 mm Hg is less than 40 mm Hg, so this is not a primary respiratory acidosis.
3. The HCO_3 of 10 mEq/L is less than 24 mEq/L, so there is a **metabolic acidosis.**

Therefore, this patient has a primary metabolic acidosis.

Q70-3: D

Anion gap acidosis and a metabolic alkalosis.

Rationale:

1. Is there evidence for a chronic acid-base disorder that requires adjustment of the patient's "normal" HCO_3? No, there is not enough evidence for a chronic acid-base disorder at baseline, so we would assume a baseline $Paco_2$ of 40 mm Hg and an HCO_3 of 24 mEq/L.

2. Expected anion gap:

$$\text{Expected Anion Gap} = 12 - (2.5) * \left[4.0\,\frac{g}{dL} - \text{Actual Serum Albumin} \right]$$
$$= 12 - (2.5 * [4.0 - 4.0])$$
$$= 12 - (2.5 * [0]) = \textbf{12 mEq/L}.$$

3. Anion gap calculation:

$$\text{Serum Anion Gap} = [Na^+] - [HCO_3^-] - [Cl^-]$$
$$= 140 - (80 + 10) = 50 \text{ mEq/L, which is} > 12 \text{ mEq/L}$$
$$\rightarrow \textbf{anion gap acidosis is present.}$$

4. Delta-delta calculation:

$$\Delta\Delta = \frac{(\text{Actual Anion Gap} - \text{Expected Anion Gap})}{(\text{Baseline HCO}_3 - \text{Actual HCO}_3)}$$
$$= (50 - 12)/(24 - 10) = \textbf{38/14, which is ~2.7.}$$

Delta-delta interpretation.	
Delta-Delta Value	**Condition Present**
< 0.4	Non-anion gap only
0.4–0.9	Anion gap *and* non-anion gap acidosis
1.0–2.0	Anion gap acidosis only
> 2.0	**Anion gap acidosis and metabolic alkalosis**

Q70-4: C
No, a concomitant respiratory acidosis is present.

Rationale: Using the Winter formula, one can calculate what the expected arterial $Paco_2$ should be for a given serum HCO_3 if the patient were completely compensated.

Respiratory Compensation for Acute Metabolic Acidosis (Winter Formula):

$$\text{Expected Paco}_2 = 1.5 * [\text{Actual HCO}_3] + 8 \pm 2 \text{ (in mm Hg)}$$
$$= (1.5 * 10) + 8 = 15 + 8 = 23 \pm 2 = (21 \text{ to } 25) \text{ mm Hg.}$$

This patient has a concomitant respiratory acidosis, with **$Paco_2$ of 34 mm Hg**, above the expected range (21 to 25 mm Hg). Therefore, a respiratory acidosis is also present.

Q70-5: G
DKA.

Rationale: The patient has an anion gap acidosis with elevated serum glucose and positive serum beta-hydroxybutyrate, indicating a ketoacidosis is present. He has a negative urine and serum drug screen, and a negative serum osmolal gap. The lactate is mildly elevated, which can occur in DKA due to altered metabolism.

Q70-6: C
CF-related lung disease.

Rationale: This patient has a relative respiratory acidosis due to underlying lung disease and an inability to appropriately compensate for the metabolic acidosis. CF is an airway-centric pulmonary process that is both an obstructive and a restrictive lung disease. Chronic airway inflammation leads to obstruction, which is the predominant issue early in the disease. As the disease progresses, with continued inflammation/infection and scarring, the lungs develop significant fibrosis leading to reduced lung compliance, or restrictive lung disease. Both obstructive and restrictive lung diseases lead to reduce pulmonary reserve. When patients with CF develop infections leading to metabolic acidosis, it is often difficult for them to adequately compensate from a respiratory standpoint. Patients with advanced CF-related lung disease often develop hypoxemic followed by chronic hypercarbic respiratory failure, leading to a chronic respiratory acidosis.

Q70-7: D
CF.

Rationale: The patient has a chloride-responsive metabolic alkalosis, with U_{Cl} less than 20 mEq/L. Based on the clinical history provided, there is no evidence of milk-alkali ingestion. Of the available answers, only hyperemesis and CF are associated with a chloride-responsive alkalosis. The patient has no report of emesis (although this might be expect in a patient with DKA, which is prone to nausea, emesis, and gastroparesis), and given the patient's diagnosis of CF this is the likely answer. CF is associated with chronic loss of chloride due to mutations in the *CFTR* gene, leading to alkalosis. This can be an acute or chronic issue, depending on the severity of the patient's mutation.

Causes of metabolic alkalosis.
History: Rule Out the Following as Causes
• Alkali load ("milk-alkali" or calcium-alkali syndrome, oral sodium bicarbonate, IV sodium bicarbonate) • Genetic causes (CF) • Presence of hypercalcemia • IV β-lactam antibiotics • Laxative abuse (may also cause a metabolic acidosis depending on diarrheal HCO_3 losses)
If None of the Above, Then…
Urine Chloride < 20 mEq/L (Chloride-Responsive Causes) • Loss of gastric acid (hyperemesis, NGT suctioning) • Prior diuretic use (in hours to days following discontinuation) • Post-hypercapnia • Villous adenoma • Congenital chloridorrhea • Chronic laxative abuse (may also cause a metabolic acidosis depending on diarrheal HCO_3 losses) • CF

(Continued)

Causes of metabolic alkalosis. (*continued*)
OR
Urine Chloride > 20 mEq/L (Chloride-Resistant Causes)
Urine Chloride > 20 mEq/L, Lack of HTN, Urine Potassium < 30 mEq/L
• Hypokalemia or hypomagnesemia • Laxative abuse (if dominated by hypokalemia) • Bartter syndrome • Gitelman syndrome
Urine Chloride > 20 mEq/L, Lack of HTN, Urine Potassium > 30 mEq/L
• Current diuretic use
Urine Chloride > 20 mEq/L, Presence of HTN, Urine Potassium Variable but Usually > 30 mEq/L
Elevated plasma renin level: • Renal artery stenosis • Renin-secreting tumor • Renovascular disease
Low plasma renin, low plasma aldosterone: • Cushing syndrome • Exogenous mineralocorticoid use • Genetic disorder (11-hydoxylase or 17-hydrolyase deficiency, 11β-HSD deficiency) • Liddle syndrome • Licorice toxicity
Low plasma renin, high plasma aldosterone: • Primary hyperaldosteronism • Adrenal adenoma • Bilateral adrenal hyperplasia

References

Abreo K, Adlakha A, Kilpatrick S, et al. The milk-alkali syndrome. A reversible form of acute renal failure. Arch Intern Med. 1993;153:1005.

Barton CH, Vaziri ND, Ness RL, et al. Cimetidine in the management of metabolic alkalosis induced by nasogastric drainage. Arch Surg. 1979;114:70.

Bates CM, Baum M, Quigley R. Cystic fibrosis presenting with hypokalemia and metabolic alkalosis in a previously healthy adolescent. J Am Soc Nephrol. 1997;8:352.

Bear R, Goldstein M, Phillipson E, et al. Effect of metabolic alkalosis on respiratory function in patients with chronic obstructive lung disease. Can Med Assoc J. 1977;117:900.

Davé S, Honney S, Raymond J, Flume PA. An unusual presentation of cystic fibrosis in an adult. Am J Kidney Dis. 2005;45:e41.

Galla JH, Gifford JD, Luke RG, Rome L. Adaptations to chloride-depletion alkalosis. Am J Physiol. 1991;261:R771.

Garella S, Chang BS, Kahn SI. Dilution acidosis and contraction alkalosis: review of a concept. Kidney Int. 1975;8:279.

Gennari FJ, Weise WJ. Acid-base disturbances in gastrointestinal disease. Clin J Am Soc Nephrol. 2008;3:1861.

Hamm LL, Nakhoul N, Hering-Smith KS. Acid-base homeostasis. Clin J Am Soc Nephrol. 2015;10:2232.

Hulter HN, Sebastian A, Toto RD, et al. Renal and systemic acid-base effects of the chronic administration of hypercalcemia-producing agents: calcitriol, PTH, and intravenous calcium. Kidney Int. 1982;21:445.

Khanna A, Kurtzman NA. Metabolic alkalosis. J Nephrol. 2006;19(suppl 9):S86.

Laski ME, Sabatini S. Metabolic alkalosis, bedside and bench. Semin Nephrol. 2006;26:404.

Luke RG, Galla JH. It is chloride depletion alkalosis, not contraction alkalosis. J Am Soc Nephrol. 2012;23:204.

Miller PD, Berns AS. Acute metabolic alkalosis perpetuating hypercarbia. A role for acetazolamide in chronic obstructive pulmonary disease. JAMA. 1977;238:2400.

Oster JR, Materson BJ, Rogers AI. Laxative abuse syndrome. Am J Gastroenterol. 1980;74:451.

Patel AM, Goldfarb S. Got calcium? Welcome to the calcium-alkali syndrome. J Am Soc Nephrol. 2010;21:1440.

Pierce NF, Fedson DS, Brigham KL, et al. The ventilatory response to acute base deficit in humans. Time course during development and correction of metabolic acidosis. Ann Intern Med. 1970;72:633.

Rose BD, Post TW. Clinical Physiology of Acid-Base and Electrolyte Disorders, 5e. New York, NY: McGraw Hill; 2001:559.

Schwartz WB, Van Ypersele de Strihou, Kassirer JP. Role of anions in metabolic alkalosis and potassium deficiency. N Engl J Med. 1968;279:630.

Scurati-Manzoni E, Fossali EF, Agostoni C, et al. Electrolyte abnormalities in cystic fibrosis: systematic review of the literature. Pediatr Nephrol. 2014;29:1015.

Sweetser LJ, Douglas JA, Riha RL, Bell SC. Clinical presentation of metabolic alkalosis in an adult patient with cystic fibrosis. Respirology. 2005;10:254.

Taki K, Mizuno K, Takahashi N, Wakusawa R. Disturbance of CO2 elimination in the lungs by carbonic anhydrase inhibition. Jpn J Physiol. 1986;36:523.

Turban S, Beutler KT, Morris RG, et al. Long-term regulation of proximal tubule acid-base transporter abundance by angiotensin II. Kidney Int. 2006;70:660.

CASE 71

An 88-year-old female nursing home resident with chronic recurrent urinary tract infections was admitted 3 days ago. You are called to consult for acute onset of altered mental status/encephalopathy and acute renal failure. The patient has a history of multidrug-resistant organisms and was started on an aminoglycoside. She takes no medications at baseline. She has a history of a prior mild stroke and dementia. She is lethargic and appears dry on examination. Her cardiac examination reveals sinus tachycardia and her pulmonary examination is unremarkable. She may have some mild flank tenderness on examination, although her responses are difficult to gauge. Her vital signs are as follows: T37.6°C, HR 104, BP 120/80, RR 17, and Sao_2 96% on room air.

Laboratory data.			
ABGs		Basic Metabolic Panel	
pH	7.27	Na	144 mEq/L
$Paco_2$	38 mm Hg	K	2.8 mEq/L
Pao_2	84 mm Hg	Cl	98 mEq/L
HCO_3	17 mEq/L	CO_2	17 mEq/L
		BUN	132 mg/dL
		Cr	4.3 mg/dL
		Glucose	89 mg/dL
		Albumin	4.0 g/dL
		EtOH	0 mg/dL

QUESTIONS

Q71-1: Define the patient's baseline acid-base status: Does this patient have an underlying chronic acid-base disorder that we need to account for in order to appropriately interpret the acute acid-base disorders?

A. There is no evidence for an underlying chronic respiratory or metabolic acid-base disorder in this patient, so we would assume a baseline $Paco_2$ of 40 mm Hg and an HCO_3 of 24 mEq/L.

B. While the patient has a condition predisposing her to a chronic acid-base disorder, there is insufficient information to estimate the patient's baseline $Paco_2$ and HCO_3 values; therefore, we will assume a baseline $Paco_2$ of 40 mm Hg and a baseline HCO_3 of 24 mEq/L.

C. The patient has an underlying acid-base condition, and we have sufficient information to estimate the patient's baseline $Paco_2$ and HCO_3 values.

Q71-2: What is/are the primary acid-base disturbance(s) occurring in this case?

A. Metabolic acidosis only
B. Respiratory acidosis only
C. Metabolic acidosis and a respiratory acidosis
D. Metabolic alkalosis and a respiratory alkalosis
E. Metabolic alkalosis only
F. Respiratory alkalosis only

Q71-3: How would the metabolic acidosis component be classified in this case?

A. Anion gap acidosis
B. Non-anion gap acidosis
C. Anion and non-anion gap acidosis
D. Anion gap acidosis and a metabolic alkalosis

Q71-4: Does the patient in this case demonstrate appropriate respiratory or metabolic compensation?

A. Yes, the respiratory compensation is appropriate.
B. No, a concomitant respiratory alkalosis is present.
C. No, a concomitant respiratory acidosis is present.
D. Yes, the metabolic compensation is appropriate.
E. No, a concomitant metabolic acidosis is present.
F. No, a concomitant metabolic alkalosis is present.

Q71-5: Additional laboratory test results are as follows:

Serum EtOH	< 3 mg/dL
Serum acetaminophen	< 5 mg/dL (ULN for therapeutic use 20 mg/dL)
Serum salicylates	< 5 mg/dL (ULN for therapeutic use 30 mg/dL)
Serum osmolality	344 mOsm/kg
Serum L-lactate	1.8 mmol/L (ULN 2.0 mmol/L venous)
Beta-hydroxybutyrate (acetone)	< 0.18 mmol/L (ULN 0.18 mmol/L)
Serum glucose	89 mg/dL
Serum phosphate	11.8 mg/dL

What is the likely cause of the patient's anion gap acidosis?

A. Aspirin toxicity
B. Lactic acidosis secondary to sepsis
C. Ethylene glycol toxicity
D. Methanol toxicity
E. Acute renal failure
F. Acetaminophen overdose
G. Diabetic ketoacidosis
H. Alcoholic ketoacidosis

Q71-6: The urine electrolytes are as follows:

U_{Na}	23 mEq/L
U_K	33 mEq/L
U_{Cl}	45 mEq/L
Urine pH	5.5

What is most likely cause of the patient's metabolic alkalosis?

A. Addison disease
B. Hyperemesis
C. Diarrhea
D. Bactrim use
E. Acetazolamide use
F. Aminoglycoside use
G. Ifosfamide chemotherapy

ANSWERS

Q71-1: A

There is no evidence for an underlying chronic respiratory or metabolic acid-base disorder in this patient, so we would assume a baseline $Paco_2$ of 40 mm Hg and an HCO_3 of 24 mEq/L. Based on the vignette it appears all the ongoing processes are acute.

Rationale: Ignoring these underlying chronic acid-base disorders can significantly alter the interpretation of a patient's acute acid-base status. This was demonstrated in the first case of the series. However, often, we do not have the necessary information (eg, prior ABG or VBG, or prior serum chemistry with an HCO_3) and are forced to assume the ongoing processes are all acute in nature. We are primarily concerned about chronic respiratory acid-base disorders, as these can significantly alter the patient's baseline or expected values for the serum HCO_3 and $Paco_2$, and we have reliable equations to predict the expected baseline values. The respiratory compensation for both chronic metabolic acidosis and alkalosis is generally poor, so there are no equations or rules to predict what the $Paco_2$ should be in these cases. While the baseline serum HCO_3 may be significantly off from our standard value of 24 mEq/L in these patients, we would assume a baseline $Paco_2$ of 40 mm Hg in patients with chronic metabolic processes. Once we identify the patient's baseline $Paco_2$ and HCO_3 values, we will need to use these values in the appropriate equations to identify the ongoing acute processes.

Q71-2: A

Metabolic acidosis only.

Rationale:

1. The pH is 7.27; therefore, the primary disorder is an **acidosis.**
2. The $Paco_2$ of 38 mm Hg is less than 40 mm Hg, so a respiratory acidosis is not present.
3. The HCO_3 of 17 mEq/L is less than 24 mEq/L, so there is a **metabolic acidosis.**

Q71-3: D

Anion gap acidosis and a metabolic alkalosis.

Rationale:

1. Is there evidence for a chronic respiratory acid-base disorder that requires adjustment of the patient's "normal" HCO_3? No, there is no evidence for a chronic respiratory acid-base disorder, so we would assume a baseline $Paco_2$ of 40 mm Hg and an HCO_3 of 24 mEq/L.
2. Expected anion gap:

$$\text{Expected Anion Gap} = 12 - (2.5) * \left[4.0 \frac{g}{dL} - \text{Actual Serum Albumin} \right]$$
$$= 12 - (2.5 * [4.0 - 4.0])$$
$$= 12 - (2.5 * [0]) = \textbf{12 mEq/L.}$$

3. Anion gap calculation:

$$\text{Serum Anion Gap} = [Na^+] - [HCO_3^-] - [Cl^-]$$
$$= 144 - (98 + 17) = 29 \text{ mEq/L, which is} > 12 \text{ mEq/L}$$
$$\rightarrow \textbf{anion gap acidosis is present.}$$

4. Delta-delta calculation:

$$\Delta\Delta = \frac{(\text{Actual Anion Gap} - \text{Expected Anion Gap})}{(\text{Baseline HCO}_3 - \text{Actual HCO}_3)}$$
$$= (29 - 12)/(24 - 17) = \textbf{17/7, which is ~2.4.}$$

Delta-delta interpretation.	
Delta-Delta Value	Condition Present
< 0.4	Non-anion gap only
0.4–0.9	Anion gap *and* non-anion gap acidosis
1.0–2.0	Anion gap acidosis only
> 2.0	**Anion gap acidosis and metabolic alkalosis**

Q71-4: C
No, a concomitant respiratory acidosis is present.

Rationale: Using the Winter formula, one can calculate what the expected arterial $Paco_2$ should be for a given serum HCO_3 if the patient were completely compensated.

Respiratory Compensation for Acute Metabolic Acidosis (Winter Formula):

$$\text{Expected Paco}_2 = 1.5 * [\text{Actual HCO}_3] + 8 \pm 2 \text{ (in mm Hg)}$$
$$= (1.5 * 17) + 8 = 25.5 + 8 = 33.5 \pm 2 = (31 \text{ to } 35) \text{ mm Hg.}$$

This patient has a concomitant respiratory acidosis, with $Paco_2$ of 38 mm Hg, above the expected range (31 to 35 mm Hg). Therefore, a respiratory acidosis is also present.

Q71-5: E
Acute renal failure.

Rationale: The patient has acute renal failure with uremia. This can lead to issues with both anion excretion as well as appropriate urinary acidification. The serum drug screen is negative, indicating no evidence of acetaminophen or aspirin toxicity, and she has no ketoacidosis. The serum osmolal gap can be calculated from the information provided using the following equation:

$$\text{Calculated Serum Osmolality} = 2 * [Na^+] + \frac{[\text{Glucose}]}{18} + \frac{[\text{BUN}]}{2.8} + \frac{[\text{EtOH}]}{3.7}.$$

The calculated serum osmolality is 340 mOsm/L, so the serum osmolal gap is 4 mOsm/L (< 10 mOsm is normal). Therefore, there is no ethylene glycol or methanol toxicity. The serum lactate is normal. However, the patient has an elevated serum Cr, a significantly elevated serum BUN, and an elevated serum phosphorus, all consistent with acute renal failure as the cause. Acute renal failure can yield an anion gap acidosis, a non-anion gap acidosis, or a mixed metabolic acidosis, depending on the mechanism of injury.

Q71-6: F
Aminoglycoside use.

Rationale: The patient has an elevated urine chloride greater than 20 mEq/L, consistent with a chloride-resistant cause of the metabolic alkalosis. She is receiving aminoglycoside therapy for the urinary tract infection. While aminoglycosides are more commonly associated with a renal tubular acidosis (type 1 > type 2 RTA), they can also be associated with a chloride-resistant metabolic alkalosis. This is also usually associated with hypomagnesemia and hypocalcemia. As is the case for this patient, the serum potassium, serum magnesium, and serum calcium levels are typically low in aminoglycoside-induced metabolic alkalosis. Aminoglycoside antibiotics can cause a reversible form of acquired Bartter syndrome, which is a chloride-resistant form of metabolic alkalosis. Recall that hyperemesis is associated with a chloride-resistant form of metabolic alkalosis. Addison disease (primary adrenal insufficiency), trimethoprim (Bactrim) use, diarrhea, acetazolamide use, and ifosfamide use are all associated with a metabolic acidosis only.

Causes of metabolic alkalosis.
History: Rule Out the Following as Causes
• Alkali load ("milk-alkali" or calcium-alkali syndrome, oral sodium bicarbonate, IV sodium bicarbonate) • Genetic causes (CF) • Presence of hypercalcemia • IV β-lactam antibiotics • Laxative abuse (may also cause a metabolic acidosis depending on diarrheal HCO_3 losses)
If None of the Above, Then. . .
Urine Chloride < 20 mEq/L (Chloride-Responsive Causes) • Loss of gastric acid (hyperemesis, NGT suctioning) • Prior diuretic use (in hours to days following discontinuation) • Post-hypercapnia • Villous adenoma • Congenital chloridorrhea • Chronic laxative abuse (may also cause a metabolic acidosis depending on diarrheal HCO_3 losses) • CF
OR

(Continued)

Causes of metabolic alkalosis. (*continued*)
Urine Chloride > 20 mEq/L (Chloride-Resistant Causes)
Urine Chloride > 20 mEq/L, Lack of HTN, Urine Potassium < 30 mEq/L
• Hypokalemia or hypomagnesemia • Laxative abuse (if dominated by hypokalemia) • Bartter syndrome (*including acquired secondary to aminoglycoside use*) • Gitelman syndrome
Urine Chloride > 20 mEq/L, Lack of HTN, Urine Potassium > 30 mEq/L
• Current diuretic use
Urine Chloride > 20 mEq/L, Presence of HTN, Urine Potassium Variable but Usually > 30 mEq/L
Elevated plasma renin level: • Renal artery stenosis • Renin-secreting tumor • Renovascular disease
Low plasma renin, low plasma aldosterone: • Cushing syndrome • Exogenous mineralocorticoid use • Genetic disorder (11-hydoxylase or 17-hydrolyase deficiency, 11β-HSD deficiency) • Liddle syndrome • Licorice toxicity
Low plasma renin, high plasma aldosterone: • Primary hyperaldosteronism • Adrenal adenoma • Bilateral adrenal hyperplasia

References

Abreo K, Adlakha A, Kilpatrick S, et al. The milk-alkali syndrome. A reversible form of acute renal failure. Arch Intern Med. 1993;153:1005.

Bailey JL. Metabolic acidosis: an unrecognized cause of morbidity in the patient with chronic kidney disease. Kidney Int Suppl. 2005:S15.

Barton CH, Vaziri ND, Ness RL, et al. Cimetidine in the management of metabolic alkalosis induced by nasogastric drainage. Arch Surg. 1979;114:70.

Bear R, Goldstein M, Phillipson E, et al. Effect of metabolic alkalosis on respiratory function in patients with chronic obstructive lung disease. Can Med Assoc J. 1977;117:900.

Chen YS, Fang HC, Chou KJ, et al. Gentamicin-induced Bartter-like syndrome. Am J Kidney Dis. 2009;54:1158.

Chou CL, Chen YH, Chau T, Lin SH. Acquired Bartter-like syndrome associated with gentamicin administration. Am J Med Sci. 2005;329:144.

Chrispal A, Boorugu H, Prabhakar AT, Moses V. Amikacin-induced type 5 Bartter-like syndrome with severe hypocalcemia. J Postgrad Med. 2009;55:208.

Galla JH, Gifford JD, Luke RG, Rome L. Adaptations to chloride-depletion alkalosis. Am J Physiol. 1991;261:R771.

Garella S, Chang BS, Kahn SI. Dilution acidosis and contraction alkalosis: review of a concept. Kidney Int. 1975;8:279.

Gennari FJ, Weise WJ. Acid-base disturbances in gastrointestinal disease. Clin J Am Soc Nephrol. 2008;3:1861.

Halperin ML, Ethier JH, Kamel KS. Ammonium excretion in chronic metabolic acidosis: benefits and risks. Am J Kidney Dis. 1989;14:267.

Hamm LL, Nakhoul N, Hering-Smith KS. Acid-base homeostasis. Clin J Am Soc Nephrol. 2015;10:2232.

Hulter HN, Sebastian A, Toto RD, et al. Renal and systemic acid-base effects of the chronic administration of hypercalcemia-producing agents: calcitriol, PTH, and intravenous calcium. Kidney Int. 1982;21:445.

Hung CC, Guh JY, Kuo MC, et al. Gentamicin-induced diffuse renal tubular dysfunction. Nephrol Dial Transplant. 2006;21:547.

Khanna A, Kurtzman NA. Metabolic alkalosis. J Nephrol. 2006;19(suppl 9):S86.

Kraut JA, Kurtz I. Metabolic acidosis of CKD: diagnosis, clinical characteristics, and treatment. Am J Kidney Dis. 2005;45:978.

Krieger NS, Frick KK, Bushinsky DA. Mechanism of acid-induced bone resorption. Curr Opin Nephrol Hypertens. 2004;13:423.

Laski ME, Sabatini S. Metabolic alkalosis, bedside and bench. Semin Nephrol. 2006;26:404.

Luke RG, Galla JH. It is chloride depletion alkalosis, not contraction alkalosis. J Am Soc Nephrol. 2012;23:204.

Melnick JZ, Baum M, Thompson JR. Aminoglycoside-induced Fanconi's syndrome. Am J Kidney Dis. 1994;23:118.

Miller PD, Berns AS. Acute metabolic alkalosis perpetuating hypercarbia. A role for acetazolamide in chronic obstructive pulmonary disease. JAMA. 1977;238:2400.

Oster JR, Materson BJ, Rogers AI. Laxative abuse syndrome. Am J Gastroenterol. 1980;74:451.

Patel AM, Goldfarb S. Got calcium? Welcome to the calcium-alkali syndrome. J Am Soc Nephrol. 2010;21:1440.

Rose BD, Post TW. Clinical Physiology of Acid-Base and Electrolyte Disorders, 5e. New York, NY: McGraw Hill; 2001:559

Schwartz JH, Schein P. Fanconi syndrome associated with cephalothin and gentamicin therapy. Cancer. 1978;41:769.

Schwartz WB, Van Ypersele de Strihou, Kassirer JP. Role of anions in metabolic alkalosis and potassium deficiency. N Engl J Med. 1968;279:630.

Sweetser LJ, Douglas JA, Riha RL, Bell SC. Clinical presentation of metabolic alkalosis in an adult patient with cystic fibrosis. Respirology. 2005;10:254.

Taki K, Mizuno K, Takahashi N, Wakusawa R. Disturbance of CO2 elimination in the lungs by carbonic anhydrase inhibition. Jpn J Physiol. 1986;36:523.

Turban S, Beutler KT, Morris RG, et al. Long-term regulation of proximal tubule acid-base transporter abundance by angiotensin II. Kidney Int. 2006;70:660.

Warnock DG. Uremic acidosis. Kidney Int. 1988;34:278.

Widmer B, Gerhardt RE, Harrington JT, Cohen JJ. Serum electrolyte and acid base composition. The influence of graded degrees of chronic renal failure. Arch Intern Med. 1979;139:1099.

CASE 72

You are working as a physician for a team of climbers at Mount Everest. At base camp, 17,600 feet above sea level, you are asked to see a climber with complaints of blurry vision, dyspnea, nausea, and anorexia. He is a 34-year-old man who is otherwise healthy. He takes no medications regularly, does not drink alcohol, and does not use illicit drugs. His vital signs are T 37.6°C, HR 121, BP 103/55, RR 19, and Sao$_2$ 85% on room air. His examination is notable for some inspiratory crackles and sinus tachycardia, but is otherwise normal. His laboratory studies are as follows:

Laboratory data.			
ABGs		Basic Metabolic Panel	
pH	7.62	Na	140 mEq/L
Paco$_2$	31 mm Hg	K	4 mEq/L
Pao$_2$	48 mm Hg	Cl	104 mEq/L
HCO$_3$	31 mEq/L	CO$_2$	31 mEq/L
		BUN	132 mg/dL
		Cr	4.3 mg/dL
		Glucose	89 mg/dL
		Albumin	4.0 g/dL
		EtOH	0 mg/dL

QUESTIONS

Q72-1: Define the patient's baseline acid-base status: Does this patient have an underlying chronic acid-base disorder that we need to account for in order to appropriately interpret the acute acid-base disorders?

A. There is no evidence for an underlying chronic respiratory or metabolic acid-base disorder in this patient, so we would assume a baseline $Paco_2$ of 40 mm Hg and an HCO_3 of 24 mEq/L.

B. While the patient has a condition predisposing him to a chronic acid-base disorder, there is insufficient information to estimate the patient's baseline $Paco_2$ and HCO_3 values; therefore, we will assume a baseline $Paco_2$ of 40 mm Hg and a baseline HCO_3 of 24 mEq/L.

C. The patient has an underlying acid-base condition, and we have sufficient information to estimate the patient's baseline $Paco_2$ and HCO_3 values.

Q72-2: What is/are the primary acid-base disturbance(s) occurring in this case?

A. Metabolic acidosis only

B. Respiratory acidosis only

C. Metabolic acidosis and a respiratory acidosis

D. Metabolic alkalosis and a respiratory alkalosis

E. Metabolic alkalosis only

F. Respiratory alkalosis only

Q72-3: What is the most likely cause of the patient's respiratory alkalosis?

A. Acetaminophen overdose

B. Aspirin overdose

C. Hypoxemia

D. Benzodiazepine overdose

E. Toluene exposure

F. Amphotericin exposure

Q72-4: The urine electrolyte values are as follows:

U_Na	23 mEq/L
U_K	10 mEq/L
U_Cl	4 mEq/L
Urine pH	5.5

Which is most likely cause of the patient's metabolic alkalosis?

A. HCO_3 infusion
B. Addison disease
C. Milk-alkali ingestion
D. Cystic fibrosis
E. Hyperemesis
F. Diarrhea
G. Bactrim use
H. Acetazolamide use
I. Aminoglycoside use
J. Ifosfamide chemotherapy

Q72-5: The patient is ordered to descend the mountain and is prescribed dexamethasone and supplemental oxygen. Which of the following drugs may be useful in the prevention of acute mountain sickness?

A. Aminoglycoside
B. Acetazolamide
C. Spironolactone
D. Furosemide
E. Augmentin

ANSWERS

Q72-1: A

There is no evidence for an underlying chronic respiratory or metabolic acid-base disorder in this patient, so we would assume a baseline $Paco_2$ of 40 mm Hg and an HCO_3 of 24 mEq/L.

Rationale: Ignoring these underlying chronic acid-base disorders can significantly alter the interpretation of a patient's acute acid-base status. This was demonstrated in the first case of the series. However, often, we do not have the necessary information (eg, prior ABG or VBG, or prior serum chemistry with an HCO_3) and are forced to assume the ongoing processes are all acute in nature. We are primarily concerned about chronic respiratory acid-base disorders, as these can significantly alter the patient's baseline or expected values for the serum HCO_3 and $Paco_2$, and we have reliable equations to predict the expected baseline values. The respiratory compensation for both chronic metabolic acidosis and alkalosis is generally poor, so there are no equations or rules to predict what the $Paco_2$ should be in these cases. While the baseline serum HCO_3 may be significantly off from our standard value of 24 mEq/L in these patients, we would assume a baseline $Paco_2$ of 40 mm Hg in patients with chronic metabolic processes. Once we identify the patient's baseline $Paco_2$ and HCO_3 values, we will need to use these values in the appropriate equations to identify the ongoing acute processes.

Q72-2: D

Metabolic alkalosis and respiratory alkalosis.

Rationale:

1. The pH is 7.62; therefore, the primary disorder is an **alkalosis.**
2. The $Paco_2$ of 31 mm Hg is less than 40 mm Hg, so there is a **respiratory alkalosis.**
3. The HCO_3 of 31 mEq/L is more than 24 mEq/L, so there is also a **metabolic alkalosis.**

Q72-3: C

Hypoxemia.

Rationale: The patient's respiratory alkalosis is due to hypoxemia caused by the reduced oxygen tension at high altitude. Additionally, due to changes in atmospheric pressure, patients are more likely to develop pulmonary edema, which further contributes.

Q72-4: E

Hyperemesis.

Rationale: The patient has hyperemesis per the vignette. This is a common symptom of altitude sickness and accounts for the patient's metabolic alkalosis. The alkalosis is a chloride-responsive alkalosis, with a urine chloride level that is less than 10 mEq/L.

Causes of metabolic alkalosis.
History: Rule Out the Following as Causes
• Alkali load ("milk-alkali" or calcium-alkali syndrome, oral sodium bicarbonate, IV sodium bicarbonate)   • Genetic causes (CF)   • Presence of hypercalcemia   • Intravenous β-lactam antibiotics   • Laxative abuse (may also cause a metabolic acidosis depending on diarrheal HCO_3 losses)
If None of the Above, Then. . .
Urine Chloride < 20 mEq/L (Chloride-Responsive Causes)   • Loss of gastric acid (hyperemesis, NGT suctioning)   • Prior diuretic use (in hours to days following discontinuation)   • Post-hypercapnia   • Villous adenoma   • Congenital chloridorrhea   • Chronic laxative abuse (may also cause a metabolic acidosis depending on diarrheal HCO_3 losses)   • CF
OR
Urine Chloride > 20 mEq/L (Chloride-Resistant Causes)
Urine Chloride > 20 mEq/L, Lack of HTN, Urine Potassium < 30 mEq/L
• Hypokalemia or hypomagnesemia   • Laxative abuse (if dominated by hypokalemia)   • Bartter syndrome   • Gitelman syndrome
Urine Chloride > 20 mEq/L, Lack of HTN, Urine Potassium > 30 mEq/L
• Current diuretic use
Urine Chloride > 20 mEq/L, Presence of HTN, Urine Potassium Variable but Usually > 30 mEq/L
Elevated plasma renin level: • Renal artery stenosis   • Renin-secreting tumor   • Renovascular disease
Low plasma renin, low plasma aldosterone: • Cushing syndrome   • Exogenous mineralocorticoid use   • Genetic disorder (11-hydoxylase or 17-hydrolyase deficiency, 11β-HSD deficiency)   • Liddle syndrome   • Licorice toxicity
Low plasma renin, high plasma aldosterone   • Primary hyperaldosteronism   • Adrenal adenoma   • Bilateral adrenal hyperplasia

Q72-5: B
Acetazolamide.

Rationale: Acetazolamide (Diamox) is commonly given to patients in high-altitude settings. It is generally used for prevention of acute mountain/altitude sickness, rather than treatment of acute sickness. The diuretic aids in the treatment of pulmonary edema and prevents the respiratory alkalosis that is induced by rapid ascent (secondary to hypoxemia), producing a non-anion gap acidosis (type 2 RTA).

Living at elevation is associated with reduced partial pressure of oxygen in the air, due to the reduced atmospheric pressure. While the arterial $Paco_2$ is typically within normal limits, mild cases of altitude sickness are due to more significant reductions in partial pressure of oxygen at end tissues. Most cases of moderate or severe altitude sickness occur during rapid ascents at high elevation, such as expeditions at Everest. The initial response to hypoxemia at altitude is an increase in minute ventilation, brought on by oxygen-sensing cells in the carotid bodies. This increased minute ventilation drives down the alveolar partial pressure of carbon dioxide ($Paco_2$), subsequently increasing the partial pressure of oxygen (Pao_2). As a consequence of the reduced arterial partial pressure of carbon dioxide ($Paco_2$), the arterial partial pressure of CO_2 ($Paco_2$) declines and the arterial pH increases, yielding a respiratory alkalosis. As discussed in Chapter 1, the kidney requires 24 hours to adjust to an acute respiratory alkalosis, but as most climbers are ascending for several days if not weeks, the respiratory alkalosis will only worsen with time. This is in large part why climbers go through the process of acclimatization, ascending a limited elevation and remaining there for several days to allow the body to compensate for the chronic respiratory alkalosis. It is thought that acetazolamide can accelerate this process by more rapidly dropping the serum HCO_3.

Causes of RTA.
Causes of Type 1 (Distal) RTA
Primary • Idiopathic or familial (may be recessive or dominant)
Secondary • Medications: Lithium, amphotericin, ifosfamide, NSAIDs • Rheumatologic disorders: Sjögren syndrome, SLE, RA • Hypercalciuria (idiopathic) or associated with vitamin D deficiency or hyperparathyroidism • Sarcoidosis • Obstructive uropathy • Wilson disease • Rejection of renal transplant allograft • Toluene toxicity
Causes of Type 2 (Proximal) RTA
Primary • Idiopathic • Familial (primarily recessive disorders) • Genetic: Fanconi syndrome, cystinosis, glycogen storage disease (type 1), Wilson disease, galactosemia
Secondary • Medications: Acetazolamide, topiramate, aminoglycoside antibiotics, ifosfamide, reverse transcriptase inhibitors (tenofovir) • Heavy metal poisoning: Lead, mercury, copper • Multiple myeloma or amyloidosis (secondary to light chain toxicity) • Sjögren syndrome • Vitamin D deficiency • Rejection of renal transplant allograft

(Continued)

Causes of RTA. (*continued*)
Causes of Type 4 RTA (Hypoaldosteronism or Aldosterone Resistance)
Primary
• Primary adrenal insufficiency
• Inherited disorders associated with hypoaldosteronism
• Pseudohypoaldosteronism (types 1 and 2)
Secondary
• Causes of hyporeninemic hypoaldosteronism such as renal disease (diabetic nephropathy), NSAID use, calcineurin inhibitors, volume expansion/volume overload
• Causes of distal tubule voltage defects such as sickle cell disease, obstructive uropathy, SLE
• Severe illness/septic shock
• Angiotensin II–associated medications: ACE inhibitors, ARBs, direct renin inhibitors
• Potassium-sparing diuretics: Spironolactone, amiloride, triamterene
• Antibiotics: Trimethoprim, pentamidine

References

Abreo K, Adlakha A, Kilpatrick S, et al. The milk-alkali syndrome. A reversible form of acute renal failure. Arch Intern Med. 1993;153:1005.

Barton CH, Vaziri ND, Ness RL, et al. Cimetidine in the management of metabolic alkalosis induced by nasogastric drainage. Arch Surg. 1979;114:70.

Bear R, Goldstein M, Phillipson E, et al. Effect of metabolic alkalosis on respiratory function in patients with chronic obstructive lung disease. Can Med Assoc J. 1977;117:900.

Davis C, Hackett P. Advances in the prevention and treatment of high altitude illness. Emerg Med Clin North Am. 2017;35:241.

Galla JH, Gifford JD, Luke RG, Rome L. Adaptations to chloride-depletion alkalosis. Am J Physiol. 1991;261:R771.

Garella S, Chang BS, Kahn SI. Dilution acidosis and contraction alkalosis: review of a concept. Kidney Int. 1975;8:279.

Gennari FJ, Weise WJ. Acid-base disturbances in gastrointestinal disease. Clin J Am Soc Nephrol. 2008;3:1861.

Hamm LL, Nakhoul N, Hering-Smith KS. Acid-base homeostasis. Clin J Am Soc Nephrol. 2015;10:2232.

Hulter HN, Sebastian A, Toto RD, et al. Renal and systemic acid-base effects of the chronic administration of hypercalcemia-producing agents: calcitriol, PTH, and intravenous calcium. Kidney Int. 1982;21:445.

Khanna A, Kurtzman NA. Metabolic alkalosis. J Nephrol. 2006;19(suppl 9):S86.

Laski ME, Sabatini S. Metabolic alkalosis, bedside and bench. Semin Nephrol. 2006;26:404.

Luke RG, Galla JH. It is chloride depletion alkalosis, not contraction alkalosis. J Am Soc Nephrol. 2012;23:204.

Miller PD, Berns AS. Acute metabolic alkalosis perpetuating hypercarbia. A role for acetazolamide in chronic obstructive pulmonary disease. JAMA. 1977;238:2400.

Oster JR, Materson BJ, Rogers AI. Laxative abuse syndrome. Am J Gastroenterol. 1980;74:451.

Patel AM, Goldfarb S. Got calcium? Welcome to the calcium-alkali syndrome. J Am Soc Nephrol. 2010;21:1440.

Rose BD, Post TW. Clinical Physiology of Acid-Base and Electrolyte Disorders, 5e. New York, NY: McGraw Hill; 2001:559.

Schwartz WB, Van Ypersele de Strihou, Kassirer JP. Role of anions in metabolic alkalosis and potassium deficiency. N Engl J Med. 1968;279:630.

Simancas-Racines D, Arevalo-Rodriguez I, Osorio D, et al. Interventions for treating acute high altitude illness. Cochrane Database Syst Rev. 2018;6:CD009567.

Sweetser LJ, Douglas JA, Riha RL, Bell SC. Clinical presentation of metabolic alkalosis in an adult patient with cystic fibrosis. Respirology. 2005;10:254.

Taki K, Mizuno K, Takahashi N, Wakusawa R. Disturbance of CO2 elimination in the lungs by carbonic anhydrase inhibition. Jpn J Physiol. 1986;36:523.

Turban S, Beutler KT, Morris RG, et al. Long-term regulation of proximal tubule acid-base transporter abundance by angiotensin II. Kidney Int. 2006;70:660.

Williamson J. Acetazolamide and altitude sickness. BMJ. 2018;361:k2153.

CASE 73

A firefighter is brought to the emergency department with tachypnea and lethargy following a large house fire. He was trapped in a smoke-filled room with a damaged and unusable oxygen tank for some time prior to being rescued. His vital signs are as follows: T 37.7°C, HR 120, BP 70/30, RR 23, and Sao_2 80% on a non-rebreather mask with estimated 95% Fio_2. He has no significant medical history, takes no medications, and does not drink alcohol, smoke tobacco, or use illicit drugs.

Laboratory data.			
ABGs		Basic Metabolic Panel	
pH	7.34	Na	138 mEq/L
$Paco_2$	19 mm Hg	K	5.5 mEq/L
Pao_2	340 mm Hg	Cl	100 mEq/L
HCO_3	10 mEq/L	CO_2	10 mEq/L
		BUN	132 mg/dL
		Cr	4.3 mg/dL
		Glucose	89 mg/dL
		Albumin	4.0 g/dL
		EtOH	0 mg/dL

QUESTIONS

Q73-1: Define the patient's baseline acid-base status: Does this patient have an underlying chronic acid-base disorder that we need to account for in order to appropriately interpret the acute acid-base disorders?

A. There is no evidence for an underlying chronic respiratory or metabolic acid-base disorder in this patient, so we would assume a baseline $Paco_2$ of 40 mm Hg and an HCO_3 of 24 mEq/L.

B. While the patient has a condition predisposing him to a chronic acid-base disorder, there is insufficient information to estimate the patient's baseline $Paco_2$ and HCO_3 values; therefore, we will assume a baseline $Paco_2$ of 40 mm Hg and a baseline HCO_3 of 24 mEq/L.

C. The patient has an underlying acid-base condition, and we have sufficient information to estimate the patient's baseline $Paco_2$ and HCO_3 values.

Q73-2: What is/are the primary acid-base disturbance(s) occurring in this case?

A. Metabolic acidosis only
B. Respiratory acidosis only
C. Metabolic acidosis and a respiratory acidosis
D. Metabolic alkalosis and a respiratory alkalosis
E. Metabolic alkalosis only
F. Respiratory alkalosis only

Q73-3: How would the metabolic acidosis component be classified in this case?

A. Anion gap acidosis
B. Non-anion gap acidosis
C. Anion and non-anion gap acidosis
D. Anion gap acidosis and a metabolic alkalosis

Q73-4: Does the patient in this case demonstrate appropriate respiratory or metabolic compensation?

A. Yes, the respiratory compensation is appropriate.
B. No, a concomitant respiratory alkalosis is present.
C. No, a concomitant respiratory acidosis is present.
D. Yes, the metabolic compensation is appropriate.
E. No, a concomitant metabolic acidosis is present.
F. No, a concomitant metabolic alkalosis is present.

Q73-5: What is the likely cause of the patient's respiratory alkalosis?

A. Aspirin toxicity
B. CNS injury
C. Smoke inhalation
D. Hypoxemia
E. Pain
F. A and B
G. B and D
H. C and D

Q73-6: Despite an elevated $Paco_2$ on the ABG, the patient's Sao_2 remains very low. The patient has a significant lactic acidosis. What is the likely cause of the patient's anion gap acidosis?

A. Aspirin toxicity
B. Cyanide poisoning
C. Ethylene glycol toxicity
D. Methanol toxicity
E. Opioid overdose
F. Toluene toxicity
G. Diabetic ketoacidosis
H. Carbon monoxide poisoning

Q73-7: The patient is intubated for airway protection and respiratory distress. He is placed on 100% Fio_2. What is the most important step in this patient's management?

A. IV methylene blue
B. Activated charcoal
C. IV fomepizole
D. Hyperbaric oxygen therapy
E. Renal replacement therapy

ANSWERS

Q73-1: A

There is no evidence for an underlying chronic respiratory or metabolic acid-base disorder in this patient, so we would assume a baseline $Paco_2$ of 40 mm Hg and an HCO_3 of 24 mEq/L.

Rationale: Ignoring these underlying chronic acid-base disorders can significantly alter the interpretation of a patient's acute acid-base status. This was demonstrated in the first case of the series. However, often, we do not have the necessary information (eg, prior ABG or VBG, or prior serum chemistry with an HCO_3) and are forced to assume the ongoing processes are all acute in nature. We are primarily concerned about chronic respiratory acid-base disorders, as these can significantly alter the patient's baseline or expected values for the serum HCO_3 and $Paco_2$, and we have reliable equations to predict the expected baseline values. The respiratory compensation for both chronic metabolic acidosis and alkalosis is generally poor, so there are no equations or rules to predict what the $Paco_2$ should be in these cases. While the baseline serum HCO_3 may be significantly off from our standard value of 24 mEq/L in these patients, we would assume a baseline $Paco_2$ of 40 mm Hg in patients with chronic metabolic processes. Once we identify the patient's baseline $Paco_2$ and HCO_3 values, we will need to use these values in the appropriate equations to identify the ongoing acute processes.

Q73-2: A

Metabolic acidosis only.

Rationale:

1. The pH is 7.34; therefore, the primary disorder is an **acidosis.**
2. The $Paco_2$ of 19 mm Hg is less than 40 mm Hg, so this is not primarily a respiratory issue.
3. The HCO_3 of 10 mEq/L is less than 24 mEq/L, so there is a **metabolic acidosis.**

Q73-3: A

Anion gap acidosis only.

Rationale:

1. Is there evidence for a chronic respiratory acid-base disorder that requires adjustment of the patient's "normal" HCO_3? No, there is no evidence for a chronic respiratory acid-base disorder, so we would assume a baseline $Paco_2$ of 40 mm Hg and an HCO_3 of 24 mEq/L.
2. Expected anion gap:

$$\text{Expected Anion Gap} = 12 - (2.5) * \left[4.0\,\frac{g}{dL} - \text{Actual Serum Albumin} \right]$$
$$= 12 - (2.5 * [4.0 - 4.0])$$
$$= 12 - (2.5 * [0]) = \textbf{12 mEq/L.}$$

3. Anion gap calculation:

$$\text{Serum Anion Gap} = [Na^+] - [HCO_3^-] - [Cl^-]$$
$$= 138 - (100 + 10) = 28 \text{ mEq/L, which is} > 12 \text{ mEq/L}$$
$$\rightarrow \textbf{anion gap acidosis is present.}$$

4. Delta-delta calculation:

$$\Delta\Delta = \frac{(\text{Actual Anion Gap} - \text{Expected Anion Gap})}{(\text{Baseline HCO}_3 - \text{Actual HCO}_3)}$$
$$= (28 - 12)/(24 - 10) = \textbf{16/14, which is} \sim \textbf{1.14.}$$

Delta-delta interpretation.	
Delta-Delta Value	Condition Present
< 0.4	Non-anion gap only
0.4–0.9	Anion gap *and* non-anion gap acidosis
1.0–2.0	**Anion gap acidosis only**
> 2.0	Anion gap acidosis and metabolic alkalosis

Q73-4: B
No, a concomitant respiratory alkalosis is present.

Rationale: Using the Winter formula, one can calculate what the expected arterial $Paco_2$ should be for a given serum HCO_3 if the patient were completely compensated.

Respiratory Compensation for Acute Metabolic Acidosis (Winter Formula):

$$\text{Expected Paco}_2 = 1.5 * [\text{Actual HCO}_3] + 8 \pm 2 \text{ (in mm Hg).}$$

So, for this patient,

$$\text{Expected Paco}_2 = (1.5 * 10) + 8 = 15 + 8 = 23 \pm 2 = (21 \text{ to } 25) \text{ mm Hg}$$

This patient has a concomitant respiratory alkalosis, with **Paco$_2$ of 19 mm Hg**, below the expected range (21 to 25 mm Hg).

Q73-5: H
C and D (smoke inhalation and hypoxemia).

Rationale: The patient had significant smoke inhalation, which can lead to both airway and alveolar injuries and tachypnea. Additionally, the patient has considerable hypoxemia (do not be fooled by the $Paco_2$—this is a measure only of dissolved oxygen), which is likely contributing as well.

Q73-6: H
Carbon monoxide poisoning.

Rationale: In addition to respiratory tract injury, carbon monoxide poisoning is a common complication following prolonged smoke inhalation. The carbon monoxide binds tightly to hemoglobin, preventing oxygen from binding. As the vast majority of oxygen is transported bound to hemoglobin (and not as dissolved gas), this can lead to an anaerobic state and the development of lactic acidosis. Although aspirin toxicity can cause the same constellation of symptoms (respiratory alkalosis with anion gap acidosis), smoke inhalation is a much more likely cause given this patient's clinical presentation.

Q73-7: D
Hyperbaric oxygen therapy.

Rationale: Hyperbaric oxygen therapy is the most important next step in this patient's management. Hyperbaric oxygen yields a two- to threefold increase in the Pa_{CO_2} in the bloodstream compared to 100% F_{IO_2} at 1 atmosphere, which drives the displacement of carbon monoxide from hemoglobin. Activated charcoal has limited use in immediate ingestions. Fomepizole is used for the treatment of methanol or ethylene glycol toxicity. Renal replacement therapy has no role here. Methylene blue is the antidote for methemoglobinemia, which is most commonly caused by the use of benzocaine (Hurricaine) anesthetic.

References

Kreisberg RA, Wood BC. Drug and chemical-induced metabolic acidosis. Clin Endocrinol Metab. 1983l;12:391.

Rose JJ, Wang L, Xu Q, et al. Carbon monoxide poisoning: pathogenesis, management, and future directions of therapy. Am J Respir Crit Care Med. 2017;195:596.

Weaver LK. Hyperbaric oxygen therapy for carbon monoxide poisoning. Undersea Hyperb Med. 2014;41:339.

Weaver LK, Hopkins RO, Chan KJ, et al. Hyperbaric oxygen for acute carbon monoxide poisoning. N Engl J Med. 2002;347:1057.

Wu PE, Juurlink DN. Carbon monoxide poisoning. CMAJ. 2014;186:611.

CASE 74

A 22-year-old man who has obesity, obstructive sleep apnea (OSA) without obesity hypoventilation syndrome (his prior ABG showed pH of 7.40 with $Paco_2$ of 42 mm Hg), and cushingoid appearance presents to the clinic with lethargy, abdominal pain, nausea, and emesis. He does not return for regular follow-up for medical care and has no other known diagnoses. He takes no medications and denies any alcohol or drug use. His vital signs are T 35.7°C, HR 130, BP 160/100, RR 26, and Sao_2 98% on room air. His abdominal imaging is negative, lipase is normal, and troponin is negative.

Laboratory data.			
ABGs		Basic Metabolic Panel	
pH	6.94	Na	131 mEq/L
$Paco_2$	24 mm Hg	K	2.2 mEq/L
Pao_2	100 mm Hg	Cl	70 mEq/L
HCO_3	5 mEq/L	CO_2	5 mEq/L
		BUN	33 mg/dL
		Cr	0.8 mg/dL
		Glucose	800 mg/dL
		Albumin	4.0 g/dL
		EtOH	0 mg/dL

QUESTIONS

Q74-1: Define the patient's baseline acid-base status: Does this patient have an underlying chronic acid-base disorder that we need to account for in order to appropriately interpret the acute acid-base disorders?

A. There is no evidence for an underlying chronic respiratory or metabolic acid-base disorder in this patient, so we would assume a baseline $Paco_2$ of 40 mm Hg and an HCO_3 of 24 mEq/L.

B. While the patient has a condition predisposing him to a chronic acid-base disorder, there is insufficient information to estimate the patient's baseline $Paco_2$ and HCO_3 values; therefore, we will assume a baseline $Paco_2$ of 40 mm Hg and a baseline HCO_3 of 24 mEq/L.

C. The patient has an underlying acid-base condition, and we have sufficient information to estimate the patient's baseline $Paco_2$ and HCO_3 values.

Q74-2: What is/are the primary acid-base disturbance(s) occurring in this case?

A. Metabolic acidosis only
B. Respiratory acidosis only
C. Metabolic acidosis and a respiratory acidosis
D. Metabolic alkalosis and a respiratory alkalosis
E. Metabolic alkalosis only
F. Respiratory alkalosis only

Q74-3: How would the metabolic acidosis component be classified in this case?

A. Anion gap acidosis
B. Non-anion gap acidosis
C. Anion and non-anion gap acidosis
D. Anion gap acidosis and a metabolic alkalosis

Q74-4: Does the patient in this case demonstrate appropriate respiratory or metabolic compensation?

A. Yes, the respiratory compensation is appropriate.
B. No, a concomitant respiratory alkalosis is present.
C. No, a concomitant respiratory acidosis is present.
D. Yes, the metabolic compensation is appropriate.
E. No, a concomitant metabolic acidosis is present.
F. No, a concomitant metabolic alkalosis is present.

Q74-5: What is the likely cause of the patient's respiratory acidosis?

A. Chest wall injury
B. Hypoxemia
C. Obesity-related hypoventilation
D. Obstructive lung disease

Q74-6: Additional laboratory test results are as follows:

Serum EtOH	< 3 mg/dL
Serum acetaminophen	< 5 mg/dL (ULN for therapeutic use 20 mg/dL)
Serum salicylates	< 5 mg/dL (ULN for therapeutic use 30 mg/dL)
Serum osmolality	330 mOsm/kg
Serum L-lactate	2.3 mmol/L (ULN 2.0 mmol/L venous)
Beta-hydroxybutyrate (acetone)	2.19 mmol/L (ULN 0.18 mmol/L)
Serum glucose	800 mg/dL
Serum phosphorus	3.4 mmol/L

Which is the likely cause of the patient's anion gap acidosis?
A. Aspirin (ASA) toxicity
B. Lactic acidosis secondary to sepsis
C. Ethylene glycol toxicity
D. Methanol toxicity
E. Opioid overdose
F. Acetaminophen overdose
G. Diabetic ketoacidosis
H. Alcoholic ketoacidosis

Q74-7: The urine electrolyte values are as follows:

Urine Na	23 mEq/L
Urine K	30 mEq/L
Urine Cl	45 mEq/L
Urine urea	NA
Urine glucose	NA
Urine osmolality	NA
Urine pH	5.5
Urine RBCs	None
Urine WBCs	None
Urine protein	None
Urine microscopic	None

What is most likely cause of the patient's metabolic alkalosis?
A. HCO_3 infusion
B. Hyperaldosteronism
C. Cystic fibrosis
D. Hyperemesis
E. Diarrhea
F. Bactrim use
G. Aminoglycoside use
H. Ifosfamide chemotherapy

ANSWERS

Q74-1: A

There is no evidence for an underlying chronic respiratory or metabolic acid-base disorder in this patient, so we would assume a baseline $Paco_2$ of 40 mm Hg and an HCO_3 of 24 mEq/L. The patient has obesity as well as known OSA, which can predispose to a chronic respiratory acidosis; however, the vignette clearly states that the patient has no known history of obesity hypoventilation syndrome, and his most recent ABG demonstrates no baseline acid-base disorder.

Rationale: Ignoring these underlying chronic acid-base disorders can significantly alter the interpretation of a patient's acute acid-base status. This was demonstrated in the first case of the series. However, often, we do not have the necessary information (eg, prior ABG or VBG, or prior serum chemistry with an HCO_3) and are forced to assume the ongoing processes are all acute in nature. We are primarily concerned about chronic respiratory acid-base disorders, as these can significantly alter the patient's baseline or expected values for the serum HCO_3 and $Paco_2$, and we have reliable equations to predict the expected baseline values. The respiratory compensation for both chronic metabolic acidosis and alkalosis is generally poor, so there are no equations or rules to predict what the $Paco_2$ should be in these cases. While the baseline serum HCO_3 may be significantly off from our standard value of 24 mEq/L in these patients, we would assume a baseline $Paco_2$ of 40 mm Hg in patients with chronic metabolic processes. Once we identify the patient's baseline $Paco_2$ and HCO_3 values, we will need to use these values in the appropriate equations to identify the ongoing acute processes.

Q74-2: A

Metabolic acidosis only.

Rationale:

1. The pH is 6.94; therefore, the primary disorder is an **acidosis.**
2. The $Paco_2$ of 24 mm Hg is less than 40 mm Hg, so this is not a primary respiratory issue.
3. The HCO_3 of 5 mEq/L is less than 24 mEq/L, so there is a **metabolic acidosis.**

Q74-3: D

Anion gap acidosis and a metabolic alkalosis.

Rationale:

1. Is there evidence for a chronic respiratory acid-base disorder that requires adjustment of the patient's "normal" HCO_3? No, there is no evidence for a chronic respiratory acid-base disorder, so we would assume a baseline $Paco_2$ of 40 mm Hg and an HCO_3 of 24 mEq/L.

2. Expected anion gap:

$$\text{Expected Anion Gap} = 12 - (2.5) * \left[4.0\,\frac{g}{dL} - \text{Actual Serum Albumin} \right]$$
$$= 12 - (2.5 * [4.0 - 4.0])$$
$$= 12 - (2.5 * [0]) = \textbf{12 mEq/L.}$$

3. Anion gap calculation:

$$\text{Serum Anion Gap} = [Na^+] - [HCO_3^-] - [Cl^-]$$
$$= 131 - (70 + 5) = 56 \text{ mEq/L, which is} > 12 \text{ mEq/L}$$
$$\rightarrow \textbf{anion gap acidosis is present.}$$

4. Delta-delta calculation:

$$\Delta\Delta = \frac{(\text{Actual Anion Gap} - \text{Expected Anion Gap})}{(\text{Baseline HCO}_3 - \text{Actual HCO}_3)}$$

$$= (56 - 12)/(24 - 5) = \textbf{44/19, which is ~2.3.}$$

Delta-delta interpretation.	
Delta-Delta Value	**Condition Present**
< 0.4	Non-anion gap only
0.4–0.9	Anion gap *and* non-anion gap acidosis
1.0–2.0	Anion gap acidosis only
> 2.0	**Anion gap acidosis and metabolic alkalosis**

Q74-4: C
No, a concomitant respiratory acidosis is present.

Rationale: Using the Winter formula, one can calculate what the expected arterial $Paco_2$ should be for a given serum HCO_3 if the patient were completely compensated.

Respiratory Compensation for Acute Metabolic Acidosis (Winter Formula):

Expected $Paco_2$ = 1.5 * [Actual HCO_3] + 8 ± 2 (in mm Hg)
Expected $Paco_2$ = (1.5 * 5) + 8 = 7.5 + 8 = 15.5 ± 2 = (13 to 17) mm Hg.

This patient has a concomitant respiratory acidosis, with **$Paco_2$ of 24 mm Hg**, above the expected range (21 to 25 mm Hg). Therefore, a respiratory acidosis is also present.

Q74-5: C
Obesity-related hypoventilation.

Rationale: The patient has obesity complicated by OSA, which indicates that the likely cause is hypoventilation. Although OSA can be isolated to an upper airway restriction, some patients with obesity can experience chest wall restriction and reduced ventilation. At rest these patients may be asymptomatic, but with activity or when in stressful situations (as described in the vignette), they are unable to compensate. There was no mention of obstructive lung disease or chest wall injury in the case description, and hypoxemia is more commonly associated with respiratory alkalosis.

Q74-6: G
Diabetic ketoacidosis.

Rationale: The patient has a blood glucose level of 800 mg/dL, an anion gap acidosis, and positive urine ketones. He has no evidence of other causes of ketoacidosis. His ASA and acetaminophen levels are negative and his lactate is near normal. The other potential cause would be an organic alcohol ingestion. The expected serum osmolality is calculated using the patient's Na, BUN, glucose, and EtOH (also sometimes K). The serum osmolal gap is calculated as the difference between the patient's measured serum osmolarity (or osmolality) and the calculated serum osmolality based on laboratory data. The calculated osmolality equation is as follows:

$$\text{Calculated Serum Osmolality} = 2*[Na^+] + \frac{[\text{Glucose}]}{18} + \frac{[\text{BUN}]}{2.8} + \frac{[\text{EtOH}]}{3.7}$$

$$\text{Calculated Osmolality} = [2*Na] + [\text{Glucose}/18]$$
$$+ [\text{BUN}/2.8] + [\text{EtOH}/3.7]$$
$$= (2*131) + (800/18) + (33/2.8) + (0/3.7)$$
$$= 321 \text{ mOsm/L}$$

$$\text{Serum Osmolal Gap} = \text{Measured Serum Osmolality} - \text{Calculated Osmolality}$$
$$= (330 - 321) = 9 \text{ mOsm/L, which is} < 10 \text{ mOsm/L}$$
$$\rightarrow \textbf{no serum osmolal gap exists.}$$

Since there is no osmolar gap, diabetic ketoacidosis is the most likely answer.

Q74-7: B
Hyperaldosteronism.

Rationale: The patient has a chloride-insensitive ($U_{Cl} > 20$) metabolic alkalosis, with a low serum K and an elevated urine potassium. He has a cushingoid appearance, with hypertension, obesity, and new-onset diabetes mellitus. This is consistent with hyperaldosteronism as a potential cause. The remaining options are not supported by the vignette.

Causes of metabolic alkalosis.
History: Rule Out the Following as Causes
• Alkali load ("milk-alkali" or calcium-alkali syndrome, oral sodium bicarbonate, IV sodium bicarbonate) • Genetic causes (CF) • Presence of hypercalcemia • IV β-lactam antibiotics • Laxative abuse (may also cause a metabolic acidosis depending on diarrheal HCO_3 losses)
If None of the Above, Then . . .
Urine Chloride < 20 mEq/L (Chloride-Responsive Causes) • Loss of gastric acid (hyperemesis, NGT suctioning) • Prior diuretic use (in hours to days following discontinuation) • Post-hypercapnia • Villous adenoma • Congenital chloridorrhea • Chronic laxative abuse (may also cause a metabolic acidosis depending on diarrheal HCO_3 losses) • CF
OR
Urine Chloride > 20 mEq/L (Chloride-Resistant Causes)
Urine Chloride > 20 mEq/L, Lack of HTN, Urine potassium < 30 mEq/L
• Hypokalemia or hypomagnesemia • Laxative abuse (if dominated by hypokalemia) • Bartter syndrome • Gitelman syndrome
Urine Chloride > 20 mEq/L, Lack of HTN, Urine Potassium > 30 mEq/L
• Current diuretic use
Urine Chloride > 20 mEq/L, Presence of HTN, Urine Potassium Variable but Usually > 30 mEq/L
Elevated plasma renin level: • Renal artery stenosis • Renin-secreting tumor • Renovascular disease
Low plasma renin, low plasma aldosterone: • Cushing syndrome • Exogenous mineralocorticoid use • Genetic disorder (11-hydoxylase or 17-hydrolyase deficiency, 11β-HSD deficiency) • Liddle syndrome • Licorice toxicity
Low plasma renin, high plasma aldosterone: • Primary hyperaldosteronism • Adrenal adenoma • Bilateral adrenal hyperplasia

References

Abreo K, Adlakha A, Kilpatrick S, et al. The milk-alkali syndrome. A reversible form of acute renal failure. Arch Intern Med. 1993;153:1005.

Barton CH, Vaziri ND, Ness RL, et al. Cimetidine in the management of metabolic alkalosis induced by nasogastric drainage. Arch Surg. 1979;114:70.

Batlle D, Grupp M, Gaviria M, Kurtzman NA. Distal renal tubular acidosis with intact capacity to lower urinary pH. Am J Med. 1982;72:751.

Batlle D, Haque SK. Genetic causes and mechanisms of distal renal tubular acidosis. Nephrol Dial Transplant. 2012;27:3691.

Batlle DC, Hizon M, Cohen E, et al. The use of the urinary anion gap in the diagnosis of hyperchloremic metabolic acidosis. N Engl J Med. 1988;318:594.

Batlle DC, von Riotte A, Schlueter W. Urinary sodium in the evaluation of hyperchloremic metabolic acidosis. N Engl J Med. 1987;316:140.

Bear R, Goldstein M, Phillipson E, et al. Effect of metabolic alkalosis on respiratory function in patients with chronic obstructive lung disease. Can Med Assoc J. 1977;117:900.

Buckalew VM Jr, McCurdy DK, Ludwig GD, et al. Incomplete renal tubular acidosis. Physiologic studies in three patients with a defect in lowering urine pH. Am J Med. 1968;45:32.

DeFronzo RA, Matzuda M, Barret E. Diabetic ketoacidosis: a combined metabolic-nephrologic approach to therapy. Diabetes Rev. 1994;2:209.

Fulop M, Murthy V, Michilli A, et al. Serum beta-hydroxybutyrate measurement in patients with uncontrolled diabetes mellitus. Arch Intern Med. 1999;159:381.

Galla JH, Gifford JD, Luke RG, Rome L. Adaptations to chloride-depletion alkalosis. Am J Physiol. 1991;261:R771.

Garella S, Chang BS, Kahn SI. Dilution acidosis and contraction alkalosis: review of a concept. Kidney Int. 1975;8:279.

Gennari FJ, Weise WJ. Acid-base disturbances in gastrointestinal disease. Clin J Am Soc Nephrol. 2008;3:1861.

Hamm LL, Nakhoul N, Hering-Smith KS. Acid-base homeostasis. Clin J Am Soc Nephrol. 2015;10:2232.

Hulter HN, Sebastian A, Toto RD, et al. Renal and systemic acid-base effects of the chronic administration of hypercalcemia-producing agents: calcitriol, PTH, and intravenous calcium. Kidney Int. 1982;21:445.

Karet FE. Mechanisms in hyperkalemic renal tubular acidosis. J Am Soc Nephrol. 2009;20:251.

Khanna A, Kurtzman NA. Metabolic alkalosis. J Nephrol. 2006;19(suppl 9):S86.

Laski ME, Sabatini S. Metabolic alkalosis, bedside and bench. Semin Nephrol. 2006;26:404.

Luke RG, Galla JH. It is chloride depletion alkalosis, not contraction alkalosis. J Am Soc Nephrol. 2012;23:204.

Miller PD, Berns AS. Acute metabolic alkalosis perpetuating hypercarbia. A role for acetazolamide in chronic obstructive pulmonary disease. JAMA. 1977;238:2400.

Oster JR, Materson BJ, Rogers AI. Laxative abuse syndrome. Am J Gastroenterol. 1980;74:451.

Patel AM, Goldfarb S. Got calcium? Welcome to the calcium-alkali syndrome. J Am Soc Nephrol. 2010;21:1440.

Porter WH, Yao HH, Karounos DG. Laboratory and clinical evaluation of assays for beta-hydroxybutyrate. Am J Clin Pathol. 1997;107:353.

Rodríguez Soriano J. Renal tubular acidosis: the clinical entity. J Am Soc Nephrol. 2002;13:2160.

Rose BD, Post TW. Clinical Physiology of Acid-Base and Electrolyte Disorders, 5e. New York, NY: McGraw Hill; 2001:559, 809-815.

Schwartz WB, Van Ypersele de Strihou, Kassirer JP. Role of anions in metabolic alkalosis and potassium deficiency. N Engl J Med. 1968;279:630.

Shen T, Braude S. Changes in serum phosphate during treatment of diabetic ketoacidosis: predictive significance of severity of acidosis on presentation. Intern Med J. 2012;42:1347.

Sweetser LJ, Douglas JA, Riha RL, Bell SC. Clinical presentation of metabolic alkalosis in an adult patient with cystic fibrosis. Respirology. 2005;10:254.

Taki K, Mizuno K, Takahashi N, Wakusawa R. Disturbance of CO2 elimination in the lungs by carbonic anhydrase inhibition. Jpn J Physiol. 1986;36:523.

Turban S, Beutler KT, Morris RG, et al. Long-term regulation of proximal tubule acid-base transporter abundance by angiotensin II. Kidney Int. 2006;70:660.

Wachtel TJ, Tetu-Mouradjian LM, Goldman DL, et al. Hyperosmolarity and acidosis in diabetes mellitus: a three-year experience in Rhode Island. J Gen Intern Med. 1991;6:495.

CASE 75

A 33-year-old woman presents to the emergency department with hematemesis. She is groggy but is able to provide a history. She has cirrhosis secondary to alcohol abuse and has known varices. Her vital signs are T 36.0C, HR 140, BP 70/30, RR 28, and Sao$_2$ 97% on room air. She has ascites on examination and her skin is pale. Her conjunctiva are pale as well. No additional information is available at this time.

Laboratory data.			
ABGs		Basic Metabolic Panel	
pH	7.33	Na	133 mEq/L
Paco$_2$	22 mm Hg	K	5.6 mEq/L
Pao$_2$	100 mm Hg	Cl	100 mEq/L
HCO$_3$	13 mEq/L	CO$_2$	13 mEq/L
		BUN	33 mg/dL
		Cr	0.5 mg/dL
		Glucose	100 mg/dL
		Albumin	4 g/dL
		EtOH	0 mg/dL

QUESTIONS

Q75-1: Define the patient's baseline acid-base status: Does this patient have an underlying chronic acid-base disorder that we need to account for in order to appropriately interpret the acute acid-base disorders?

A. There is no evidence for an underlying chronic respiratory or metabolic acid-base disorder in this patient, so we would assume a baseline $Paco_2$ of 40 mm Hg and an HCO_3 of 24 mEq/L.

B. While the patient has a condition predisposing her to a chronic acid-base disorder, there is insufficient information to estimate the patient's baseline $Paco_2$ and HCO_3 values; therefore, we will assume a baseline $Paco_2$ of 40 mm Hg and a baseline HCO_3 of 24 mEq/L.

C. The patient has an underlying acid-base condition, and we have sufficient information to estimate the patient's baseline $Paco_2$ and HCO_3 values.

Q75-2: What is/are the primary acid-base disturbance(s) occurring in this case?

A. Metabolic acidosis only
B. Respiratory acidosis only
C. Metabolic acidosis and a respiratory acidosis
D. Metabolic alkalosis and a respiratory alkalosis
E. Metabolic alkalosis only
F. Respiratory alkalosis only

Q75-3: How would the metabolic acidosis component be classified in this case?

A. Anion gap acidosis
B. Non-anion gap acidosis
C. Anion and non-anion gap acidosis
D. Anion gap acidosis and a metabolic alkalosis

Q75-4: Does the patient in this case demonstrate appropriate respiratory or metabolic compensation?

A. Yes, the respiratory compensation is appropriate.
B. No, a concomitant respiratory alkalosis is present.
C. No, a concomitant respiratory acidosis is present.
D. Yes, the metabolic compensation is appropriate.
E. No, a concomitant metabolic acidosis is present.
F. No, a concomitant metabolic alkalosis is present.

Q75-5: Results of the patient's serum and urine studies are as follows:

Serum Studies	
Serum EtOH	< 3 mg/dL
Serum acetaminophen	< 5 mg/dL (ULN for therapeutic use 20 mg/dL)
Serum salicylates	< 5 mg/dL (ULN for therapeutic use 30 mg/dL)
Serum osmolar gap	8 mOsm/L
Serum L-lactate	8.0 mmol/L (ULN 2.0 mmol/L venous)
Beta-hydroxybutyrate (acetone)	< 0.18 mmol/L (ULN 0.18 mmol/L)
Serum glucose	100 mg/dL
Serum K	5.6 mEq/L
Urine Studies	
Urine Na	40 mEq/L
Urine K	30 mEq/L
Urine Cl	30 mEq/L
Urine pH	5.5

Match the acid-base disorders in this patient to the most likely etiology from the list below. (Choose only one answer per disorder.)

A. Cirrhosis
B. COPD
C. Lactic acidosis
D. Aspirin overdose
E. Diuresis
F. Spironolactone
G. Acetazolamide
— Anion gap acidosis
— Non-anion gap acidosis
— Respiratory alkalosis

ANSWERS

Q75-1: B

While the patient has a condition predisposing her to a chronic acid-base disorder, there is insufficient information to estimate the patient's baseline $Paco_2$ and HCO_3 values; therefore, we will assume a baseline $Paco_2$ of 40 mm Hg and a baseline HCO_3 of 24 mEq/L. The patient has cirrhosis, which can predispose to a chronic acid-base disorder. However, no information is provided in the vignette to confirm this possibility.

Rationale: Ignoring these underlying chronic acid-base disorders can significantly alter the interpretation of a patient's acute acid-base status. This was demonstrated in the first case of the series. However, often, we do not have the necessary information (eg, prior ABG or VBG, or prior serum chemistry with an HCO_3) and are forced to assume the ongoing processes are all acute in nature. We are primarily concerned about chronic respiratory acid-base disorders, as these can significantly alter the patient's baseline or expected values for the serum HCO_3 and $Paco_2$, and we have reliable equations to predict the expected baseline values. The respiratory compensation for both chronic metabolic acidosis and alkalosis is generally poor, so there are no equations or rules to predict what the $Paco_2$ should be in these cases. While the baseline serum HCO_3 may be significantly off from our standard value of 24 mEq/L in these patients, we would assume a baseline $Paco_2$ of 40 mm Hg in patients with chronic metabolic processes. Once we identify the patient's baseline $Paco_2$ and HCO_3 values, we will need to use these values in the appropriate equations to identify the ongoing acute processes.

Q75-2: A

Metabolic acidosis only.

Rationale:

1. The pH is 7.33; therefore, the primary disorder is an **acidosis.**
2. The $Paco_2$ of 22 mm Hg is less than 40 mm Hg, so this is not a primary respiratory acidosis.
3. The HCO_3 of 13 mEq/L is less than 24 mEq/L, so there is a **metabolic acidosis.**

Q75-3: C

Anion and non-anion gap acidosis.

Rationale:

1. Is there evidence for a chronic acid-base disorder that requires adjustment of the patient's "normal" HCO_3? No, there is no evidence for a chronic acid-base disorder, so we would assume a baseline $Paco_2$ of 40 mm Hg and an HCO_3 of 24 mEq/L.

2. Expected anion gap:

$$\text{Expected Anion Gap} = 12 - (2.5) * \left[4.0 \, \frac{g}{dL} - \text{Actual Serum Albumin} \right]$$
$$= 12 - (2.5 * [4.0 - 4.0])$$
$$= 12 - (2.5 * [0]) = \textbf{12 mEq/L.}$$

3. Anion gap calculation:

$$\text{Serum Anion Gap} = [Na^+] - [HCO_3^-] - [Cl^-]$$
$$= 133 - (100 + 13) = 20 \text{ mEq/L, which is} > 12 \text{ mEq/L}$$
$$\rightarrow \textbf{anion gap acidosis is present.}$$

4. Delta-delta calculation:

$$\Delta\Delta = \frac{(\text{Actual Anion Gap} - \text{Expected Anion Gap})}{(\text{Baseline HCO}_3 - \text{Actual HCO}_3)}$$
$$= (20 - 12)/(24 - 13) = \textbf{8/11, which is ~0.73.}$$

Delta-delta interpretation.	
Delta-Delta Value	Condition Present
< 0.4	Non-anion gap only
0.4–0.9	**Anion gap *and* non-anion gap acidosis**
1.0–2.0	Anion gap acidosis only
> 2.0	Anion gap acidosis and metabolic alkalosis

Q75-4: B
No, a concomitant respiratory alkalosis is present.

Rationale: Using the Winter formula, one can calculate what the expected arterial $Paco_2$ should be for a given serum HCO_3 if the patient were completely compensated.

Respiratory Compensation for Acute Metabolic Acidosis (Winter Formula):

Expected $Paco_2 = 1.5 * [\text{Actual HCO}_3] + 8 \pm 2$ (in mm Hg)
Expected $Paco_2 = (1.5 * 13) + 8 = 19.5 + 8 = 27.5 \pm 2 = (25 \text{ to } 29)$ mm Hg.

This patient has a **concomitant respiratory alkalosis**, with $Paco_2$ **of 22 mm Hg**, less than the expected range (25 to 29 mm Hg).

Q75-5: A; B; C
Lactic acidosis; Spironolactone; Cirrhosis.

Rationale: This patient has a triple acid-base disorder. The anion gap acidosis is due to a significant lactic acidosis secondary to acute blood loss. The remaining causes are generally ruled out by the additional laboratory tests. Cirrhosis is the likely cause of the patient's respiratory alkalosis, as no ASA is present and the patient does not have a history of congestive heart failure, pulmonary embolism, or CNS insult.

The non-anion gap acidosis is likely due to spironolactone use (common in patients who have cirrhosis with ascites), as the urine anion gap is positive, the urine pH is low, and the serum K is high, consistent with a type 4 RTA. Although ideally we would use the serum osmolal gap here, we lack the needed information to calculate this value.

Urine Anion Gap:

$$\text{Urine Anion Gap} = [U_{Na}] + [U_K] - [U_{Cl}].$$

Therefore, for this patient,

$$\text{Urine Anion Gap} = U_{Na} + U_K - U_{Cl} = (30 + 40) - 30 = (+40) \text{ mEq/L}.$$

Interpretation:

- A urine anion gap that is greater than 20 mEq/L $\rightarrow$ reduced renal acid excretion (RTA).
- A urine anion gap that is -20 mEq/L $\rightarrow$ GI loss of HCO_3 (eg, diarrhea), although type II RTA is possible.
- A urine anion gap between -20 and $+10$ mEq/L is generally considered inconclusive.

Limitation: The urine anion gap can be inappropriately elevated in anion gap acidosis, a situation in which multiple unmeasured anions may be present in the urine (beta-hydroxybutyrate/acetoacetate [ketoacidosis], hippurate [toluene], HCO_3 [proximal RTA], D-lactate [D-lactic acidosis], L-lactate, 5-oxoproline [acetaminophen toxicity]). Therefore, in patients with a significant anion gap, the urine osmolar gap is typically more useful.

Evaluation of RTA.			
	Type 1 RTA	**Type 2 RTA**	**Type 4 RTA**
Severity of metabolic acidosis, (HCO_3)	Severe (< 10–12 mEq/L typically)	Intermediate (12–20 mEq/L)	Mild (15–20 mEq/L)
Associated urine abnormalities	Urinary phosphate, calcium are increased; bone disease often present	Urine glucose, amino acids, phosphate, calcium may be elevated	
Urine pH	HIGH (> 5.5)	Low (acidic), until serum HCO_3 level exceeds the resorptive ability of the proximal tubule; then becomes alkalotic once reabsorptive threshold is crossed	Low (acidic)
Serum K^+	Low to normal; should correct with oral HCO_3 therapy	Classically low, although may be normal or even high with rare genetic defects; worsens with oral HCO_3 therapy	HIGH
Renal stones	Often	No	No

(Continued)

Evaluation of RTA. (*continued*)

Renal tubular defect	Reduced NH$_4$ secretion in distal tubule	Reduced HCO$_3$ resorption in proximal tubule	Reduced H$^+$/K$^+$ exchange in distal and collecting tubule due to decreased aldosterone or aldosterone resistance
Urine anion gap	> 10	Negative	> 10
Urine osmolal gap	Reduced during acute acidosis		Reduced during acute acidosis

Causes of RTA.

Causes of Type 1 (Distal) RTA

Primary
- Idiopathic or familial (may be recessive or dominant)

Secondary
- Medications: Lithium, amphotericin, ifosfamide, NSAIDs
- Rheumatologic disorders: Sjögren syndrome, SLE, RA
- Hypercalciuria (idiopathic) or associated with vitamin D deficiency or hyperparathyroidism
- Sarcoidosis
- Obstructive uropathy
- Wilson disease
- Rejection of renal transplant allograft
- Toluene toxicity

Causes of Type 2 (Proximal) RTA

Primary
- Idiopathic
- Familial (primarily recessive disorders)
- Genetic: Fanconi syndrome, cystinosis, glycogen storage disease (type 1), Wilson disease, galactosemia

Secondary
- Medications: Acetazolamide, topiramate, aminoglycoside antibiotics, ifosfamide, reverse transcriptase inhibitors (tenofovir)
- Heavy metal poisoning: Lead, mercury, copper
- Multiple myeloma or amyloidosis (secondary to light chain toxicity)
- Sjögren syndrome
- Vitamin D deficiency
- Rejection of renal transplant allograft

Causes of Type 4 RTA (Hypoaldosteronism or Aldosterone Resistance)

Primary
- Primary adrenal insufficiency
- Inherited disorders associated with hypoaldosteronism
- Pseudohypoaldosteronism (types 1 and 2)

Secondary
- Causes of hyporeninemic hypoaldosteronism such as renal disease (diabetic nephropathy), NSAID use, calcineurin inhibitors, volume expansion/volume overload
- Causes of distal tubule voltage defects such as sickle cell disease, obstructive uropathy, SLE
- Severe illness/septic shock
- Angiotensin II–associated medications: ACE inhibitors, ARBs, direct renin inhibitors
- Potassium-sparing diuretics: Spironolactone, amiloride, triamterene
- Antibiotics: Trimethoprim, pentamidine

References

Adeva-Anandy M, López-Ojén M, Funcasta-Calderón R, et al. Comprehensive review on lactate metabolism in human health. Mitochondrion. 2014;17:76.

Arbus GS, Herbert LA, Levesque PR, et al. Characterization and clinical application of the "significance band" for acute respiratory alkalosis. N Engl J Med. 1969;280:117.

Batlle D, Grupp M, Gaviria M, Kurtzman NA. Distal renal tubular acidosis with intact capacity to lower urinary pH. Am J Med. 1982;72:751.

Batlle D, Haque SK. Genetic causes and mechanisms of distal renal tubular acidosis. Nephrol Dial Transplant. 2012;27:3691.

Batlle DC, Hizon M, Cohen E, et al. The use of the urinary anion gap in the diagnosis of hyperchloremic metabolic acidosis. N Engl J Med. 1988;318:594.

Batlle DC, von Riotte A, Schlueter W. Urinary sodium in the evaluation of hyperchloremic metabolic acidosis. N Engl J Med. 1987;316:140.

Buckalew VM Jr, McCurdy DK, Ludwig GD, et al. Incomplete renal tubular acidosis. Physiologic studies in three patients with a defect in lowering urine pH. Am J Med. 1968;45:32.

Demeter SL, Cordasco EM. Hyperventilation syndrome and asthma. Am J Med. 1986;81:989.

Gardner WN. The pathophysiology of hyperventilation disorders. Chest. 1996;109:516.

Karet FE. Mechanisms in hyperkalemic renal tubular acidosis. J Am Soc Nephrol. 2009;20:251.

Krapf R, Beeler I, Hertner D, Hulter HN. Chronic respiratory alkalosis. The effect of sustained hyperventilation on renal regulation of acid-base equilibrium. N Engl J Med. 1991;324:1394.

Lee Hamm L, Hering-Smith KS, Nakhoul NL. Acid-base and potassium homeostasis. Semin Nephrol. 2013;33:257.

Levy B. Lactate and shock state: the metabolic view. Curr Opin Crit Care. 2006;12:315.

Madias NE. Lactic acidosis. Kidney Int. 1986;29:752.

Martinu T, Menzies D, Dial S. Re-evaluation of acid-base prediction rules in patients with chronic respiratory acidosis. Can Respir J. 2003;10:311.

Mikkelsen ME, Miltiades AN, Gaieski DF, et al. Serum lactate is associated with mortality in severe sepsis independent of organ failure and shock. Crit Care Med. 2009;37:1670.

Nardi AE, Freire RC, Zin WA. Panic disorder and control of breathing. Respir Physiol Neurobiol. 2009;167:133.

Oh M, Carroll HJ. Value and determinants of urine anion gap. Nephron. 2002;90:252.

Rodríguez Soriano J. Renal tubular acidosis: the clinical entity. J Am Soc Nephrol. 2002;13:2160.

Saisch SG, Wessely S, Gardner WN. Patients with acute hyperventilation presenting to an inner-city emergency department. Chest. 1996;110:952.

INDEX

Page references followed by "f" denote figures; "t" denote tables.